Westmead
Anaesthetic Manual

This manual is dedicated to my loving and ever patient wife Tracey and to our three wonderful sons, Max, Angus and Hugo, who deserve much more of my time.

Westmead
Anaesthetic Manual

Third Edition

Dr Anthony P. Padley

MBBS (UNSW), FANZCA

The McGraw-Hill Companies

Mc Graw Hill **Medical**

The McGraw·Hill Companies

First published 2000
Second edition published 2004
Third edition published 2009

Text © 2009 Anthony Padley
Illustrations and design © 2009 McGraw-Hill Australia Pty Ltd
Additional owners of copyright are acknowledged in on-page credits

National Library of Australia Cataloguing-in-Publication data:

Padley, Anthony P.
Westmead anaesthetic manual [electronic resource] /
Anthony P. Padley
3rd ed.
ISBN 97800 70159204
ISBN 97800 70271920 (Scherung-Plough edition)
Anaesthetics—Handbooks, manuals, etc
Anaesthesia—Handbooks, manuals, etc
617.96

Published in Australia by
McGraw-Hill Australia Pty Ltd
Level 2, 82 Waterloo Road, North Ryde NSW 2113
Publisher: Elizabeth Walton
Managing editor: Kathryn Fairfax
Production editor: Eleanna Raissis
Copy editor: Tina Allen
Art director: Astred Hicks
Cover design: Blue Cork
Internal design: Peta Nugent
Illustrator: Lorenzo Lucia
Proofreader: Tim Learner
Typeset in 8/10.5 pt Zapf Humans 601 by Midland Typesetters, Australia
Printed on 80 gsm matt art by 1010 Printing International Limited, China

Preface to the third edition

This book is intended to be a comprehensive, concise 'use at the bedside' manual for anaesthetic consultants, registrars, GP anaesthetists, intensivists and anaesthetic nurses. The aim of this manual is to provide rapidly accessible essential anaesthetic information on a comprehensive array of topics including the management of anaesthetic crises and medical emergencies. Included in this manual are dosage guidelines for hundreds of drugs used in anaesthesia and intensive care with listed advantages and disadvantages of each therapy. This manual also provides step-by-step descriptions of numerous anaesthetic-related procedures such as ultrasound-guided brachial plexus block and the use of video/optical laryngoscopes including the Airtraq. Also contained in this book are many interesting and complex comorbidities which confront anaesthetists from time to time, sometimes in the anaesthetic bay, such as carcinoid tumour and long Q-T syndrome. There are also the latest guidelines on many important areas including cardiac arrest management, bacterial endocarditic prophylaxis, malignant hyperthermia and difficult airway management.

Now in its third edition, it is the author's hope that this book will continue to be an invaluable aid to the practice of anaesthesia and for registrars preparing for anaesthetic exams. No other anaesthetic manual offers so much essential anaesthetic information in such a compact and portable form with an instant access alphabetical layout.

Contents

Q

R

Abbreviations

AAA	abdominal aortic aneurysm
ABG	arterial blood gas
ACEI	angiotensin converting enzyme inhibitor
ANH	acute normovolaemic haemodilution
AEC	airway exchange catheter
AED	automated external defibrillator
AF	atrial fibrillation
ALS	advanced life support
AP	anterior-posterior
AS	aortic stenosis
ASD	atrial septal defect
ASIS	anterior superior iliac spine
ATE	arterial thromboembolism
AV	atrioventricular
BE	bacterial endocarditis
BIS	Bispectral Index
BLS	basic life support
BLM	bleomycin
BMI	body mass index
BPF	bronchopleural fistula
bpm	beats or breaths per minute (depending on context)
BSL	blood sugar level
C	cervical vertebra
CABG	coronary artery bypass grafting
CAD	coronary artery disease
CEA	carotid endarterectomy
CCF	congestive cardiac failure
CHD	congenital heart disease
CK	creatine kinase
CMV	cytomegalovirus
CNS	central nervous system
COMT	catechol-O-methyl transferase
CO	carbon monoxide
COX	cyclo-oxygenase
CP	cervical plexus
CPAP	continuous positive airway pressure
CPP	cerebral perfusion pressure
CPR	cardio-pulmonary resuscitation
CS	Caesarean section
CSF	cerebrospinal fluid
CT	computerised tomogram/ tomography
CVA	cerebrovascular accident
CVS	cardiovascular system
CXR	chest X-ray
DA	dopamine receptor
DC	direct current
DIC	disseminated intravascular coagulation
DLT	double lumen tube
DTA	distal thoracic aorta
DVT	deep venous thrombosis
ECC	external cardiac compression
ECG	electrocardiography, electrocardiograph
ECMO	extra-corporeal membrane oxygenation
EDBP	epidural blood patch
EDLA	extended duration local anaesthetic
EEG	electroencephalogram/ electroencephalograph
EF	ejection fraction

EMLA	eutectic mixture of local anaesthetic agents	**IDDM**	insulin dependent diabetes mellitus
ET	endotracheal	**IM**	intramuscular
FBC	full blood count	**IO**	interosseous
FDP	fibrin degradation products	**IOP**	intra-ocular pressure
FEV$_1$	forced expiratory volume in the first second	**IPPV**	intermittent positive pressure ventilation
FFP	fresh frozen plasma	**IV**	intravenous
FGF	fresh gas flow	**JW**	Jehovah's Witness
FiO$_2$	fractional concentration of inspired O_2	**KCL**	potassium chloride
		L	lumbar vertebra
FOB	fibre-optic bronchoscope	**LA**	local anaesthetic
FVC	forced vital capacity	**LBBB**	left bundle branch block
GA	general anaesthesia	**LD**	loading dose
GCS	Glasgow coma score	**LED**	light emitting diode
GEB	gum elastic bougie	**LFTs**	liver function tests
G6PD	glucose-6-phosphate dehydrogenase	**LMA**	laryngeal mask airway
		LMWH	low molecular weight heparin
GTN	glyceryl trinitrate	**LOR**	loss of resistance
HB	heart block	**LQTS**	long QT syndrome
Hb	haemoglobin	**LV**	left ventricle
HbA	normal adult haemoglobin with 2 α and 2 β chains	**min**	minute
HbA$_2$	2.5% of adult haemoglobin with 2 α and 2 δ chains	**MAC**	minimum alveolar concentration (of anaesthetic drug in O_2 preventing movement in response to skin incision in 50% of subjects studied)
HbF	fetal haemoglobin with 2 α and 2 γ chains		
HbS	sickle cell haemoglobin with 2 α chains and 2 abnormal β chains		
		MOA	monoamine oxidase
Hct	haematocrit	**MAP**	mean arterial pressure
HITS	heparin induced thrombocytopenia	**MCL**	midclavicular line
		MET	metabolic equivalent
HCM	hypertrophic cardiomyopathy	**MG**	myasthenia gravis
		MH	malignant hyperthermia
HR	heart rate	**MI**	myocardial infarction
HRT	hormone replacement therapy	**min**	minute
		MRI	magnetic resonance imaging
5-HT$_3$	5-hydroxytryptamine 3 (receptor)	**N**	Newton
		NAC	N-acetyl cysteine
ICP	intracranial pressure	**NDNMBD**	
ICS	intercostal space		non-depolarising neuromuscular blocking drug
ICU	intensive care unit		

NIDDM
non-insulin dependent diabetes mellitus
NG nasogastric
NMDA N-methyl-D-aspartate
NMS neuroleptic malignant syndrome
NR normal range
N/S normal saline
NSAIDs
non-steroidal anti-inflammatory drugs
OCP oral contraceptive pill
OSA obstructive sleep apnoea
PAC/PA catheter
pulmonary artery catheter
PAP pulmonary artery pressure
PCA patient controlled analgesia
PCEA patient controlled epidural analgesia
PDE III phosphodiesterase type III inhibitors
PDPH postdural puncture headache
PE pulmonary embolism
PEA pulseless electrical activity
PEEP positive end expiratory pressure
PEFR peak expiratory flow rate
PONV postoperative nausea and vomiting
PTCA percutaneous transluminal coronary angioplasty
PV per vaginam
PVR pulmonary vascular resistance
rFVIIa recombinant activated factor VII
Rh Rhesus factor
ROSC return of spontaneous circulation

R-R R-R interval (time in s between two R waves on the ECG)
RSI rapid sequence induction
s second
SA sinoatrial node
SAB subarachnoid block
SAH subarachnoid haemorrhage
SB sternal border or short bevelled
SCA sickle cell anaemia
SLIPA streamlined liner of the pharynx airway
SNP sodium nitroprusside
subcut subcutaneous
SVC superior vena cava
SVR systemic vascular resistance
SVT supraventricular tachycardia
T thoracic vertebra
TBSA total body surface area
TBV total blood volume
TCP transcutaneous cardiac pacing
TF tissue factor
TIVA total intravenous anaesthesia
TL/TR therapeutic level/therapeutic range
TOE transoesophageal echocardiography
TPN total parenteral nutrition
TPW temporary pacing wire
U, u units
UEC urea, electrolytes and creatinine
URTI upper respiratory tract infection
VF ventricular fibrillation
VSD ventricular septal defect
VT ventricular tachycardia
VTE venous thromboembolism
WCC white cell count
WPW Wolff-Parkinson-White syndrome

Acknowledgements

I would like to thank the anaesthetic consultants and registrars at Westmead Hospital for their invaluable advice and assistance. In particular I would like to thank Associate Professor Peter Klineberg for his ongoing support and guidance and Dr Alwin Chuan for his invaluable ultrasound expertise and illustrations. Many thanks also go to my father Terence Padley for assisting with proofreading this manuscript.

Comments

Criticisms, comments and suggestions are welcome for subsequent editions of this book and can be e-mailed to: Anthonypadley@bigpond.com or posted to: PO Box 2748 North Parramatta, NSW 1750, Australia.

○ Abciximab

Antiplatelet drug that works by inhibiting glycoprotein IIb/IIIa on the platelet surface. Effects last for 12–24 h. ***See*** *Platelet IIb/IIIa Receptor Antagonists*.

○ Abdominal Aortic Aneurysm (AAA) Surgery

Topics Covered in this Section
▶ Elective Open Abdominal Aortic Aneurysm Repair
▶ Endoluminal Abdominal Aortic Aneurysm Repair
▶ Ruptured Abdominal Aortic Aneurysm Repair

See also *Thoraco Abdominal and Thoracic Aortic Aneurysm and Dissection Repair*.

Elective Open Abdominal Aortic Aneurysm (AAA) Repair

Morbidity and Mortality of Elective AAA Repair

The overall mortality rate for elective surgery is about 2–5%, usually due to cardiac events such as myocardial infarction. Peri-operative renal failure is another serious complication, usually due to acute tubular necrosis secondary to renal ischaemia. The incidence of renal failure with infrarenal cross-clamping is about 5%. Renal failure occurs in up to 17% of cases with suprarenal cross-clamping.[1] Spinal cord ischaemia occurs in between 1 and 11% of distal aortic aneurysm repairs.

Anaesthetic Aims

1 Maintain optimal intravascular volume and cardiovascular stability throughout the peri-operative period.
2 Prepare for potentially massive blood loss.
3 Prevent/detect/treat myocardial ischaemia. Ischaemic heart disease is usually present.
4 Maintain renal function. There is often underlying renal disease.

Patient Assessment and Preparation Prior to the Day of Surgery

1 Evaluate cardiovascular function and optimise management of cardiovascular disease. ***See*** *Cardiovascular Peri-operative Risk Prediction for Non-cardiac surgery*.
2 Organise blood cross-match or group and save if the hospital blood bank is able to provide cross-matched blood rapidly.

3 Some researchers have suggested commencing the patient on β blocker therapy such as atenolol to decrease the incidence of cardiac events in the first 6 months after surgery.[2] This approach has been challenged recently by the POISE trial. *See Beta-blocker Therapy and Reduction of Cardiac Risk*.

Pre-operative Management

1 Prepare for potentially massive blood loss using such equipment as a Cell Saver, Alton Dean™ rapid infusion systems, rapid infusion device catheters™ and/or pulmonary artery catheter introducer sheaths. *See Rapid Infusion Catheter Exchanger Set*.

2 Establish appropriate monitoring including arterial line, triple lumen central venous line or pulmonary artery catheter and 5-lead ECG monitoring with ST segment analysis (*see ST Segment Analysis*). Also monitor urine output and body temperature. Transoesophageal echocardiography has an increasingly important role in intra-operative cardiac monitoring.

3 Consider utilisation of a thoracic epidural sited at about the T8–9 level for intra-operative and postoperative analgesia.

4 Maintain body temperature with devices such as an upper body Bair Hugger™. The legs must not be actively warmed while the aorta is clamped, as this will worsen the effects of leg ischaemia.

5 Prepare an infusion of glyceryl trinitrate (GTN), 50 mg in 100 mL 5% glucose, to be used as a vasodilator.

Intra-operative Management up to the Time of Cross-clamping (Including Renal Protective Strategies)

1 Aim for the smooth induction of anaesthesia with cardiovascular stability using e.g. fentanyl, propofol or thiopentone and rocuronium.

2 Maintain anaesthesia with O_2, air, isoflurane or sevoflurane.

3 Provide prophylactic antibiotic 'cover' e.g. cephazolin 1 g IV.

4 There is little evidence that any drugs provide renal protective effects. However consider the following strategies to attempt to protect renal function:[3]

a) Maintain optimal intravascular volume and perfusion pressure. This is the most important strategy.

b) Give mannitol before cross-clamping. The optimal dose of mannitol is unclear from the literature but 10–25 g would appear to be reasonable.[4] Mannitol may act by reducing renal cell oedema and increasing glomerular filtration helping to 'flush out' tubular debris. It may also scavenge oxygen free radicals.

c) Frusemide may be of benefit by decreasing the resorption of solute thus reducing cellular metabolic activity and giving some protection against cellular ischaemia. In addition, frusemide may stimulate prostaglandin E_1 release, improving renal blood flow. Evidence for this effect is weak.[5]

QUICK FLICK **A**

d) Dopamine does not appear to provide any renal protection effect.[5]

e) Fenoldopam is a systemic vasodilator drug with selective agonist activity at dopamine 1 receptors. This drug causes a significant increase in renal blood flow and decreases renal vascular resistance, and may be of use in aortic surgery. Two studies have indicated fenoldopam provided a measure of renal protection during infrarenal cross-clamping.[6,7] However a study by Oliver et al. showed no difference in renal protective qualities between fenoldopam and a combination of sodium nitroprusside and dopamine during AAA surgery with infrarenal cross-clamping.[8]

f) N-acetyl cysteine (NAC) has been used successfully to reduce the incidence of IV contrast induced renal failure in some studies. *See N-acetyl cysteine (NAC)*. However a study by Hynninen using NAC to prevent renal injury during AAA surgery showed no benefit compared with placebo.[9]

6 Give heparin prior to clamping of the aorta. Discuss the heparin dose with the surgeon.

7 Give sufficient IV fluid to maintain pulmonary capillary wedge pressure at 10–15 mm Hg and a urine output of > 60 mL/h.

Physiological Effects of Aortic Cross-clamping

These effects depend in part on how proximally the aorta is clamped. The haemodynamic responses include:

1 An increase in systemic vascular resistance with increased left ventricular end diastolic wall stress.

2 Increased mean arterial pressure.

3 No significant change in heart rate.

4 Cardiac preload increases especially with supracoeliac cross-clamping but it may decrease or not change. This effect depends on several factors such as prevailing sympathetic tone. With infracoeliac cross-clamping there are inconsistent effects on preload. Compression of the inferior vena cava and other factors may interfere with blood volume redistribution and preload.

5 Filling pressures (central venous pressure, pulmonary capillary wedge pressure) are likely to increase in patients with significant coronary artery disease and decrease in patients without coronary artery disease.

6 Cardiac output and stroke volume may decrease.

7 With increased duration of aortic cross-clamping, systemic vascular resistance increases and cardiac output decreases.

8 Infrarenal cross-clamping causes a 75% increase in renovascular resistance and a 30% decrease in renal blood flow.

Strategies to Minimise the Physiological Effects of Cross-clamping

1 Aim for slightly reduced filling pressures for the half hour prior to clamp placement.

2 Vasodilator therapy e.g. a glyceryl trinitrate (GTN) infusion can reduce or reverse the decrease in cardiac output due to the increase in afterload resulting from cross-clamping.

3 GTN is particularly indicated if there is myocardial ischaemia or hypertension during cross-clamping.

4 If more aggressive afterload reduction is required commence sodium nitroprusside (SNP).

5 If mean arterial pressure cannot be maintained, commence inotropic support. If impaired myocardial contractility is suspected consider a dobutamine infusion.

6 The greatest blood loss usually occurs at the time when the aneurysm is open and there is back bleeding from the lumbar arteries.

Physiological Effects of Unclamping the Aorta

1 Systemic vascular resistance is suddenly decreased with a decrease in mean arterial pressure. Reactive hyperaemia of the lower body and washout of accumulated vasodilator substances contributes to the fall in mean arterial pressure. This effect begins after 10 s and a maximal response occurs 15 min after unclamping.

2 Accumulation of myocardial depressant substances may occur.

Strategies to Minimise the Physiological Effects of Unclamping

1 Prior to unclamping, fluid load the patient to a central venous pressure (or pulmonary capillary wedge pressure) of ≈ 16 mm Hg or at least slightly greater than pre-clamping pulmonary capillary wedge pressure.

2 Replace blood loss appropriately. ***See*** *Blood Loss Assessment and Initial Management* and *Blood Transfusion.*

3 Cease vasodilator therapy prior to unclamping.

4 Releasing the clamp gradually may allow for smoother cardiovascular control. Consider reapplying the clamp if sustained hypotension occurs. Inotropic support may be required.

Endoluminal Abdominal Aortic Aneurysm Repair

Endoluminal aortic aneurysm repair involves placing an aortic graft into the lumen of the aneurysm via the femoral arteries.

Advantages

1 Less haemodynamic changes with less morbidity/mortality.

2 Much less blood loss.

3 Can be done without general anaesthesia.

4 ICU admission postoperatively is much less likely.

5 Endoluminal repair has an increasing role in the management of ruptured AAA.

Disadvantages

1 Graft (endo) leaks can occur requiring further surgery in about 15% of patients.[10]
2 Conversion to open repair may be required but is rare.
3 Renal dysfunction may occur due to significant intravenous dye load especially in patients with pre-existing renal disease. A recent study showed no benefit from N-acetyl cysteine in preventing contrast-induced nephropathy in endoluminal AAA repair.[11]
4 Bowel, pelvic or spinal cord ischaemia can occur due to vascular exclusion by the graft.

Preparation for Surgery

Preparation for potentially massive blood loss must be made. Positioning on the operating table must be extremely precise and requires the assistance of the radiographer.

Anaesthetic requirements include:
1 rapid infusion catheter (7 or 8.5 Fr)
2 intra-arterial blood pressure monitoring
3 5-lead ECG monitoring
4 urinary catheter, temperature probe
5 warming blanket over upper body.

Induction and Maintenance Phase

1 Aim for cardiovascular stability as for an open procedure. Haemodynamic stability is significantly greater with endoluminal repair compared with open repair.[12]
2 The patient must be heparinised at the time of femoral or iliac artery instrumentation.
3 Stent grafts are usually self-expanding. Some require balloon dilatation to obtain an endo-seal. During the phase of balloon inflation or placement of the self-expanding graft, hypotension may be required.[11] This is to reduce the force pushing the stent distally. Hypotension can be achieved by increasing the inspired concentration of sevoflurane, or boluses of propofol.

Ruptured Abdominal Aortic Aneurysm Repair

Between 30% and 60% of patients with ruptured abdominal aortic aneurysm die before reaching hospital. Of the patients who survive to hospital admission about 50% die in the peri-operative period.

Principles of Management—Pre-anaesthetic Phase

1 Transfer the patient to the operating theatre with minimal delay. Diagnostic procedures should be kept to a minimum. The aggressiveness of initial fluid resuscitation prior to surgery is a controversial issue.[13] Some

clinicians argue that fluid resuscitation leads to more bleeding, and a systolic BP of 50–70 mm Hg should be accepted and maintained with minimum transfusion of blood or colloid.[14,15] Other researchers believe a more conventional approach should be taken aiming for a mean blood pressure of around 65 mm Hg.[13]

2 After ensuring a clear airway and ventilation the next priority is the insertion of several large bore IV cannulas so that adequate intravascular resuscitation can occur. *See Blood Loss Assessment and Initial Management* and *Blood Transfusion*.

3 Obtain cross matched blood as soon as possible.

4 Obtaining intra-arterial blood pressure monitoring is the next priority. Other invasive pressure monitoring devices can be placed after the aorta is clamped.

Induction and Maintenance of Anaesthesia

1 Prepare the abdomen surgically and drape the patient prior to induction of anaesthesia to minimise anaesthesia to aortic clamp time.

2 There is no evidence to support one choice of anaesthetic agents over another as long as the drugs are used appropriately to minimise cardiovascular instability.[13] A rapid sequence induction should be used but recommended induction agents include combinations of fentanyl, thiopentone (in small doses), midazolam and ketamine. One or more of these drugs is combined with a rapidly acting muscle relaxant such as rocuronium or suxamethonium. For a discussion of anaesthetic options in the presence of severe blood loss *see Blood Loss Assessment and Initial Management*.

3 Rapid attainment of aortic cross-clamping is the next aim, to reduce haemorrhage. When bleeding is controlled and the patient stabilised, ongoing management is as described for elective repair.

◇ Abdominal Pregnancy

In this condition fertilisation takes place outside the uterine adnexae or a tubal pregnancy ruptures and survives in the abdominal cavity. Implantation can occur on organs such as the external uterine wall, liver or spleen and the pregnancy progresses. The incidence is about 1 per 10 000 live births.[16] This situation can result in massive haemorrhage at any time during pregnancy due to detachment of the placenta with a high maternal (up to 30%) and fetal (40–90%) mortality.[17] Fetal congenital abnormalities are also common.[17]

Diagnosis

Surprisingly only about 50% of cases are diagnosed prior to rupture, usually by ultrasound and clinical evaluation.[18] Suggestive symptoms and signs are:

1 persistent transverse or oblique lie
2 abdominal pain and tenderness
3 palpable fetal parts.

Management of Diagnosed Abdominal Pregnancy

If the condition is diagnosed before 24 weeks gestation, surgery to remove the fetus and placenta is recommended. If diagnosed after 24 weeks gestation and the fetus is viable, management is similar to placenta praevia. Management includes:

1 Admit the patient to a tertiary obstetric hospital with advanced neonatal care facilities.
2 Prepare for massive blood loss at any time.
3 Surgical delivery at an appropriate time decided upon by the mother and obstetrician. Preparation must be made for massive intra-operative haemorrhage. **See** *Blood Loss Assessment and Initial Management* and *Blood Transfusion*.

Management of Undiagnosed Abdominal Pregnancy

The patient will either present with torrential haemorrhage or the diagnosis will be made at Caesarean section. Management is as for other situations involving massive haemorrhage. Arterial embolisation by an interventional radiologist may assist in the ongoing management of these patients.

�‣ Abruptio Placentae

This condition is defined as the separation of the placenta from its attachment to the decidua basalis prior to delivery of the fetus resulting in haemorrhage. It occurs in 0.66% of deliveries[19] and accounts for 15–20% of all perinatal deaths.[20] About 90% of abruptions are mild to moderate and well tolerated by fetus and mother.

Symptoms and Signs

1 Severely painful unrelenting uterine contractions with incomplete uterine relaxation.
2 Non-reassuring fetal heart trace/fetal death.
3 Concealed or revealed blood loss which may cause various degrees of shock.
4 Coagulopathy, DIC.

Anaesthetic Management

1 Ensure patient has adequate airway and ventilation.
2 Resuscitate the patient's intravascular volume with appropriate fluids (crystalloid, colloid, blood). **See** *Blood Loss Assessment and Initial Management*.
3 Identify and treat coagulopathy.

4 Consider invasive monitoring such as CVP and direct arterial blood pressure measurement.

5 Aim for a urine output of 0.5–1 mL/kg/h and a haematocrit of 30%.

6 Delivery may be vaginal in mild cases or in some cases of fetal death.

7 Epidural or spinal anaesthesia can be used cautiously in controlled situations where the patient is cardiovascularly stable and has been fully resuscitated, there is not significant fetal distress, and coagulopathy is not present.[20]

8 For patients with coagulopathy or uncontrolled haemorrhage or fetal distress GA will usually be required.[21]

◑ Activated Clotting Time (ACT)

Tests the intrinsic and common clotting pathways. Used for such purposes as monitoring heparin therapy during cardiac surgery. NR for ACT 90–120 s. For full heparinisation aim for ACT > 400 s, preferably > 500 s.

◑ Activated Factor VIIa (NovoSeven)

See Recombinant Activated Factor VII.

◑ Activated Partial Thromboplastin Time (APTT)

Tests the intrinsic clotting pathway. NR 25–36 s. Prolonged APTT occurs with heparin therapy and a decrease in the activity of clotting factors; V, X, XI, XII and fibrinogen. *See* Heparin (Unfractionated and Low Molecular Weight Heparins).

◑ Acute Dystonic Reaction

See Dystonic Reaction, Acute.

◑ Acute Fatty Liver of Pregnancy

See Fatty Liver of Pregnancy, Acute.

◑ Acute Intermittent Porphyria

See Porphyria.

◑ Acute Normovolaemic Haemodilution (ANH)

The aim of ANH is to reduce the need for homologous blood transfusion. In this technique the patient's blood is collected after anaesthesia, but before significant blood loss has occurred. The blood is then re-infused after surgical blood loss ceases. ANH can be used in surgery where significant blood loss is expected (> 1000 mL) and the patient can tolerate the technique.

Technique

1 After induction of anaesthesia, 2–3 units of blood (or possibly more) are collected from an arterial line or large venous line.

2 The blood is stored in anticoagulated blood bags that are appropriately labelled. These can be stored without refrigeration for up to 6 h.

3 As the blood is withdrawn, IV fluids are given to replace the volume lost e.g. 1.2 mL gelofusine/1 mL blood.

4 Transfuse the collected blood once the period of significant blood loss is over or Hb < 7–8 g/100 mL.

Rationale

1 Blood lost intra-operatively will be at a lower Hct

2 Blood returned to the patient is fresh whole blood rich in platelets and clotting factors

Evidence for this Technique

ANH is difficult to study because the optimal amount of blood that should be removed, the lowest acceptable Hct for a given patient and how much blood a patient will lose intra-operatively are all unknown or speculative. ANH gambles on the premise that surgical blood loss with ANH will be less in total than without ANH, reducing the amount of homologous blood required. It is difficult to prove this argument clinically. Numerous mathematical models have been proposed and these suggest that for ANH to reduce the need for autologous blood:[22,23,24]

1 A significantly greater amount of blood than 2–3 units needs to be withdrawn (i.e. perhaps > 6 units).

2 Surgical blood needs to be substantial (4–6 L or more).

3 The patient must be able to tolerate a low Hct (e.g. 0.2).

If the above conditions are not met then the amount of autologous blood saved is very modest (< 1 unit). Boldt et al. found that for patients having radical prostatectomy the transfusion rate for homologous blood was reduced by about 15% in the ANH group compared to controls and an average of 0.35 units of homologous blood was saved per patient.[25]

Goodnough et al. estimated that for patients having a radical prostatectomy and ANH, an average of 95 mL of homologous blood was saved per patient.[26] Sanders et al. found in a prospective randomised control trial that ANH did not affect the homologous transfusion rate compared with controls in major gastrointestinal surgery.[27]

▷ Adenosine

Adenosine is a naturally occurring purine nucleoside which is used therapeutically as an antiarrhythmic and hypotensive drug. Adenosine acts mainly at the SA and AV nodes, by stimulating adenosine receptors. It causes reduced automaticity in the SA node and slowed conduction through the AV node.

Indications

1 Used for reverting paroxysmal supraventricular tachycardia (SVT) to sinus rhythm. ***See*** *Supraventricular Tachycardias*.
2 Useful in the management of supraventricular and broad complex tachycardia associated with Wolff-Parkinson-White syndrome. ***See*** *Wolff-Parkinson-White (WPW) Syndrome*.
3 Can be used to help diagnose supraventricular dysrhythmias by providing transcient AV nodal block to enable the atrial rhythm to be clearly visualised on ECG.
4 Has also been used to provide temporary asystole. One report describes the use of adenosine 48 mg to provide asystole for 35 s to enable the repair of a massively bleeding ruptured subclavian artery.[28]

Dose

Dose in Adult for SVT 6 mg IV given as rapidly as possible, flushed through with 20 mL of N/S. If no effect after 2 min give 12 mg then 18 mg if SVT persists. A brief period of asystole lasting up to 15 s is common.

Dose in Child for SVT 0.1 mg/kg IV (max 6 mg), then 0.2 mg/kg (max 12 mg). A third dose of 0.3 mg/kg (max 18 mg) can be considered if necessary.

Dose for Controlled Hypotension 40 μg/kg/min up to 500 μg/kg/min.

Contraindications

Adenosine contraindicated in patients with:

1 asthma
2 sick sinus syndrome or second and third degree heart block unless a pacemaker is present.

Notes

1 Adenosine may cause bronchospasm and profound bradycardia with ventricular excitability. Rarely ventricular tachycardia or fibrillation may occur.
2 Patients on xanthines which block adenosine receptors (e.g. theophylline) and patients on dipyridamole may require an increased dose of adenosine.
3 Patients with denervated hearts, or who are on dipyridamole or carbamazepine, may have an exaggerated response to adenosine that may be hazardous. ***See*** *Heart Transplant Patients, Anaesthetic Consideration for Non-cardiac Surgery*.
4 Adenosine may produce a dangerously rapid ventricular rate if given for a supraventricular tachycardia in patients with Wolff-Parkinson-White syndrome.
5 The effects of adenosine last 20–30 s.

◯ Adrenaline

A catecholamine sympathomimetic drug. Agonist at α and β adrenergic receptors (*see Adrenergic Receptors* below). The degree of stimulation of the various receptors depends on the dose. In adults β-1 and β-2 actions predominate at IV infusion doses less than 2 μg/min. α and β actions occur at IV infusion doses of 2–10 μg/min. Predominantly α actions occur at IV infusion doses greater than 10 μg/min.

Indications

Adrenaline is used in the treatment of:

1 cardiac arrest
2 anaphylaxis
3 low cardiac output states
4 severe bradycardia
5 As a vasoconstrictor to reduce bleeding at the site of surgery and to increase the duration of LA agents
6 to reduce upper airway obstruction secondary to inflammation
7 bronchospasm.

Dose

IV Infusion Add 6 mg of adrenaline to 100 mL N/S (60 μg/mL). The usual dose range for inotropic support 0.01–0.1 μg/kg/min. Start at 5 mL/h, titrate to clinical effect.

IV Bolus Dose Depends on the situation. Do not give a dose > 10 μg in an adult except in extremis.

Adult Cardiac Arrest 1 mg IV boluses for every 3 minutes of arrest time. *See Cardiac Arrest*.

Paediatric Cardiac Arrest 10 μg/kg IV/IO (0.1 mL/kg of 1:10 000 solution). If IV/IO access is not available give 100 μg/kg down the ET tube.

Anaphylaxis The dose for adults is 0.25–0.75 mg IM and for children 10 μg/ kg up to 0.5 mg IM.[29] For life-threatening anaphylaxis administer adrenaline intravenously. Give 5 μg/kg slowly (for a 70 kg patient give 350 μg). Repeat this dose at 5 minute intervals depending on the response. If ongoing adrenaline is required, commence an adrenaline infusion (6 mg in 100 mL N/S). Commence this at 0.25 μg/kg/min (for a 70 kg patient start the infusion at 17 mL/h). Titrate as required to restore CVS stability. *See Anaphylaxis/ Anaphylactoid Reactions*.

Dose via Nebuliser Useful for the treatment of croup and postextubation stridor. Administer 0.5 mL/kg of 1:1000 adrenaline up to 5 mL.[30] 1 mg is reported to be effective in the adult.[31]

Adding Adrenaline to LA Solutions

For a solution containing 1:200 000 adrenaline add 0.1 mL of 1:1000 solution (100 µg) to 20 mL of LA.

Topical Adrenaline (used as a vasoconstrictor)

Use the 1:10 000 solution. Apply liberally to the site, e.g. to skin graft donor site. There is very little systemic absorption of topical adrenaline.[32]

Note: Adrenaline is inactivated if mixed with sodium bicarbonate.

◗ Adrenergic Receptors

These are divided into α1, α2, β1 and β2 adreno-receptors.

α1 Adreno-receptor Stimulation Effects:

Positive inotropy and arterial and venous vasoconstriction.

α2 Adreno-receptor Stimulation Effects:

1 decreased noradrenaline release from sympathetic nerve endings (presynaptic action)
2 decreased sympathetic outflow (central action).

β1 Adreno-receptor Stimulation Effects:

1 positive inotropy and chronotropy
2 increased renin release.

β2 Adreno-receptor Stimulation Effects:

1 vasodilatation of skeletal muscle, coronary and splanchnic vascular beds
2 relaxation of bronchial smooth muscle
3 insulin and glucagon secretion.

◗ Air Embolism

See *Gas Embolism, Venous*.

◗ Airtraq

The Airtraq is a new type of disposable optical laryngoscope developed in Spain and released in 2006 which may assist in the management of the difficult airway. It features:

1 A high-resolution angled optical system allowing indirect wide-angle visualisation of the larynx.
2 A self-contained light system and distal lens warming system to prevent fogging.
3 A guiding channel through which the ET tube can be held and inserted. Once in position the ET tube is passed through the guiding channel into the trachea while visualising the larynx.
4 The device can be used with an optional camera attachment so that the view can be displayed on a screen.

Note: The patient must be able to open their mouth a minimum of about 3 cm.

Indications for the Airtraq

1   Failure of direct laryngoscopy to visualise the larynx. A grade 1 view is usual with the Airtraq. Dhonneur et al. published a report in which 2 morbidly obese patients for CS could not be intubated due to failure of direct laryngoscopy to visualise the larynx. The Airtraq was then used and intubation easily achieved. The time taken from activating the device to securing the airway was less than 1 minute.[33]

2   Awake intubation after suitable LA topicalisation of the oral airway and larynx.[34]

3   Intubation of patients with actual or suspected cervical spine injury. No head/neck manipulation is required with the Airtraq.

4   Intubation by minimally trained staff.[35]

5   Intubation in any position from which access to the oral cavity can be obtained.

6   Inspection of the larynx and periglottic structures prior to extubation for difficult to intubate patients.[36]

Technique for Using the Airtraq

The Airtraq is a single-use device and involves the following steps:

1   Activate the switch on the left side of the eye-piece to turn the light on.

2   Allow a warm-up time of 30–45 sec. This is to warm the lenses to prevent fogging. In an emergency this warm-up time can be ignored.

3   Insert the well-lubricated ET tube into the lateral channel, with the tip of the ET tube aligned with the distal end of the lateral channel. Use a size 3 Airtraq for ET tube sizes 7–8.5, and a size 2 Airtraq for ET tube sizes 6–7.5.

4   Position the patient in the 'neutral' head and neck position (without extending the head or flexing the neck). It is not necessary to align the oral and pharyngeal axes. Jaw thrust may aid positioning of the device.

5   Lubricate the inner curve of the device and insert into the oral cavity over the tongue in the midline.

6   Look through the eyepiece and position the tip just anterior to the base of the epiglottis (in the vallecula).

7   Use the device to elevate the pharynx and expose the larynx and vocal cords. The vocal cords should be in the centre of the field of view.

8   Insert the ET tube under vision through the larynx and into the trachea.

9   Detach the ET tube from the device by carefully moving the device towards the left side of the patient while fixating the ET tube. Then remove the device from the patient.

QUICK FLICK **A**

◗ Airway Anaesthesia

See Awake Fibre-optic Intubation.

◗ Airway Exchange Catheters (AEC)

These devices are very useful for the following situations:

1 Trial of extubation in intubated patients who are difficult to intubate

2 Changing ET tubes in intubated patients who are difficult to intubate

AECs consist of long narrow tubes with multiple openings at the tracheal end and a connection at the proximal end for jet ventilation, circuit ventilation or bag ventilation.

Directions for Use

1 Insert the airway exchange catheter through the endotracheal tube aligning the distance markers.

2 Remove the proximal connector from the AEC.

3 Extubate the patient over the AEC ensuring that the tip of the AEC remains well into the trachea.

4 If required, the patient can be oxygenated via the AEC either by providing supplementary oxygen to the spontaneously breathing patient or by jet ventilation in the paralysed patient.

5 If re-intubation is required, railroad an ET over the AEC using optimal patient positioning and laryngoscopy to assist the intubation.

6 If the tip of the ET tube 'catches' at the level of the laryngeal inlet, rotate the ET tube 90° counterclockwise.

7 There is a significant risk of barotrauma if jet ventilation is used.[37]

◗ Airway Fire

See Tracheostomy, Elective.

◗ Airway Haemorrhage

See Haemoptysis, Massive.

◗ Airway Injury

See Tracheal Rupture.

◗ Airway Scope

See Pentax-AWS Video Laryngoscope.

◗ Albumin Solution

Intravenous colloid solution derived from pooled human plasma. It is sterilised by heat treatment and ultrafiltration and the risk of disease transmission is extremely low. A stabiliser such as sodium caprylate may be added. Albumin has a molecular weight of 69 000 (69 kDa) and is used for:

1 Plasma volume expansion.
2 Cardiopulmonary bypass.
3 Plasma exchange therapy.
4 Treatment and prevention of hepatorenal syndrome. ***See*** *Hepatorenal Syndrome*.

Albumin is presented as a 4% solution and a 25% solution in saline. The 25% solution is hypotonic but hyperoncotic and is used to provide albumin in situations where patients may be unable to cope with a fluid and/or electrolyte load, e.g. renal failure. The half life of albumin in the plasma is > 24 h. Albumin 4% solution also contains sodium 140 mmol/L, chloride 128 mmol/L and octanoate 6.4 mmol/L.

Albumin Studies

The SAFE study reported that there was no increase or decrease in mortality with the use of 4% albumin for intravascular resuscitation of critically ill patients compared to N/S.[38]

A review by Barron et al. indicated that albumin had a lower incidence of adverse side effects (such as anaphylactic/anaphylactoid reactions, renal dysfunction and coagulopathy) compared with artificial colloid solutions.[39]

❯ Alfentanil

Potent short-acting opioid with a peak effect 1 min after injection. Duration of action ≈ 10 min.

Dose

Dose for Spontaneously Breathing Patient 7 μg/kg IV bolus, maintenance dose 2–3 μg/kg IV at 10–15 min intervals.

IV Bolus and Infusion Dose for Controlled Ventilation Patients For procedures lasting 10–30 min use 20–40 μg/kg. For procedures lasting 30–60 min use 40–80 μg/kg. For procedures lasting longer than 60 min use an infusion of 0.5–1 μg/kg/min.

Dose for Reducing the Hypertensive Response to Intubation 20–50 μg/kg IV. Effects last 30–45 min.

❯ Allergic Reaction Prevention

Required for situations such as radiological contrast studies in patients with a history of allergy to contrast media. Although reactions cannot always be prevented, pretreatment does appear to reduce the incidence and severity of reactions.[40]

Based on the Westmead Department of Radiology Protocol (1999):
1 Prednisone 25 mg PO night before and morning of procedure.
2 Promethazine 25 mg PO night before and morning of procedure.

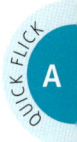

3 Cimetidine 400 mg PO the night before and the morning of procedure.

In addition Have equipment and drugs ready to deal with an allergic reaction. **See** *Anaphylaxis/Anaphylactoid Reactions*.

Note: Allergic reactions are more common with older ionic contrast agents compared with newer agents, and more common with venography compared with arteriography.

◘ American Society of Anesthesiologists Grading

See *ASA (American Society of Anesthesiologists) Grading*.

◘ Aminocaproic Acid

An anti-fibrinolytic drug which acts by inhibiting binding of plasmin to fibrin by blocking the lysine binding sites. It can be used to reduce blood loss during surgery.

Dose
1–15 g IV as a loading dose followed by an infusion of 1–2 g/h for the duration of surgery.

◘ Aminophylline

Methylated xanthine derivative used to treat bronchospasm.

Loading Dose
5 mg/kg over 20 min followed by an infusion of 0.5 mg/kg/h. Mix 500 mg aminophylline with 500 mL N/S. For a 70 kg man give a bolus of 350 mL over 20 min then run an infusion at 35 mL/h.

Note: Do not give a loading dose if the patient is on oral theophylline. TR 10–20 µg/mL.

◘ Amiodarone

Iodinated benzofuran drug which is a predominantly class III antiarrhythmic medication. The pharmacology of amiodarone is extremely complex. Amiodarone is useful for the treatment of
1 Tachydysrhythmias, in particular recurrent ventricular tachycardia and fibrillation, atrial fibrillation and atrial flutter.
2 Ventricular fibrillation resistant to DC cardioversion. Amiodarone is currently the drug of choice for this indication.[41,42]

Dose for Treatment of Tachydysrhythmias Not Associated with Cardiac Arrest
IV Dose Adult 5 mg/kg in 250 mL 5% glucose IV over 20 min to 2 h then 10–15 mg/kg IV in 500 mL 5% glucose over 24 h (infusions of amiodarone over longer periods than 2 h must be contained in glass or polyfine bottles

and a non-PVC giving set must be used, because amiodarone absorbs to PVC). Give preferably via a central line as the drug carrier is highly irritant. Amiodarone is not compatible with normal saline.

Oral Dose 200–400 mg 8 h. After 1 week reduce the oral dose to 200–400 mg daily.

Dose for Shock Resistant VF or VT Associated with Cardiac Arrest or Pre-arrest

IV Dose Adult 5 mg/kg or 300 mg in 20 mL 5% glucose IV bolus. If the initial dose is ineffective give a second dose of 150 mg IV.

IV Dose Child Give 5 mg/kg in 10 mL 5% glucose IV bolus. Give a second dose of 5 mg/kg if required.

Precautions/Contraindications

1 Patients on amiodarone given metoprolol or propranolol may suffer severe bradycardia, cardiac arrest or ventricular fibrillation.[43]
2 There is an increased risk of severe cardiac dysfunction including dysrhythmia for patients on amiodarone exposed to inhalational anaesthetic agents.[43]
3 Amiodarone is contraindicated in patients with iodine hypersensitivity, pregnancy (except for cardiac arrest), thyroid dysfunction, sinus node dysfunction with marked bradycardia and second and third degree AV node block.

◑ Amniotic Fluid Embolus (AFE)

Pathophysiology

This syndrome is due to amniotic fluid components entering the maternal circulation and producing a potentially fatal reaction with severe hypoxia, cardiovascular collapse and coagulopathy. There is thought to be both obstruction and vasoconstriction in the pulmonary vasculature. Mortality is high (> 80%) with about 50% of deaths occurring in the first hour.[44] The incidence is between 1:8000 and 1:80 000 pregnancies. The diagnosis is a clinical one and other causes of sudden collapse must be considered e.g. anaphylaxis. There is no specific test for AFE although the presence of fetal squames in the pulmonary circulation/alveoli is suggestive. There are no specific risk factors for AFE except pregnancy itself.[45] AFE is the fifth most common cause of maternal death.[46]

Clinical Manifestations

Most episodes of AFE occur during labour, particularly during the first stage.[45] Typically there is:

1 dyspnoea, bronchospasm, cyanosis.
2 headache, loss of consciousness, seizure.

3 disseminated intravascular coagulopathy and haemorrhage.
4 hypotension, tachycardia.
5 cardiopulmonary arrest.

If the patient survives the initial episode, subsequent complications may include non-cardiogenic pulmonary oedema, renal failure and permanent brain damage.

Management

Treatment involves the following:

1 Protecting the airway and optimising ventilation.
2 Maintaining intravascular volume with appropriate fluids including blood.
3 Providing circulatory support with inotropes.
4 Correcting coagulopathy (**see** *Disseminated Intravascular Coagulopathy* and *Cardiac Arrest*).
5 Delivering the fetus immediately if resuscitation from cardiac arrest is not successful within 4 minutes.

▷ Amrinone

Bipyridine derivative phosphodiesterase III inhibitor useful for its positive inotropic and vasodilator actions. It is indicated for the treatment of low cardiac output states of cardiac cause.

Dose

Mix 100 mg in 250 mL N/S (not glucose). Give LD of 750 μg/kg ($\approx$ 130 mL in 70 kg patient). Follow this with an infusion of 5–20 μg/kg/min ($\approx$ 50–200 mL/h in 70 kg patient).

Advantages

1 Cardiac output increases without a significant increase in myocardial O_2 consumption. There is little increase in heart rate.
2 Has positive lusiotropic effects (aids myocardial relaxation).
3 Amrinone's pulmonary vasodilator action is useful in the setting of pulmonary hypertension and right ventricular failure.

Disadvantages

1 Vasodilation may result in hypotension.
2 Can cause thrombocytopenia if used for more than 24 h, due to the metabolite N-acetyl amrinone.
3 High doses may cause tachycardia.

▷ Anaphylaxis/Anaphylactoid Reactions

Topics Covered in this Section

▶ Definition
▶ Pathophysiology of Anaphylaxis
▶ Incidence and Causes

- ▶ Clinical Manifestations
- ▶ Treatment—First-line Therapy
- ▶ Treatment—Second-line Therapy
- ▶ Investigations
- ▶ Special Points

Definition

Anaphylaxis (Type 1 hypersensitivity reaction) results from an IgE mediated degranulation of mast cells and basophils in response to a triggering agent such as a drug. For a diagnosis of anaphylaxis the reaction should be 'life-threatening' i.e. respiratory compromise and/or hypotension, rapid in onset and IgE mediated. Anaphylactoid reactions are clinically indistinguishable from anaphylaxis and also involve mast cell and basophil degranulation but the process does not involve IgE antibody. The term 'non-IgE mediated anaphylaxis' is replacing the term 'anaphylactoid'.

Pathophysiology of Anaphylaxis

The steps in this process begin with exposure to a substance resulting in IgE antibodies being produced by plasma cells. The IgE then binds to tissue mast cells and circulating basophils. Re-exposure to the substance, now called an antigen, leads to cross-linkage between the antigen and 2 specific IgE antibodies. This in turn causes mast cells and circulating basophils to degranulate and release vasoactive substances such as histamine, proteases, proteoglycans and leukotrienes. These substances cause profound vasodilatation, increased vascular permeability, and transudation of fluid into the tissues. This results in profound hypovolaemia, falling blood pressure and decreased myocardial perfusion.

Anaphylaxis can occur despite no previous exposure to a triggering substance. It is presumed that this is due to cross-sensitisation with substances of similar structure in food, cosmetics, industrial exposure or some other sources.

Incidence and Causes

The incidence of anaphylaxis is about 1:6000–1:20 000 anaesthetics.[47] Anaphylaxis is most frequently due to muscle relaxants (~60%), especially suxamethonium and rocuronium.[48] Vecuronium and pancuronium are the next most frequent triggers followed by atracurium.[48] Antibiotics account for about 15% of cases.[49] Latex also accounts for about 15% of reactions.

Clinical Manifestations

These include:

1 rash, erythema, urticaria
2 soft tissue swelling (angio-oedeoma) with potential or actual airway compromise
3 cramping abdominal pain, vomiting

4 anxiety, dysphoria
5 cough, bronchospasm
6 tachycardia, bradycardia or other dysrhythmias
7 hypotension and circulatory collapse
8 cardiac arrest.

Note: About 10% of cases present with cardiac arrest or profound hypotension only.[49]

Treatment: First-line Therapy

1 Notify the surgeon and summon skilled assistance.
2 Cease administration of the causative substance e.g. vancomycin infusion, contact with latex.
3 Ensure adequate airway and ventilation. Emergency intubation may be required.
4 Adrenaline must be given and is the most important therapy (together with IV fluids) in the treatment of anaphylaxis. Dose depends on the severity of the reaction:
   a) *Mild-to-moderate Reaction (Early in the Course of Anaphylaxis)* The IM route is preferred for reactions of mild-to-moderate severity due to the risks of IV therapy. *For adults* give 0.25–0.75 mg (0.25–0.75 mL of 1:1000 solution) IM and *for children* 10 µg/kg up to 0.5 mg (0.01 mL/kg of 1:1000 adrenaline up to 0.5 mL) IM.[49] If an *IV line is already in place* consider IV adrenaline. *In adults with mild reactions* use 5–10 µg and for *moderate reactions* give 50–100 µg. For children give 5–10 µg/kg IV.
   b) *Immediately Life Threatening Anaphylaxis* Administer adrenaline IV. *In adults* give 5 µg/kg IV (for a 70 kg patient give 350 µg). *In children* give 10 µg/kg IV. In both adults and children repeat doses of 5 µg/kg can be given 3–5 minutely. If ongoing adrenaline is required, commence an adrenaline infusion (6 mg in 100 mL N/S). Commence this at 0.25 µg/kg/min (for a 70 kg patient start the infusion at 17 mL/h). Titrate as required to restore CVS stability.
   c) *Cardiac Arrest—Adult* 1 mg every 3 min, *Child* 10 µg/kg IV every 3 min. **See** *Cardiac Arrest*.
5 Patients on β blocker drugs may be resistant to adrenaline. Adrenaline dosages may need to be increased or other inotropes, such as noradrenaline, added or substituted. Glucagon 1–2 mg IV every 5 min may be of benefit in adult patients unresponsive to adrenaline.[50]
6 Metaraminol or other pure α agonist has been used successfully in adrenaline resistant anaphylaxis.[51,52]
7 Vasopressin should also be considered. Kill et al. reported the successful use of vasopressin 10 IU–40 IU in 2 patients with adrenaline resistant anaphylaxis.[53]

8 Give liberal N/S. Large volumes may be required (2–4 L). Colloids (e.g. gelatin solutions) can be used in addition to or instead of crystalloids but there is no evidence of improved outcome.[54] Note that gelatin infusions themselves can cause anaphylaxis.

9 Consider the use of a MAST suite for refractory hypotension. **See** Mast Suite.

10 If the patient becomes pulseless, initiate external cardiac compression regardless of ECG rhythm.

Treatment: Second-line Therapy

See Bronchospasm.

1 Antihistamines: give both histamine 1 and 2 receptor blockers intravenously. For H_1 blockade give promethazine 0.5–1 mg/kg and for H_2 blockade give ranitidine 1 mg/kg or famotidine 0.4 mg/kg or cimetidine 4 mg/kg.

2 Hydrocortisone 2–6 mg/kg IV 6h.

3 Nebulised adrenaline (5 mL of 1:1000) may be effective in treating laryngeal oedema but intubate early if airway obstruction is progressive.

4 If intubation is required, induce anaesthesia cautiously as anaesthetic drugs may exacerbate hypotension.

5 Consider using fentanyl 1–10 µg/kg + suxamethonium 1–2 mg/kg.

6 Referral to ICU for ongoing care. Note that in up to 20% of cases there is a recurrence of symptoms from 1–72 h after the initial reaction. This is termed a bi-phasic reaction.

Investigations

1 Serum tryptase 1–3 h after the reaction. The normal value is 5 µg/L and an elevated value (> 25 µg/L) is strongly indicative of an anaphylactic reaction having occurred. Collection up to 8 h after the reaction may still be useful.

2 Referral to an appropriate clinic for further testing after a period of 4–6 weeks. Useful investigations at this time include:
   a) skin tests (intradermal and prick tests).
   b) allergen specific IgE testing (RAST).
   The aim of testing is to identify which drugs are 'safe' or 'unsafe'. The patient should carry a relevant letter and should wear a MedicAlert® bracelet. Information should be added to the letter each time the patient has an anaesthetic or other relevant drug for the first time.

Special Points

1 Patients on histamine 2 receptor blocking drugs such as ranitidine may suffer A–V node block in the presence of massive histamine release.

2 In patients who die from presumed anaphylaxis, serum tryptase and detection of drug reactive IgE antibodies in blood taken after death can help confirm or exclude diagnosis of an allergic reaction.[55]

◐ Angiotensin Related Antihypertensive Drugs and Anaesthesia

Angiotensin converting enzyme inhibitors (ACEI) and angiotensin II antagonists are used to treat hypertension. Several investigators have noted hypotension on induction in patients treated with these drugs.[56,57] This hypotension may be relatively resistant to vasopressor therapy and related to bradykinin activity.[56] Powell et al. reported that gelofusine may make hypotension associated with ACEI and anaesthetic agents worse.[58]

It is therefore recommended to cease angiotensin converting enzyme inhibitors and angiotensin II antagonists on the day before surgery. If intra-operative hypotension does occur in this setting and is refractory to ephedrine and phenylephrine, consider vasopressin therapy.[59]

◐ Ankle Blocks and Innervation of the Foot

The foot is innervated almost entirely by the sciatic nerve except for the skin on the medial side of the lower leg and foot and the arch of the sole. These areas are innervated by the saphenous nerve. This is a branch of the posterior division of the femoral nerve. Sciatic branches are the:

1 *Sural Nerve* Supplies the skin on the back of the lower leg and lateral foot.
2 *Medial Plantar Nerve* Innervates the skin on the medial sole of the foot and the plantar surface of first $3\frac{1}{2}$ toes.
3 *Lateral Plantar Nerve* Supplies the lateral sole.
4 *Superficial Peroneal Nerve* Supplies the medial side of the great toe and most of the dorsum of the foot.
5 *Deep Peroneal Nerve* Innervates the skin between the great and second toe.

Ankle Block Technique

Requires 5 separate injection sites.

Tibial (Medial Popliteal, Posterior Tibial) Nerve Block

This gives rise to the medial and lateral plantar and the medial calcaneal nerves. The nerve runs behind the medial malleolus, crossing the posterior tibial artery posteriorly.

1 Place the patient prone with the ankle supported on a pillow. Insert a 22 G needle, just behind the pulsation of the posterior tibial artery. The nerve lies adjacent to the artery. Direct the needle 45° anteriorly, seeking paraesthesia in the sole of the foot.
2 If paraesthesia is obtained, inject 5 mL of LA (e.g. lignocaine 2%). If paraesthesia is not obtained, inject 10 mL of LA in a fan-like pattern between the posterior tibial artery and the Achilles tendon.

Sural Nerve Block (runs behind lateral malleolus)
Insert the needle into the groove between the lateral malleolus and the calcaneus. Inject 5 mL of LA.

Saphenous Nerve Block (runs in front of the medial malleolus)
Infiltrate LA around the long saphenous vein just anterior to the medial malleolus.

Deep Peroneal Nerve Block
Insert the needle just lateral to the anterior tibial artery (which continues on as the dorsalis pedis artery) at the distal end of the tibia at the level of the skin crease. Inject 5 mL of LA.

Superficial Peroneal Nerve Block
Infiltrate a ridge of LA from the anterior tibia to lateral malleolus, using ≈ 10 mL of LA.

◑ Anticholinergic Crisis

See *Myasthenia Gravis*.

◑ Anticholinergic Syndrome

See *Central Anticholinergic Syndrome*.

◑ Anticoagulation Therapy and Epidurals

See *Epidural Anaesthesia (Anticoagulant Therapy and Epidurals)*.

◑ Anticoagulation Therapy and Surgery

Anticoagulant drugs can be divided into:
1 indirect thrombin inhibitors e.g. heparin.
2 direct thrombin inhibitors e.g. hirudin, argatroban. *See* *Direct Acting Thrombin Inhibitors (DTI)*.
3 vitamin K antagonists such as warfarin. *See* *Warfarin*.
The following recommendations are based on balancing the risk of peri-operative anticoagulation with the risk of thromboembolism.[60] Contact the patient's haematologist for advice.

Topics Covered in this Section
▶ Oral Anticoagulation and Elective Surgery
▶ Oral Anticoagulation and Emergency Surgery
▶ For a discussion of heparin therapy and surgery *see* *Heparin (Unfractionated and Low Molecular Weight Heparins)*.
▶ For a discussion of regional anaesthesia and anticoagulant therapy *see* *Epidural Anaesthesia*.

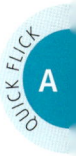

Oral Anticoagulation and Elective Surgery

Patients on warfarin fall into 5 main groups:
1 deep venous thrombosis/pulmonary embolus (DVT/PE)
2 acute arterial embolism e.g. CVA
3 atrial fibrillation
4 mechanical heart valves
5 congestive cardiac failure.

For some types of surgery it is unnecessary to cease warfarin e.g. excision of superficial skin lesions, cataract surgery, some vascular surgery. Check with the surgeon if in any doubt. If anticoagulation therapy needs to be stopped, omit warfarin for 4 days prior to surgery. Measure the INR on the day before surgery. If INR > 1.5 give Vit K 1 mg IV. If INR < 1.5 surgery can safely proceed.

Table A1 Oral anticoagulation and surgery

Condition	Preop	Postop
DVT/PE < 1 month	Full	Full
DVT/PE > 1 month < 3 months	Nil	Full
Recurrent DVT/PE	Nil	Prophylactic
Arterial embolism < 1 month	Full	Full (see below)
Atrial fibrillation (non valvular)	Nil	Prophylactic
Mechanical heart valve	Full	Prophylactic
Congestive heart failure	Nil	Prophylactic

Full = Full Anticoagulation Therapy

If full anticoagulation therapy is required preoperatively start LMW heparin when the INR < 2. Cease LMW heparin therapy at least 24 h before surgery. If full dose therapy is required postoperatively commence at least 24 h after major surgery and possibly longer. Discuss this issue with the surgeon and haematologist.

The subcut doses for full anticoagulation are:
1 enoxaparin (clexane) 1 mg/kg 12 h or 1.5 mg/kg daily
2 dalteparin (fragmin) 100 u/kg 12 h.

Do not use LMW heparins in patients with renal failure. If patients have renal impairment, reduce the quoted doses by 50%. IV heparin can be used instead of LMW heparin. **See** *Heparin (Unfractionated and Low Molecular Weight Heparins)*. Cease heparin infusion 6–8 h before surgery. Recommence heparin infusion at least 24 h after major surgery, or longer in some circumstances, without a loading dose. Discuss the timing of restarting heparin with the surgeon.

Prophylactic = Prophylactic Anticoagulation Therapy

Start prophylactic anticoagulant therapy at least 6 h after surgery.
The prophylactic doses are:

1 enoxaparin 40 mg daily
2 dalteparin 5000 u daily
3 heparin 5000 u 8 h.

Recommencing Warfarin Therapy

Warfarin should be restarted on the evening of surgery, if possible, at the patient's regular dose without a loading dose. Warfarin therapy should be overlapped with LMW heparin or heparin for at least 5 days and until the INR has been in the therapeutic range for at least 2 days. *See Warfarin*.

Oral Anticoagulation and Emergency Surgery

If surgery is urgent and the patient is fully warfarinised, the anticoagulant effects of warfarin can be reversed by:

1 vitamin K 5 mg IV
2 prothrombinex-HT 25 u/kg
3 fresh frozen plasma 1 or more units
4 recombinant Activated Factor VII.

See Warfarin.

◗ Antiplatelet Drugs

Drugs that inhibit platelet function include:

1 Aspirin. *See Aspirin*.
2 NSAIDs. *See Non-steroidal Anti-inflammatory Drugs (NSAIDs)*.
3 Platelet adenosine diphosphate receptor antagonists. These include clopidogrel (Plavix), ticlopidine and prasugrel. *See Platelet Adenosine Diphosphate (ADP) Receptor Antagonists*.
4 Platelet glycoprotein IIb/IIIa receptor antagonists. Examples include abciximab and tirofiban. *See Platelet Glycoprotein IIb/IIIa Receptor Antagonists*.

◗ Aortic Valve Incompetence (Chronic)

Chronic aortic valve incompetence or regurgitation (AI) is usually much better tolerated than aortic valve stenosis. Chronic AI results in left ventricular dilatation and hypertrophy, eventually leading to left ventricular failure with reduced exercise tolerance and dyspnoea. An ejection fraction of < 55% and atrial fibrillation are associated with increased risk of cardiac morbidity and mortality.[61]

Management Aims During Anaesthesia

For chronic AI only:

1 Avoid bradycardia as this can result in acute left ventricular overload. A mild tachycardia may be beneficial.
2 Avoid increases in systemic vascular resistance which can result in an increase in the regurgitant fraction and left ventricular failure. Afterload reduction may be beneficial.

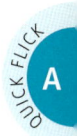

3 Maintain myocardial contractility. Avoid drugs which are myocardial depressants.

4 Consider bacterial endocarditic prophylaxis. Currently the American Heart Association does not advocate antibiotics for this lesion unless there has been a history of endocarditis. *See Bacterial Endocarditis (BE) Prophylaxis*.

○ Aortic Valve Stenosis (AS)

Severe aortic stenosis is a major predictor of cardiac risk for non-cardiac surgery. *See Cardiovascular Peri-operative Risk Prediction for Non-cardiac Surgery*.

Patients with suspected severe aortic stenosis should have elective surgery delayed and be referred to a cardiologist for assessment and/or aortic valve replacement, especially if they are symptomatic.[62] The estimated mortality for non-cardiac surgery in patients with severe symptomatic AS is about 10%.[62] Percutaneous balloon aortic valvulotomy should be considered for patients with severe stenosis who have refused valve replacement or who are at high risk for valve replacement.

Clinical Picture

Symptoms include:

1 Dyspnoea, especially shortness of breath on exertion.

2 Angina due to the hypertrophied myocardium being vulnerable to ischaemia.

3 Syncope, usually with effort, due to the heart being unable to maintain adequate output and blood pressure during the period of vasodilatation associated with exercise.

Note: Sudden death may occur.

Examination and Investigation Findings

1 A pulse pressure < 30 mm Hg suggests severe disease.

2 CXR may show left atrial enlargement and dilatation of the aortic root. Pulmonary oedema can occur acutely.

3 ECG may show LV hypertrophy, LV strain pattern and LBBB.

4 Echocardiography to calculate valve area and transvalvular pressure gradient.

Table A2 Aortic valve area as an indication of AS severity[63]

Severity of AS	Aortic Valve Area
Normal Valve Area	2.5–3.5 cm^2
Mild AS	> 1.5 cm^2
Moderate AS	0.8–1.5 cm^2
Severe AS	< 0.7 cm^2

Note: Transvalvular pressure gradient across the aortic valve greater than 50 mm Hg is consistent with severe disease. A transvalvular gradient of < 20 mm Hg indicates mild disease.

Management Aims During Anaesthesia

1. Maintain sinus rhythm to preserve the contribution of atrial contraction to preload. Always have a defibrillator immediately available.
2. Ensure adequate preload and maintain normovolaemia.
3. Maintain systemic vascular resistance as a decrease may result in a decreased mean arterial pressure with decreased coronary blood flow and subsequent myocardial depression. A vicious cycle can thus be created as myocardial depression leads to further decreases in coronary blood flow and cardiac output.
4. Optimise heart rate to 70–80 bpm. Avoid bradycardia which may result in decreased cardiac output and overdistension of the left ventricle.
5. Avoid tachycardia which can result in decreased left ventricular filling and ejection.
6. Consider invasive monitoring including use of an arterial line and a PA catheter. CVP measurement may be an unreliable measure of preload in patients with reduced left ventricular compliance.
7. Consider bacterial endocarditis prophylaxis. Currently the American Heart Association does not advocate antibiotics for this lesion unless there has been a history of endocarditis. *See Bacterial Endocarditis (BE) Prophlylaxis*.
8. Treat hypotension with vasoconstrictor agent. Use ephedrine if heart rate is low or metaraminol if heart rate is high.
9. If cardiac arrest occurs, external heart massage may be ineffective and internal heart massage should be considered early.

Aortic Stenosis and Obsteric Anaesthesia

The issue of whether regional anaesthesia or general anaesthesia is used for CS is highly debatable.[64,65] In either case extreme caution must be exercised and appropriate monitoring used.

CS Under GA

In addition to the precautions outlined above, Orme et al. recommend:[66]

1. Induction with etomidate 0.1–0.2 mg/kg, remifentanil 2–4 µg/kg and suxamethonium.
2. Maintenance with remifentanil 0.05–0.15 µg/kg/min plus isoflurane.

Regional Anaesthesia and AS

There are numerous reports of the successful use of epidural anaesthesia for labour and delivery in patients with AS.[64] A single shot spinal should not be used. Epidural anaesthesia should be used slowly and carefully. Incremental SAB has been successfully used for CS utilising a spinal microcatheter and 1 mL doses of heavy bupivacaine.[67]

◖ Apgar Score

See Neonatal Resuscitation.

◗ Aprepitant

Anti-nausea drug that acts by antagonising the neurokinin-1 receptor. For the prevention of PONV give 40 mg PO 1–3 h before surgery. **See** *Nausea and Vomiting, Postoperative (PONV)*.

◗ Aprotinin

Naturally occurring serine protease inhibitor which inhibits trypsin, plasmin and plasma and tissue kallikreins thus inhibiting fibrinolysis and promoting haemostasis. It is the most potent of the antifibrinolytic drugs.

Uses

Aprotinin is used for reduction of blood loss during operations such as cardiac, orthopaedic, vascular, liver and prostate surgery.

Dose

Adult Loading Dose 500 000–1 000 000 kallikrein inhibition units (KIU) IV slowly followed by an infusion of 200 000 KIU/h until bleeding stops.

Risks

Although more studies are required, Mangano et al. found that aprotinin use in cardiac surgery significantly increased the risk of renal failure, myocardial infarction, heart failure and stroke.[68] In November 2007 the BART (Blood Conservation using Antifibrinolytics: A Randomised Trial) was halted because of an excess number of deaths in the aprotinin treatment arm compared with aminocaproic acid or tranexamic acid. Aprotinin sales were suspended that same month.

◗ Argatroban

Direct acting thrombin inhibitor which is excreted in bile and is therefore useful in patients with renal failure. It is given by IV infusion and monitored by APTT.

◗ Arrow MAC™ Two Lumen Central Venous Access Device

The MAC™ is a 2 lumen central venous access kit from Arrow International. The device provides multilumen large bore central venous access and is inserted in an identical way to a pulmonary artery catheter introducer sheath using a Seldinger technique. The distal lumen of the MAC is 9 Fr and there are 2 large side lumens of 12 G each. A MAC compatible triple lumen central line can be passed through the MAC and locked into place with a Luer-Lock fitting. Alternatively a PA catheter can also be inserted through the MAC™.

○ Arterial Blood Gas (ABG) Analysis

Normal range (NR) of arterial blood gas values:

pH	7.36–7.44
PaO_2	85–100 mm Hg (11.3–13.3 kPa)
$PaCO_2$	36–44 mm Hg (4.8–5.9 kPa)
Bicarbonate	22–26 mmol/L. This is the plasma bicarbonate concentration calculated from the pH and pCO_2 values using the Henderson-Hasselbalch equation.
Standard Bicarbonate	22–26 mmol/L. This is the bicarbonate concentration when $PaCO_2$ = 40 mm Hg and the blood is fully oxygenated at $37°C$.
Base excess	0 +/– 4. Defined as the amount of strong acid needed to titrate 1 L of fully saturated blood at $37°C$ to a pH of 7.4 when the $PaCO_2$ is 40 mm Hg.

'Rules of Thumb' for ABG Interpretation[69]

1 If PaO_2 + $PaCO_2$ > 140 mm Hg the patient is receiving supplemental oxygen.
2 PaO_2 decreases with age.
   $PaO_2 ≈ 100 – age/3$.
3 With a respiratory acidosis, for every 10 mm Hg increase in $PaCO_2$, bicarbonate increases by 1 mmol/L acutely and by 3–4 mmol/L chronically.
4 With a respiratory alkalosis bicarbonate decreases by 2.5 mmol/L per 10 mm Hg fall in $PaCO_2$ down to a minimum of 18 mmol/L.
5 With a metabolic acidosis the $PaCO_2$ is usually within +/– 5 mm Hg of the last 2 digits of the pH value down to a pH of 7.15.
6 In a metabolic alkalosis the $PaCO_2$ is usually within +/– 5 mm Hg of the last 2 digits of the pH value up to a pH value of 7.60.

Table A3 Direction of changes in pH, $PaCO_2$ and bicarbonate in the following pathological conditions

Pathological state	pH	$PaCO_2$	Bicarb	BE
Metab acidosis	↓	↓	↓	–ve
Metab alkalosis	↑	↑	↑	+ve
Resp acidosis	↓	↑	↑	+ve
Resp alkalosis	↑	↓	↓	–ve

○ Arterial Injection

See *Intra-arterial Injection*.

○ Arterial Switch Procedure

See *Transposition of the Great Vessels*.

◯ ASA (American Society of Anesthesiologists) Grading

I – Healthy patient
II – Mild systemic illness
III – Severe systemic illness that is not incapacitating
IV – Severe systemic illness which is a constant threat to life
V – Patient moribund and unlikely to survive 24 h with or without surgery
E – Emergency surgery
T – Trauma

◯ Aspiration, Prevention and Treatment

The incidence of aspiration is about 1:4000 for elective surgery and 1:900 for emergency surgery.[70] Patients are unlikely to suffer pulmonary complications from aspiration if they do not have symptoms or signs of pulmonary pathology within 2 h of the aspiration episode.[71] Of patients who aspirate, about 50% suffer major morbidity, about 20% require ventilation in ICU for > 6 h, and approx 4% die.[70,72]

Patients at Risk

1 Pregnant patients. Aspiration risk may begin as early as 12th week and continues until 2–3 days post delivery. *See Pregnancy and Non-obstetric Surgery—Anaesthetic Considerations*.
2 Obese patients. *See Body Mass Index (BMI) and Obesity*.
3 Patients with a history of reflux and/or hiatus hernia.
4 Patients with oesophageal strictures or stents.
5 Patient with a full, or potentially full, stomach due to such situations as:
   a) Inadequate pre-operative fasting. *See Fasting Pre-operatively*.
   b) Less than 6 h between the time of a significant injury (e.g. limb bone fracture) and time of last solid food.
   c) Emergency abdominal surgery.
6 Many other pre-existing illnesses can predispose to aspiration such as diabetes mellitus, burns and decreased level of consciousness.

Strategies to Prevent Aspiration and/or Minimise its Effects

1 Adequate fasting pre-operatively.
2 Ranitidine 150 mg or omeprazole 40 mg PO the night before and the morning of surgery.
3 Sodium citrate 0.3 M 30 mL within 30 min before induction of anaesthesia.
4 Consider metoclopramide 10 mg IV or IM to increase the rate of gastric emptying and increase lower oesophageal sphincter tone.
5 Placement of a nasogastric tube and sucking out of gastric contents prior to induction of anaesthesia. This is strongly recommended in patients with intestinal obstruction and/or abdominal distension.

6 Use of 'rapid sequence induction' technique. **See** *Rapid Sequence Induction (RSI)*.

7 Extubate patient in the lateral position when the patient is 'awake' and able to protect their own airway.

QUICK FLICK A

Management of Aspiration

This is a life-threatening emergency. Inform the surgeon.

1 Put patient immediately in left lateral position with 30° of head down tilt ('tilt and turn') and vigorously suck out the pharynx and larynx. Apply cricoid pressure immediately unless patient is actively vomiting. This is because cricoid pressure can result in oesophageal rupture in the vomiting patient. **See** *Cricoid Pressure*.

2 If the patient is conscious supply oxygen by face mask in the recovery position. Further management depends on the clinical effects of the aspiration.

3 If the patient is unconscious and breathing provide 100% oxygen via the anaesthetic circuit and mask with cricoid pressure. Decide whether intubation is required or whether the patient should be allowed to wake up, depending on the perceived severity of the aspiration and the patient's clinical condition. For trivial aspiration consider deepening anaesthesia to aid suctioning of the larynx and bag mask ventilation.

4 If the patient is unconscious and apnoeic or hypoxic intubate immediately using suxamethonium and cricoid pressure. Suction through the ET tube to remove aspirated material prior to ventilation unless the patient is hypoxic, in which case ventilate immediately. The appropriate size 'Y' cath suction catheter = 2 × the ET tube internal diameter.

5 Ventilate with 100% oxygen and pass an oropharyngeal tube to empty the stomach.

6 If there is clinical/radiological evidence of airway obstruction by aspirated material, perform bronchoscopy and remove the obstruction. Bronchial lavage may be helpful.

7 Decide whether:

   a) Aspiration is significant or not. The lower the pH of the aspirate and the greater the volume, the greater the potential for lung injury. Patients are at risk if pH of aspirate < 2.5 and volume aspirated is > 25 mL.[73]

   b) Decide whether surgery should be abandoned or must continue.

   c) If surgery abandoned or completed decide whether patient should remain intubated or should be extubated. This decision is based on the perceived severity of the aspiration.

8 Anticipate/treat bronchospasm. **See** *Bronchospasm*.

9 Do not give antibiotics unless signs and symptoms of infection develop or unless aspiration of feculent material, in which case consider cefotaxime or clindamycin, plus gentamicin + metronidazole.[74,75]

10 Alter antibiotics appropriately depending on available sensitivities.

11 Commence/continue antacid therapy (e.g. H_2 blocker drug).

12 In patients who have aspirated and are to remain intubated and ventilated, consider early application of PEEP.[75]

▷ **Aspirin**

Acetylsalicylic acid used for its anti-inflammatory, antipyretic, antiplatelet and analgesic effects. Aspirin inhibits cyclo-oxygenase type 1 irreversibly in platelets and its antiplatelet effects last for about 7 days.

Dose

For an antiplatelet effect in adults e.g. to prevent TIAs or recurrence of MI use 100–150 mg daily PO. For analgesia, anti-inflammatory antiantipyretic effects in adults use 300–600 mg PO.

Special Points

1 Aspirin should not be used in children under 12 yrs due to the risk of Reye's syndrome.

2 Can cause exacerbation of asthma.

3 Can increase blood loss in cardiac, orthopaedic and other types of surgery.

4 Aspirin use in itself up to 300 mg/day is not a contraindication to epidural or spinal anaesthesia.[76]

5 If patients are on aspirin for prevention of stent thrombosis it should be continued peri-operatively.[76]

▷ **Asthma**

Pre-operative Preparation of the Asthmatic Patient

1 Optimise the patient's anti-asthma medication and continue therapy up to the time of surgery.

2 If the patient is asymptomatic, tests of respiratory function are usually not required.

3 If the patient is suffering from an acute exacerbation of their asthma, elective surgery should be postponed because of the increased anaesthetic risk.

4 If the optimal condition of the patient is in doubt, or the patient has moderate-to-severe asthma, lung function tests are indicated. The most helpful are spirometry, in particular Forced Expiratory Volume in 1 second (FEV$_1$), Forced Vital Capacity (FVC), Peak Expiratory Flow Rate (PEFR), and arterial blood gas analysis. For adults, a PEFR of < 120 L/min, FEV$_1$ of <1 L, and hypercapnia are indicative of severe disease.[77,78] FEV$_1$ will usually be less than 50% of FVC in severe disease.

5 If the patient has been on steroid therapy for a significant period of time, steroids must be continued and extra steroid dosage given to cover the stress of surgery. **See** *Steroid 'Cover' for Surgery/Anaesthesia*. For patients with moderate-to-severe asthma, consider initiating a course of steroid therapy to cover the peri-operative period e.g. prednisone 40 mg daily started 3 days prior to surgery, or hydrocortisone 1–3 mg/kg IV daily.[79]

6 Cancel elective surgery if the patient is suffering from an acute URTI or chest infection. Wait for 2–3 weeks after clinical recovery before elective surgery.[80]

7 Always consider regional anaesthesia.

Premedication
If premedication is required consider a benzodiazepine such as diazepam.

Induction
Suitable drugs include propofol and ketamine. Thiopentone may cause increased airway constriction.[78] Prior to intubation, the patient should be deeply anaesthetised. Consider lignocaine 1–2 mg/kg IV to help prevent bronchoconstriction.[80] Topical lignocaine is not effective and may induce bronchoconstriction in asthmatics.[81] Avoid intubation if possible. LMA is tolerated much better in asthmatics than intubation.[82]

Maintenance
Sevoflurane, isoflurane and halothane cause bronchodilation. Sevoflurane is probably the inhalational agent of choice.[83] Desflurane can cause bronchoconstriction and should be avoided in the asthmatic.[83] Use a non-histamine releasing neuromuscular blocking drug e.g. rocuronium.

Treatment of Intra-operative Bronchospasm
See *Bronchospasm*.

Emergence
Extubate the patient 'deep' if possible. If patient must be extubated awake consider lignocaine 1–2 mg/kg IV 5 minutes before extubation.

Postoperative Management
1 Restart patient's anti-asthma therapy as soon as possible after surgery.

2 Consider chest physiotherapy e.g. incentive spirometry.

Analgesic Considerations
1 **Opioids**

It is probably preferable to use opioids which cause minimal histamine release such as fentanyl. Morphine does cause some histamine release and is traditionally avoided.[78] All opioid drugs may cause respiratory depression.

2 **Non-steroidal Anti-inflammatory Drugs (NSAIDs)**

An acute exacerbation of asthma can be precipitated by NSAIDs, especially in patients who are hypersensitive to aspirin.[84]

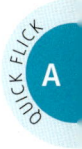

Note:
1   β blocker drugs should be avoided in asthmatics
2   Halothane can interact with aminophylline to produce life-threatening dysrhythmias.[77]
3   H_2 receptor antagonists such as cimetidine should be avoided as they enhance histamine-induced bronchospasm and slow the metabolism of theophylline.

○ Atenolol

Selective β1 adreno-receptor blocker useful for the treatment of hypertension, angina and tachydysrhythmias. The routine use of atenolol in patients at risk of cardiac complications may significantly reduce cardiac-related morbidity and mortality associated with major surgery.[2] Manufacture of IV atenolol in Australia was ceased in June 2003. At the time of writing this book, IV atenolol is still being manufactured in the USA. ***See*** *Beta-blocker Therapy and Reduction of Cardiac Risk*.

Dose for Hypertension
Adult 2.5–10 mg IV. Give in 1 mg/min increments. Oral dose 50–100 mg/day.

Child 0.05 mg/kg/dose IV every 5 min until desired response, maximum of 4 doses. Oral dose 1–2 mg/kg 12–24 h.

○ Atrial Fibrillation (AF), Acute

Identify and Treat Cause if Possible
The most common causes are:[85]
1   ischaemic and valvular heart disease
2   hypertension
3   thyrotoxicosis
4   pneumonia
5   electrolyte and acid–base disturbances.

Patients Requiring Immediate Treatment
This can be defined as patients with heart rate >150 bpm, chest pain or evidence of shock. Cardioversion may also be required urgently if there is severe aortic stenosis or hypertrophic cardiomyopathy.
1   Seek urgent expert assistance.
2   Heparinise the patient.
3   Provide DC cardioversion under sedation or anaesthesia. If a monophasic defibrillator is used, give 25–100 J initially. The shock must be synchronised with the QRS complex. Up to 200 J may be required. Biphasic defibrillation is more effective than monophasic shock and requires less energy.[86] Start with 70–100 J.
4   Correct possible causes or exacerbating factors e.g. hypokalaemia.

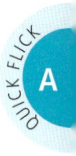

5 If cardioversion fails or AF recurs give amiodarone. *See Amiodarone*.
6 Repeat cardioversion after amiodarone and if this is not successful or AF recurs consider a second dose of amiodarone.

Patients Not Requiring Immediate Treatment AND Known to Have AF < 24 h

Seek expert advice. Patients without CVS compromise can be treated with:
1 Heparin + warfarin.
2 Amiodarone for rate control and chemical cardioversion. Flecainide 100–150 mg over 30 min is an alternative.[87]
3 Consider DC cardioversion if chemical cardioversion unsuccessful or patient may suffer eventual compromise from AF. Do not cardiovert if there is digoxin toxicity or a history of sick sinus syndrome or bradycardia.[85]

Patients Known to Have AF > 24 h

In patients with sub-optimal perfusion or structural heart disease treat with:
1 heparinisation
2 amiodarone

DC cardioversion in 3–4 weeks. Do not cardiovert without either 3 weeks of anticoagulation or exclusion of intracardiac thrombus by transoesophageal echocardiography. Continue anticoagulation for 4 weeks after successful cardioversion.

Low-risk patients can be treated as follows:
1 If ventricular rate 100–150, provide rate control with β blockers or verapamil or diltiazem.
2 Heparinisation, warfarin and DC cardioversion in 3–4 weeks (or earlier after intracardiac clot excluded by TOE) as described above. Consider chemical cardioversion with e.g. amiodarone but with the same precautions as for electrical cardioversion.

▷ Atrial Fibrillation, Chronic

For patients with chronic AF, the aim is to control ventricular response either chronically or acutely. The optimal ventricular rate for patients in AF is 90 bpm.[85]

Therapy for Slowing Ventricular Response to AF

1 Digoxin

Oral Dose Adult Give loading dose of 0.5–1 mg, followed by 0.25–0.5 mg every 6 h to a maximum dose of 1.5–2 mg in the first 24 h. Usual maintenance dose in adult is 62.5–250 μg/day depending on such factors as age and renal function.[88]

IV Dose Adult Loading dose 500 μg over 30 min, repeat after 6 h if required. Give up to ≈ 20 μg/kg total LD.

Oral Dose Child 15 μg/kg loading dose, then 5 μg/kg/dose 12 h.

IV Dose Child 15 μg/kg over 30 min, then 5 μg/kg 6 h later, then 5 μg/kg/ dose 12 h.

Note: Peak effect occurs at ≈ 2 h. TR 1–2 ng/mL.

2 Verapamil *Adult* 1 mg/min IV to a total dose of 15 mg.

3 β Beta-blocker e.g. esmolol or metoprolol. (**See** *Beta–blocker Therapy and Reduction of Cardiac Risk*).

4 Anticoagulation with warfarin is usually required with chronic AF due to the risk of stroke.

◖ Atrial Flutter, Acute

With atrial flutter the heart rate is often exactly 150/min due to an atrial rate of 300 with a 2:1 heart block. This rate can thus be a clue for the diagnosis.

Electrical Cardioversion

Electrical cardioversion will be required urgently if there is cardiovascular compromise. Use monophasic synchronised shock starting with 25–50 J in the adult, or a biphasic shock of 25–50 J. Atrial overdrive pacing may also be effective. Patients may be converted to sinus rhythm or AF (see above).[89]

Chemical Cardioversion

Acute atrial flutter is usually unresponsive to drug therapy.[85] Ibutilide appears to be the most effective drug.[89]

Drugs to Slow the Ventricular Rate

These drugs are the same as those used for chronic AF.

◖ Atrial Septal Defect (ASD)

ASDs account for about 10% of congenital heart disease. Unrepaired large ASDs can cause pulmonary hypertension but more slowly than VSDs. If repaired the long-term prognosis for ASD is excellent. Endocarditis does not occur in the repaired defect unless there are other abnormalities such as a cleft mitral valve. Arrythmias usually do not occur post repair unless present prior to repair.

◖ Atrial Switch Procedure

See *Transposition of the Great Vessels*.

◖ Atrio-ventricular Block

See *Heart Block (HB)*.

◖ Atropine

An anticholinergic drug which acts as a competitive antagonist at muscarinic receptors. Used for:

1 Drying airway secretions.

2 Treating bradycardia by opposing vagal tone.

3 Countering the muscarinic stimulatory effects of the acetylcholinesterase inhibitor drugs.

Dose

15–20 µg/kg IV or IM. In adults the max dose is 3 mg which causes complete vagal blockade.

Note: Atropine can induce anticholinergic syndrome (**see** *Central Anticholinergic Syndrome*). It can also cause blurred vision.

◯ Automated External Defibrillators

See *Defibrillators*.

◯ Autonomic Dysreflexia

See *Spinal Cord Injury (Chronic) and Anaesthesia*.

◯ AutoPulse

This device from the Revivant Corporation is an automated chest compression machine useful in the management of cardiac arrest. The AutoPulse resembles a short surfboard and utilises a load distributing band which compresses the chest evenly and effectively during CPR. It is unlikely that ECC performed by human rescuers can achieve sufficient coronary perfusion pressure (>15 mm Hg) to maintain cardiac viability during prolonged cardiac arrest (> 3–4 min).[90] This may partially explain why survival from cardiac arrest is so poor. However automated ECC with the AutoPulse does achieve a CPP averaging 21 mm Hg and short- and long-term cardiac arrest survival may be improved.[91] Such devices may therefore represent a major advance in cardiac arrest management. The device is intended for adults up to 136 kg but if the band will fit without an error message (large paediatric patients or adults > 136 kg) then use the device.

Instructions for Use

1 Place the cardiac arrest victim onto the AutoPulse orientated as per the line markings on the machine.
2 Switch the machine on.
3 Fully extend the compression band over the victim's chest.
4 As the band winds in release the band which will then size itself around the victim's chest.
5 The AutoPulse can then be set for continuous compression at a rate of 100 compressions per min or with a pause after every 30 compressions for 2 ventilations.

Advantages

1 Chest compressions are uniformly effective without the deterioration in performance that occurs with human external cardiac compression (ECC).

2 Cerebral and myocardial blood flow are improved compared with human ECC.

3 There is little risk of sternal or rib fracture.[90]

4 Survival from cardiac arrest may be improved. A study by Casner et al. showed a 15% increase in survival to hospital admission in cardiac arrest patients with an initial diagnosis of asystole or PEA.[92]

5 At least one rescuer is freed up for other duties.

6 ECC can be provided while the patient is transported or tilted (as for cardiac arrest in pregnancy).

7 Paramedics do not have to stand in the back of a moving ambulance to perform manual ECC.

Disadvantages

1 The device is bulky, heavy and expensive.

2 Battery life is limited to about 20–30 minutes, although spare charged batteries can be easily carried.

3 Head and arm movement may be excessive.

◐ Awake Fibre-optic Intubation

1 Premedicate with an antisialogogue agent e.g. glycopyrrolate 0.2 mg IV on entering the anaesthetic bay.

2 Sedate with agents such as midazolam, fentanyl and propofol during the procedure +/– a propofol infusion at a sedating dose. *See Propofol*.

3 Topically anaesthetise the airway. There are many ways of doing this, including:

   a) Use 3 mL of 2% lignocaine nebulised in a salbutamol type nebuliser and inhaled by the patient. Alternatively a Devilvis nebuliser can be used with topical 4% lignocaine.

   b) For nasal intubation, soak 4 cotton pledgets in 4% cocaine solution. Insert a cotton pledget gently and gradually along the floor of the nose on each side. The nasal mucosa will be anaesthetised as the pledget is advanced. Insert the other pledgets between the inferior and middle turbinates bilaterally to anaesthetise the sphenopalatine ganglion. Alternatively use 2% lignocaine with adrenaline 1:200 000 or cophenylcaine forte on the pledgets.

   c) 2 mL of 4% lignocaine topical dripped onto the back of the pharynx and larynx with a Cass needle. This may be gargled by the patient.

   d) Cricothyroid puncture is then performed. *See Cricothyroid Puncture and Cricothyrotomy*.
   To perform this procedure:

   i) Anaesthetise the skin over the cricothyroid membrane with a bleb of LA.

ii) Attach a 22 G cannula to a 5 mL syringe containing 2 mL of 2% plain lignocaine.

iii) Insert the cannula through the cricothyroid membrane and confirm tracheal puncture by aspirating air.

iv) Remove the needle stylet and re-attach the syringe to the cannula then inject lignocaine. Warn the patient that this will cause coughing.

e) Consider bilateral superior laryngeal nerve blocks, although these are not usually necessary. **See** *Superior Laryngeal Nerve Block*.

4 A very successful alternative technique to airway anaesthesia relies almost entirely on nebulised lignocaine (adapted from Jenkins and Marshall).[93] For this method:

a) Obtain a 3-way tap, 22 G cannula and green O_2 tubing. A maximum of 20 mL of lignocaine with adrenaline is used.

b) Attach the 3-way tap to the cannula and the green O_2 tubing.

c) Connect the tubing to an O_2 source delivering 2 L/m.

d) Inject through the third port of the 3-way tap 2% lignocaine with adrenaline 0.5–1 mL at a time in a 5 mL syringe.

e) Start by nebulising the LA into nostril (for a nasal intubation) using enough LA (5–10 mL) so that a size 6 nasopharyngeal airway covered with lignocaine jelly is tolerated when inserted through the nostril.

f) Nebulise more LA down the nasopharyngeal tube timed with slow deep inspiration until the voice changes.

g) Remove the nasopharyngeal airway and perform intubation as described below.

h) For oral intubation gargle with 3–5 mL of 1% lignocaine and use 10% lignocaine spray on the tongue and or pharynx.

i) Insert a Burman airway covered with lignocaine jelly and nebulise lignocaine through this airway until the voice changes. Perform FOB and intubation as described below.

5 *Prepare Fibre-optic Bronchoscope (FOB)* Ensure the FOB is correctly focused and orientated. Form a cylinder with the fingers of the right hand and inspect this 'tunnel' through the FOB to check orientation and focus. Apply demisting solution to the tip of the instrument.

6 *For nasal intubation* soften the endotracheal (ET) tube tip by immersing it in hot water. Load the ET tube onto the FOB (size 7–7.5 for an adult male, size 6.5–7.0 for an adult female) ensuring the tube is well lubricated and the Murphy eye is orientated anteriorly facing the epiglottis. Place the patient in the same position as for conventional intubation and ask the patient to protrude the tongue and/or ask an assistant to gently grasp the tongue with gauze and pull it forward. Give supplementary O_2 via a nasal catheter in the contralateral nostril. Consider passing the ET tube through

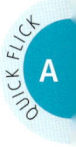

QUICK FLICK **A**

the nose first into the nasopharynx, then passing the tip of the FOB throught the ET tube and then into the larynx.

7 For *oral intubation* use a Burman or Ovassapian airway as a guide, placed exactly in the midline. These airways prevent biting of the FOB and can be removed around the FOB without displacing it.

8 Airway anaesthesia can be supplemented by inserting an epidural catheter down the suction port of the FOB and injecting 4% lignocaine directly onto the site to be anaesthetised. The FOB suction port is of little use for suctioning. It is more effective to suck out secretions with a Yanker sucker, or suction catheter placed blindly into pharynx.

9 Intubate the larynx and trachea with the FOB and identify the carina. Pass the ET tube over the FOB while the view of carina is maintained. As the FOB is removed ensure the ET tube tip is well into the trachea but above the carina. For nasal intubations the ET tube should be at about 26–28 cm at the nares in adults.

�‣ **Awake Intubation without a Fibre-optic Bronchoscope**

Several other devices can be used for awake intubation if the patient is able to open their mouth sufficiently and the oral airway can be adequately topicalised with LA. Also consider the use of analgesia and sedation.

These include:

1 Airtraq
2 Glidescope
3 C-Trach™ and Fastrach™
4 Retrograde intubation
5 Lightwand.

See Airtraq, Glidescope, Fastrach™ Device, Retrograde Intubation and *Lightwand Intubation*.

◖ **Awareness**

Awareness is a surprisingly common and potentially devastating complication of anaesthesia. As stated by one patient:

'… The pain was so acute I couldn't move a finger. My screams stayed in my head … the pain was overwhelming'.[94]

Incidence

The risk of conscious awareness with explicit recall and severe pain is estimated to be < 1:3000 general anaesthetics.[95] Conscious awareness with explicit recall but without severe pain is estimated to be 3:1000 general anaesthetics.[96]

Implicit memory refers to subconscious processing of information while anaesthetised and can be revealed by hypnosis or behavioural suggestions. The risk of awareness is highest in patients undergoing cardiac and obstetric anaesthesia, and is usually due to drug error such as failure of delivery of volatile agent.[97]

The incidence of awareness is also increased in patients undergoing opioid-based anaesthetics.[96]

Detection of Awareness

Signs suggesting awareness (and light anaesthesia) include:

1 tachycardia and hypertension
2 diaphoresis and lacrimation
3 movement.

These signs are very unreliable and frequently do not occur in patients with awareness.[98]

Fortunately there are now available specific monitors for 'wakefulness', including the BIS monitor and the M-Entropy monitor. **See** *Bispectral Index (BIS) EEG Monitor* and *Entropy*.

Management of Significant Awareness

1 Treat the patient with appropriate concern and respect. Believe the patient's account.
2 Post traumatic stress disorder (PTSD) and other physiological conditions may result from awareness under anaesthesia and every effort must be made to appropriately refer and manage patients who have undergone this complication.
3 Notify your Medical Defence Organisation (MDO).

REFERENCES

1 Gelman S. The pathophysiology of aortic cross-clamping and unclamping. *Anesthesiology* 1995; 82: 1026–60.
2 Wallace A, Layug B, Tateo I et al. Prophylactic atenolol reduces postoperative myocardial ischaemia. *Anesthesiology* 1998; 88: 7–17.
3 Mahon P, Shorten G. Perioperative acute renal failure. *Curr Opin Anaesthesiol* 2006; 19: 332–8.
4 Walker GV, Beattie C. Abdominal Aortic Aneurysm Repair. In Roizen MF, Fleisher LA eds. *Essence of Anesthesia Practice*. WB Saunders, Philadelphia 1997: 337.
5 Playford H, Sladen RN. What is the best means of preventing perioperative renal dysfunction? In Fleischer LA ed. *Evidence-Based Practice of Anesthesiology*. Saunders, Philadelphia 2004: 181–90.
6 Halfpenny M, Rushe C, Breen P et al. The effects of fenoldopam on renal function in patients undergoing elective aortic surgery. *Eur J Anesthesiol* 2002; 19: 32–9.

7   Gilbert TB, Hasnain JU, Flinn WR et al. Fenoldopam infusion associated with preserving renal function after aortic cross-clamping for aneurysm repair. *J Cardiovasc Pharmacol Ther* 2001; 6: 31–6.

8   Oliver WC, Nuttall GA, Cherry KJ, Decker PA, Bower T. A comparison of fenoldopam with dopamine and sodium nitroprusside in patients undergoing cross-clamping of the abdominal aorta. *Anesth Analg* 2006; 103: 833–40.

9   Hynninen MS, Niemi TT, Poyhia R et al. N-acetyl cysteine for the prevention of kidney injury in abdominal aortic surgery: a randomized, double-blind, placebo-controlled trial. *Anesth Analg* 2006; 102: 1638–45.

10 Hinchliffe RJ, Hopkinson BR. Current concepts and controversies in endovascular repair of abdominal aortic aneurysms. *J Cardiovasc Surg* 2003; 44: 437–42.

11 Moore NN, Lapsley M, Norden AG et al. Does N-acetyl cysteine prevent contrast induced nephropathy during endovascular AAA repair? A randomized controlled pilot study. *J Endovasc Ther* 2006; 13: 660–6.

12 Baxendale BR, Baker DM, Hutchinson A et al. Haemodynamic and metabolic response to endovascular repair of infra-renal aortic aneurysms. *Br J Anaesth* 1996; 77: 581–5.

13 Brimacombe J, Berry A. A review of anaesthesia for ruptured abdominal aortic aneurysm with special emphasis on preclamping fluid resuscitation. *Anaesth Intensive Care* 1993; 21: 311–23.

14 Ernst CB. Abdominal aortic aneurysm. *New Eng J Med* 1993; 328: 1167–72.

15 Crawford ES. Ruptured abdominal aortic aneurysm: an editorial. *J Vasc Surg* 1991; 13: 348–50.

16 Atrash HK, Friede A, Hogue CJ. Abdominal pregnancy in the United States: frequency and maternal mortality. *Obstet Gynecol* 1987; 69: 333–7.

17 Ramachran K, Kirk P. Massive hemorrhage in a previously undiagnosed abdominal pregnancy presenting for elective Cesarean delivery. *Can J Anesth* 2004; 51: 57–61.

18 Costa SD, Presley J, Bastert G. Advanced abdominal pregnancy. *Obstet Gynecol Surv* 1991; 46: 515–25.

19 Obstetrical Haemorrhage. In Cunningham FG, MacDonald PC, Gant NF et al. eds. *Williams Obstetrics*, 20th edn. Stamford, CT: Appleton and Lange;1997: 746.

20 Ross BK. Critical care issues in obstetric anesthesia. *Audio Digest Anesthesiology* 1999: 41.

21 Terui K. Antepartum Haemorrhage. In Birnbach DJ, Gatt SP, Datta S. *Textbook of Obstetric Anesthesia*. Churchill Livingstone, Philadelphia 2000: 401.

22 Feldman JM, Roth JV, Bjoraker DG. Maximum blood savings by acute normovolaemic hemodilution. *Anesth Analg* 1995; 80: 108–13.

23 Weiskopf RB. Efficacy of acute normovolaemic hemodilution assessed as a function of fraction of blood volume lost. *Anesthesiol* 2001; 94: 439–6.

24 Brechner ME, Rosenfeld M. Mathematical and computer modeling of acute normovolaemic hemo dilution. *Transfusion* 1994; 34: 176–9.

25 Boldt J, Weber A, Mailer K et al. Acute normovolaemic haemodilution vs. controlled hypotension for reducing the use of allergenic blood in patients undergoing radical prostatectomy. *Br J Anaesth* 1999; 82: 170–4.

26 Goodnough LT, Grishaber JE, Monk TG et al. Acute preoperative hemodilution in patients undergoing radical prostatectomy: a case study analysis of efficacy. *Anesth Analg* 1994; 78: 932–7.

27 Sanders G, Mellor N, Rickards K et al. Prospective randomized controlled trial of acute normovolaemic haemodilution in major gastrointestinal surgery. *Br J Anaesth* 2004; 93: 775–81.

28 Schwarte LA, Hartmann M. Intentional circulatory arrest to facilitate surgical repair of a massively bleeding artery. *Anesth Analg* 2003; 97: 339–40.

29 *Australian Prescriber* 2001; 24: Wall Chart Insert.

30 McDonogh AJ. The use of steroids and nebulized adrenaline in the treatment of viral croup over a seven year period in a district hospital. *Anaesth Intensive Care* 1994; 22: 175–8.

31 MacDonnell SPJ, Timmins AC, Watson JD. Adrenaline administered via a nebulizer in adult patients with upper airway obstruction. *Anaesthesia* 1995; 50: 35–6.

32 O'Connell AJ, Keneally JP. Paediatric burns. *Curr Anaesth Crit Care* 1994; 5: 209–17.

33 Dhonneur G, Ndoko S, Amathieu R et al. Tracheal intubation using the Airtraq® in morbid obese patients undergoing emergency Cesarean delivery. *Anesthesiol* 2007; 106: 629–30.

34 Suzuki A, Toyama Y, Iwasaki H. Airtraq® for awake tracheal intubation (Letter). *Anaesthesia* 2007; 62: 744–5.

35 Woollard M, Lighton D, Mannion W et al. Airtraq vs. standard laryngoscopy by student paramedics and experienced prehospital laryngoscopes managing a model of difficult intubation. *Anesthesia* 2008; 63: 26–31.

36 Mort CT. Laryngoscopy vs. optical stylet vs. optical laryngoscopy (Airtraq®) for extubation evaluation (Abstract). *Anesthesiology* 2006; 105: A823.

37 Benumof JL. Airway exchange catheters: Simple concept, potentially great danger (Editorial). *Anesthesiology* 1999; 91: 342–4.

38 The SAFE study Investigations. A comparison of albumin and saline for fluid resuscitation in the intensive care unit. *N Eng J Med* 2004; 350: 2247–56.

QUICK FLICK A

39 Barron ME, Wilkes MM, Navickis RJ. A systemic review of the comparative safety of colloids. *Arch Sur* 2004; 139: 552–63.

40 Levy JH. *Anaphylactic Reactions in Anesthesia and Intensive Care*, 2nd edn. Butterworth–Heinemann, Boston 1992: 33.

41 Kudenchuk PJ, Cobb LA, Copass MK et al. Amiodarone for resuscitation after out of hospital cardiac arrest due to ventricular fibrillation. *N Eng J Med* 1999; 341: 871–8.

42 Silfast T, Pettila V. Amiodarone versus lidocaine for shock resistant ventricular fibrillation. *N. Eng J Med* 2002; 347: 368–70.

43 Stern R. *Drugs, Diseases and Anaesthesia*. Lippincott-Raven, Philadelphia 1997: 9–10.

44 Davies MG, Harrison JC. Amniotic fluid embolism: maternal mortality revisited. *Br J Hosp Med* 1992; 47: 775–6.

45 Cattaneo AN. Air and amniotic fluid embolus. In: Birnbach DJ, Gatt SP, Datta S eds. *Textbook of Obstetric Anaesthesia*. Churchill Livingstone, Philadelphia, 2000: 435–54.

46 Clarke J, Butt M. Maternal collapse. *Curr Opin Gynecol* 2005; 17: 157–60.

47 Fisher M. Clinical observations on the pathophysiology and treatment of anaphylactic cardiovascular collapse. *Anaesth Intensive Care* 1986; 14: 17–21.

48 Mertes PM. Anaphylactic reactions during anaesthesia—let us treat the problem rather than debating its existence. *Acta Anaesthesiol Scand* 2005; 49: 431–3.

49 Axon AD, Hunter JM. Editorial III: Anaphylaxis and anaesthesia—all clear now? *Br J Anaesth* 2004; 93: 501–4.

50 Guidelines 2000 for cardiopulmonary resuscitation and emergency cardiovascular care. *Circulation* 2000; 102(suppl): 1241–3.

51 Heytman M, Rainbird A. Use of alpha-agonists for the management of anaphylaxis occurring under anaesthesia: case studies and review. *Anaesthesia* 2004; 59: 1210–15.

52 McBrien ME, Breslin DS, Atkinson S, Johnston JR. Use of methoxamine in the resuscitation of epinephrine-resistant electromechanical dissociation. *Anaesthesia* 2001; 56: 1085–9.

53 Kill C, Wranze E, Wulf H. Successful treatment of severe anaphylactic shock with vasopressin. *Int Arch Allergy Immunol* 2004; 134: 260–1.

54 Fisher MM. Anaphylaxis. In Bersten AD, Soni N, Oh TE eds. *Oh's Intensive Care Manual* 5th edn. Butterworth–Heinemann, Edinburgh 2003; 617–20.

55 Fischer M, Baldo BA. The diagnosis of fatal anaphylactic reactions during anaesthesia: employment of immunoassays for mast cell tryptase and drug reactive IgE antibodies. *Anaesth Intens Care* 1993; 21: 353–7.

56 Brabant SM, Bertrand M, Eyraud D et al. The haemodynamic effects of anesthetic induction in vascular surgical patients chronically treated with angiotensin II receptor antagonists. *Anesth Analg* 1999; 88: 1388–92.

57 Bertrand M, Godet G, Meersscharet K et al. Should the angiotensin II agonists be discontinued before surgery? *Anesth Analg* 2001; 92: 26–30.

58 Powell CG, Unsworth DJ, McVey FK. Severe hypotension associated with angiotensin-converting enzyme inhibition in anaesthesia. *Anaesth Intensive Care* 1998; 26: 107–9.

59 Duke J. Blood pressure disturbances. In Duke J ed. *Anesthesia Secrets*, 3rd edn. Mosby Philadelphia 2006: 196–202.

60 *Guidelines for Anticoagulation* Version 6—June 2005 for the Central and Eastern Cluster. Sydney Western Area Health Service.

61 Dujardin KS, Enriquez-Sarano M, Schaff HV et al. Mortality and morbidity of aortic regurgitation in clinical practice. A long term follow-up study. *Circulation* 1999; 99: 1851–7.

62 *ACC/AHA 2007 guidelines on perioperative cardiovascular evaluation and care for non cardiac surgery*. A report of the American College of Cardiology/American Heart Association Task Force on Practice.

63 Mason R. *Anaesthesia Databook,* 3rd edn. Greenwich Medical Media Limited, London 2001: 46.

64 Brighouse D. Anaesthesia for Caesarean section in patients with aortic stenosis: the case for regional anaesthesia. *Anaesthesia* 1998: 53: 107–9.

65 Whitfield A, Holdcroft A. Anaesthesia for Caesarean section in patients with aortic stenosis: the case for general anaesthesia. *Anesthesia* 1998; 53: 109–112.

66 Orme RMLE, Grange CS, Ainsworth QP et al. General anaesthesia using remifentanil for caesarean section in patient with critical aortic stenosis: a series of four cases. *Internat J Obstet Anesth* 2004; 13: 183–7.

67 Pittard A, Vucevic M. Regional anaesthesia with a subarachnoid micro catheter for Caesarean section in a patient with aortic stenosis. *Anaesthesia* 1998; 53: 69–73.

68 Mangano DT, Tudor IC, Dietzel C. The risk associated with aprotinin in cardiac surgery. *N Engl J Med* 2006; 354: 353–65.

69 Kirby RR, Taylor RW, Civetta JM. *Pocket Companion of Critical Care: Immediate Concerns*, JB Lippincott Company, Philadelphia, 1990: 35–7.

70 Vanner R. Preventing regurgitation and aspiration. *Anaesthesia and Intensive Care Med* 2004; 5: 293–7.

71 Sakai T, Planinsic RM, Quinlan JJ et al. The incidence and outcome of perioperative pulmonary aspiration in a university hospital: a 4-year retrospective analysis. *Anesth Analg* 2006; 103: 941–7.

72 *Crisis Management Manual*. Australian Patient Safety Foundation, 2nd edn. 2006: 19.

73 Teabeault JR. Aspiration of gastric contents: experimental study. *Am J Pathol* 1952; 28: 51–67.

74 Tuxon DV. Aspiration syndromes. In Oh TE ed. *Intensive Care Manual*, 3rd edn. Butterworths, Oxford, 1990: 216.

75 Yao F-S F. Aspiration Pneumonitis and Acute Respiratory Failure. In Yao F-S F ed. *Yao and Artusio's Anesthesiology: Problem Orientated Patient Management* 4th edition. Lippincott-Raven, Philadelphia 1998: 53–85.

76 Chassot P-G, Delabys A, Spahn DR. Perioperative antiplatelet therapy: the case for continuing therapy in patients at risk of myocardial infarction. *Br J Anaesth* 2007; 99: 316–28.

77 Mason R. *Anaesthesia Databook*, 3rd edn. Greenwich Medical Media Limited, London 2001: 54–9.

78 Hirshman C. Perioperative management of the asthmatic patient. *Can J Anaesth* 1991; 38: 4: 26–32.

79 Kablin CS, Yarnold PR, Grammer LC. Low complication rate of corticosteroid treated asthmatics undergoing surgical procedures. *Arch Intern Med* 1995; 155: 1379–84.

80 Tait AR, Knight PR. Intraoperative respiratory complications in patients with upper respiratory tract infections. *Can J Anaesth* 1987; 34: 300–3.

81 McAlpine LG, Thomson NC. Lidocaine-induced bronchoconstriction in asthmatic patients. Relation to histamine airway responsiveness and effect of preservatives. *Chest* 1989; 96: 1012–15.

82 Kim ES, Bishop MI. Endotracheal intubation, but not laryngeal mask airway insertion, produces reversible bronchoconstriction. *Anesthesiology* 1999; 90: 391–4.

83 Goff MJ, Shahbaz RA, Ficke DJ, Uhrich TD, Ebert TJ. Absence of bronchodilation during desflurane anaesthesia. *Anesthesiology* 2000; 93: 404–8.

84 Mashford ML, Cosolo W, Day RO et al. *Therapeutic Guidelines: Analgesic*, 3rd edn. Therapeutic Guidelines Limited on behalf of the Victorian Drug Use Advisory Committee Melbourne 1997: 61.

85 Nathanson MH, Gajraj NM. Review Article: The perioperative management of atrial fibrillation. *Anaesthesia* 1998; 53: 665–76.

86 Mittal S, Ayati S, Stein KM et al. Transthoracic cardioversion of atrial fibrillation. Comparison of rectilinear biphasic versus damped sine wave monophasic shocks. *Circulation* 2000; 101: 1282–7.

87 Sanghavi S, Rayner-Klein J. Management of peri-arrest arrhythmia. *Br J Anaesth CEPD Reviews* 2002; 4: 104–112.

88 *Cardiovascular Drug Guidelines*, 2nd edn. Victorian Medical Post Graduate Foundation Inc. Australia 1995: 115.

89 Holt A. Management of Cardiac Arrhythmias. In Bersten AD, Soni N, Oh TE eds. *Oh's Intensive Care Manual*, 5th edn. Butterworth–Heinemann, Edinburgh 2003: 157–205.

90 Ikeno F, Kaneda H, Hongo Y et al. Augmentation of tissue perfusion by a novel compression device increases neurological intact survival in a porcine model of prolonged cardiac arrest. *Resuscitation* 2006; 68: 109–18.

91 Ong ME, Ornatio JP, Edwards DP et al. Use of an automated, load-distributing band chest compression device for out-of-hospital cardiac arrest resuscitation. *JAMA* 2006; 295: 2629–37.

92 Casner M, Anderson D, Isaacs SM. The impact of a new CPR assist device on rate of return of spontaneous circulation in out-of-hospital cardiac arrest. *Prehospital Emerg Care* 2005; 9: 61–7.

93 Jenkins SA, Marshall CF. Awake intubation made easy and acceptable. *Aneasth Intens Care* 2000; 28: 556–61.

94 Cobcroft MD, Forsdick C. Awareness under anaesthesia: the patient's point of view. *Anaesth Intens Care* 1993; 21: 837–43.

95 Schwender D, Klasing S, Daunderer M et al. Awareness during general anesthesia. Definition, incidence, clinical relevance, causes, avoidance and medicolegal aspects. *Anaesthetist* 1995; 44: 743–54.

96 Ottevaere JA. Awareness During Anaesthesia. In Duke J ed. *Anesthesia Secrets*, 2nd edn. Hanley and Belfus Inc, Philadelphia, 2000; 165–8.

97 Jenkins K, Baker AB. Review Article: Consent and anaesthetic risk. *Anaesthesia* 2003; 58: 962–84.

98 Bailey AR, Jones JG. Patient's memories of events during general anaesthesia. *Anaesthesia* 1997; 52: 460–76.

QUICK FLICK A

○ **Bacterial Endocarditis (BE) Prophylaxis**

The following guidelines are based on recommendations from the American Heart Association published in *Circulation* in 2007.[1] These guidelines recommend that antibiotic prophylaxis is only required for the lesions listed below. According to the AHA working party, while antibiotic prophylaxis appears to be justified for invasive dental procedures, they do not recommend prophylaxis for genitourinary or gastrointestinal procedures unless infection is already present. The British Society of Antimicrobial Chemotherapy recommend a more traditional approach in their 2006 guidelines.[2] Both approaches are presented here. Ultimately it is the decision of the patient's treatment team and cardiologist whether prophylactic antibiotics are used or not.

Topics Covered in this Section
▶ Lesions Predisposing to Bacterial Endocarditis (BE)
▶ Procedures for Which Antibiotic Prophylaxis is Recommended
▶ Procedures for which Antibiotic Prophylaxis is Not Recommended
▶ Antibiotic Prophylaxis Regimens

Lesions Predisposing to Bacterial Endocarditis (BE)
1 Prosthetic heart valves or prosthetic material used in valve repair.
2 Previous endocarditis.
3 Congenital heart disease (CHD) either unrepaired or with palliative shunts or conduits.
4 CHD completely repaired with prosthetic material for the first 6 months post procedure.
5 CHD repaired with residual defects at the site of prosthetic material.
6 Cardiac transplant recipients with valve disease.

Procedures for which Antibiotic Prophylaxis is Recommended
Oral and Respiratory Tract
1 Dental extractions, scaling, root planning, implants and dental procedures associated with bleeding.
2 Tonsillectomy/adenoidectomy, surgical operations on the respiratory mucosa.
3 Rigid bronchoscopy.
4 Surgical operations involving respiratory mucosa.
5 Nasotracheal intubation.

Gastrointestinal Tract

The AHA guidelines do not recommend prophylactic antibiotics unless infection is already present.[1] The 2006 guidelines from British Society of Antimicrobial Chemotherapy recommend prophylactic antibiotics for:[2]

1 sclerotherapy of oesophageal varices and stricture dilatation.
2 oesophageal laser therapy.
3 endoscopic retrograde cholangiography with biliary obstruction.
4 biliary tract surgery.
5 operations involving intestinal mucosa.
6 panendoscopy in high-risk patients.
7 percutaneous gastrostomy, liver biopsy in high-risk patients.
8 gall stone lithotripsy.

Genitourinary Tract

The 2007 AHA guidelines do not recommend prophylactic antibiotics for genitourinary procedures unless infection is already present. The 2006 British Society of Antimicrobial Chemotherapy recommends antibiotic prophylaxis for:

1 prostate surgery
2 cystoscopy
3 urethral dilatation
4 ureteric stone lithotripsy
5 vaginal hysterectomy
6 Caesarean section.

Other Procedures

1 Any procedure involving infected material. Use antibiotics specific to infecting organism.
2 Urinary tract instrumentation in the presence of a urinary tract infection (UTI).

Procedures for which Antibiotic Prophylaxis is Not Recommended (Unless Infection is Already Present)

1 flexible bronchoscopy
2 orotracheal intubation
3 panendoscopy (unless high risk)
4 colonoscopy/polypectomy/sphincterotomy
5 transoesophageal echocardiography
6 endoscopic banding or ligation of varices
7 vaginal delivery
8 urethral catheterisation
9 uterine dilatation and curettage
10 cervical biopsy
11 sterilisation procedures

12 incision or biopsy of surgically scrubbed skin
13 circumcision.

Antibiotic Prophylaxis Regimens

Take oral therapy 30–60 min before procedure and IV or IM therapy within 30 min of procedure. The total dose for children should not exceed the adult dose.

Dental, Oral, Respiratory Tract or Oesophageal Procedures

Adult Amoxicillin 2 g PO or Ampicillin 2 g IV/IM.
Child Amoxicillin 50 mg/kg PO or ampicillin 50 mg/kg IV/IM.

If Penicillin Allergy

Adult Oral Therapy Clindamycin 600 mg or cephalexin 2 g or cefadroxil 2 g or clarithromycin 500 mg.
Adult IV Therapy Clindamycin 600 mg or cefazolin 1 g (note that patients with anaphylaxis to penicillin should not be given cephalosporins).
Child Oral Therapy Clindamycin 20 mg/kg, cephalexin 50 mg/kg, cefadroxil 50 mg/kg, clarithromycin 15 mg/kg
Child IV Therapy Clindamycin 20 mg/kg, cefazolin 25 mg/kg

If Already Taking Penicillin

Delay the procedure for 10 days after completing the penicillin therapy if possible. If this is not practical use clindamycin, azithromycin or clarithromycin.

Genitourinary/Gastrointestinal/Obstetric/Gynaecological Procedures (*Note:* AHA Recommends No Prophylaxis)

Adult Ampicillin 2 g IV and gentamicin 1.5 mg/kg up to 120 mg. Give amoxicillin 1 g PO or ampicillin 1 g IV/IM 6 h after procedure.
Child Ampicillin 50 mg/kg IV plus gentamicin 1.5 mg/kg. Give ampicillin 25 mg/kg IV/IM or amoxicillin 25 mg/kg PO 6 h after procedure.

If Penicillin Allergy

Adult Vancomycin 1 g IV over 1–2 h and gentamicin. Complete infusion within 30 min of procedure.
Child Vancomycin 20 mg/kg over 1–2 h, and gentamicin. Complete infusion within 30 min of procedure.

◖ Beta-blocker Therapy and Reduction of Cardiac Risk

Several studies have concluded that peri-operative beta-blocker therapy reduces the incidence of cardiac complications in patients with ischaemic heart disease.[3] Cardioselective β blockers such as bisoprolol and metoprolol are the drugs of choice. The dose should be titrated to a pre-operative heart rate of 50–60 bpm.[4]

Patients with Clear Indications for β blockers

These include patients with:

1 the need for β blockers to control angina
2 symptomatic arrhythmias
3 hypertension
4 patients at high risk for cardiac complications based on cardiac testing.

These patients should start β blocker therapy at first contact and continue therapy postoperatively indefinitely.[5]

Results of the POISE Trial[6]

This blinded randomised controlled trial examined 8351 patients having non-cardiac surgery who received either metoprolol or placebo. Although the incidence of myocardial infarction was reduced in the metoprolol group the overall mortality was higher in this group and there was an increased incidence of strokes. This study has therefore indicated that β blocker therapy is not without significant risk. The initiation of β blocker therapy without a specific indication unrelated to planned surgery must be seriously questioned.

Absolute Contraindications to β blockers

1 symptomatic bradycardia (rate < 50–60)
2 symptomatic hypotension (systolic < 90–100 mm Hg)
3 severe heart failure/cardiogenic shock
4 asthma
5 second or third degree heart block.

◗ Bier Block

IV regional anaesthetic technique which can be used for surgery of the upper or lower limb.

Technique for Upper Limb Anaesthesia

1 Insert an IV cannula in each arm. Place the cannula distally in the limb to be anaesthetised.
2 Apply a single cuffed surgical tourniquet to the arm to be blocked. Prior to inflation, drain blood from the venous system by either:
   a) applying an Esmach bandage from distal to proximal; or
   b) occluding the brachial artery at the elbow and elevate the limb for 1 min.
3 Inflate the tourniquet to 100 mm Hg above the measured systolic blood pressure or a maximum of 300 mmHg.
4 Inject LA solution over at least 90 s. Use lignocaine 0.5% 3 mg/ kg. *Do not use adrenaline containing solutions*. For a 70 kg person use ≈ 40 mL of LA solution. Onset of block takes ≈ 5–10 min.
5 *Deflation of Tourniquet* Do not release the tourniquet if less than 20 min has elapsed. If 45 min has elapsed, the tourniquet can be released as a

QUICK FLICK B

1-step procedure. Between 20 and 45 min, release the tourniquet cuff pressure for 10 s then reinflate cuff for 1 min. Repeat this cycle 3 times before final release.

◑ Biphasic Defibrillators

See *Defibrillators*.

◑ Bispectral Index (BIS) EEG Monitor

This monitor is a continuous highly processed electroencephalograph which measures changes in interfrequency coupling. BIS is used to provide a measure of hypnosis during anaesthesia and thus diminish the risk of awareness.

Underlying Principles of BIS

Part of the cortical EEG is influenced by neuronal activity of subcortical structures, and this interaction is reflected in harmonic and phase relationships in the EEG signal called biocoherence.[7] Broadly speaking EEG measurements change from low-amplitude, high-frequency signals while awake to large amplitude low-frequency signals when anaesthetised. Biocoherence patterns also change with increasing concentrations of hypnotic drugs. The BIS monitor analyses these EEG pattern changes using measurement algorithms which were derived empirically. This involved applying a stepwise regression analysis to EEGs from over 2000 subjects in various phases of anaesthesia, sedation and wakefulness. The regression equation obtained combines several features such as burst suppression and β wave activation. This regression equation is converted to a 1–100 scale where:

100	Awake
70	Light Hypnosis/Sedation
60	Moderate Hypnosis (aim for a BIS level of < 60 to prevent awareness).
40	Deep Hypnosis (excessive hypnosis for routine anaesthesia).
0	Isoelectric EEG.

Advantages of BIS

1. By using BIS monitoring there is the potential to safely minimise anaesthetic dosage, resulting in fewer unwanted anaesthetic drug side effects, faster wake up time and earlier discharge.[8]
2. BIS monitoring may enable a reduced possibility of patient awareness under anaesthesia. The B-Aware trial concluded that BIS monitoring reduced the risk of awareness in high risk patients by 82%.[9] High-risk patients were those having general anaesthesia with muscle relaxation and another risk factor such as coronary artery bypass surgery or Caesarean section.

Disadvantages of BIS

1 BIS monitoring can be affected by brain ischaemia or hypoxia and hypothermia. BIS is also affected by forehead muscle activity which must be considered in evaluating the non-paralysed patient.[10]
2 BIS values must be interpreted in the light of other patient monitors and clinical evaluation of the patient.

The equipment, including electrode costs, is expensive.[10]

Practical Aspects of Using BIS

A typical device is the Aspect A-1000 EEG monitor®. To use this device:

1 Attach 4 Zipprep™ or other suitable electrodes to the head. Two of these are positioned over both temporal bones, laterally from the eyes. A reference electrode is placed on the centre of the forehead between the eyebrows. A 4th ground electrode is placed on the forehead.
2 BIS values are calculated by the Aspect monitor and displayed.
3 BIS values between 40 and 60 are recommended as optimal to prevent awareness while avoiding excessive anaesthesia.[9]

◌ Blalock-Taussig Shunts

See *Tetralogy of Fallot*.

◌ Bleomycin (BLM)

See *Immunosuppressive Drugs, Anaesthetic Implications*.

◌ Blind Nasal Intubation

1 If patient is to be awake, anaesthetise the nasal and pharyngeal airway and provide sedation. *See* *Awake Fibre-optic Intubation*.
2 If the patient is undergoing GA, maintain spontaneous ventilation.
3 Use a mucosal vasoconstrictor in nose e.g. cocaine, oxymetazoline or co-phenylcaine.
4 Place the patient in the usual intubation position.
5 Soften the endotracheal (ET) tube tip in hot water prior to use. Allow the tube to cool to an acceptable temperature before insertion.
6 Gently introduce well-lubricated ET tube (7–7.5 for male, 6.5–7 for female) into the nose with its concave side facing the feet. If the patient is breathing spontaneously, occlude the other nostril to increase the volume of breath sounds audible through the ET tube. Listen for breath sounds and monitor capnography as the tube is advanced.
7 If breathing sounds disappear look for a visible bulge in the neck which may indicate in which direction to manipulate the tube. Advance the tube during inspiration or coughing.
8 Methods to increase likelihood of successful placement include:
    a) Inflate the ET tube cuff in the oropharynx. Advance tube until slight

resistance is felt at which point the cuff may be against the vocal cords. Deflate the cuff and advance the ET tube into the trachea.[11]

b) If the oesophagus is intubated reattempt intubation with increased neck flexion.

c) Rotation of the ET tube and manipulation of the larynx may also be helpful.

Contraindications

1 CSF leak

2 Le Fort facial fractures or base of skull fractures.

▷ Blood

See *Red Cells* and *Whole Blood*.

▷ Blood Loss Assessment and Initial Management

Topics Covered in this Section

▶ Grading Blood Loss

▶ Initial Management of Severe Blood Loss

▶ Anaesthesia in the Presence of Severe Blood Loss

Grading Blood Loss

Graded into 4 classes based on blood loss as a percentage of total blood volume (TBV).[12] Figures quoted for blood loss assume a TBV of 5 L.

Class 1 (Up to 15% TBV) (≈ 800 mL) Associated with minimal clinical symptoms/signs.

Class 2 (15–30% TBV) (≈ 800–1500 mL) Usually see tachycardia, tachypnoea and narrowing of the pulse pressure with increased diastolic blood pressure. The patient is usually anxious/agitated. Urine output is reasonably well maintained.

Class 3 (30–40% TBV) (≈ 1500–2000 mL) Clinically see marked tachycardia and tachypnoea, a fall in systolic blood pressure, and the patient may become confused. Urine output is reduced.

Class 4 (> 40% TBV) (> 2000 mL) A marked tachycardia occurs with a very depressed systolic blood pressure and narrow pulse pressure. There is little or no urine output. The patient's skin is pale and cool with decreased capillary return. There is also marked depression of the central nervous system usually with loss of consciousness if > 50% of TBV is lost.

Initial Management of Severe Blood Loss

1 Secure the airway and ensure adequate ventilation. Give high concentration O_2.

2 Control haemorrhage e.g. direct pressure to the wound site, suturing of skin bleeders. Elevate the site of bleeding if possible. The patient may require immediate surgical intervention.

3 Secure large bore IV access i.e. insert a Rapid Infusion Device™. **See** *Rapid Infusion Catheter Exchanger Set*. Insert a second large bore IV cannula. A pulmonary artery (PA) catheter introducer sheath can also be used. A useful device for large bore central venous access is the Arrow Mac™. (**See** *Arrow Mac™ Two Lumen Central Venous Access Device*.)

4 Send blood specimens off for urgent full blood count, coagulation studies and cross-match.

5 Give IV fluids as follows:
   a) *In adults* give 1–2 L of colloid (e.g. gelofusine) rapidly and assess response. If the patient is still cardiovascularly unstable, he/she will probably need blood urgently +/– urgent surgery.
   b) *In children* give 20 mL/kg of Hartmann's solution. If the patient is still cardiovascularly unstable give a second bolus of crystalloid 20 mL/kg. If there are persistent signs of shock, give 10 mL/kg of type specific or O –ve blood (packed cells).

6 Establish intra-arterial blood pressure monitoring and central venous pressure monitoring.

7 For ongoing management **see** *Blood Transfusion*.

Anaesthesia in the Presence of Severe Blood Loss

The general principles are:

1 Ensure adequate airway and ventilation.

2 Establish large bore IV access as described above. Resuscitate the patient with intravenous crystalloid, colloid, blood as required.

3 Insert an arterial line to measure blood pressure accurately and enable frequent blood sampling.

4 Prep and drape the surgical area prior to the induction of anaesthesia if possible. This is because anaesthesia may cause:
   a) A reduction in sympatho-adrenal stimulation.[1]
   b) Loss of the tamponading effect of abdominal musculature that may occur in the awake patient.[13]

5 Perform a rapid sequence induction but induce anaesthesia cautiously. For example use:
   a) fentanyl 100–200 µg plus thiopentone in a reduced dose (e.g. 50–100 mg depending on the severity of haemorrhagic shock) *or*
   b) ketamine 1.5–2.5 mg/kg *or*
   c) etomidate 0.3 mg/kg *plus*
   d) a rapidly acting muscle relaxant such as suxamethonium or rocuronium.

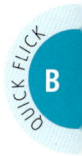

QUICK FLICK **B**

6 Maintain anaesthesia with O_2 + a low concentration of isoflurane or sevoflurane as tolerated by the patient.
7 As soon as practically possible organise:
   a) 2 or more blood warmers and/or a rapid warmed fluid delivery system such as the Level One™
   b) urinary catheter insertion
   c) patient warming devices such as a Bair Hugger
   d) naso-pharyngeal temperature probe
   e) blood scavenging device such as a Cell Saver.
8 Insert a CVP line to aid in the estimation of intravascular filling.
9 It is essential to prevent or minimise hypothermia and prevent the deleterious effects of hypothermia on coagulation.[14]
10 Ensure there are adequate numbers of trained theatre staff in attendance. Call more staff in if required.
11 Communicate with blood bank and haematologist early regarding:
   a) Number of units required and urgency of request.
   b) Need for other blood products such as fresh frozen plasma (FFP) and platelets.
12 Consider the use of an anti-shock suite (military anti-shock trousers—MAST). **See** *Mast Suite*.

Blood Loss Prevention

Pre-operative Measures

1 Identify/investigate patients with possible bleeding tendencies.
2 Cease drugs which may cause increased bleeding prior to surgery or reverse their effects. These include the following:
   a) *Aspirin* Aspirin irreversibly inhibits platelet function (i.e. for the life-time of the platelet ≈ 7–10 days) by inhibiting cyclo-oxygenase 1 (COX1) enzyme. Cease 1 week before surgery. If aspirin is ingested within 5 days of surgery, and surgery is urgent and likely to be associated with severe blood loss, consider the use of desmopressin (DDAVP) and/or platelet transfusion. **See** *Desmopressin (DDAVP)*.
   b) *Heparin, Low Molecular Weight Heparin and Warfarin.* **See** *Anticoagulation Therapy and Surgery*.
   c) *Non-steroidal Anti-inflammatory Drugs* (other than aspirin) NSAIDs are of 2 types, non-selective inhibiting both COX1 and COX2 enzymes, and selective COX 2 inhibitors.The non selective NSAIDs reversibly inhibit platelet aggregation only while effective plasma concentration is maintained. Cease the drug 3 days before surgery if the intra-operative bleeding risk is of particular concern.
   d) *New Antiplatelet Drugs*. These include platelet glycoprotein IIb/IIIa receptor antagonists (such as abciximab, tirofiban and eptifibatide)

and platelet adenosine diphosphate (ADP) receptor antagonists (e.g. ticlopidine and clopidogrel). These drugs cause profound platelet inhibition making surgery hazardous. *See Platelet Glycoprotein IIb/IIIa Receptor Antagonists* and *Platelet Adenosine Denosine Diphosphate (ADP) Receptor Antagonists* for specific recommendations.

e) *Recombinant Activated Factor VIIa* (*see Recombinant Activated Factor VII (RFVIIa)*) has been used prophylactically to reduce bleeding prior to high-risk surgery, such as open prostatectomy. It may be acceptable to JW patients.

QUICK FLICK B

Intra-operative Measures

1 Meticulous surgical technique.
2 Modest hypotension and avoidance of hypertension.
3 Maintain normal body temperature to prevent the adverse effects of hypothermia on coagulation.[14]
4 Use of a tourniquet during limb surgery.
5 Position surgical site uppermost.
6 Use of regional anaesthesia.[15]
7 Use of pharmacological agents such as:
   a) DDAVP (*see Desmopressin*).
   b) Antifibrinolytic agents such as epsilon aminocaproic acid or tranexamic acid. *See Tranexamic Acid.*
   d) recombinant activated factor VIIa. *See Recombinant Activated Factor VIIa (RFVIIa).*

◆ Blood Patching

See Epidural Anaesthesia.

◆ Blood Substitutes

There are several artificial oxygen carrying solutions under development. They include:

Haemoglobin Raffimer
Purified cross linked human haemoglobin. *See Haemoglobin Raffimer.*

Perfluorocarbons (PFC)
Marketed as Fluosol DA in Japan, this product has been shown to reduce the need for erythrocytes in patients with severe blood loss.

Diaspirin cross-linked Haemoglobin This has been trialled but has been found to be an ineffective blood substitute.[16]

Polymerised Human Haemoglobin Marketed in the US as PolyHem, this substance has been reported to reduce erythrocyte requirements in patients requiring blood transfusion.

Polyethylene Glycol Haemoglobin

Has been studied in pigs and shows promise but has not been evaluated in humans.[17]

Cattle Haemoglobin

Although the use of cattle haemoglobin has been shown to reduce transfusion requirements by 27% in abdominal aortic aneurysm repair, there is concern regarding transmission of diseases such as bovine spongiform encephalomyopathy.[16]

◐ Blood Transfusion

Topics Covered in this Section
▶ Risks of Allogenic Blood Transfusion
▶ Strategies to Avoid Allogenic Blood Transfusion
▶ Haemoglobin Level as a Transfusion 'Trigger'
▶ Decision to Transfuse Based on Volume of Blood Loss
▶ Massive Blood Transfusion Management

Risks of Allogenic Blood Transfusion

Acute Risks

1 incompatability related haemolytic reaction
2 bacterial contamination leading to sepsis
3 allergic reaction
4 TRALI—transfusion related acute lung injury due to the presence of HLA antibodies or leukocytes in the donor plasma. ***See*** *Transfusion Related Acute Lung Injury (TRALI).*

See also Problems Associated with Massive Blood Transfusion below.

Non-acute Risks

1 transmission of illnesses such as HIV, Hep C
2 immunosuppression
3 graft vs host disease.

Strategies to Avoid Allogenic Blood Transfusion

1 Pre-operative autologous blood donation. This technique is associated with poor cost effectiveness and high wastage rates.[18] This method is particularly useful when cross-match is difficult due to multiple antibodies. Blood can be collected up to 6 weeks before surgery with a unit collected every 3–7 days.
2 Pre-operative use of iron therapy and/or erythropoietin to increase haemoglobin levels. This treatment can be combined with preoperative autologous blood donation.[19]
3 Acute normovolaemic haemodilution (***see*** *Acute Normovolaemic Haemodilution*).

4   Intra-operative blood salvage through such devices as a cell saver.
5   Intra-operative blood loss prevention strategies (**see** *Blood Loss Prevention*).
6   Postoperative blood recovery e.g. from surgical drains.
7   Blood substitutes. These include O_2 carrying perflurochemicals (e.g. Fluosol DA®) and cell free haemoglobin based substances (**see** *Blood Substitutes*).

Haemoglobin Level as a Transfusion 'Trigger'

There is little evidence-based medicine supporting a decision to transfuse based solely on a haemoglobin (Hb) level.[20] Blood transfusion is rarely indicated if the Hb > 10 g/100 mL and almost always indicated if Hb < 7 g/100 mL.[20] Transfusing 1 unit of blood will increase the Hb by ≈ 1 g/100 mL in the adult.

The following guidelines are suggested transfusion 'triggers' based on measured Hb and assuming that intra-vascular volume is maintained.

Healthy Young Patients

Tolerate Hb > 7–8 g/100 mL provided that intravascular volume is well maintained.[21] Transfusion is probably indicated if Hb < 7 g/100 mL in these partients.[22] Jehovah's Witnesses do not usually die from anaemia alone if the Hb level is > 3 g/100 mL.[19]

Patients Requiring a Minimum Hb of 10 g/100 mL

1   Patients older than 60 yrs.[21]
2   Significant systemic disease.
3   Known or possible coronary artery disease.
4   Cerebrovascular disease or severe lung disease.

Decision to Transfuse Based on Volume of Blood Loss

1   *Loss of up to 15% Total Blood Volume (TBV)* (≈ 700 mL in a 70 kg patient) In young healthy patients, this amount of loss is usually well tolerated with little or no haemodynamic effects.
2   *Loss of 15–30% TBV* (≈ 800–1500 mL) Blood transfusion likely to be required in unfit or elderly patient but can be tolerated by young fit patient as long as intravascular volume is maintained.
3   *Loss of 30–40% TBV* (≈ 1500–2000 mL) In a young fit patient can be treated adequately with crystalloid therapy.[23] Blood transfusion will almost certainly be required in all other patients.
4   *Loss of > 40% TBV* (> 2000 mL) Severe life-threatening haemorrhage requiring blood transfusion in almost all circumstances.

Massive Blood Transfusion Management

See *Blood Loss Assessment and Initial Management*. Massive blood transfusion is defined as acute administration of greater than 1 total blood

volume within a 24 h period.[24] In a 70 kg patient this equates to about
12 units of blood.[24] Ongoing severe haemorrhage treated with transfusion
of packed cells will lead to coagulopathy and thrombocytopenia. However
these clotting deficits are multifactorial in origin and are not just due to the
amount of blood lost and replaced. Other factors such as hypothermia and
prolonged periods of hypotension are also important.[21]

1 Involve a haematologist early in resuscitation for advice on the type and
   quantity of clotting factors to give. Measure FBC and clotting factors after
   every 4–6 units of blood.

2 Obtain fully cross-matched blood as quickly as possible. Use O Rh –ve
   blood until fully cross-matched blood can be obtained. If the O Rh –ve
   blood supply is exhausted and patient's life is threatened give O Rh +ve
   blood (but O Rh –ve blood is preferable particularly in women of child
   bearing age or younger).[23] If O Rh +ve blood or platelets are given to an
   O Rh –ve female with child bearing potential give anti-D if the patient
   does not already have an anti-D antibody detected. All blood given for
   massive haemorrhage should preferably be < 10 days old.

3 If bleeding is ongoing after 6 units of blood have been transfused give
   4 units of fresh frozen plasma (FFP).

4 If blood loss is continuing after 8 units of blood give platelets (2–4 units).
   Significant thrombocytopenia due to transfusion tends to occur after
   1.5–2 blood volumes have been transfused.

5 Give 1 g of calcium gluconate 10% solution (10 mL) per 5 units of
   rapidly transfused blood or FFP. See Problems Associated with Massive
   Transfusion below.

6 Give more FFP if PT or APTT > 1.5 × normal[20] or INR > 2. Use
   10–15 mL/kg.

7 Give more platelets if platelet count drops below 50/mm^3 (50 × 10^9/L) or
   on clinical grounds if the wound looks 'oozy'.

8 Cryoprecipitate is indicated if fibrinogen concentrations fall below
   80–100 mg/100 mL (0.8–1 g/L).[20] Give 10 units. **See** *Cryoprecipitate* (and
   Cryodepleted Plasma).

9 Other clotting factor products to consider are prothrombinex-HT, factor
   VIII, factor IX.

10 Recombinant activated factor VII is a major advance in the treatment of
   ongoing severe blood loss associated with coagulopathy. **See** *Recombinant
   Activated Factor VII (RFVIIa)*.

11 Ongoing requirements of blood products and clotting factors depend on
   clinical judgement and advice from the haematologist.

12 Prevent/reverse hypothermia which inhibits platelet function and
   increases bleeding times.

13 Consider embolisation of bleeding vessels under radiological control.

14 Pneumatic anti-shock trousers may help reduce bleeding and centralise remaining blood volume especially in certain groups of patients e.g. pelvic fractures and ruptured abdominal aortic aneurysm (**see** *MAST Suite*).[16]

Problems Associated with Massive Blood Transfusion

1 Anticipate/treat 'citrate toxicity' due to citrate binding to calcium in the serum leading to low levels of ionised calcium. **See** *Calcium*. This occurs when blood is being given so rapidly that the liver has insufficient time to metabolise the citrate i.e. > 1 unit of blood per 5 min. Effects of citrate induced ionised hypocalcaemia include hypotension, decreased cardiac output, electromechanical dissociation and prolongation of the Q-T interval. To prevent/treat citrate toxicity give 1 g calcium gluconate IV 10% solution (10 mL) for every 5 units of blood. Give the same amount of calcium gluconate if FFP is given at 5 units per min or faster. Patients with liver disease have an increased susceptibility to citrate toxicity.

2 Anticipate/treat hyperkalaemia due to high potassium content of stored blood (e.g. 40 mmol/L at 4 weeks).[17] Monitor the ECG closely for evidence of hyperkalaemia. For a description of the ECG changes seen with hyperkalaemia **see** *Electrocardiography*.

3 Coagulopathy may occur due to low levels of clotting factors and platelets in the transfused blood plus the underlying process leading to the requirement of massive transfusion e.g. severe trauma.

◑ Blood Volume

Table B1 Total blood volume in mL/kg at various ages

Age	Blood volume
Premature infant	100 mL/kg
Term infant	90 mL/kg
6–8 yrs	Adult Levels
Adult male	70 mL/kg
Adult female	60 mL/kg

Table B2 Distribution of 5 L of blood in a 70 kg patient

Volume	Site
1000 mL	Heart, arterial circulation and capillaries
1000 mL	Pulmonary circulation
3000 mL	Venous circulation

◑ Blunt Airway Trauma

See *Tracheal Rupture*.

◊ Body Mass Index and Obesity

$$BMI = \frac{Weight\ (kg)}{Height\ (m)^2}$$

Ideal body weight in kg ≈ for men height in cm – 100, and for women height in cm – 105.

Normal BMI 23–26.

Table B3 Obesity classification and BMI

Weight description	BMI
Anorexic	<17.5
Underweight	17.6–20
Overweight	27–29
Obesity	30–35
Morbidly Obese	>35
Super Morbidly Obese	>50

Obesity can be defined as a body weight more than 20% greater than ideal body weight (IBW).

Obesity corresponds to a BMI > 27 for men and > 25 for women.

Morbid obesity is a body weight > 2 × IBW or a BMI > 35.[25]

◊ Bone Cement Implantation Syndrome

See *Fat Embolism Syndrome and Bone Cement Implantation Syndrome*.

◊ Brachial Plexus Block

Topics Covered in this Section

▶ Introductory Comments
▶ Anatomy of the Brachial Plexus
▶ Interscalene Approach
▶ Supraclavicular Approach
▶ Infraclavicular Approach
▶ Axillary Approach
▶ Continuous Axillary Blockade (Adults)

There are many different methods for providing a brachial plexus block. A selection of these is presented.

With all the blocks described below:

1 The patient should be awake or lightly sedated.
2 Use strict aseptic technique.
3 Place an IV cannula in the non-block limb.
4 Place a bleb of LA in the skin prior to insertion of the short bevelled block needle.

5 Aspirate prior to injecting LA to ensure the needle is not in a blood vessel or subarachnoid.

6 Inject a test dose of 1–2 mL. There should be little resistance to injection and the injection should not be painful. Pain on injection suggests intraneural placement of the needle tip.

7 Inject the LA incrementally in 5 mL boluses, aspirating after each injection. Observe the patient closely for any side effects.

The interscalene block is useful for surgery on the upper arm and shoulder. The supraclavicular block can be used for surgery on the forearm and upper arm. The infraclavicular block is useful for surgery on the elbow, forearm, wrist and hand but not the shoulder. The axillary block is suitable for surgery on the wrist and hand. As a rough guide lignocaine with adrenaline will provide reasonable anaesthesia for up to 3 h and analgesia for up to 6 h. Ropivacaine (up to 30 mL of 0.75%) will provide anaesthesia for 6–8 h and analgesia for 9–16 h.[26] Bupivacaine provides similar durations of anaesthesia/analgesia to ropivacaine at equivalent dosages.[27]

Anatomy of the Brachial Plexus

The brachial plexus is formed from the anterior rami of C5–T1 nerve roots. It is the main sensory, motor and sympathetic innervation of the upper limb. Some of the important anatomical features of the brachial plexus are discussed in the descriptions of the various types of brachial plexus blocks. See Figure B1.

Interscalene Approach

The interscalene block is recommended for surgery on the upper arm and shoulder. The block is most dense in the C4–C7 root distribution. Interscalene blocks tend to be of shorter duration than axillary or supraclavicular blocks due to increased LA absorption in this area.[26] The 5 roots of the brachial plexus form 3 trunks (upper, middle and lower). These trunks are sandwiched between scalenus anterior and scalenus medius. The fasciae of these muscles form a sheath around the plexus.

Technique

1 Position the patient supine, with the head turned away slightly, with a small folded towel as a pillow. The ipsilateral shoulder is depressed by reaching for knee.

2 Identify the cricoid cartilage at the level of C6. At this level identify the interscalene groove behind the lateral edge of the sternomastoid muscle. The external jugular vein almost always crosses the interscalene groove at the level of C6. The transverse process of C6 (Chassaignac's tubercle) may be palpated in the interscalene groove. At the base of the groove the pulsations of the subclavian artery may be palpable. The roots of the brachial plexus lie closer to middle than the anterior scalenus muscle.

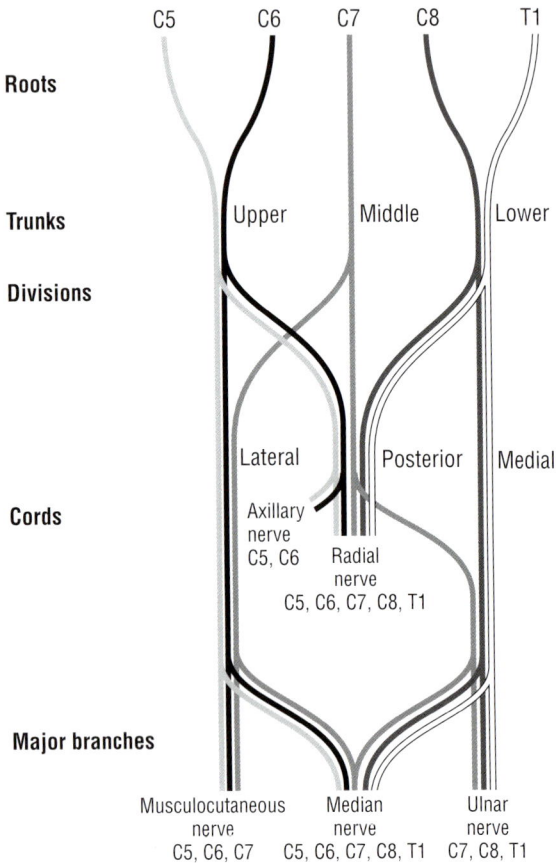

Figure B1 The brachial plexus illustrated schematically

3 Insert a short bevelled 22 G block needle into the groove, closer to the scalenus medius, in a direction that is ≈ perpendicular to the skin in every plane. The direction of placement is slightly caudad, medial and posterior angling towards Chassaignac's tubercle. If bone is contacted, redirect the needle slightly anteriorly or posteriorly but never cephalad or directly medially.

4 Elicit paraesthesia or use a nerve stimulator to identify the brachial plexus. To use a nerve stimulator:

a) Use an insulated short bevelled block needle such as a Stimuplex®

needle. Attach this to a suitable nerve stimulator via the black electrode (negative electrode). Attach the red electrode to an ECG dot positioned on the ipsilateral shoulder.

b) Stimulate with a current of 2 mA initially at 1 Hz.

c) When contractions are seen in either biceps or a muscle group in the forearm, reduce the current strength gradually, aiming for contractions at 0.2–0.4 mA.

5 Once paraesthesia or satisfactory nerve stimulation is obtained, inject a 2 mL test dose of LA. If pain occurs with injection of the test dose withdraw needle slightly (to avoid intraneural injection) and repeat the test dose injection.

6 Use a LA volume of ≈ 30 mL in a 70 kg patient. Suitable anaesthetic agents include lignocaine 1.5% with adrenaline 1:200 000 or lignocaine 2% with adrenaline mixed with an equal volume of bupivacaine 0.5% with adrenaline. Alternatively 30–40 mL of ropivacaine 5 mg/mL can be used. Inject the LA cautiously in 5 mL increments. Aspirate for blood or cerebrospinal fluid before each injection.

Ultrasound Guided Approach

1 First, identify the brachial plexus in the supraclavicular region as described for the ultrasound approach to the supraclavicular block.

2 Follow the brachial plexus up the neck for a short distance with the probe orientated 90° to the skin and at right angles to the neck (short axis approach).

3 The brachial plexus changes in appearance from a bundle of nerves to a compressed bundle with the nerves 'lining up' vertically in a stack. The nerves look round with a hollowed out appearance. This is the level at which the injections should be made. This level is slightly lower than if a non ultrasound technique is used.

4 Make the first injection between the nerve bundle and scalenus medius and the second injection between scalenus anterior and the nerve bundle. The needle is inserted 'out of plane' (the centre of the broadside of the probe). Inject a test dose of 0.5 mL to confirm needle position then a further 9.5 mL of LA at these two sites.

5 The nerve bundle will start to appear more circular as the volume of LA pushes apart the scalene muscles.

Complications of Interscalene Block

1 Block of the phrenic nerve is expected.[26]

2 Inadvertent epidural or subarachnoid injection can occur. **See** *Brainstem Anaesthesia*.

3 Vertebral artery injection. Seizures are likely with this complication. The incidence of vertebral artery injection was 0.3% in one series.[26]

QUICK FLICK **B**

SCM	– Sternocleidomastoid muscle	A	– superior trunk	} of brachial plexus
SA	– Scalenus anterior	B	– middle trunk	
SM	– Scalenus medius	C	– inferior trunk	

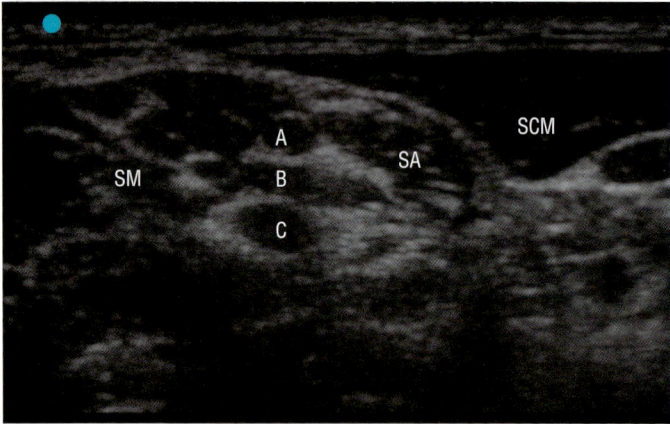

Figure B2 Ultrasound image of the brachial plexus in the neck

4 Nerve damage particularly associated with sharp needles and repeated stabs.
5 Horner's syndrome which has an incidence of about 60%.[28]
6 Hoarse voice.
7 Bronchospasm.
8 CVS instability including hypotension, bradycardia and asystole. The mechanism of these episodes may be due to the Bezold-Jarisch reflex and may be resistant to atropine. Ephedrine appears to be an effective treatment.

Supraclavicular Approach

The 3 trunks emerge from between the scalenus anterior and medius and pass in a closely grouped cluster downwards and laterally across the base of the posterior triangle of the neck and across the first rib. See Figure B3.

Technique

1 Position the patient supine, with the head turned slightly to the opposite side.
2 Identify the lateral edge of the sternomastoid muscle, then the interscalene groove behind this muscle. Palpate groove as caudally as possible. Attempt to palpate the subclavian artery overlying the first rib.
3 From behind the top of the patient's head insert a 22 G short bevelled needle in a caudad direction parallel to the floor and just behind the

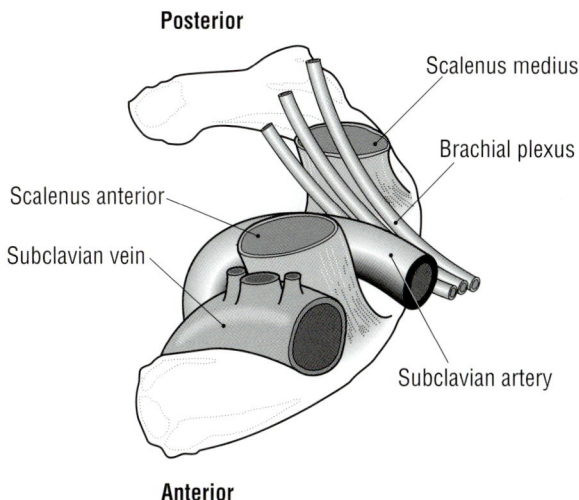

Figure B3 Anatomical relations of the superior surface of the first rib

subclavian artery. Insert the needle closer to the edge of the scalenus medius than the scalenus anterior. Obtain paraesthesia or use a nerve stimulator (see above). Inject a test dose then the full dose of LA as described for interscalene block.

Technique Using Ultrasound

1 Sit the patient semi-upright.
2 Hold the ultrasound probe in the non-dominant hand in a plane transverse to the subclavian artery (short axis view) and identify this vessel by its pulsation.
3 The brachial plexus bundle is situated slightly superficial and slightly posterior to the artery and lies < 2.0 cm below the skin surface. The nerves of the brachial plexus appear as 3–4 dark (hypoechoic) circular structures in a group just touching the artery.
4 When the tip of your needle is adjacent to the brachial plexus inject a test dose of 0.5 mL which should inject easily and the area of injection will be visible on the ultrasound screen. Reposition needle tip if necessary.
5 Inject the rest of the dose slowly ensuring an even distribution of LA around the brachial plexus.

Complications of Supraclavicular Block

1 Pneumothorax may occur. A pneumothorax rate of 2–5% is quoted.[26]
2 Phrenic nerve block occurs in a majority of patients.[26]

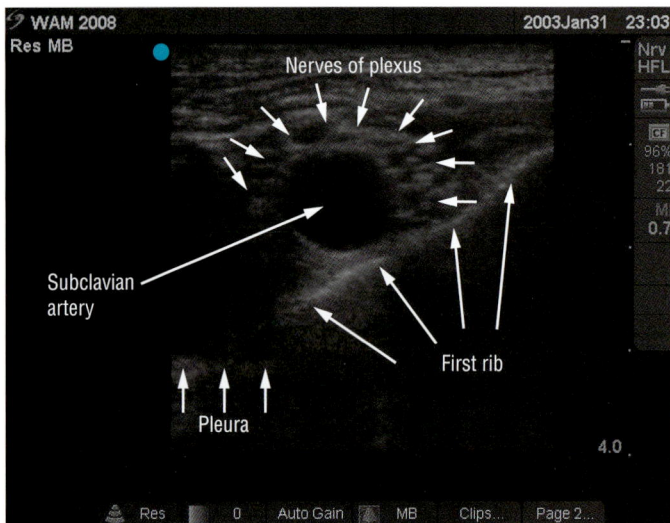

Figure B4 Ultrasound image of the brachial plexus in the supraclavicular region

3   Nerve damage.
4   Intravascular injection.

Infraclavicular Approach

This block is suitable for arm surgery below the mid-humerus, but not the shoulder.

Technique Using a Nerve Stimulator

This particular approach is described by Poon.[29] It is a proximal axillary block and is easy to perform. Note that a long (10 cm) needle is needed. The steps in the block are:

1   Identify the coracoid process (the part of the scapula which protrudes just superior and medial to the humeral head).The point of entry is 2 cm medial and 2 cm caudad to the tip of the coracoid process.

2   Using a suitable stimulating block needle (e.g. a 10 cm 22 G Braun Stimuplex needle), direct the needle at 90° to the long access of the patient in a parasaggital direction ('plumb bob').

3   Use an initial stimulation current of 1 mA at 1–2 Hz.

4   The average depth of insertion required is 4–4.25 cm. If stimulation is not achieved after reaching a depth of 6 cm, redirect the needle more

cephalad. If still unsuccessful redirect the needle more caudad. Do not use any medial or lateral direction on the needle.

5 When stimulation of the medial cord (wrist flexion, ulnar deviation) or lateral cord (elbow flexion) is achieved, reduce the current to 0.4 mA. Inject if stimulation is still present. (The lateral cord is seldom touched but would produce elbow extension.)[30]

Note: This block is a right angle approach to the plexus and is unsuitable for passing catheters.

Technique Using Ultrasound

The brachial plexus winds around the subclavian artery as it travels into the axilla. See Figure B5.

1 Position the patient supine with the arm by the side.
2 Position the probe over the delto-pectoral groove at right angles to the groove (short axis view).
3 Identify the medial, lateral and posterior cord.
4 Inject 5 mL of LA around each cord.
5 This approach has a risk of puncturing the pleura which is about 1 cm from the target.

The following approach has less risk of pleural puncture:

1 Position the patient supine with the arm abducted 110° and externally rotated. The elbow is flexed to 90°.

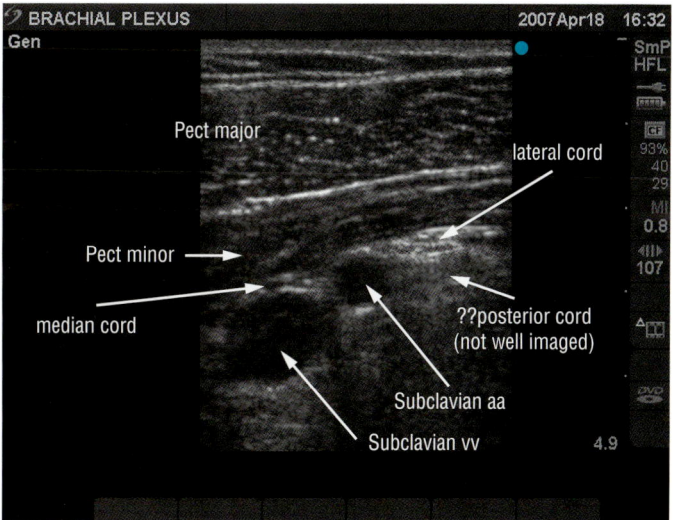

Figure B5 Ultrasound image of the brachial plexus in the infraclavicular region

2　Feel along the delto-pectoral groove to its apex. This is the insertion site.

3　Use the ultrasound probe placed over the delto-pectoral groove to visualise the axillary artery, vein and medial, lateral and posterior cords of the brachial plexus. The medial cord is the most difficult to identify.

4　Anaesthetise the skin and pectoral muscles prior to insertion of the block needle.

5　Insert the block needle at the apex of the delto-pectoral groove, superior to the probe and 45° to the skin. Pass the needle caudally in the saggital plane. The average depth of insertion is 3.7 cm.

6　Inject 10 mL of LA around each cord aiming to surround each cord with a ring of fluid.

7　If cords are difficult to identify, aim to inject cephalo-posterior to the subclavian artery.

Complications of Infraclavicular Block

1　Pneumothorax (but risk is very low).

2　Vascular puncture is reasonably common (10%).

Axillary Approach

After crossing the first rib the trunks divide into 6 divisions. These divisions stream into the axilla and then rejoin to form 3 cords (medial, lateral and posterior). The cords then divide into terminal branches. The fascial layers from the scalene muscles that envelop the brachial plexus extend into the axilla to form a tubular sheath that includes the axillary artery (see Figure B6). A multiple injection technique may improve success rate up to 97%.[26]

Technique Using a Nerve Stimulator

1　Position patient supine with forearm pronated, shoulder abducted to 90° and elbow flexed to 90°.

2　Palpate the axillary artery as proximally as possible.

3　The musculocutaneous nerve is sought first. Insert the block needle aiming to position the tip just above and deep to the axillary artery. Stimulation of the musculocutaneous nerve causes arm flexion. Use a current of 2 mA initially reducing the current to 0.3–0.5 mA with ongoing arm flexion confirming good position. Inject 5 mL of LA if aspiration is negative.

4　The needle is then repositioned so that the tip lies just superior and anterior to the axillary artery aiming for the ulnar and median nerves indicated by wrist and finger flexion. Again 2 mA is used initially reducing to 0.3–0.5 mA. Inject 15 mL of LA incrementally (after –ve aspiration).

5　For the third injection the needle point is redirected to just inferior to the axillary artery aiming for the radial nerve. With stimulation using the same pattern as above extension of fingers and thumb is seen. Inject 10 mL of LA after –ve aspiration.

6　Onset of block with lignocaine will take 10–20 min.

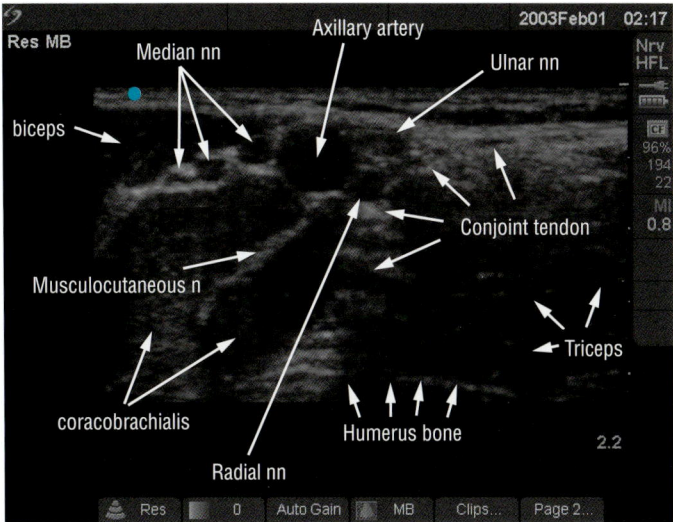

Figure B6 Ultrasound image of the brachial plexus in the axillary region

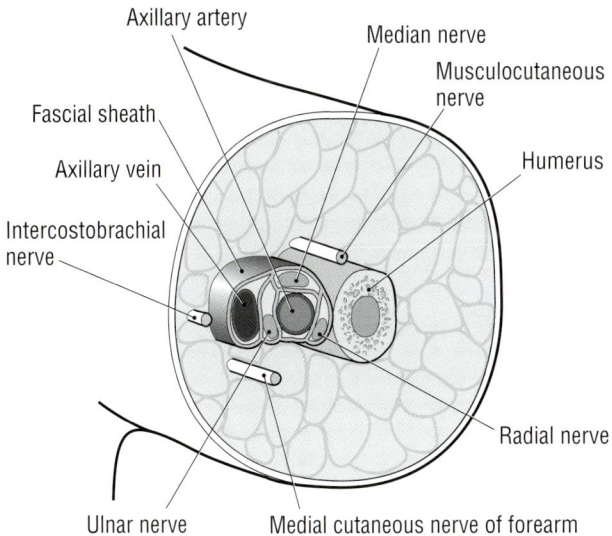

Figure B7 Brachial plexus anatomy in the axilla

Technique with Ultrasound

As described above the median, radial and ulnar nerves are in close proximity to the axillary artery.

1 Position the patient as described above.
2 Place the ultrasound probe just below the axilla at right angles to the long axis of the arm (short axis view) over the axillary artery.
3 The image obtained will show veins (compressible) and the axillary artery (pulsatile and compressible only with force against the humerus). The median and ulnar nerves are easier to locate than the radial nerve which is usually deep to the radial artery. The musculocutaneous nerve is situated beneath the bulk of the biceps muscle and is usually clearly visible.
4 The nerves can be approached with the needle in the longitudinal plane of the probe from the chest side of the probe and/or perpendicular to the longitudinal plane of the probe.
5 Instill 5 mL of LA around each nerve.

Complications of Axillary Block

1 There is less risk of major complications than with the other techniques.
2 May get nerve damage.
3 Risk of intravascular injection and haematoma if the artery is punctured.

Continuous Axillary Blockade (Adults)

This can be achieved by passing a catheter into the brachial plexus sheath. The steps in placement of the catheter are the same as for axillary brachial plexus block except that a catheter through needle technique is used. Kits are available for this technique such as the Contiplex® Katheterset. Insert the catheter 1–3 cm beyond the needle tip then remove the needle. Give a standard bolus dose as described above. Wait 1 h then run an infusion of bupivacaine 0.25% at 10 mL/h. Ropivacaine can also be used. A suggested regimen is 0.2% run at 10 mL/h. If pain occurs give a bolus of 10 mL and increase infusion rate by 3 mL/h to a maximum of 15 mL/h.

◗ Bradycardia

Defined as a pulse rate < 60 beats/min. Causes include:

1 *Physiological Derangements* e.g. hypoxia.
2 *Pharmacological Causes* e.g. suxamethonium.
3 *Surgical Causes* e.g. traction on the eye muscles.
4 *Pathological Causes* e.g. heart disease.

Bradycardia may or may not be associated with signs of poor perfusion which include:

1 altered mental state
2 chest pain

3 hypotension (SBP < 90 mm Hg)
4 heart failure or other signs of shock
5 HR < 40 bpm.

If there is no evidence of poor perfusion bradycardia treatment is not urgent. If poor perfusion is diagnosed the bradycardia must be treated urgently as follows:

1 Ensure adequate airway and ventilation.
2 Measure pulse-rate and blood pressure. If the patient is in extremus commence CPR. *See Cardiac Arrest*.
3 Diagnose the type of bradycardia. If sinus bradycardia give atropine up to 20 μg/kg IV. The maximum IV dose for an adult is 3 mg. Do not give atropine if the patient has third degree heart block or Morbitz type II second degree heart block as ventricular escape rates may be slowed. *See Heart Block (HB)*.
4 If bradycardia is due to heart block:
  a) Commence pacing either transvenous, oesophageal or transcutaneous approach. *See Pacing, Pacemakers and Anaesthesia*.
  b) If pacing is delayed, consider fist pacing—50–70 rhythmic blows per minute to the left lower edge of the sternum. *See Pacing, Pacemakers and Anaesthesia*.
  c) If pacing is delayed, pharmacological pacing can also be considered with an adrenaline infusion 2–10 μg/min or a dopamine infusion 2–10 μg/kg/min. Isoprenaline can also be considered. Give a bolus dose of 1–10 μg then infusion of 1–8 μg/min.
  d) For patients with bradycardia associated with drug-induced bradycardia from e.g. β blockers or calcium antagonists that does not respond to atropine give glucagon 3 mg IV then an infusion run at 3 mg/h.[31]

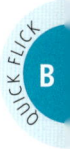

◗ Brainstem Anaesthesia

Aetiology

Brainstem anaesthesia is due to accidental intrathecal injection or intrathecal spread of a local anaesthetic drug to the region of the brainstem. This condition has has been associated with various types of regional anaesthetic blocks performed around the head and neck including:[32]

1 deep cervical plexus block
2 stellate ganglion block
3 interscalene brachial plexus block
4 retrobulbar block with accidental subarachnoid injection.

Diagnosis

This syndrome is characterised by the rapid (over 2–10 min)[32] appearance of:

1 restlessness, drowsiness and confusion

QUICK FLICK **B**

2 vomiting
3 cardiac depression
4 respiratory arrest
5 absence of brainstem reflexes on laryngoscopy.

Treatment

Supportive measures are required until the LA effect wears off. These include:

1 intubation of the airway and ventilation.
2 circulatory support with IV fluids and vasopressor agents.

◑ Breast Feeding and Anaesthesia

Patients who require anaesthesia while breast feeding should be advised as follows:

1 Continue breast feeding up until the time of anaesthesia and surgery.
2 After surgery when the next feed is due, express and discard the first breast milk that has accumulated and provide formula feed for the infant.
3 Resume breast feeding at the usual intervals.

◑ Broad Complex Tachycardia

Diagnosis

Differential diagnosis is between ventricular tachycardia (VT) and supraventricular tachycardia (SVT) with left bundle branch block (LBBB). Diagnostic features on the ECG to distinguish between these 2 dysrhythmias include:

1 *P Waves*—If P waves present before each QRS, this favours SVT whereas atrio-ventricular (AV) dissociation favours VT.
2 *QRS Axis*—A bizarre axis or a change in axis from the patient's usual ECG favours VT.
3 *QRS Duration*—A QRS duration < 0.14 s favours SVT, whereas a duration > 0.14 s favours VT.
4 *Lead V1*—A monophasic positive QRS in V1 favours VT, but a right bundle branch block (RBBB) pattern in V1 favours SVT. If QRS in V1 is biphasic and the first R wave is taller than the second r wave, this favours VT.
5 *Lead V6*—A deep S in V6 strongly favours VT. A positive QRS in V6 favours SVT especially if the QRS is double peaked and the R (first) peak is smaller than the r (second) peak.
6 *Concordance*—favours VT (all the QRS complexes look similar in shape).
7 *Fusion Beats*—favour VT (QRS complexes that look half way between a normal QRS and the broadened QRS complexes).
8 *Capture Beats*—also favour VT (a normal looking QRS between 2 broad QRS complexes).
9 Always consider the clinical picture. An elderly patient with ischaemic

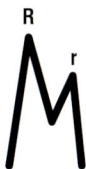

This pattern in V1 favours VT.

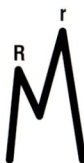

This pattern in V1 favours SVT with LBBB.

Figure B8 Lead V1 QRS morphology in the differentiation of broad complex tachycardia

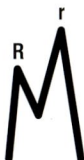

This pattern in lead V6 favours SVT.

Figure B9 Lead V6 QRS morphology in the differentiation of broad complex tachycardia

heart disease is much more likely to have VT than SVT. Young patients without heart disease are more likely to have SVT.

10 *Cannon Waves*—visible in the jugular venous pulse wave indicate AV dissociation. These waves support the diagnosis of VT.

Management of Broad Complex Tachycardia

1 If unstable cardiovascularly, DC cardioversion.
2 If stable, it is much safer to treat as VT than SVT. If a patient with VT is treated with verapamil on the assumption that the patient has SVT with LBBB, the result could be fatal. If there is a strong suspicion of SVT with LBBB the safest course of action is to treat with adenosine. *See Adenosine, Supraventricular Tachycardias* and *Ventricular Tachycardia*. Adenosine may reverse SVT but will have little effect on VT and has a high safety profile.
3 If the origin of the haemodynamically stable broad complex tachycardia remains obscure treat with amiodarone, procainamide or sotalol.

◐ Bronchial Blockers

See One Lung Ventilation.

○ Bronchopleural Fistula (BPF)

This condition can result from a wide variety of causes including:

1 post-thoracic surgery with breakdown of a suture line
2 ruptured lung abscess, bulla or cyst
3 erosion by malignancy
4 barotrauma.

Diagnosis

The lesion may be small, chronic and have little clinical impact. Clinical symptoms and signs for acute large bronchopleural fistulas include:

1 sudden dyspnoea, cyanosis, respiratory distress
2 subcutaneous emphysema
3 deviation of the trachea
4 tension pneumothorax
5 failure of a chest tube to drain a pneumothorax, often with a massive air-leak.[33]

Treatment

1 *Airway*—Optimise airway.
2 *Breathing*—Ensure adequate ventilation.
3 *Circulation*—Ensure adequate pulse and blood pressure. Tension pneumothorax can cause pulse-less electrical activity. If tension pneumothorax is suspected insert a chest tube. ***See*** *Chest Drain*.
4 Provide adequate IV fluid resuscitation.
5 Establish usual non-invasive monitoring plus consider insertion of an arterial line to detect early peri-cardial tamponade.
6 Pre-anaesthetic bronchoscopy should be performed if possible and may provide information regarding the site and extent of the BPF.
7 Options for induction of anaesthesia include:
   a) rapid sequence induction if patient is in extremus.
   b) awake fibre-optic bronchoscopy and intubation.
   c) inhalational induction.
8 A double lumen tube is usually required to isolate the lung with the BPF.

○ Bronchospasm

Topics Covered in this Section

▶ Treatment Strategies to Alleviate Causes of Bronchospasm
▶ Treatment Strategies to Reverse Bronchospasm
▶ Ventilation Strategies for Patients with Severe Bronchospasm
▶ Drug Dosages in Children

For strategies to prevent bronchospasm ***see*** *Asthma*.

Treatment Strategies to Alleviate Causes of Bronchospasm

1. Notify the surgeon, cease stimulation/surgery if possible.
2. Obtain skilled assistance early if serious bronchospasm.
3. Identify the cause. **See** *COVER ABCD A SWIFT CHECK Crisis Management Algorithm*. Always consider aspiration, asthma, anaphylaxis and pneumothorax as possible causes.
4. Assess airway, breathing and circulation.
5. Increase FiO_2 to 100% if oxygen saturation is reduced.
6. Remove any airway irritation e.g. secretions, endotracheal tube tip touching carina.
7. Suck out the endotracheal tube and consider withdrawing it slightly. If desflurane is being used change to sevoflurane.
8. If an LMA is being used, check for aspiration, laryngospasm and oral secretions and treat appropriately. **See** *Aspiration, Prevention and Treatment* and *Laryngospasm*.
9. Cease surgical stimulation and deepen anaesthesia if it is suspected that the patient is 'too light'.

Treatment Strategies to Reverse Bronchospasm

1. Give salbutamol aerosolised down the endotracheal tube via a 'spacer' device attached between the endotracheal tube and the breathing system. If no spacer device is available give the aerosolised salbutamol directly down the tube.
2. Give salbutamol 200–300 µg IV over 5 min then infusion run at 2–20 µg/min. Mix 15 mg salbutamol in 250 mL N/S, run at 2–20 mL/h.
3. Give adrenaline if bronchospasm is severe and not responding to the above measures. The dose depends on the urgency of the situation. In general give between 1 µg/kg boluses and 0.5 mg IV (the higher dose for imminent cardiorespiratory arrest). Follow up with an infusion of adrenaline. Mix 6 mg in 100 mL N/S and titrate to effect starting with 5 mL/h. If IV access is not available give 0.3 mg subcut. Repeat at 20 minute intervals $\times$ 2 if required.[34]
4. Aminophylline may also be useful. Give a loading dose of 5 mg/kg over 15–30 min (unless the patient is on oral theophylline, in which case a loading dose is contraindicated). Then give an aminophylline infusion of 0.5 mg/kg/h.
5. Give hydrocortisone 200 mg IV.
6. Be aware of the constant risk of tension pneumothorax in patients with severe bronchospasm. This condition may be bilateral and may result in cardiac arrest.

Other Treatments of Bronchospasm to Consider

1. Give ipratropium bromide (inhaled anticholinergic drug) which can be used in combination with nebulised salbutamol. *Dose in Adult 2 mL of 0.025% solution 2 h initially then 4–6 h.*

QUICK FLICK B

2 Consider ketamine. For non-intubated patients, give 0.1–0.2 mg/kg followed by an infusion of 0.5 mg/kg/h.[34] Atropine 0.1 mg or more should be given with ketamine to prevent excessive oral secretions. For intubated, ventilated patients a ketamine infusion of 1–5 mg/kg/h can be considered.[35]

3 A lignocaine infusion can be tried, run at 1–3 mg/kg/h.[36]

4 Magnesium sulphate IV. Give 2–3 g IV over 3 minutes.[34]

5 Sevoflurane has significant bronchodilating effects, and is superior to halothane in this regard. It can also be considered for therapy.[37]

6 Sodium bicarbonate in ventilated patients to normalise pH. Acidosis is thought to oppose the bronchodilator effects of sympathomimetic drugs.

7 External chest compression to assist expiration. At the end of inflation firmly squeeze the lower chest wall bilaterally until the next inflation.

8 Intratracheal injection of recombinant human deoxyribonuclease, which acts as a mucolytic agent, has produced dramatic improvement in some cases.[38]

9 Heliox (helium/oxygen) mixture reduces airflow resistance and decreases the work of breathing. A 60:40 mixture of helium and O_2 is commonly used and may be of some benefit with severe bronchospasm.[39]

10 Cardiopulmonary bypass.

Ventilation Strategies for Patients with Severe Bronchospasm

The overall principles are small tidal volumes, slow respiratory rate and a long expiratory time.

1 Aim for adequate oxygenation at acceptable airway pressures. Allow permissive hypercapnoea up to 80 mm Hg if necessary.[34]

2 Aim for a ventilation rate of 8–10 breaths per minute (bpm) and a tidal volume of 5–7 mL/kg.

3 Peak flow should be 60 L/min.

4 If this pattern still results in unacceptably high airway pressures, decrease ventilation rate to 6–8 bpm and reduce tidal volume to 3–5 mL/kg. Increase peak flow to 90–120 L/min to further decrease the inspired to expired time ratio. Also ensure that the patient is fully paralysed and adequately sedated.

5 A pneumothorax can occur and tension with hypotension and desaturation.

6 Massive auto-PEEP buildup can cause profound hypotension. Treat by disconnecting the patient from the ventilation device for a brief period to allow auto-PEEP to dissipate.

7 An ICU ventilator will be more effective than an anaesthetic ventilator due to its higher driving power and less tubing compliance.

Dosages in Children

1 Salbutamol IV bolus 5–10 µg/kg slowly (max 250 µg) then infusion 5–7.5 µg/kg/h.

2 Aminophylline 5 mg/kg over 1 h IV, then infusion. No loading dose if on oral theophylline. Rate of infusion depends on age. Age 1–9 yrs 1 mg/kg/h, 10–16 yrs 0.8 mg/kg/h.

3 Hydrocortisone IV 4 mg/kg 6 h.

◐ **Bupivacaine**

Amide type local anaesthetic agent. Suitable for all types of local and regional anaesthesia except for intravenous regional blockade and obstetric paracervical block.

Advantages
1 Longer acting than lignocaine.
2 Due to tissue binding, adding adrenaline is not needed to prolong bupivacaine's duration of action.

Disadvantages
1 More cardiotoxic than lignocaine, levobupivacaine or ropivacaine.
2 Cardiovascular collapse due to bupivacaine is much more difficult to treat successfully than CVS collapse due to ropivacaine or lignocaine.[40]

Maximum Dose
Adult 2–2.5 mg/kg. Maximum dose per 24 h 400 mg.
Child 3 mg/kg. This is almost equivalent to 1 mL/kg of the 0.25% solution or 0.5 mL/kg of the 0.5% solution.

Effects of Accidental IV Injection
As blood bupivacaine levels increase the following effects may be seen:
1 Tingling in the lips and tongue, dysphoria, tinnitus.
2 Loss of consciousness/seizure.
3 Respiratory arrest.
4 Hypotension, cardiac dysrhythmia, cardiovascular collapse, cardiac arrest.

Treatment of IV Bupivacaine Toxicity
1 If the patient becomes incoherent or loses consciousness seizures are imminent. Ventilate with 100% O_2.
2 Moore recommends adrenaline 0.3–0.5 mg IV in the adult if the HR drops below 60 bpm in the non-athlete, and cardiac compression if the HR drops below 25 bpm.[41]
3 If cardiac arrest occurs provide basic and advanced life support as described in *Cardiac Arrest*.
4 For cases in which all conventional resuscitative measures fail to produce a return of spontaneous circulation begin intralipid therapy. **See** *Intralipid for the Treatment of Bupivacaine/Ropivacaine Toxicity*.
5 Evidence for this treatment comes from researchers such as Weinberg et al.[42] and has been used successfully in at least one patient.[43]

◐ **Buprenorphine**

Buprenorphine is an opioid drug with agonist-antagonist properties. It is a thebaine derivative with a similar structure to morphine. It is $35\times$ more potent than morphine and it has a prolonged duration of action (up to 10 h).[44]

Dose

Adult IM 0.3 mg 6 h; *Sublingual* 0.4–0.8 mg.
Child 3–12 µg/kg/dose sublingual, IM or slow IV.[45]

Advantages

1 Does not cause significant histamine release hence is a useful opioid in conditions where histamine release is undesirable e.g. asthma, phaeochromocytoma surgery.[46]
2 Effective sublingually.
3 Does not stimulate the sigma receptor and does not cause hallucinations or dysphoria.

Disadvantages

1 Onset of analgesia is slow i.e. 30 min after IM injection.
2 Like other agonist/antagonist drugs, increasing dosages result in a plateau effect. Respiratory depression does not increase linearly with increasing dosage and the drug may partially antagonise itself. If respiratory depression requiring treatment does occur, it is difficult to reverse due to high opioid receptor affinity. Naloxone may be ineffective and doxapram may be helpful.[44]
3 Side effects such as nausea and vomiting and sedation can be marked and long lasting.[44]

◐ **Burns**

Topics Covered in this Section

▶ Initial Management and Assessment in the Emergency Department
▶ Calculating Area of Burns as a Percentage of Body Surface Area
▶ Definition of Major Burns
▶ Fluid Management for Major Burns
▶ Management of Carbon Monoxide Poisoning
▶ Anaesthetic Considerations for Burns Patients

Initial Management and Assessment in the Emergency Department

1 Provide immediate resuscitative measures if airway, breathing or circulation are compromised.

2 Obtain a detailed history of the injury which may provide an indication of additional injuries and the likelihood of airway burns and carbon monoxide poisoning.

3 Ensure the burning process is stopped e.g. removal of burning clothing.

4 As for all traumas, assess for other less obvious injuries.

5 Inspect the airway for any evidence of inhalational injury, such as pharyngeal burns, sooty sputum, a hoarse voice and singed nasal hair. Intubate early if the airway is compromised or is likely to become compromised e.g. severe neck/facial burns. The options to be considered are:

   a) Rapid sequence induction. Suxamethonium does not cause a significant hyperkalaemic response in burn patients for at least 24 h, and probably for a few days post burn.[47] After this time suxamethonium is contraindicated until several months after burns have completely healed.[47]

   b) Awake fibre-optic intubation.

   c) Inhalational induction and direct laryngoscopy and/or fibre-optic intubation or Airtraq intubation. *See Difficult Airway Management*.

6 Establish large bore IV access. Take bloods for FBC, electrolytes and creatinine, ABG, blood group and save, coagulation studies and CO levels. Obtain a CXR.

7 The burnt area should be irrigated with tepid H_2O (15°C) for 20–30 min if possible to minimise the eventual depth and area of burn.[48]

8 Exclude/manage associated trauma. Immobilise the cervical spine if neck injury is possible. If the patient is unconscious consider head trauma, drug/alcohol use, carbon monoxide (CO) poisoning and/or smoke inhalation. Always log roll the patient to identify injuries on the back.

9 Provide tetanus prophylaxis.

10 Hypovolaemic shock if present will not usually be due to the burn itself in the early stages, but due to other injuries, which must be identified.[48]

11 Give adequate analgesia (usually opioids) only when all other injuries are identified.

12 The next step is to calculate the percentage of skin area burnt.

13 Early escharotomy may be required for circumferential burns to areas such as the chest. This procedure may be urgent and life saving.

14 Cling film can be used as an initial dressing.

Calculating Area of Burns as a Percentage of Body Surface Area

The percentage of total body surface area (TBSA) burnt in adults and children can be calculated from the following tables. Only areas of skin with partial or full thickness burns should be included.

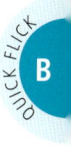

Table B4 Calculating area of burns (rule of nines) in the adult

Region	% OF TBSA
Arm	9
Trunk	36
Head	9
Leg	18
Perineum	1

Table B5 Calculating % burns in the child

Region	% OF TBSA	
	0–3Yrs	>3Yrs
Head & neck	18	12
Trunk & groin	32	38
Both arms	20	20
Both legs	30	30

Definition of Major Burns

Major Burns Defined as:

Adult > 15% TBSA having partial and full thickness burns or > 10% TBSA full thickness burns.

Child > 10% TBSA full thickness burn or > 20% partial and/or full thickness burns.

Fluid Management for Major Burns

1 Commence fluid resuscitation. Various formulae are used which in general aim at providing about 2–4 mL/kg per % TBSA burns in the first 24 h post burn. The most widely used is the Parkland formula and its modifications.[49] Give Hartmann's 4 mL/kg per % TBSA burn over first 24 h (from time of burn). Give half this over the first 8 h and the rest over the next 16 h. For example a 70 kg patient with 40% burns would receive 11.2 L in the first 24 h with 5.6 L given in the first 8 h after the burn.

2 Aim for at least 0.5–1 mL/kg/h urine output in adults and at least 1 mL/kg/h in children.[48] If oliguria occurs increase IV fluids by 50%.[50]

3 Fluid requirements over the second 24 h period depend on the patient's condition and local burn unit policies. This may include 5% glucose and colloid 0.3–0.5 mL/kg/%TBSA burns.[51]

Management of Carbon Monoxide (CO) Poisoning

Haemoglobin has 240 × more affinity for CO than O_2. The oxygen–haemoglobin dissociation curve is shifted to the left and O_2 content of the blood is severely reduced with significant poisoning. CO also binds to mitochondrial cytochrome oxidase inhibiting cellular respiration. CO binding to myoglobin reduces its O_2 storage function.

Clinical Effects of CO Poisoning

Effects of CO poisoning include:

1 Confusion, fitting or coma and death.
2 Cherry pink skin and mucosa can occur but cyanosis is more common.
3 Cerebral irritability may persist for weeks.[52]
4 Cardiac dysrhythmias may occur and cardiac output may fall.[53]

Relevant Investigations

ECG may show ST segment changes. Pulse oximetry is misleading because only oxyhaemoglobin and deoxyhaemoglobin are detected. In the presence of carboxyhaemoglobin (COHb) a falsely elevated O_2 saturation reading will be obtained.[52] A low co-oximeter O_2 with raised COHb levels is diagnostic.[54]

Table B6 Significance of various COHb levels[53,55]

COHb level	Significance
< 2%	Normal
Up to 12%	Heavy smokers
15%	Monitor closely
30%	Life-threatening hypoxia
> 50%	Lethal

Treatment

In addition to general supportive measures, treat CO poisoning with 100% O_2. This reduces the half-life of COHb from 240 min to 30–40 min. Hyperbaric O_2 therapy is recommended but its management value is doubted by some researchers.[50]

Table B7 Half-life of CO in blood under various conditions of FiO_2 and pressure[56]

CO half-life in blood	Pressure & concent. of inhaled O_2 (%)
250 min	21% at 1 atm
50 min	100% at 1 atm
22 min	100% at 2.5 atm

Anaesthetic Considerations for Burns Patients

1 Suxamethonium can be used in the first 24–48 hrs post burn. After this time, suxamethonium is contraindicated due to the risk of severe hyperkalaemia. Suxamethonium remains contraindicated until well after the burns have healed, some authorities recommending a period of

2 years after the burn injury.[57] Burns patients are resistant to the effects of non-depolarising neuromuscular blocking drugs.

2 Pay meticulous attention to maintaining the patient's body temperature peri-operatively.

3 Prepare for moderate to severe blood loss during grafting procedures. Try to limit the area excised at each debridement to less than 20% of TBSA and blood loss to < 50% of total blood volume. Encourage the surgeon to use vasoconstrictor infiltration, such as:

a) POR 8 diluted to 0.1–0.2 units/mL (use a maximum dose of 0.5 units/kg).[58]

b) Adrenaline can also be used topically on skin donor sites. Use 1:10 000 solution liberally as there is very little systemic absorption.[58]

REFERENCES

1 Wilson W, Taubert KA, Gewitz M, et al. Prevention of infective endocarditis: guidelines from the American Heart Association (see journal for full title). *Circulation* 2007; 116: 1736–54.

2 Gould FK, Elliott TS, Foweraker J, et al. Guidelines for the prevention of endocarditis: report of the Working Party of the British Society for Antimicrobial Chemotherapy. *J Antimicrobial Chemoth* 2006; 57: 1035–42.

3 Mangano DT, Layug EL, Wallace A, Tateo I, for the Multicenter Study of Perioperative Ischaemia Research Group. Effect of atenolol on mortality and cardiovascular morbidity after noncardiac surgery: Multicenter Study of Perioperative Ischaemia Research Group. *N Engl J Med* 1996; 335: 1713–20.

4 Eagle KA, Berger PB, Calkins H, et al. ACC/AHA guideline update for perioperative cardiovascular evaluation for noncardiac surgery: A report of the American College of Cardiology/American Heart Association Task Force on Practice Guidelines (Committee to Update the 1996 Guidelines on Perioperative Cardiovascular Evaluation for Noncardiac Surgery). 2002. American College of Cardiology website: http://www.acc.org/ (accessed June 2008).

5 Priebe H-J. Review article. Perioperative myocardial infarction — aetiology and prevention. *Br J Anaesth* 2005; 95: 3–19.

6 POISE Study Group. Effects of extended-release metropolol succinate in patients undergoing non-cardiac surgery (POISE trial): a randomised controlled trial. *Lancet* 2008; 371:1839–47.

7 Roscow CE. Can we measure the depth of anaesthesia? American Society of Anesthesiologists 50th Annual Refresher Course lectures 1999; 114: 1–7.

8 Gan TJ, Glass PS, Windsor A, Payne F, Roscow C, Sebel P, Manberg P and the BIS Utility Study Group. Bispectral index monitoring allows faster

emergence and improved recovery from propofol, alfentanil, and nitrous oxide anaesthesia. *Anesthesiology* 1997; 87: 808–15.

9 Myles PS, Leslie K, McNeil J, Forbes A, Chan MTV. Bispectral Index monitoring to prevent awareness during anaesthesia: the B-Aware randomized controlled trial. *Lancet* 2004; 363: 1757–63.

10 Yli-Hankala A, Vakkuri A, Annila P, Korttila K. EEG bispectral index monitoring in sevoflurane or propofol anaesthesia: analysis of direct costs and immediate recovery. *Acta Anaesthesiol Scand* 1999; 43: 545–9.

11 Gorbock MS. Inflation of the endotracheal tube cuff as an aid to blind nasal intubation.(Letter) *Anesth Analg* 1987; 66: 913.

12 American College of Surgeons, Committee on Trauma: *Advanced Life Support Course Manual*. Chicago, American College of Surgeons, 1989.

13 Brimacombe J, Berry A. A review of anaesthesia for ruptured abdominal aortic aneurysm with special emphasis on preclamping fluid resuscitation. *Anaesth Intensive Care* 1993; 21: 311–23.

14 Sessler DI. Symposium article; deliberate mild hypothermia. *J Neurosurg Anesthesiology* 1995; 7: 38–46.

15 Ramsa JG. Methods of reducing blood loss and non blood substitutes. *Can J Anaesth* 1991; 38: 592–612.

16 Monk TG. Alternatives to allogenic blood transfusions. *Can J Anesth* 1999; 46: R3–R6.

17 Goodnough LT, Monk TG, Andriole GL. Erythropoietin therapy. *N Engl J Med* 1997; 336: 933–8.

18 Report by the ASA task force on blood component therapy. Practice guidelines for blood component therapy. *Anesthesiology* 1996; 84: 732–47.

19 Crosby ET. Review article: Perioperative haemotherapy part 1, indications for blood component transfusion. *Can J Anaesth* 1992; 39: 695–707.

20 Goodnough LT, Brecher ME, Kanter MH, Aubuchon JP. Transfusion Medicine (first of two parts) Blood Transfusion. *N Eng J Med* 1999; 340: 438–47.

21 Trauma committee of the Royal Australian College of Surgeons. Early Management of Severe Trauma Course Manual. 1992; 61.

22 Goskowicz R. Massive transfusion: problems and solutions in blood conservation/massive transfusion. *Audio Digest Anesthesiology* 1996; 38: 23.

23 Heier HE, Bugge W, Hjelmeland K, Søreide E, Sørlie D, Håheim LL. Transfusion vs. alternative treatment modalities in acute bleeding: a systemic review. *Acta Anaesthesiol Scand* 2006; 50: 920–31.

24 Lovric VA. Alterations in blood components during storage and their clinical significance. *Anesth Intensive Care* 1984; 12: 246–51.

25 Benumof JL. Sleep apnoea and the obese patient. Audio Digest: *Anesthesiology* 2000; 42.

QUICK FLICK B

26 Al-Haddad MF, Coventry DM. Brachial plexus blockade. *Br J Anaesth CEPD Reviews* 2002: 33–6.

27 Klein SM, Greengrass RA, Steele SM et al. A comparison of 0.5% bupivacaine, 0.5% ropivacaine, and 0.75% ropivacaine for interscalene brachial plexus block. *Anesth Analg* 1998; 87: 1316–19.

28 Sukhani R, Barclay J, Aasen M. Prolonged Horner's syndrome after interscalene block: a management dilemma. *Anesth and Analg* 1994; 79: 601–3.

29 Poon A. The use of naropin (ropivacaine HCL) infraclavicular block for distal limb surgery. Block of the Month 2002: AstraZeneca Educational material.

30 Raw R. Brachial plexus blocks below the clavicle. *The Specialist Forum* 2003; February: 20–8.

31 American Heart Association. Part 7.3: Management of Symptomatic Bradycardia and Tachycardia. *Circulation* 2005; 112: IV67–IV77.

32 Carling A, Simmonds M. Complications from regional anaesthesia for carotid endarterectomy. *Br J Anaesthesia* 2000; 84: 797–800.

33 Devitt JH. Refresher Course Outline: Blunt thoracic trauma: anaesthesia, assessment and management. *Can J Anaesth* 1993; 40: R29–R34.

34 Guidelines 2000 for cardiopulmonary resuscitation and emergency cardiovascular care. *Circulation* 2000; 102(suppl): I237–I240.

35 Hemmingsen C, Kielson P, Ordorico J. Ketamine in the treatment of bronchospasm during mechanical ventilation. *Am J Emerg Med* 1994; 12: 417–20.

36 Hirshman CA. Perioperative management of the asthmatic patient. *Can J Anaesth* 1991; 38: R26–R32.

37 Goff MJ, Shahbaz RA, Ficke DJ, Uhrich TD, Ebert TJ. Absence of bronchodilation during desflurane anaesthesia. *Anesthesiology* 2000; 93: 404–8.

38 Patel A, Harrison E, Durward A, Murdoch IA. Intrathecal recombinant human deoxyribonuclease in acute life-threatening asthma refractory to conventional treatment. *Br J Anaesth* 2000; 84: 505–7.

39 Manthous CA, Hall JB, Caputo MA, et al. Heliox improves pulsus paradoxus and peak expiratory flow in nonintubated patients with severe asthma. *Am J Respir Crit Care Med* 1995; 151: 310–14.

40 Covino BG. Recent advances in local anaesthesia. *Can J Anaesth* 1991; 38: R26–R32.

41 Moore DC. Lipid rescue from bupivacaine cardiac arrest: a result of failure to ventilate and maintain cardiac perfusion (Letter). *Anesthesiol* 2007; 106: 636.

42 Weinberg G, Hertz P, Newman J. Lipid, not propofol, treats bupivacaine overdose (letter). *Anesth Analg* 2004; 99: 1875.

43 Rosenblatt MA, Abel M, Fischer GR, Itzkovich C, Eisenkraft JB. Successful use of a 20% lipid emulsion to resuscitate a patient after presumed bupivacaine-related cardiac arrest. *Anesthesiol* 2006;105: 217–18.

44 Wilkinson DJ. Opioid agonist/antagonists in general anaesthesia. *Br J H Med* 1987 (Aug): 130–3.

45 Shann F. *Drug Doses*. 11th edn 2001. Collective Pty Ltd: 10.

46 Singh G, Kam P. An overview of anaesthetic issues in phaeochromocytomas. *Annals Academy of Medicine* 1998; 27: 843–8.

47 Juels AN. Anesthesia and burns. In: Duke J, Rosenberg SG, eds. *Anesthesia Secrets*. Hanley & Belfus, Inc, Philadelphia, Mosby, St Louis,1996; 352–5.

48 Shaw A, Anderson J, et al. The early management of large burns. *Br J Hosp Med* 1995; 53: 247–50.

49 Warden GD. Burn shock resuscitation. *World J Surg* 1992; 16: 16–23.

50 Hilton PJ, Hepp M. The immediate care of the burned patient. *Br J Anaesth CEPD Reviews* 2001; 1; 113–16.

51 Tjeuw M. Burns. In Yao F-S, Fontes ML, Malhotra V, eds. *Yao and Artusio's Anesthesiology: Problem-Oriented Patient Management*, 6th ed. Lippincott Williams and Wilkins, Philadelphia, Pennsylvania 2008: 1113–33.

52 Brogan TV, Sharar SR. Toxic gas, fume, and smoke inhalation. In: Parrillo JE, ed. *Current Therapy in Clinical Care Medicine*, 3rd edn. Mosby, St Louis 1997: 258–63.

53 Atkinson RS, Rushman GB, Davies NJH. *Lee's Synopsis of Anesthesia*, 11th edn. Butterworth–Heinemann, Oxford 1993, 851–2.

54 Oxer HF. Hyperbaric oxygen—an interest for anaesthetists? *Australasian Anaesthesia* 1992; 25–33.

55 Sykes MK, Vickers MD, Hull CJ, Winterburn PJ, Shepstone BJ. *Principles of Measurement and Monitoring in Anaesthesia and Intensive Care*, 3rd edn. Blackwell Scientific Publications, Oxford 1991; 265.

56 Pace N, Strajman E, Walker EL. Acceleration of carbon monoxide elimination in man by high pressure oxygen. *Science* 1950; 111: 652.

57 Hartmann GS. Burns. In Yao F-S F, ed. *Anesthesiology Problem-Orientated Patient Management*, 4th edn, Lippincott-Raven, Philadelphia 1998; 898–918.

58 O'Connel AJ, Keneally JP. Paediatric burns. *Curr Anaesth Crit Care* 1994; 5:209–17.

C

◯ Caesarean Section (CS)

Topics Covered in this Section
- ▶ Choice of Anaesthetic Technique
- ▶ Pre-operative Assessment and Preparation
- ▶ Minimising Fetal Compromise Prior to CS
- ▶ General Anaesthesia—Induction and Intubation Phase and Failed Intubation Drill
- ▶ Epidural Anaesthesia
- ▶ Subarachnoid Block Anaesthesia

Choice of Anaesthetic Technique

Regional anaesthesia has a lower maternal risk than general anaesthesia.[1] Hawkins et al. calculated that the relative risk of maternal mortality is 16.7 × greater with GA compared with a regional technique.[2] The risk of failed intubation in the obstetric population is estimated to be about 0.4%.[3] The majority of anaesthesia-related maternal deaths are due to failed intubation and/or aspiration.[4]

General anaesthesia is still often required for failed regional anaesthesia, patient refusal of regional anaesthesia and for some obstetric emergencies. Although tracheal intubation for CS has long been thought to be the 'gold standard' the laryngeal mask airway has been used successfully in at least one large trial in selected patients.[5]

Pre-operative Assessment and Preparation

In addition to routine history and examination:
1. Carefully assess the airway to identify possibly difficult intubation. Prepare for unanticipated difficult intubation. *See Difficult Airway Management*.
2. Acid aspiration prophylaxis:
   a) Ranitidine 150 mg PO the night before and morning of surgery.
   b) Sodium citrate 0.3 M 30 mL on call to op-suite, or in op-suite.
   c) Metoclopramide. Consider 10 mg IV or IM if the patient has had a recent meal, to increase gastric emptying.

Minimising Fetal Compromise Prior to CS

There are several strategies that can be used to optimise the condition of the compromised fetus. These include:
1. Treat maternal hypotension aggressively with IV (non glucose containing) fluids and vasoconstrictor drugs.

2 Alleviate aortocaval compression e.g. left lateral tilt or other change in maternal position such as right lateral tilt and the knee-chest position.

3 If uterine atony is suspected stop the syntocinon infusion. Consider a uterine relaxant agent such as nitroglycerine. **See** *Uterine Relaxation for Retained Placenta*.

4 Increase fetal oxygenation with high concentration oxygen administered to the mother by facemask.

General Anaesthesia–Induction and Intubation Phase and Failed Intubation Drill

1 Position the patient in left lateral tilt with a wedge placed under the right buttock to prevent aortocaval compression. **See** *Supine Hypotensive Syndrome*.

2 If the patient's airway appears to be 'difficult' consider an awake fibre-optic intubation or revisiting the use of regional anaesthesia.

3 If the patient's airway looks acceptable a rapid sequence induction is performed.
   a) Preoxygenate patient for 3–5 min.
   b) Give thiopentone 4–5 mg/kg followed immediately by suxamethonium 1–1.5 mg/kg (or rocuronium 0.6 mg/kg if suxamethonium is contraindicated).

   Note: Assistant must apply cricoid pressure as the patient begins to lose consciousness and does not release cricoid pressure until trachea is intubated and the anaesthetist requests its release.

   For a more detailed discussion of this manoeuvre **see** *Rapid Sequence Induction*.

4 Always be prepared for the possibility of failed intubation and be familiar with an appropriate failed intubation drill.

Suggested Failed Intubation Drill for CS

1 Send for help and alert the surgeon. Maintain cricoid pressure. Consider the immediate insertion of the Airtraq if available and you are skilled in its use. Dhonneur et al. describe the incorporation of the Airtraq into their hospital's failed intubation management algorithm. In their report two morbidly obese parturients could not be intubated with direct laryngoscopy due to inability to visualise the larynx. The Airtraq provided a grade 1 view and enabled intubation in less than 60 s.[6]

2 Oxygenation must be maintained via mask and bag + an oral or nasal airway as required. If unable to maintain oxygenation insert a laryngeal mask airway (LMA) or ProSeal LMA. It may be necessary to release cricoid pressure temporarily while placing the LMA/ProSeal™.[7] **See** *Difficult Airway Management*.

3   If able to maintain oxygenation consider reattempting intubation with whatever aids are available (e.g. teflon introducer, McCoy blade, Airtraq). Do not attempt intubation more than 3 times in total.

4   If able to maintain oxygenation but unable to intubate, decide whether CS *must proceed immediately* to save the life of the baby (fetal distress) and/or the mother (e.g. bleeding placenta praevia or ruptured uterus). If CS must proceed immediately it is very controversial as to what to do next. Perhaps the best option is to use the ProSeal™ as recommended by Awan:[8]

   a) Insert the ProSeal™. It may be necessary to release cricoid pressure to allow correct positioning.

   b) Inflate the ProSeal™ cuff and test ventilate.

   c) If successful release cricoid pressure and insert a gastric tube through the gastric lumen of the ProSeal™ and empty the stomach.

   d) Maintain paralysis and allow the patient to awaken in the left lateral position at the end of the procedure.

   The LMA is the next best option. Cricoid pressure should be momentarily removed to allow correct positioning of the LMA and then reapplied until the patient awakens.

5   Another possible approach is to maintain anaesthesia with bag-mask ventilation and constant cricoid pressure. It is probably best to keep the patient paralysed so that surgery is expedited and bag/mask ventilation may be easier to perform.[9]

6   If able to maintain oxygenation and *CS is not urgent* allow the patient to 'wake up' and use epidural, spinal or awake intubation technique. CS using LA infiltration is another option.

7   If unable to maintain oxygenation using an LMA or ProSeal™ obtain a surgical airway via cricothyrotomy or cricothyroid membrane needle puncture. ***See*** *Cricothyroid Puncture and Cricothyrotomy*.

8   When maternal oxygenation is obtained wake the patient up and formulate a new anaesthetic plan. Although this may delay delivery, the anaesthetist's first duty of care is to the mother.

Anaesthetic Management after Intubation

1   Maintain anaesthesia with O_2, air and volatile agent.

2   Maintain muscle relaxation with intermediate acting muscle relaxant such as rocuronium.

3   Avoid hypocapnia which may result in decreased placental perfusion.

4   Give 5–10 IU oxytocin IV + opioid (e.g. morphine 5–10 mg) once baby is delivered. The surgeon may request an oxytocin infusion (40 IU in 1000 mL of Hartmann's solution run over 4–6 h). Instead of oxytocin (bolus and infusion) carbetocin 100 µg IV over 1 min can be used.

5   Extubate the patient in the left lateral position 'awake' i.e. when she is

able to protect her own airway. Selecting the optimum time to extubate is a matter of experience but usually a patient can be extubated when she has a vigorous cough and shows evidence of voluntary muscle control e.g. opening eyes to voice, trying to self extubate.

Epidural Anaesthesia

Aortocaval compression must be prevented at all times using left lateral tilt or positioning the patient on each side sequentially. During the procedure preload the patient with 500–1000 mL of Hartmann's solution or N/S. Use lignocaine 2% + 1:200 000 adrenaline with fentanyl 5 µg/mL. Give 20–25 mL slowly titrating dose to effect. It is necessary to block to a dermatomal level T4–6. About 1.5–2 mL of LA is required per dermatomal segment. If the epidural block fails to provide adequate anaesthesia for surgery, consider:

1 General anaesthesia.
2 Repeat epidural with cautious loading of LA solution.
3 CSE technique with a conservative initial spinal dose e.g. 1 mL hyperbaric bupivacaine.[10]

Note: Do not perform a single shot spinal with a 'full dose' of LA e.g. 2.2 mL hyperbaric bupivacaine on top of a failed epidural, as this may produce a very high block and is inherently unsafe.[10]

Subarachnoid Block Anaesthesia

Anticipate hypotension which may be of a more rapid onset than with epidural. Preload patient with 1–1.5 L of crystalloid (not 5% glucose) during the administration of the block. Consider using a bolus of vasopressor prophylactically immediately after injection of LA. For the subarachnoid block use 'heavy' bupivacaine 0.5 % (contains glucose 80 mg/mL). Use 2.2–2.4 mL for the average sized patient with fentany 25 µg + 150 µg morphine. Position the patient to avoid aortocaval compression at all times (e.g. left lateral tilt). Consider tilting the patient 5° head down for 5 minutes to enhance spread of the block. Treat any hypotension aggressively with boluses of phenylephrine, metaraminol or ephedrine. Note that nausea and lightheadedness may pre-empt hypotension and should be treated with a bolus of vasopressor.[10] Also treat bradycardia immediately with glycopyrrolate or atropine. *See Subarachnoid Block Anaesthesia*. If, despite adequate dosing and time to allow onset, the block is inadequate for surgery to proceed, consider performing an epidural and cautiously dosing the patient with LA. Even small volumes of LA e.g. 5 mL in the epidural space may improve the quality of SAB sufficiently for surgery to occur successfully.

Combined Spinal Epidural (CSE) Anaesthesia

This technique is enjoying increasing popularity for CS. *See Subarachnoid Block (SAB)*.

○ Calcium

Calcium is an essential electrolyte for body metabolism. It is particularly important for nerve conduction and skeletal, cardiac and smooth muscle contraction and in many enzymatic processes such as coagulation.
NR 2.25–2.6 mmol/L. To correct for the serum albumin level, actual Ca^{2+} level equals measured Ca^{2+} + (40 – measured albumin) × 0.024. It is the ionised calcium level that is clinically significant.

Hypercalcaemia
Severe if Ca > 3.5 mmol/L.

Causes of Hypercalcaemia
1 malignancy e.g. boney mets, myeloma
2 hyperparathyroidism
3 iatrogenic e.g. TPN
4 endocrine disorders—phaeochromocytoma, acromegaly.

Clinical Effects
1 Drowsiness, lethargy, weakness
2 Nausea and vomiting
3 Abdominal pain
4 Pancreatitis
5 Polydypsia, polyuria and dehydration
6 Dysrrhythmias including bradycardia, tachycardia, heart block
7 Hypertension
8 ECG may show a shortened Q-T interval, a prolonged PR and QRS intervals, and T wave flattening and widening.
9 AV nodal block progressing to complete heart block may occur.
10 Coma, cardiac arrest.

Treatment
1 Rehydrate with N/S.
2 Establish forced saline diuresis with 1000 mL N/S over 4 h then 1000 mL N/S + 20 mEq KCl + 20 mg frusemide 4 h. Monitor the following:
   a) Potassium, calcium and magnesium levels.
   b) Intravascular volume status (including use of CVP measurement).
   c) Urine output and urinary sodium. Aim to keep urinary Na^+ greater than 100 mmol/L.
3 If the hypercalcaemia is due to myeloproliferative disorder give mithramycin (plicamycin) 25 μg/kg by infusion over 3 h. Administer one dose only.
4 Calcitonin is effective for hypercalcaemia associated with cancer. Give 3–4 u/kg IV, then 4 u/kg subcutaneously 12–24 h.
5 Hydrocortisone 200–400 mg/day IV.

6 EDTA 15–50 mg/kg.
7 Dialysis.

Hypocalcaemia

Causes

1. pancreatitis
2. hypoparathyroidism
3. lack of Vitamin D
4. elderly/cachexia/malnutrition
5. drugs e.g. phenytoin, cis-platinum.

Clinical Effects of Hypocalcaemia

Clinical manifestations occur when serum $Ca^{2+} < 2$ mmol/L. These include:

1. tetany, cramps, carpo-pedal spasm
2. positive Chvostek and Trousseau's signs
3. mental changes
4. reduced cardiac output, hypotension
5. perioral and peripheral paraesthesia.

Treatment

1. Provide adequate airway and ventilation.
2. Provide circulatory support if cardiac output is inadequate.
3. Give IV calcium either calcium chloride 10% 10 mL (6.8 mmol) or calcium gluconate 20 mL (4.4 mmol). The final dose depends on the degree of deficiency although the maximum daily dose should not exceed 15 g. See below.

Calcium Gluconate

Calcium gluconate is presented in 10 mL ampoules containing 1 g (2.2 mmol) of calcium. Calcium gluconate is useful in the treatment of:

1. hypocalcaemia
2. hyperkalaemia
3. hypermagnesaemia
4. calcium channel blocker overdose.

Adult Dose

Hyperkalaemia/Hypermagnesaemia 2.2 mmol by slow IV injection (over 5 min), repeat if required.

Hypocalcaemia **see** *Calcium*.

Calcium Channel Blocker Poisoning 2.2–4.4 mmol by slow IV injection (over 5 min).

Precautions

Do not give in the presence of digoxin toxicity.

QUICK FLICK C

◑ Carbetocin

This drug is a long acting oxytocic useful for the routine prevention of postpartum haemorrhage by promoting uterine contraction post delivery. It can be used as an alternative to an oxytocin bolus and infusion post Caesarean section delivery or post-vaginal delivery in women at high risk of post-partum haemorrhage. It may be more effective than an oxytocin infusion.[11]

Dose
100 µg IV (over 1 min) or IM.
It is well tolerated with relatively minor side effects such as metallic taste and flushing.

◑ Carbon Monoxide Poisoning

See *Burns*.

◑ Carcinoid Tumours and Carcinoid Syndrome

Carcinoid tumours are derived from enterochromaffin tissue or Kulchitsky cells. They occur most commonly in the gut especially the appendix. About 8–20% of tumours cause carcinoid syndrome which results from secretion of serotonin, kallikrein (which generates bradykinin), histamine, prostaglandins and other substances. The liver inactivates these substances so gut carcinoid usually does not produce the syndrome. When carcinoid syndrome occurs there are usually liver metastases or the tumours arise from non-gut tissue such as ovary/testicle, pancreas or bronchi.

Clinical Features of Carcinoid Syndrome
1 Diarrhoea, abdominal pain, gastrointestinal bleeding.
2 Tachycardia, tachydysrhythmias and hypertension (due to serotonin).
3 Hypotension and bronchospasm (due to bradykinin).
4 Mild hyperglycaemia.
5 Flushing.
6 Oedema.
7 Heart failure.
8 Vitamin B12, folate deficiency.
9 Clotting abnormalities can result from malabsorption of fat soluble vitamins.
10 Pellagra may develop due to dietary tryptophan being converted to serotonin instead of niacin.

Diagnostic Tests and Biochemical Abnormalities
1 Raised urinary 5-hydroxyindoleacetic acid (5-HIAA) levels. Prognosis is poor if this value is greater than 1000 µg/day.

2 Hyperglycaemia, hypoproteinaemia, elevated liver enzymes, electrolyte abnormalities.

3 Abnormalities of the pulmonary or tricuspid valves. The valves of the left side of the heart are at less risk due to lung tissue inactivating tumour secretions. Carcinoid induced heart disease is associated with a poorer prognosis.[12]

Treatment of Carcinoid Syndrome

Octreotide 200 µg 8 h can be tried and if successful a longer acting somatostatin analogue (lanreotide) can be used.

Anaesthesia for Carcinoid Syndrome

The main aims of anaesthesia are to:

1 Reduce the risk of mediator release.

2 Anticipate/treat peri-operative carcinoid crisis (hypotension/bronchospasm).

Peri-operative octreotide therapy results in a decreased incidence of intra-operative complications and death.[12]

Pre-operative Phase

1 Assess patients carefully for the presence of carcinoid syndrome.

2 Look for any evidence of heart failure and valve disease especially tricuspid and pulmonary valves.

3 Correct electrolyte abnormalities.

4 Consider pre-operative octreotide 100 µg subcut 6–8 h prior to surgery. Alternatively consider cyproheptadine 4 mg 8 h or ketanserin 40 mg 12 h. Use both for 3 days prior to surgery.

5 Patients with significant valve lesions should have appropriate endocarditis prophylaxis. **See** *Bacterial Endocarditis (BE) Prophylaxis*.

6 Keep patients well hydrated.

Intra-operative Phase

1 Premedicate with octreotide 50–150 µg subcut.

2 Avoid suxamethonium which may increase intra-abdominal pressure and tumour secretion.

3 Intraoperatively consider an infusion of octreotide 100 µg/h.

4 Avoid catecholamines which may induce a carcinoid crisis (adrenaline, noradrenaline, dopamine)

5 Ketamine is probably best avoided.

6 Avoid histamine releasing drugs such as morphine and pethidine.

7 Treat carcinoid crisis (hypotension and/or bronchospasm) with IV fluid loading and octreotide 20 µg IV. Do not use adrenaline.

8 If hypertension occurs use a β blocker (e.g. esmolol) or ketanserin 10 mg IV over 3 min then an infusion run at 3 mg/h.

Postoperative Phase
Patients may be excessively drowsy postoperatively due to the effects of serotonin.

◯ Cardiac Arrest

Topics Covered in this Section
▶ Basic Life Support—Adult
▶ Advanced Life Support—Adult
▶ Basic Life Support—Infant and Child
▶ Advanced Life Support—Infant and Child
▶ Cardiac Arrest in Pregnancy
▶ Administration of Drugs by the Endotracheal Route

For management of neonatal cardiac arrest *see* *Neonatal Resuscitation*.
   The following guidelines are based mainly on the recommendations of:
1 The Australian Resuscitation Council (2008 guidelines).
2 2005 International Consensus on Cardiopulmonary Resuscitation (CPR) and Emergency Cardiovascular Care (ECC) Science with Treatment Recommendations—*Circulation* (Supplement) 2005: 112.
Survival to hospital discharge for out of hospital cardiac arrest is about 5%, and for in-hospital cardiac arrest victims is about 20%.

Basic Life Support (BLS)–Adult
The steps in BLS are summarised by DRABCD:
1 *Danger* Ensure the safety of the rescuer, victim and bystanders. For example the victim may be in a wet area such as a shower, posing a risk to rescuers during defibrillation.
2 *Response* Establish patient response via simple commands e.g. 'open your eyes' and non-injurious physical stimulation e.g. squeezing the shoulders.
3 If the patient is unresponsive activate the *Advanced Life Support (ALS) service* for that area. The aim is to get a defibrillator to the patient with minimal delay. For patients with a shockable rhythm, early defibrillation and BLS provides the best chance of survival.
4 *Airway* Establish a clear airway by backward head tilt (extending the head on the neck), jaw thrust, opening the mouth slightly (jaw support) and removal of any obvious loose foreign body in the mouth such as loose dentures. Well-fitting dentures should be left in place.
5 *Breathing* Look for evidence of breathing by listening for breath sounds and feeling for exhaled gas. If the patient is not breathing, commence artificial ventilation by mouth-to-mouth, mouth-to-mask or bag-mask ventilation. Give 2 initial breaths allowing 1 second for inspiration per breath and ensure that the chest rises. Provide oxygen supplementation if

possible e.g. mouth to mask technique with oxygen tubing attached to a suitable port on the mask.

6 *Circulation* Rather than feeling for a carotid pulse, the ARC recommends commencing ECC if there are no signs of life i.e. patient is unconscious, unresponsive, not moving, not breathing. The basis of this recommendation is that checking for a carotid pulse is an inaccurate way of identifying the presence of a circulation.[13] In addition, there is little risk of injury to compression of a beating heart whereas withholding compression to a patient in cardiac arrest will greatly decrease or negate the patient's chances of survival. The exception to this advice may be the presence of staff highly trained in resuscitation that are competent at detecting the presence or absence of a pulse. ECC should be applied to the lower half of the sternum with the dominant hand lowermost and the fingers parallel to the ribs. If uncertain where to compress the chest, compress the perceived 'middle of the chest'. Compress at a rate of 100 per minute. The depth of compression should be $\frac{1}{3}$ the anterior to posterior diameter of the chest ($\approx$ 5 cm in the average adult). The ratio of ECC to ventilation is 30:2 for 1 or more rescuers. The ratio of compression to relaxation time (the 'duty cycle') should be 1:1. Allow for complete chest recoil. If more than 1 rescuer is present, alternate the role of ECC every 2 minutes. Continue CPR until:

a) the patient shows signs of life e.g. movement, moaning
b) the ALS service arrives and instructs you to cease
c) you are too exhausted to continue

Note: Do not interrupt CPR to check for a pulse.

7 *Defibrillation* Defibrillation takes precedence over BLS if a defibrillator is immediately available and the patient is in a shockable rhythm. However if cardiac arrest has occurred longer than 4 minutes without BLS, 2 minutes of BLS should be provided prior to defibrillation.

Points to Note Regarding BLS

1 If an automated external defibrillator is available (AED) apply the pads to the patient's chest and follow the voice prompts. ***See*** *Defibrillators*.
2 For a witnessed monitored arrest due to VF or pulseless VT, or a witnessed cardiac arrest due to electrocution, and a defibrillator is not immediately available, give a precordial thump. This manoeuvre consists of a blow to the mid-sternum with the ulnar surface of the clenched fist. This may revert these dysrhythmias. This technique is more effective for pulseless VT than VF. A precordial thump is contraindicated if there has been a recent sternotomy for coronary artery grafts or valve replacement or recent chest trauma.
3 ECC produces a cardiac output that is only 25–35% of normal.[14] Brain blood flow is 50–90% of normal and myocardial blood flow is 20–50%

of normal. Although a systolic blood pressure of 40–80 mm Hg can be achieved, diastolic blood pressure is very low. Automated chest compression devices are becoming increasingly available and provide more effective ECC than human rescuers. **See** *AutoPulse*.

4 Once the patient is intubated provide 8–10 ventilations per minute and 100 ECC per minute. Do not co-coordinate ventilation and ECC. Do not hyperventilate the patient as this will reduce venous return to the heart and therefore reduce ECC induced cardiac output.

5 The Resuscitation Council of the United Kingdom in their 2005 guidelines recommends performing ECC before rescue breaths.

Advanced Life Support (ALS)—Adult

ALS is BLS plus invasive techniques including defibrillation and IV drug therapy. ALS management of cardiac arrest depends on diagnosing the underlying cardiac rhythm. The rhythm will either be shockable (VF/ pulseless VT) or non shockable (asystole or pulseless electrical activity).

VF or Pulseless VT

Early defibrillation is the most important aspect of management. Defibrillation within the first 3 minutes of VF cardiac arrest is associated with a survival of > 50% in out-of-hospital cardiac arrest. Without CPR survival from VF arrest decreases by 7–10% per minute.

Witnessed Arrest

The ARC recommends giving up to 3 'stacked' shocks initially. This means giving the shocks as rapidly as possible. The ECG is checked between shocks and the shocks are ceased if an organised rhythm on the ECG is seen. The energy used depends on the type of defibrillator.

1 Monophasic defibrillator 360 J. Use same energy for all subsequent shocks.

2 Biphasic defibrillator 200 J. If relevant clinical data is known about the particular biphasic defibrillator being used supporting a different energy level, use of this level is acceptable. Use the same energy for all subsequent shocks.

Unwitnessed Arrest

Give a *single* shock of 360 J (monophasic) or 200 J (biphasic). If relevant clinical data is known about the particular biphasic defibrillator being used supporting a different energy level, use of this level is acceptable. Use the same energy for all subsequent shocks.

Subsequent Management

Immediate resumption of CPR for 2 min and establish IV access.
(Intubate the patient if you have the skills to do so.)
↓

Check rhythm/pulse—if still VF/ pulseless VT,
adrenaline 1 mg IV, circulate with 1–2 min of ECC
(repeat adrenaline every 3 min of arrest time)
and repeat shock × 1
↓
Immediate resumption of CPR for 2 min
↓
Check rhythm/pulse—if still VF/ pulseless VT
amiodarone 300 mg or lignocaine 1 mg/kg (inferior choice)
circulate with 1–2 min of ECC
and repeat shock × 1
↓
immediate resumption of CPR for 2 min
↓
Check rhythm/pulse—if still VF/ pulseless VT
amiodarone 150 mg or lignocaine 0.5 mg/kg
circulate with 1–2 min of ECC
and repeat shock × 1
↓
Check rhythm/pulse— if still VF/ pulseless VT
↓
Repeat shock × 1
immediate resumption of CPR for 2 min
↓
Identify and treat reversible causes (see below)
Send blood for urgent ABG analysis
Consider other drug therapy if indicated (see below)
Consider an amiodarone and/or adrenaline infusion if indicated

Other Drug Therapy to Consider for VF/pulseless VT

1 *Sodium bicarbonate* is indicated for cardiac arrest associated with:
    a) prolonged arrest (> 15 min)
    b) documented metabolic acidosis prior to arrest
    c) hyperkalaemia
    d) overdose of tricyclic antidepressants
    e) hyponatraemia.
    Use a dose of 50–100 mmol IV.
2 *Magnesium Sulphate* is useful for the treatment of cardiac arrest associated with:
    a) hypokalaemia/hypomagnesaemia
    b) Torsades de pointes. **See** *Torsades de Pointes*.
    c) digoxin toxicity related dysrhythmias
    d) VF/pulseless VT refractory to defibrillator shocks and vasopressor.

Dilute 10 mmol in 20 mL N/S, give 10 mL (5 mmol) IV as an initial bolus which can be repeated × 1. If required give an infusion of magnesium 20 mmol over 4 h. ***See*** *Magnesium Sulphate*.

3 *Calcium* is indicated for cardiac arrest due to, or complicated by:
   a) hypocalcaemia
   b) hyperkalaemia
   c) overdose of calcium channel blocker drugs
   d) magnesium toxicity.
   Give 5–10 mL calcium chloride 10% solution IV.
4 *Potassium* is indicated for hypokalaemia. Give 5 mmol IV.
5 *Fibrinolytic therapy* should be considered for cardiac arrest associated with known or suspected pulmonary embolus induced cardiac arrest. ***See*** *Pulmonary Embolus (PE)*.

Points to Note Regarding VF/Pulseless VT
1 Do not use lignocaine and amiodarone together.
2 The rate of successful defibrillation of VF/pulseless VT decreases rapidly over time.
3 Effective BLS increases the likelihood of successful defibrillation.[15]
4 Give IV drug therapy while preparing to defibrillate.
5 The Resuscitation Council of the United Kingdom in their 2005 guidelines recommends single shocks only (no stacked shocks). For biphasic defibrillators the initial shock should be 150–200 J. Subsequent shocks should be 150–360 J. For monophasic defibrillators all shocks should be 360 J.

Non-shockable Rhythms
In the management of non-shockable rhythms in cardiac arrest, identification and treatment of the cause of the cardiac arrest provides the only avenue of survival.

Causes of Cardiac Arrest
The causes of cardiac arrest can be divided into:
1 Cardiac chamber related causes:
   a) inadequate cardiac filling (haemorrhage, anaphylaxis)
   b) embolus (pulmonary, amniotic fluid, bone marrow, gas).
2 Cardiac muscle related causes:
   a) hypoxia (global or regional due to e.g. coronary artery thrombosis)
   b) metabolic abnormalities e.g. hyperkalaemia, acidosis
   c) hypothermia/hyperthermia
   d) drug effects e.g. digoxin toxicity.
3 Cardiac compression related causes:
   a) pericardial effusion with tamponade
   b) tension pneumothorax.

4 Another approach to diagnosis is the 4 Hs and 4 Ts

1) Hypoxia
2) Hypovolaemia
3) Hypo/Hypothermia
4) Hypo/Hyperkalaemia

1) Tamponade: pericardial
2) Tension pneumothorax
3) Toxins/poisons
4) Thrombosis: pulmonary/coronary artery

While identifying and treating a specific cause, supportive measures that can be used include:

Asystole
Effective BLS—ECC may convert asystole to VF
↓
adrenaline 1 mg IV initially
then for every 3 minutes of arrest time
↓
atropine 1 mg boluses up to 3 mg IV
↓
transcutaneous pacing if p waves present
(no evidence of benefit for pacing true asystole)
↓
reassess rhythm after every 2 minutes

Note: The Resuscitation Council of the United Kingdom in their 2005 guidelines recommends giving a single dose of atropine 3 mg for asystole resistant to adrenaline.

Pulseless Electrical Activity (PEA)
Defined as organised cardiac electrical activity (other than pulseless VT) without a palpable pulse. Cardiac output may or may not be present but there is no palpable pulse. Supportive treatment includes:

Effective BLS
↓
Adrenaline 1 mg IV initially then for every 3 minutes of arrest time
↓
IV Fluids—Gelofusine 1 L
↓
Atropine 1 mg boluses up to 3 mg if rate of PEA is less than 60 bpm
Consider transcutaneous pacing
↓
Pericardiocentesis if cardiac tamponade possible. ***See*** *Cardiac Tamponade.*

Note: The Resuscitation Council of the United Kingdom in their 2005 guidelines recommends giving a single dose of atropine 3 mg for PEA with a rate less than 60 bpm.

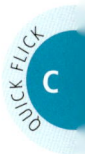

QUICK FLICK **C**

Postresuscitation Care after Adult Cardiac Arrest

Patients who remain unconscious despite return of spontaneous circulation have a high incidence of death or severe neurological deficit if they survive. Several studies have shown that if these patients are cooled for 12–24 h to a core temperature of 32–34° C their prognosis and neurological recovery is significantly improved.[16]

Basic Life Support–Infant and Child

Most cardiac arrests in children result from hypoxia, hypotension or both. The initial cardiac rhythm is usually asystole or severe bradycardia. However VF may also be encountered especially associated with congenital heart disease, poisoning and during the course of resuscitation. If a cardiac cause appears obvious e.g. sudden collapse of a child in a running race, then obtaining a defibrillator is a top priority.

Basic Life Support—Older Child (9–14 Years)

The same approach to BLS in the adult applies also to the older child but with the following qualifications:

1 Compress the chest approximately one third of the antero-posterior (AP) diameter of the chest.
2 The rate of compression is 100 compressions per minute.
3 The ratio of ECC to ventilation is 30:2 with one rescuer. If 2 rescuers are present use a ratio of 15:2.

Basic Life Support—Younger Child (1–8 Years)

As above.

Basic Life Support—Infant (1 Month–1 Year Old)

The same approach to BLS in the adult applies also to the infant but with the following qualifications:

1 Head tilt should not be used to optimise the airway.
2 The brachial pulse is easier to feel and locate than the carotid pulse, in the infant.
3 Compress the chest by placing two fingers one finger's breadth beneath a line joining the nipples.
4 Compress the chest approximately one third of the AP diameter of the chest.
5 The compression rate is 100 compressions per minute.
6 The ratio of ECC to ventilation is 30:2 with one rescuer. If 2 rescuers are present use a ratio of 15:2.

Basic Life Support—Neonate

See *Neonatal Resuscitation.*

Advanced Life Support—Infant and Child

Asystole or Severe Bradycardia

1   Adrenaline 10 µg/kg (0.1 mL/kg of 1:10 000 solution) IV or interosseous (IO). *See Interosseous Puncture*. If unable to obtain IV or IO access give 100 µg/kg via the endotracheal (ET) tube. Repeat this dose of adrenaline every 3 min of resuscitation.

2   If still unsuccessful give sodium bicarbonate 1 mmol/kg IV. *Do not give sodium bicarbonate via the ET tube or IO route.*

3   Atropine 20 µg/kg IV, IO or 30 µg/kg via the ET tube.

4   Attempt pacing (oesophageal, transcutaneous or transvenous).

5   If hypovolaemia is suspected give crystalloid 20 mL/kg and repeat this dose until hypovolaemia is reversed.

6   Identify and treat underlying cause if possible.

Ventricular Fibrillation/Pulseless Ventricular Tachycardia

All shock energies are for monophasic or biphasic defibrillators

1   For a witnessed arrest DC shock give 3 stacked shocks: 2 J/kg then 4 J/kg then 4 J/kg.

2   For an unwitnessed arrest give a single shock of 2 J/kg.

3   Provide 2 minutes of CPR.

4   If no response give adrenaline 10 µg/kg IV or IO or 100 µg/kg via the ET tube. Repeat this dose every 3 min of arrest time. Circulate with 1–2 min of ECC.

5   Repeat DC shock. Use 4 J/kg for this and all subsequent shocks. Give 2 min CPR.

6   If still unsuccessful give amiodarone 5 mg/kg IV or IO. Alternatively lignocaine 1 mg/kg can be used but is inferior.

7   Circulate with 1–2 min of ECC.

8   Repeat DC shock. Give 2 min CPR.

9   Repeat amiodarone dose 5mg/kg.

10 Repeat DC shock. Give 2 min CPR.

11 Consider sodium bicarbonate 1 mmol/kg IV.

12 Identify and treat underlying cause if possible.

Pulseless Electrical Activity (Electromechanical Dissociation)

1   As in the adult identify/treat the cause.

2   Adrenaline 10 µg/kg IV or IO or give 100 µg/kg via ET tube. Repeat dose every 3 min of arrest time.

3   IV fluid bolus 20 mL/kg (colloid or crystalloid).

4   Consider sodium bicarbonate 1 mmol/kg.

Supraventricular Tachycardia

1   If severe hypotension or no palpable pulse administer a DC shock 0.5–1 J/kg (monophasic or biphasic).

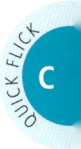

QUICK FLICK C

2 If the patient's circulation is adequate treat with pharmacotherapy. Adenosine is the drug of choice (*see Adenosine*). *Do not use Verapamil or other Ca²⁺ channel blocker to treat SVT in the infant.* Other options to consider are:

a) Carotid sinus massage (never perform bilaterally at the same time).
b) Valsalva during mechanical ventilation.
c) Ice pack applied to face.
d) Overdrive pacing.

Defibrillation in Children
Small paddles are used with a cross sectional area of 12–20 cm².

Cardiac Arrest in Pregnancy

Cardiac arrest in pregnancy is rare with an incidence of about 1 in 30 000 pregnancies and mortality is high.[17] The usual causes are pulmonary embolus, amniotic fluid embolus, haemorrhage, pre-eclampsia and eclampsia and sepsis. These patients are very difficult to resuscitate due to the high percentage of cardiac output that is diverted to the uterus (10–30%), and aortocaval compression by the gravid uterus. Treatment is the same as adult cardiac arrest described above with the following caveats:

1 Summon personnel capable of performing a Caesarean section.
2 Left lateral tilt to prevent/reduce aortocaval compression. This makes ECC more difficult. The AutoPulse automated chest compressor may be advantageous in this situation. *See AutoPulse*.
3 ECC should be applied slightly higher up the sternum.
4 Intubation should be done immediately due to the increased aspiration risk, higher oxygen demands and reduced lung reserve associated with pregnancy.
5 If after 4 minutes resuscitation is unsuccessful, CS should be performed in the best interests of mother and fetus. No sterile precautions or special equipment other than a scalpel is required. Many case reports indicate rapid return of spontaneous circulation in arrested pregnant patients after surgical delivery of the fetus.[18]

Administration of Drugs by the Endotracheal Route

The endotracheal route can be used for the administration of adrenaline, lignocaine and atropine. These should be given at 2–2.5 × the recommended IV dose and diluted in 10 mL of N/S. A catheter should be passed beyond the tip of the ET tube and chest compression is stopped as the drug solution is sprayed quickly through the catheter. Give 2–3 quick insufflations to aerosolise the medication and hasten absorption.

◐ Cardiac Arrest in the Newborn

See Neonatal Resuscitation.

Cardiac Conduction Abnormalities

See *Heart Block (HB).*

Cardiac Failure

See *Congestive Cardiac Failure (CCF).*

Cardiac Investigations

Can be divided into non-invasive and invasive tests.

Non-invasive Tests

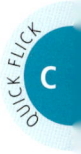

1. *Exercise Tolerance* This gives a good indication of peri-operative risk. A patient with normal exercise tolerance is at much less risk of peri-operative ischaemia than a patient with angina/dyspnoea on mild exertion.
2. *Electrocardiogragh (ECG)* The resting ECG is normal in 25–50% of patients with coronary artery disease.[19] Patients with a previous Q-wave myocardial infarct (MI) may be at less anaesthetic risk than patients with a previous non-Q-wave MI.[20]
3. *Chest X-ray.*
4. *Exercise Stress Test.* A positive stress test is indicative of an increased anaesthetic risk but a negative stress test may not exclude an increased risk.[20]
5. *Transthoracic Echocardiography* This is able to show wall motion, chamber size and valvular function. This test also gives a semi-quantitative estimate of left ventricular ejection fraction (LVEF). This measurement gives an indication of the effectiveness of myocardial contraction. Normal left ventricular ejection fraction is 50–75%. A left ventricular ejection fraction of < 40% indicates significant left ventricular impairment.
6. *Ambulatory ST Segment Analysis.*
7. *Dobutamine Stress and Exercise Stress Echocardiography* These tests are thought to be highly predictive of significant ischaemic heart disease if positive. Regional wall abnormalities especially at low heart rates are thought to be highly suggestive.[21]
8. *Dipyridamole and Exercise Thallium Isotope Scan (Nuclear Stress Test).* Thallium 201 is a potassium analogue which penetrates into the myocardium. Exercise (or dipyridamole if patient unable to exercise) causes coronary vasodilatation. Dobutamine can also be used to increase myocardial O_2 demand. Ischaemic myocardium takes up little thallium and appears as a cold spot on gamma imaging. A second scan is performed after 3–4 h and may show delayed uptake indicating ischaemic myocardium (thallium redistribution). Failure to take up thallium suggests an area of infarction.
9. *Sesta—MIBI Scan* Similar principle to above.

Invasive Tests

1 *Transoesophageal Echocardiography* is more sensitive than transthoracic echocardiography for the detection of prosthetic valve dysfunction, atrial thrombus, atrial septal defect, aortic dissection and infective endocarditis.

2 *Coronary Angiography* is the 'gold standard' for elucidating coronary vascular disease. Coronary angiography enables study of ventricular contraction and pressure measurements in chambers and across valves. It also provides the opportunity for intervention with angioplasty or stent placement in coronary vessels. This test has a mortality of < 0.1% and a coronary dissection or embolism rate of 0.2%.[22] In patients with peripheral vascular disease mortality is up to 2.5%.[23] The indications for coronary angiography are:

   a) evidence of high risk for significant coronary artery disease (CAD) based on non-invasive tests

   b) angina unresponsive to adequate medical therapy

   c) unstable angina

   d) equivocal non-invasive test results in patients at high risk of CAD undergoing high-risk surgery

⊃ Cardiac Ischaemia

See Myocardial Ischaemia, Peri-operative.

⊃ Cardiac Risk Factors

See Cardiovascular Peri-operative Risk Prediction for Non-cardiac Surgery.

⊃ Cardiac Tamponade

General Measures

1 Ensure the airway is patent and that ventilation is optimal.

2 Give IV fluid loading to optimise ventricular diastolic filling and improve cardiac output.

3 Inotropic support may be required.

4 Maintain systemic vascular resistance to support coronary perfusion.

5 Maintain a heart rate of 90–140 bpm.

6 Perform emergency pericardiocentesis if pericardial fluid results in a life-threatening reduction in cardiac output. Opening of the chest by a trained cardiothoracic surgeon may be required for patients who have had recent heart surgery.

Technique for Pericardiocentesis

1 Position patient sitting at 45° in bed.

2 Connect the limb leads of the ECG monitor to patient's limbs and a chest lead to a 16 FG aspiration needle (or other suitable needle such as an 18 g spinal needle).

3 Insert the needle between the xiphisternum and the seventh costal cartilage on the left side, at an angle of $\approx 35°$ to the midline and $\approx 45°$ to the skin.[24] Aim for the left shoulder. Aspirate constantly with a syringe while inserting the needle.

4 Elevation of the ST segments or ectopic beats suggests the needle is entering the myocardium and that it needs to be pulled back.

5 Drain fluid using a 3-way tap. If possible consider leaving a plastic cannula in place for continuous or repeated pericardial sac drainage. This can be done by a Seldinger technique utilising a guide wire passed through the drainage needle.

◑ Cardiac Transplant and Subsequent Non-cardiac Surgery

See *Heart Transplant Patients, Anaesthetic Consideration for Non-cardiac Surgery*.

◑ Cardiogenic Shock

See *Congestive Cardiac Failure (CCF)*.

◑ Cardiomyopathy of Pregnancy

See *Peripartum Cardiomyopathy*.

◑ Cardiovascular Peri-operative Risk Prediction for Non-cardiac Surgery

This topic is undergoing intense review and discussion with recommendations undergoing constant refinement.

The following information is based on recommendations from the American College of Cardiology and the American Heart Association (ACC–AHA guidelines).[25]

There are 4 issues to consider:

1 What are the patient's cardiac risk factors?
2 What is the patient's functional capacity?
3 What is the risk of the surgery?
4 How to proceed?

Patient's Risk of Cardiac Morbidity/Mortality

Patients at highest risk are those with Active Cardiac Conditions for which the patient should be pre-operatively referred to a cardiologist, investigated and treated. These are:

1 Unstable coronary syndromes—unstable or severe angina, recent MI (> 7 days < 4 weeks).
2 Decompensated heart failure—NYHA IV or new onset CCF or worsening CCF.

3 Significant arrhythmia—high-grade AV block (Morbitz II, CHB), symptomatic ventricular arrhythmia, SVT with uncontrolled ventricular rate (> 100 bpm), symptomatic bradycardia, newly recognised VT.

4 Severe valvular disease—severe aortic stenosis, symptomatic mitral stenosis.

The next category of risk indicators to consider are termed *Clinical Risk Factors* which are:

1 history of IHD

2 history of compensated or prior CCF

3 history of CVA

4 diabetes mellitus

5 renal impairment.

The third category of risk factors are termed *Minor Predictors*. These include:

1 age > 70 years

2 abnormal ECG

3 rhythm other than sinus

4 uncontrolled hypertension.

Independently these minor predictors do not predict adverse cardiac outcomes but are markers of cardiac disease.

Evaluating the Patient's Functional Capacity

In patients with excellent functional capacity without symptoms, management will rarely be changed based on further testing. A patient's exercise function can be divided into:

1 Poor—unable to climb 2 flights of stairs

2 Moderate—unlimited walking, run short distances

3 Excellent—able to exercise strenuously

The MET concept is also useful, MET standing for metabolic equivalent. This is another measure of exercise function. 1 MET = the O_2 consumption of a resting male 70 kg 40-yr-old (3.5 mL/kg/min).

Table C1 MET exercise equivalents[26]

1–4 MET	Walk around house; walk on flat surface 200 m; slow dancing.
5–9 MET	Walk 6 km; run short distances; ride a bike
> 10 MET	Strenuous exercise

Type of Surgery and Cardiac Risk

High Risk (> 5% peri-operative risk of a cardiac event such as MI)

1 major emergency surgery especially in the elderly.

2 aortic and other major vascular surgery.

3 peripheral vascular surgery.

4 surgery associated with large fluid shifts or blood loss.

Intermediate Risk (1–5% peri-operative risk of a cardiac event)
1 intraperitoneal and intrathoracic surgery
2 carotid surgery
3 head and neck procedures
4 prostate surgery
5 orthopaedic surgery
6 endovascular AAA repair.

Low Risk
1 breast surgery and superficial procedures
2 endoscopic procedures
3 cataract surgery
4 ambulatory surgery.

Using the Above Predictors to Plan Management
If emergency surgery is indicated proceed to surgery. If non-emergency surgery proceed as follows:

Active Cardiac Condition Present
Refer to a cardiologist, investigate and treat *prior to surgery*.

Active Cardiac Condition Not Present
1 Low-risk surgery—proceed with surgery.
2 Intermediate and high-risk surgery with good functional capacity (> 4 METs)—proceed with surgery.

Active Cardiac Condition Not Present But Poor Functional Capacity
1 > 3 clinical risk factors and vascular surgery consider cardiologist referral/investigation prior to surgery.
2 > 3 clinical risk factors and intermediate surgery—consider non invasive testing and β blocker before proceeding.
3 1–2 clinical risk factors and vascular surgery or intermediate surgery—consider non invasive testing and β blocker before proceeding.
4 No clinical risk factors—proceed with surgery.

Points to Note
1 In general patients who have had coronary revascularisation within 5 years or cardiac evaluation within 2 years, with stable symptomatology, do not require cardiology review prior to noncardiac surgery.[27]
2 It is unclear from the literature whether coronary revascularisation procedures performed pre-operatively are superior to optimal medical therapy in preventing myocardial ischaemia and infarction, except for very high-risk patients.
3 Coronary revascularisation is recommended if there is significant left main coronary artery stenosis, 3 vessel disease, high-risk unstable angina

or acute MI. ***See*** *Coronary Artery Revascularisation Procedures and Subsequent Non-cardiac Surgery*.

4   When optimising the patient's medical therapy consider:
   a) β blocker therapy. Findings from the POISE study suggest β blocker therapy may actually increase mortality. ***See*** *Beta-blocker Therapy and Reduction of Cardiac Risk*.
   b) Alpha 2 agonists.[28]
   c) Peri-operative statin therapy.[29]

▷ Cardioversion

Adult-sized cardioversion paddles have an area of 50–80 cm^2 (14 cm diameter) whereas the paediatric type have an area of 12– 20 cm^2 (5–8 cm diameter). Increasingly paddles are being superseded by gel electrode pads.

Paddle Positions
a) Right paddle or pad placed to the right of the sternum below the clavicle over the second intercostal space.
b) Left paddle or pad placed laterally to the left nipple and centred over the mid-axillary line and the sixth intercostal space.

Alternative Paddle Position
1   Anterior paddle or pad placed over the precordium.
2   Posterior paddle or pad placed behind the heart.

Table C2 DC monophasic cardioversion electrical energy for the various dysrhythmias

Dysrhythmia	Suggested initial electrical energy for cardioversion
Atrial fibrillation	Adult—100, 200 J
Atrial flutter	Adult—50, 100 J
Supraventricular	Adult—30, 50 J
Tachycardia (with pulse)	Child—0.5–1 J/kg
Supraventricular	Adult—100, 200, 360 J
Tachycardia (pulseless)	Child—0.5–1, 2, 4 J/kg
Ventricular tachycardia (with pulse)	
Monomorphic	Adult—100 J
Polymorphic	Adult—200 J
Ventricular fibrillation	Adult—360 J
Ventricular tachycardia (pulseless)	Child—2–4 J/kg

Table C3 DC biphasic cardioversion electrical energy for the various dysrhythmias

Dysrhythmia	Suggested initial electrical energy for cardioversion
Atrial fibrillation	Adult–100 J
Atrial flutter	Adult–50 J
Supraventricular tachycardia	Adult–25-50 J
Ventricular tachycardia (with pulse)	Adult–100 J
Ventricular	Adult–200 J
Tachycardia (pulseless)	Child–1-2 J/kg
Ventricular fibrillation	Adult–200 J Child–1-2 J/kg

Points to Note

1. Cardiovert during expiration to minimise impedance.
2. Synchronise shock with the R wave when cardioverting a supraventricular dysrhythmia (SVT, AF or atrial flutter) or ventricular tachycardia with a palpable pulse. Do *not* synchronise the shock if pulseless VT or VF is present.
3. Do not defibrillate over ECG electrodes or nitrate patches, or over implanted devices such as pacemakers.
4. Ensure the patient is not in contact with metal.
5. Use conductive gel pads and ensure these are not touching each other.
6. Digoxin toxicity reduces the threshold for inducing ventricular arrythmias with cardioversion shocks.
7. Cardioversion in pregnancy appears to be relatively safe for the fetus.
8. Biphasic defibrillation/cardioversion in children requires about 50% of the monophasic energy dose.

Carotid Endarterectomy (CEA)

The most feared complications of CEA are myocardial infarction and stroke. The 30-day mortality of CEA is about 1% and the incidence of myocardial infarction is about 2%.[30] About 3.4% of patients suffer a stroke within 30 days of CEA.[30]

A major area of controversy is whether it is better to perform CEA under regional or general anaesthesia. Advantages of regional anaesthesia are:

1. An awake patient is the best cerebral monitor.
2. Unnecessary shunting is avoided.
3. Hospital stay may be shortened.[31]
4. Hospital costs may be reduced.[31]

Advantages of GA are:

1. Patient cooperation is not required.

2 Conversion from regional to GA will not be required if complications occur. The conversion rate is about 1–3%.[32]

Overall morbidity and mortality appear to be unaffected by the choice of anaesthetic.[33] Ultimately the choice between regional and GA depends on the preference of the surgeon, patient and anaesthetist.

Pre-operative Evaluation and Assessment

1 CEA patients have a high incidence of ischaemic heart disease. **See** *Cardiac Investigations* and *Cardiovascular Peri-operative Risk Prediction for Non-cardiac Surgery*.

2 CEA surgery is considered to be an intermediate risk operation for myocardial infarction. However there is little evidence that CABG surgery performed either before or in combination with CEA lowers the overall risk of stroke and MI.[34]

3 Patients requiring both CEA and CABG are usually operated on sequentially with the most urgent surgery performed first.[35]

4 Hypertension is common and should be controlled between reasonable limits. Aim for a preoperative blood pressure less than 180 mm Hg systolic.

5 Document pre-existing neurological deficits.

6 Assess patient's respiratory function carefully, especially if cervical plexus block is planned as this will affect phrenic nerve function.

7 Consider commencing the patient on β blocker therapy pre-operatively if there are no contraindications to reduce the incidence of tachycardia and myocardial ischaemia and improve long-term prognosis. The recently published POISE study has questioned this approach. **See** *Beta-blocker Therapy and Reduction of Cardiac Risk*.

Anaesthesia Aims

1 Aim for cardiovascular stability erring on the side of slight hypertension throughout the peri-operative period.

2 Prevent/identify/treat cerebral and/or myocardial ischaemia.

3 Aim for prompt awakening at the end of surgery if GA is used.

4 Hyperglycaemia must be avoided as it can increase the incidence of cerebral cellular damage.[36] Similarly glucose containing solutions should be avoided.

5 Consider pre-operative evaluation of vocal cord function if the patient has had previous contralateral carotid surgery, to detect recurrent laryngeal nerve injury. Bilateral nerve injury may cause acute airway compromise.[36]

General Anaesthesia Technique
Pre-induction Phase

1 In addition to routine monitoring use a 5-lead ECG system displaying leads II and V. **See** *St Segment Analysis*. Invasive arterial blood pressure measurement is also required.

2 Monitoring of cerebral function and perfusion must be undertaken. No technique is ideal in patients receiving general anaesthesia. Options include:

a) *Internal Carotid Artery Stump Pressure.* The artery is temporarily occluded and the back pressure in the artery upstream from the clamp is measured. A mean arterial stump pressure of > 50–60 mm Hg is generally accepted (by surgeons who measure stump pressure) as indicative of adequate perfusion.[36] Stump pressures do not correlate consistently with other measures of cerebral perfusion such as assessment of the awake patient.[37]

b) *EEG monitoring.* Variations of EEG techniques include Compressed Spectral Array and Density Spectral Array. EEG techniques reflect cortical activity only and do not indicate ischaemia in deeper structures. The BIS monitor is not useful for cerebral ischaemia monitoring.[30]

c) *Somatosensory Evoked Potentials.*

d) Regional Cerebral Blood Flow Studies. Utilise a radioactive tracer such as Xenon 133 or Krypton 85 and an external array of scintillation monitors.

e) *Transcranial Doppler Ultrasonography.* Measures middle cerebral artery blood flow. One advantage of this technique is that it can detect emboli.

f) *Near Infrared Spectroscopy.* This technique provides a measure of regional cerebral oxygenation.

g) *Jugular Venous Oximetry.*

Induction and Maintenance Phase

1 Appropriate induction drugs include:

a) midazolam 3 mg.

b) fentanyl 100–250 µg.

c) thiopentone or propofol.

d) rocuronium 0.6 mg/kg.

e) consider lignocaine 1.5 mg/kg IV 1 minute prior to intubation to blunt the haemodynamic response to intubation.

2 Maintain anaesthesia with oxygen air and isoflurane or sevoflurane. N_2O should not be used due to its cerebral vascular effects.[30] Maintain normocarbia.

3 Consider a cervical plexus block prior to incision to reduce intraoperative nociceptive stimulation and Postoperative pain. **See** *Cervical Plexus (CP) Block*.

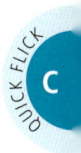

4 Stretching of the carotid baro-receptor can result in severe bradycardia and hypotension. This can be avoided by the surgeon infiltrating around the carotid bifurcation with 1% lignocaine. However this technique has been associated with postoperative hypertension and is not recommended routinely.[38]

5 Maintain MAP about 20% above the patient's usual blood pressure but < 160 mm Hg systolic. Use light anaesthesia rather than vasoconstrictors to achieve this as the use of sympathomimetics such as metaraminol is associated with an increased risk of myocardial ischaemia and infarction.[37]

6 Prior to clamping of the common carotid artery give heparin (100 u/kg or about 5000 IU). The surgeon may choose to insert a shunt between the common carotid artery and the internal carotid artery upstream from the clamp.

7 Adjust ventilation to ensure normocarbia.[36] Both hypocarbia (causing cerebral vasoconstriction) and hypercarbia (causing cerebral vasodilation and potentially 'steal' phenomenon) are undersirable.[36]

8 Consider the use of mild hypothermia ($\approx 35°C$) up until the point of completion of the carotid endarterectomy which may reduce ischaemic brain injury.[36] Begin active rewarming after the clamp is removed.

9 If severe hypertension occurs with carotid clamping notify the surgeon immediately. This may indicate cerebral ischaemia and the need for clamp release and shunt insertion.

10 The surgeon may request a dose of protamine to reverse the effects of heparin at completion of surgery.

Emergence and Immediate Postoperative Phase

1 Aim for smooth emergence with minimal CVS disturbance. Consider using a drug to reduce the hypotensive response to extubation such as IV lignocaine 1.5 mg/kg 1–2 min before extubation or esmolol 2–3 mg/kg IV.

2 Aggressively treat Postoperative hyper/hypotensioin, tachycardia or bradycardia. Aim for values within the patient's usual pre-operative range for pulse rate and blood pressure.

Regional Anaesthesia Technique

Perform a deep and superficial cervical plexus block. Surgery can be done with the superficial cervical plexus block only.[30] ***See*** *Cervical Plexus (CP) Block*.

1 Monitoring used is identical to that used for GA except that patient assessment is used for neurological evaluation.

2 Give O_2 by facemask throughout the procedure.

3 Sedation can be provided with midazolam. Fentanyl can be added if midazolam is inadequate.[39] However the sedation must not impair patient cooperation.

4   An inadequate cervical plexus block can be supplemented by LA infiltration by the surgeon.
5   Phrenic nerve block occurs commonly with cervical plexus block. It is well tolerated in patients with normal respiratory function but may cause severe respiratory compromise in patients with underlying respiratory disease.[40]

Postoperative Complications

1   Airway compromise can occur due to oedema, haemorrhage and recurrent laryngeal nerve palsy (if previous contralateral recurrent laryngeal nerve injury). *See Neck Haematoma* for management of airway compromise due to haemorrhage.
2   Neurological deterioration is a surgical emergency and the surgeon must be notified immediately. In addition to thromboembolic phenomena, the hyperperfusion syndrome can also cause neurological dysfunction. This syndrome is usally associated with surgery on severely stenotic lesions and may cause ipsilateral headache, seizures and/or intracranial haemorrhage.[40] Treatment includes aggressive correction of hypertension to a blood pressure < 140 mm Hg. Agents that can be used include clonidine, esmolol, hydralazine and/or glyceryl trinitrate depending on its severity.
3   Bilateral carotid body dysfunction can result if surgery on both sides of the neck has occurred, leading to a decreased ventilatory response to hypoxia.[36]

◗ Carotid Sinus Massage

See Supraventricular Tachycardias (SVT).

◗ Caudal Anaesthesia

Useful for analgesia during and after surgery to areas supplied by the sacral segments. Appropriate operations include haemorrhoidectomy and circumcision.

Anatomy

The dural sac terminates at S2 and the extradural space terminates at the sacral hiatus.

This triangular shaped hiatus is formed by the unfused lamina of S5 and lies at the posterior aspect of the lower end of sacrum. The sacral cornua are part of the S5 lamina remnants. It is roofed by the sacrococcygeal ligament which is equivalent to the ligamentum flavum. This site thus provides an access point to the epidural space.

Technique

1   Establish IV access.

2   Position the patient laterally with the legs drawn up towards the chest. Palpate the posterior superior iliac spines (PSISs). An imaginary line drawn between the PSISs forms the base of an inverted equilateral triangle. At the caudal apex of this triangle is the sacral hiatus at the lower end of the sacrum. As stated above the triangular shaped sacral hiatus is formed by the deficient laminae of S5 which bears the sacral cornua and the spinous process of S4 or S3 above.

3   Using aseptic technique and a suitable needle such as a 22 G short bevelled needle, penetrate the skin and subcutaneous tissue at an angle of about 45° to the skin.

4   Next, penetrate the posterior sacrococcygeal ligament and then flatten the needle to insert the tip 2–3 mm into the sacral canal. Use a syringe and extension tubing to aspirate on the needle to check for CSF or blood. If no fluid is aspirated inject 0.5 mL of air. There should be no resistance to injection. By placing a stethoscope over the sacrum, injected air can be heard entering the epidural space in the sacral canal (called the 'whoosh' test).[41]

Dose of LA

Adult For surgery such as circumcision, inject bupivacaine 0.5% with adrenaline 1:200 000 10 mL + 5 mL N/S.

Child For surgery such as circumcision, inject bupivacaine 0.25% with adrenaline 0.5 mL/kg up to 20 mL. To cover upper lumbar and lower thoracic segments e.g. for hip surgery, inject 0.75 mL/kg of bupivacaine 0.25% with adrenaline. Do not exceed 3 mg/kg of bupivacaine in the child. Ropivacaine can also be used. For a block below T12 use 0.2% 2 mg/kg up to 25 kg.

Complications

1   Dural puncture with total spinal anaesthesia.
2   Intravascular or interosseous injection of LA and adrenaline with dysrhythmias and cardiac arrest has been reported.[42] The risk of this complication may be reduced by the 'whoosh' test described above plus careful aspiration.
3   Injection into the fetal scalp has been described with fatal results.[43]
4   Periosteal injection or haematoma with postoperative pain that may last weeks.
5   Urinary retention.
6   Infection.
7   Neurological injury.

◑ Cell Saver

These devices consist of suction tubing, filter, reservoir and a washing bowl that is centrifuge driven. Heparinised saline (30 000 units of Heparin per litre of N/S) is added to blood sucked from the surgical site to prevent clotting. The heparinised blood is washed in saline and the final product consists of RBCs suspended in saline (without heparin) which is retransfused back into the patient. The haematocrit of the recollected blood is 50–60%. About 75% of shed blood can be collected and retransfused, provided that blood loss does not exceed the rate at which it can be sucked up. Suction pressure should be < 150 mm Hg.

Problems with this Technique
Most of the platelets and clotting factors are lost in this process.

Contraindications to Cell Saver Use
1 *Infected material* at operative site e.g. bowel contents.
2 *Malignancy.* Tumour cells may not be removed by standard washing techniques, but limited studies do not suggest a reduced patient survival rate.[44] This may therefore be a relative contraindication. A leucocyte filter, and gamma irradiation, can be used to remove malignant cells.[45] Irradiation of the salvaged blood takes 1–2 h.
3 *Amniotic fluid.* This should be sucked away before blood is sucked into the cell saver. Laboratory investigations have suggested that while there is effective clearance of solute proteins there is incomplete clearance of fetal squames even with leucodepleting filtration.[46]

◗ Celecoxib

Cyclo-oxygenase (COX)-2 inhibitor non-steroidal anti-inflammatory analgesic drug without COX-1 effects at clinical doses. Useful for the treatment of osteo- and rheumatoid arthritis.

Dose
Adult 100 mg–200 mg 12 h.

Points to Note
Celecoxib is contraindicated in patients who have a history of sulfonamide allergy. ***See*** *Non-steroidal Anti-inflammatory Drugs (NSAIDs)*.

◗ Cement Implantation Syndrome

See *Fat Embolism Syndrome and Bone Cement Implantation Syndrome*.

◗ Central Anticholinergic Syndrome

Confusional state due to effects of anticholinergic drugs, such as atropine and scopolamine, on the brain.

Treatment
Adult Give physostigmine 1 mg IV

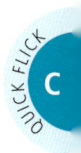

Prevention

Avoid anticholinergics that cross the blood–brain barrier (scopolamine, atropine) especially in patients over 60 yrs. Use glycopyrronium as an alternative drug. **See** *Glycopyrronium (Glycopyrrolate).*

○ Cerebral Aneurysm Surgery

Topics Covered in this Section

▶ Clinical Effects of Subarachnoid Haemorrhage (SAH)

▶ Grading the Severity of SAH

▶ Pre-anaesthetic Considerations for Cerebral Aneurysm Repair or Coiling

▶ Anaesthetic Management up to the Time of Aneurysmal Clipping

▶ Aneurysmal Clipping and Subsequent Anaesthetic Management

▶ Intra-operative Aneurysm Rupture

▶ Cerebral Vasospasm Treatment

▶ Cerebral Aneurysm Coiling

Clinical Effects of Subarachnoid Haemorrhage (SAH)

About of 75% of cases of subarachnoid haemorrhage are due to cerebral aneurysm rupture.[47] The other causes are arteriovenous malformations, extension of an intracerebral haemorrhage and haemorrhage into an infarct or tumour.

Clinical symptoms and signs include:

1 sudden severe headache
2 loss of consciousness, which may be transient or prolonged
3 neck stiffness
4 hypertension
5 seizures
6 focal neurological signs
7 cardiac dysrhythmias
8 vasogenic pulmonary oedema.

SAH has a poor prognosis with a 30-day mortality of about 45%.[48] The main predictors of mortality or poor neurological outcome are:[49]

1 impaired level of consciousness on admission
2 advanced age
3 a large amount of intracranial blood on the initial CT scan.

The main complications after the initial SAH are:

1 rebleeding—20% of aneurysms rebleed within the first 14 days
2 cerebral vasospasm can occur possibly due to the irritant effects of intracranial blood, leading to cerebral ischaemia
3 raised ICP
4 cardiopulmonary dysfunction, hypertension or hypotension
5 electrolyte abnormalities especially hyponatraemia
6 hyperglycaemia.

Grading the Severity of SAH

Table C4 Severity scale for subarachnoid haemorrhage – World Federation of Neurosurgeons grade[50]

World Federation of Neurosurgeons grade	Glasgow coma score	Motor deficit
0 (unruptured aneurysm)	15	Nil
I	15	Nil
II	13–14	Nil
III	13–14	Present
IV	7–12	Present or Absent
V	3–6	Present or Absent

Table C5 Classification of SAH: Hunt and Hess modified clinical grades[51]

Clinical presentation	Grade
Unruptured aneurysm	0
Asymptomatic or minimal headache	1
Moderate/severe headache, nuchal rigidity +/− cranial nerve palsy	2
Drowsy, confused +/− mild focal deficit	3
Stupor, mild or severe hemiparesis, early decerebrate rigidity	4
Deep coma, moribund	5

Pre-anaesthetic Considerations for Cerebral Aneurysm Repair or Coiling

The diagnosis of cerebral aneurysm causing SAH is usually made by CT scan followed by 4 vessel cerebral angiography.

Surgery or coiling is usually undertaken within 72 h. Preparation includes:

1 *Nimodipine* is given to prevent vasospasm. The dose is 60 mg PO 4 h for 3 weeks. Oral therapy is no less effective than IV therapy which is more likely to cause hypotension. IV nimodipine must be given via a central line due to its irritant effects. The infusion system must be protected from light. The IV dose is 1 mg/h for 2 h, increase to 2 mg/h if the patient's SBP > 130 mm Hg. Continue IV nimodipine for at least 5 days after surgery. For treatment of established cerebral vasospasm see below.

2 Ensure patients are well hydrated and electrolytes are normalised.

3 Correct hyper or hypoglycaemia.

4 Assess cardiopulmonary function for possible myocardial ischaemia and neurogenic pulmonary oedema. Cardiology consultation and cardiac echo may be required but surgery should not be delayed.

Anaesthetic Management Up to the Time of Aneurysmal Clipping

The anaesthetic aims are to maintain a stable haemodynamic profile, an optimal physiological environment for the brain and favourable operating conditions for the surgeon.

1 Establish invasive blood pressure monitoring via arterial cannulation. Measure the arterial pressure at the level of the brain. Establish central venous access, although this can be done after induction. Use 5-lead ECG monitoring. Ensure that the patient's bladder is catheterised after induction. Have a sodium nitroprusside infusion readily available. *See Sodium Nitroprusside (SNP)*.

2 Continue or commence a nimodipine infusion.

3 It is essential to attenuate the hypertensive response to laryngoscopy and intubation. *See Hypertensive Response to Intubation (Attenuation of)*. Anaesthesia can be induced with:

   a) Fentanyl 2–5 µg/kg IV + thiopentone 3–5 mg/kg or propofol 2–2.5 mg/kg.

   b) Rocuronium 0.6 mg/kg: ensure the patient is fully relaxed prior to intubation.

   c) Prior to intubation consider lignocaine 1.5 mg/kg or esmolol 0.5 mg/kg or remifentanil infusion 1–1.5 µg/kg/min run for 60–90 s prior to induction.

   d) Spray the cords with 3 mL of 4% topical lignocaine.

4 Use of a rapid sequence induction is controversial because of the risk of aneurysmal rupture (if the sympathetic responses to laryngoscopy and intubation are inadequately controlled) may exceed the risk of aspiration.[52] Give repeated boluses of thiopentone if hypertension occurs with laryngoscopy, intubation or at other times during surgery.

5 Maintain anaesthesia with O_2/air and isoflurane or sevoflurane. Alternatively a propofol infusion can be used instead of a volatile agent. Desflurane should not be used.[52] *See Desflurane*. A remifentanil infusion is also useful.

6 Application of the head-pin holder can be associated with marked hypertension. This can be attenuated by LA injection at the pin sites prior to their insertion.

7 Position the patient with 10° of reverse Trendelenburg to help control ICP. The neurosurgeon may request mannitol, dexamethasone and/ or phenytoin. *See Neuroanaesthesia*. If mannitol is given, begin the infusion after the dura is opened. This is to avoid reduction of ICP causing increased transmural pressure, resulting in aneurysmal rupture.

8 Discuss arterial blood pressure requirements with the neurosurgeon. In general aim to maintain blood pressure at pre-operative levels.[49]

9 In some institutions and situations intracranial pressure (ICP) may be reduced through the use of a lumbar drain or a ventricular drain. Cerebrospinal fluid must not be drained before removal of the cranial flap.[47] The amount of acutely drained CSF should be < 30 mL.[49] In patients with an intracerebral haematoma lumbar CSF drainage is contraindicated due to the risk of brainstem herniation.[49]

10 Modest intra-operative hypothermia (35°C) may be beneficial, with active rewarming of the patient undertaken during wound closure.[53] Hyperthermia must not occur. The International Hypothermia Aneurysm Trial did not find any benefit from intra-operative hypothermia to 33°C.[54]

11 Maintain adequate cerebral perfusion pressure and circulating volume as guided by central venous pressure, urine output and mean arterial pressure (MAP). Use N/S as replacement fluid.

Aneurysmal Clipping and Subsequent Anaesthetic Management

1 The neurosurgeon may temporarily occlude the aneurysm's parent blood vessel to lower pressure stress within the aneurysm. Consider increasing MAP by 10–15% to improve collateral blood flow.[53] Some neurosurgeons may request a bolus of thiopentone (2–3 mg/kg) at this point to suppress brain EEG activity.

2 After the cerebral aneurysm is clipped consider increasing MAP to the high normal range, moderate hypervolaemia, and haemodilution (i.e. Hb ≈ 10 g/dL to reduce viscosity). This is referred to as 'Triple H Therapy'. These measures are intended to decrease the incidence of cerebral artery vasospasm.[53]

3 Give prophylactic anti-nausea medication e.g. ondansetron.

4 During emergence, aim to avoid coughing, straining, hypercarbia, hypertension and hypotension. Give 1.5 mg/kg lignocaine ≈ 2 min prior to planned extubation. Attempt to extubate the patient 'deep' i.e. as soon as the patient is breathing effectively. Patients with a Hunt and Hess Grade IV and V SAH usually require postoperative ventilation.[55]

5 Patients who do not wake up within a reasonable period or who have a new neurological deficit should have urgent CT scanning + angiography. If cerebral vasospasm is suspected see below.

Intra-operative Aneurysm Rupture

The incidence of this anaesthetic and surgical emergency is about 11% of previously ruptured cerebral aneurysms.[56] Rupture is suggested by:

1 sudden sustained hypertension

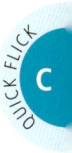

2 massive brain swelling

3 bradycardia or other arrhythmias

4 haemorrhagic shock.

Mortality approaches 75%.[55] The risk of aneurysm rupture on induction is 1–2% and has a higher mortality than rupture during surgical dissection.[55] Treatment includes:

1 Control blood pressure. For hypertension give boluses of thiopentone. If the patient is hypotensive management is controversial. A MAP of 50 mm Hg may offer benefits of decreased bleeding but may result in cerebral ischaemia.

2 Maintain normovolaemia.

3 Lower ICP with mannitol and frusemide.

4 Once the dura is open consider SNP infusion to maintain a MAP of 50 mm Hg to help decrease bleeding and improve surgical exposure.[56]

5 The surgeon may consider a cut down onto the cervical internal carotid artery and/or compression of the ipsilateral common carotid artery may be required.[53]

Cerebral Vasospasm Treatment

Cerebral vasospasm may occur pre or postoperatively. It can be diagnosed clinically, via angiography and by trans-cranial Doppler studies indicating increased flow rates.

In addition to nimodipine, treatment includes triple H therapy:[49]

1 Hypertension—to a MAP 120–150 mm Hg presurgery and 160–200 mm Hg post clipping.

2 Hypervolaemia—CVP 8–12 mm Hg.

3 Haemodilution—Hct 0.3–0.35.

4 Other measures include balloon angioplasty and intra-arterial papaverine.

Cerebral Aneurysm Coiling

Although these procedures can be done under sedation GA is usually preferred.[57] These patients tend to get less aggressive monitoring and the risk of bleeding is much less than with surgery.[57]

◑ Cerebral Blood Flow

50 mL/100 g/min—normal cerebral blood flow

25 mL/100 g/min—threshold for cerebral ischaemia and neuronal impairment

20 mL/100 g/min—EEG becomes isoelectric

15 mL/100 g/min—below this level evoked potentials become unrecordable

10 mL/100 g/min—neuronal death will occur if flow is maintained at this level or less.

○ Cerebral Oedema

See *Intracranial Pressure (ICP) and Treatment of Raised ICP*.

○ Cerebral Perfusion Pressure (CPP)

Cerebral perfusion pressure is the difference between mean arterial pressure and jugular venous pressure *or* intracranial pressure, whichever is the greater. CPP = MAP – (CVP *or* ICP). Aim for a CPP of at least 70 mm Hg.

○ Cerebro-spinal Fluid

Normal values:

pH	7.32
Glucose	2.8–4.4 mmol/L
Protein	0.45 g/L
PCO_2	50 mm Hg
Sodium	144–152 mmol/L
Potassium	2–3 mmol/L
Bicarbonate	24–32 mmol/L.

Normal CSF pressure is 10–13 cm H_2O or 10 mm Hg.

○ Cervical Plexus (CP) Block

Anatomy

The cervical plexus (CP) is made up of the anterior rami of C1–4 and supplies sensory and motor innervation to the neck and posterior scalp. The CP can be divided into superficial cutaneous branches and deep motor branches, the most important of which is the phrenic nerve (C3, C4, C5). The superficial cutaneous branches are:

1 lesser occipital nerve (C2)
2 greater auricular nerve (C2, C3)
3 anterior cutaneous nerve of the neck, or transverse cervical nerve (C2, C3)
4 supraclavicular nerves (C3, C4).

Superficial CP Block

May provide analgesia for surgery such as thyroidectomy, tracheostomy, cervical lymph node biopsy and carotid endarterectomy.

Technique for Superficial CP Block

1 Establish IV access. Identify the midpoint of the posterior border of the sternocleidomastoid muscle (SCM). This point corresponds to the junction of the external jugular vein and the posterior border of the SCM.
2 Insert a 4 cm 22 G needle just behind and deep to the SCM muscle.
3 Inject 10–15 mL of local anaesthetic solution e.g. ropivacaine 1%. The injection is made in a fan-like pattern along the posterior border of the SCM 4 cm caudally and 4 cm cranially from the entry point.

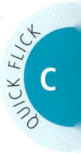

QUICK FLICK C

Technique for Deep CP Block

The indications for this block are the same as for the superficial cervical plexus block.

1 The patient lies supine with the face turned to the contralateral side. Palpate the mastoid process and the transverse process of C6 vertebrae (tubercle of Chassaignac) which lies at the level of the cricoid cartilage. Draw a line between these 2 landmarks.

2 Draw a second line 0.5–0.75 cm behind and parallel to this first line.

3 Identify the transverse process of C2 which will lie 1.5 cm (≈ 1 finger's breadth) caudal to the mastoid process on the second more posterior line. Mark this point. C3 and C4 transverse processes will be at 1.5 cm intervals from C2 along this same line. The C4 transverse process underlies the point where the external jugular vein crosses the posterior border of the SCM. Clearly mark all three injection points.

4 Using a 4 cm 22 G needle, penetrate the skin over each point, directing the needle in a slightly caudad direction to contact each transverse process. Confirm the position by 'walking' the needle off the tip of the transverse process caudally and/or cranially.

5 Ensure that neither blood nor CSF can be aspirated.

6 Cautiously inject 3–5 mL of LA solution adjacent to the transverse processes of C2, C3 & C4.

7 Anticipate phrenic nerve block on the side of the injections. The incidence of phrenic nerve block is 50–60%.[58]

Complications of Deep Cervical Plexus Block

1 Recurrent laryngeal nerve blockade causing hoarseness, paroxysmal coughing, impaired cough reflex

2 Dyspnoea due to phrenic nerve anaesthesia

3 Airway obstruction

4 Seizures and tachycardia from intravascular injection

5 Dysphagia

6 Stellate ganglion block

7 Horner's syndrome

8 Brainstem anaesthesia (due to intrathecal injection or spread). *See* *Brainstem Anaesthesia*.

◖ Chest Drain

Site of Insertion

Insert in the 'triangle of safety' i.e. the area bounded by the anterior axillary line, midaxillary line and a line passing dorsally at the level of the nipple. The catheter should be inserted in the fifth or sixth intercostal space. *Alternatively*—insert catheter in the second intercostal space in the midclavicular line.

Table C6 Suggested chest drain sizes[58]

Adult	Pneumothorax	26–28 FG
	Pleural effusion or haemothorax	36–40 FG
Child	Small child	6–10 FG
	Child up to 30 kg	14–20 FG
	Adolescent >30 kg	20–28 FG

Technique

1 Insert IV cannula and sit patient up 30°. Sterilise site of insertion and infiltrate with a generous amount of 1% lignocaine.
2 With a scalpel make an incision long enough to just allow passage of the appropriate size chest drain.
3 Blunt dissect with heavy forceps through the subcutaneous tissues and intercostal muscles to the pleura ensuring that the route taken is over the top of the rib below and *NOT* under the rib above.
4 Break through the pleura with a finger, then introduce the chest tube with the trocar removed and the tip held with forceps. Clamp the tube unless air is under pressure in the pleural space, in which case allow the air to escape before clamping.
5 Direct the tube posteriorly and basally if fluid is to be drained and apically if air is to be drained.
6 Suture the wound with 3.0 silk so that it is closed snugly around the tube and tie the tube securely.
7 Place a separate suture which is to be tied when the chest tube is removed.
8 Connect the tube to an underwater sealed drain with 2 cm of water above the distal end of the drainage tube.[59]
9 Consider application of low suction (15–20 cm H_2O of negative pressure).[59]

For Tension Pneumothorax

If tension pneumothorax is causing respiratory or cardiovascular embarrassment it can be relieved rapidly by inserting a 14 G cannula into one of the sites described above and releasing the air. Then insert a chest tube as described above.

◐ Cholesterol Lowering Drugs

See Statin Therapy.

◐ Cholinergic Crisis

See Myasthenia Gravis.

QUICK FLICK C

◌ **Cholinergic Receptors**

These are acetylcholine receptors classified into nicotinic and muscarinic receptors which are divided into the following subtypes:

1   *N1* is a receptor in autonomic ganglia, adrenal medulla and also in the central nervous system. Stimulation causes activation of autonomic ganglia (parasympathetic and sympathetic) and has diverse effects such as vasoconstriction.

2   *N2* receptors are present at the neuromuscular junction, and are blocked by the neuromuscular blocking drugs. Stimulation of these receptors causes skeletal muscle contraction.

3   *M1* receptors are also present in autonomic ganglia and the central nervous system, and in gastric parietal cells. Stimulation of these receptors causes increased gastric acid secretion. These receptors are inhibited by pirenzepine.

4   *M2* receptors are present mainly in the heart and salivary glands. Stimulation causes bradycardia, increased salivation and pupillary constriction.

◌ **Cinchocaine**

See *Subarachnoid Block (SAB)*.

◌ **Cisatracurium**

Non-depolarising neuromuscular blocking drug. Cisatracurium is one of the 10 isomers of atracurium. It is 3 × more potent than atracurium and is broken down almost entirely by Hofmann elimination.

Advantages

1   It can be used in patients with liver and/or renal failure.

2   Unlike atracurium, cisatracurium does not cause significant histamine release.

Disadvantages

1   As for atracurium, cisatracurium metabolism results in the production of laudanosine which can cause excitement and seizure activity. However levels of laudanosine produced are less with cisatracurium than atracurium.

2   Cisatracurium should be refrigerated during storage. Once removed from refrigeration it should be discarded after 30 days.

3   It has a relatively slow onset.

Dose

The dose is 0.15 mg/kg. Its onset of action is slightly slower than atracurium. Effects last ≈ 45 min.

Repeat Bolus Injections Give 0.03 mg/kg, lasts ≈ 20–25 min.

Continuous IV Infusion Mean infusion rate to maintain steady state block is 1.4 μg/kg/min (0.084 mg/kg/h).

⬤ Citrate Toxicity

See *Blood Transfusion (Massive Blood Transfusion Management.)*

⬤ Clonidine

A selective α2 presynaptic adrenoreceptor agonist (selectivity for α2:α1 ratio 200:1). Stimulation of these receptors results in decreased noradrenaline release from sympathetic nerve endings and a decreased sympathetic outflow via a central action.

Useful for:
1 Treatment of hypertension.
2 Analgesia when used epidurally or intrathecally.
3 Sedative/anaesthetic sparing properties.

Dose for Hypertension
IV Dose in Adult 150–300 μg, the maximum dose is 750 μg/24 h. May get transient increase in blood pressure prior to the hypotensive effect which takes about 10 min to come on.

IV Dose in Child 5 μg/kg.

Epidural Dose for Analgesia
Adult 150 μg. Clonidine enhances both sensory and motor blockade produced by local anaesthetic agents and has sedating effects. Although clonidine does not enhance the hypotensive effects of LA agents, it greatly prolongs the duration of analgesia.[60]

Child 2 μg/kg

Premedication Dose
5 μg/kg PO provides effective sedation and reduces intraoperative anaesthetic requirements.

Points to Note
1 Rapid withdrawal of clonidine in patients on long term clonidine therapy may result in severe rebound hypertension.
2 Clonidine has a long duration of action with a half life of 6–10 h.
3 Clonidine has also been used intrathecally.

⬤ Clopidogrel

Potent thienopyridine antiplatelet drug with significant anaesthetic and surgical implications. Irreversibly inhibits platelet function. It has fewer side effects than ticlodipine. **See** *Platelet Adenosine Diphosphate Receptor Antagonists* and *Coronary Artery Revascularisation Procedures and Subsequent Non-cardiac Surgery*.

◗ CM5 ECG Monitoring

See *Electrocardiography*.

◗ Cocaine

Amino-ester type local anaesthetic and vasoconstricting agent, used for these purposes in nasal surgery and for awake nasal intubation. Presented as pastes and solutions in concentrations of 1–10%.

Maximum Topical Dose To Mucosa
3 mg/kg. Effects last 20–30 min.

◗ Codeine Phosphate

Methylated morphine derivative analgesic drug suitable for mild-to-moderate pain. Codeine acts primarily by conversion to morphine.

Indications
Codeine is used for:

1 Analgesic for pain of mild-to-moderate severity.
2 Constipating and antitussive agent.

Use in Neurosurgery
Codeine is traditionally recommended for patients requiring neurological assessment due to a reputedly lower incidence of opioid side effects compared with more potent opioids such as morphine. This lower incidence of side effects is most likely due to codeine's lower potency (about 10% as potent as morphine). It has variable efficacy and is ineffective in about 20% of patients following neurosurgery.[49] Morphine is a superior analgesic drug for neurosurgical patients and does not cause confusion between neurological deterioration and opioid side effects.[61] Hirsch argues that the use of codeine in neurosurgical patients should be abandoned.[62]

Use in Paediatrics
Codeine is frequently used in paediatrics due to a perceived low incidence of side effects. As for its use in neurosurgery this low incidence of side effects is at the cost of poor and variable effectiveness.

Dose
Adult Oral/IM 30–60 mg 4–6 h.

Child Oral 0.5–1 mg/kg 4–6 h or
Subcutaneously 1 mg/kg up to 4 hrly. Maximum paediatric dose 3 mg/kg/day.[63]

Advantages

Relatively low incidence of opioid related side effects unless used in high doses.[63]

Disadvantages

1   Codeine has a relatively low analgesic potency and its effectiveness is variable and unpredictable.[63]
2   IV codeine is not recommended due to the risk of hypotension probably related to histamine release.[63]

◑ Combined Spinal/Epidural Technique

See *Subarachnoid Block (SAB)*.

◑ Combitube™

This device is a plastic double lumen tube and can be considered for use in patients in whom other forms of ventilation (bag-mask, LMA, intubation) fail. The lumens are joined together for most of their length except for the proximal portion. One lumen has 8 openings in the supraglottic region and is occluded at its tip. This is termed the 'oesophageal channel'. The second lumen is a simple tube open at each end and is termed the 'tracheal channel'. There are 2 cuffs, a larger one to occlude the oropharynx and a smaller one to occlude the oesophagus or trachea. The patient's head and neck can be in the neutral position for insertion. The device comes in 2 sizes: 37F for a small adult and 41F for an adult.

Technique for Insertion of Combitube™ [64]

1   Insert the device gently into the mouth. Placement is almost always into the oesophagus. Insert to the depth indicated on the device.
2   Inflate the oropharyngeal balloon with 100 mL of air using the enclosed large syringe. This cuff presses against the base of the tongue and the soft palate thus sealing the hypopharynx from the oral and nasal cavities. Then inflate the distal cuff with 10–15 mL of air. This cuff seals the oesophagus.
3   Attempt ventilation via the 'oesophageal' lumen (which has the supraglottic openings). If successful the 'tracheal' channel can be used for gastric fluid aspiration.
4   If attempted ventilation via the 'oesophageal' lumen is unsuccessful, attempt ventilation via the 'tracheal' lumen as the Combitube™ may be in trachea.
5   If still unable to ventilate the patient's lungs consider pulling the device back slightly as the pharyngeal balloon may be obstructing the larynx.
6   One study showed a complication rate of 29.7% with the use of the combitube including oesophageal laceration, perforation and vocal cord injury.[65]

QUICK FLICK C

○ Common Peroneal Nerve Block

See Popliteal Fossa Block.

○ Confusion, Agitation, Decreased Level of Consciousness Postanaesthetic

There are numerous causes of postanaesthetic confusion/decreased level of consciousness. These can be divided into:

1 *Pharmacological Causes.* All drugs given to the patient should be considered as a possible cause particularly opioids, benzodiazepines, atropine/scopolamine (*see* Central Anticholinergic Syndrome), ketamine and droperidol. Also consider drugs the patient may be taking such as alcohol and amphetamines. Other causes to consider are toxins and poisons such as carbon monoxide.

2 *Metabolic/Physiological Causes.* These include hypoxia, hypercarbia, hypotension, electrolyte disorders such as hyponatraemia and hypoglycaemia. Also consider severe pain, bladder distension and hypothermia as possible causes.

3 *Pathological Causes.* These include cerebral injury due to CVA, embolism or tumour and encephalopathy due to such causes as liver failure. Look for systemic causes such as overwhelming sepsis, malignant hyperthermia, haemorrhage and endocrinopathies such as thyrotoxicosis. Consider an acute exacerbation of dementia in the elderly patient. Fat embolism should also be considered.

4 *Psychiatric Causes.* Only consider psychiatric causes when organic causes have been excluded.

Management of Postoperative Confusion

1 Check the patient's response to verbal and tactile stimulation.

2 The combative or aggressive patient must be restrained to prevent self injury and injury to staff.

3 Ensure patient's airway is patent and that ventilation is adequate. Exclude hypoxia and check patient's pulse oximetry.

4 Check patient's pulse and blood pressure. Exclude a significant dysrhythmia, hypotension or hypertension.

5 Examine the patient carefully for causes of postoperative confusion looking in particular for any neurological signs, bladder distension or evidence of haemorrhage. Check patient's temperature looking for hypothermia or hyperthermia (sepsis, MH).

6 Review the patient's history and preanaesthetic state.

7 Review all drugs given to the patient and dosages, and consider the possibility of a drug error. Consider antagonists such as naloxone, flumazenil. Consider central anticholinergic syndrome.

8   Inform the surgeon of the patient's condition.
9   Check arterial blood gas (hypoxia/hypercarbia/acidosis), electrolytes and blood sugar level. Exclude hypoglycaemia. Check FBC for anaemia and raised WCC (sepsis). Consider blood and urine screen for illicit drugs.
10 Consider cerebral CT/MRI scan, neurological/geriatric consultation and ICU transfer.
11 If significant correctable causes are ruled out or unlikely, consider small doses of opioid (if pain suspected) and/or midazolam. Consider haloperidol 2–10 mg IV for on-going severe agitation. Keep the patient warm. Attempt to verbally calm and reassure the patient and keep him/her orientated.
12 Droperidol has been reported as being useful for the prevention and treatment of severe emergence agitation. Hatzakorzian et al. reported using droperidol 5 mg intraoperatively to successful prevent emergence agitation in a patient who had this problem after 3 previous anaesthetics.[66] A second patient weighing 218 kg received droperidol 8 mg IV for severe, violent emergence agitation.[66] He became calm over a few minutes.

◑ Congenital Heart Disease (CHD) in Adults and Non-cardiac Surgery

This is a vast topic and only a brief description of this subject is provided. Readers are advised to consult larger texts. About 1% of newborns suffer from congenital heart disease or abnormalities of the great vessels and an increasing number of these patients are surviving to adult life due to advances in surgical and medical care. These conditions are usually but not invariably corrected either fully or partially by adult life. For pregnant patients, functional deterioration occurs in 50% of patients with cyanotic CHD and 15% of those with acyanotic heart disease.[67]

Main Anaesthetic Concerns with Congenital Heart Disease and Repair Procedures

The skill, experience and knowledge of the anaesthetist, invasive monitoring and gradual controlled anaesthesia are more important considerations than the specific drugs or techniques used. Factors to consider are:

1   Hypoxaemia—when persistent right-to-left shunting occurs or with pulmonary hyperperfusion due to left-to-right shunts. Hypoxaemia also leads to polycythaemia, increased blood viscosity and an increased tendency to thrombosis. Hyperviscosity syndrome may occur consisting of headache, visual impairment and dizziness. Paradoxically polycythaemia can be associated with bleeding abnormalities due to thrombocytopenia, platelet dysfunction and abnormal fibrinolysis. *See Polycythaemia*.
2   There may be myocardial ischaemia and fibrosis.
3   Pulmonary hypertension. *See Pulmonary Hypertension*.

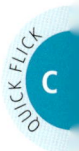

4 Dysrhythmias—atrial surgery predisposes to atrial dysrhythmias while ventricular septal surgery leads to abnormal conduction.

5 Valve dysfunction.

6 Deleterious alterations to shunt flow or shunt reversal.

7 Endocarditis prophylaxis. ***See*** *Bacterial Endocarditis (BE) Prophylaxis.*

8 Airway compression due to conduits, dilated atria or pulmonary arteries.

9 Do not allow air to enter IV lines. This may result in paradoxical embolus.

Optimising Pulmonary Blood Flow with Right-to-left Shunts
To avoid further hypoxaemia during anaesthesia:

1 Ensure adequate intravascular filling at all times e.g. provide pre-operative IV fluid hydration.

2 Maintain adequate systemic blood pressure to prevent increased right-to-left shunting.

3 Avoid increases in pulmonary vascular resistance due to hypercapnia, acidosis, hypoxia and high airway pressures. If GA is used intubate the patient and control ventilation meticulously.

4 Use invasive monitoring (arterial line, CVP).

Physiological Effects of Left-to-right Shunting

1 Decreased pulmonary compliance with increased work of breathing.

2 Enlarged pulmonary arteries with the potential for bronchial compression, atelectasis, chest infection and localised emphysema.

Optimising CVS Parameters with Left-to-right Shunts
Increased blood flow from the pulmonary circulation to the systemic circulation leads to increased left ventricular workload and left ventricular failure if systemic circulation requirements can not be met. These patients are also predisposed to chest infections. Anaesthetic aims include:

1 Avoid myocardial depression.

2 Avoid vasodilatation/hypotension. If neuroaxial block is used introduce the block slowly and incrementally.

3 To optimise intravascular filling use invasive monitoring (arterial line, CVP).

Congenital Heart Disease and Pregnancy
In general normal vaginal delivery should be aimed for with CS reserved for obstetric indications or if the patient's CVS is unable to cope with labour. Other aims are:

1 Preserve ventricular function avoiding anaesthetic induced myocardial depression.

2 Maintain adequate preload.

3 Prevent undesirable changes in shunt flow (see above).

4 If epidural anaesthesia is used induce the block very slowly with invasive monitoring with the aim of preventing sudden fluctuations in cardiac output, pre-load and systemic blood pressure. Consider extradural or subarachnoid morphine for labour analgesia in particularly brittle patients.

5 Provide endocarditis prophylaxis.

Specific Types of Congenital Heart Disease

For a very brief description of these conditions and the effects of corrective procedures *see Atrial Septal Defect (ASD), Ebstein's Anomaly, Eisenmenger's Syndrome, Fontan Procedure, Glenn Shunt, Tetralogy of Fallot, Pulmonary Hypertension* and *Ventricular Septal Defect (VSD).*

◐ Congestive Cardiac Failure (CCF)

(**See also** *Pulmonary Oedema*)

CCF is usually secondary to ischaemic heart disease. Other causes include cardiomyopathy and hypertensive and valvular heart disease. Ejection fraction (EF) is an important prognostic indicator. An EF < 40% is indicative of significant cardiac impairment.

Treatment of Mild-to-moderate CCF

1 Dietary modification including salt and water restriction and correction of excess weight.
2 Diuretic therapy. This results in a loss of sodium and water from the body decreasing preload and thus ventricular volume overload.
3 ACE inhibitors, such as enalapril (Vasotec) are beneficial by decreasing systemic vascular resistance and ventricular filling. Angiotensin receptor blocker drugs can be used in patients intolerant of ACE inhibitors.
4 Digoxin. Marginally improves EF (≈ 4–5%) and is the only oral positive inotropic agent available.
5 β blockers. These improve survival in patients with CCF after myocardial infarction.[68]
6 Aldosterone antagonists e.g. spirinolactone and eplerenone.
7 Cardiac resynchronisation therapy via biventricular pacing. **See** *Pacing, Pacemakers and Anaesthesia*.

Severe CCF/Cardiogenic Shock

Treat the cause of cardiogenic shock (e.g. myocardial ischaemia, hypertensive heart failure, dysrhythmias) if possible. Invasive monitoring with a pulmonary artery catheter and arterial line will usually be required. In addition to general supportive measures such as O_2 therapy and sitting the patient up, the basic principles of management are to optimise preload, contractility and afterload.

Preload Optimisation

A PCWP of 15–18 mm Hg is usually optimal. If the initial PCWP is < 18 mm Hg provide plasma volume expansion incrementally.[69] If PCWP > 18 mm Hg preload needs to be reduced. Reducing excessive preload

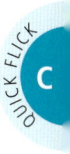

decreases left ventricular wall stress and O_2 consumption and enables resolution of pulmonary congestion through reduced right atrial pressure. Reduced preload also enables more effective ventricular contraction, lessens physiological mitral regurgitation and improves myocardial perfusion during diastole. Preload can be reduced by:

1 *Loop Diuretic* e.g. frusemide 40–120 mg IV.
2 *Vasodilators* e.g. glyceryl trinitrate (GTN) or sodium nitroprusside (see below). GTN is predominantly a venodilator at lower dosages and decreases ventricular filling pressure and ventricular dilatation. As many patients with ventricular overload have functional mitral + tricuspid regurgitation, reduced ventricular volume decreases the regurgitant fraction and improves forward cardiac output.[70] Nitrates can be given sublingually for a more immediate effect while a GTN infusion is prepared.

Inotropes and Other Drugs to Improve Contractility

1 *Dobutamine* acts on β1 adrenoreceptors leading to increased contractility and heart rate. In addition dobutamine stimulates β2 adrenoreceptors leading to decreased systemic vascular resistance. Its use is most appropriate when there is mild-to-moderate hypotension and severe congestive heart failure.[71] Dobutamine is not the inotrope of choice if there is profound hypotension/shock as it lacks significant α effects.[69,71] ***See*** *Dobutamine*.
2 *Dopamine* is used for its ability to increase coronary blood flow and positive inotropic effects with a slight decrease in systemic vascular resistance at a dose of < 15 μg/kg/min. At doses > 15 μg/kg/min α adrenoreceptor effects predominate ***See*** *Dopamine*.
3 *Adrenaline—**see** Adrenaline*.
4 *Phosphodiesterase Inhibitors **see** Amrinone* and *Milrinone*. Milrinone may be preferable to inotropic drugs in patients with critical coronary artery disease[71] due to its ability to increase cardiac output without increasing myocardial O_2 demand.
5 *Levosimendan* increases contractility by enhancing the sensivity of myocardial cells to calcium. ***See*** *Levosimendan*.

Afterload Reduction with an arterial vasodilator such as sodium nitroprusside or phosphodiesterase inhibitor such as milrinone. These drugs may be particularly effective in patients with heart failure due to hypertensive disease.

Ventilation Strategies such as positive pressure ventilation with positive end-expiratory pressure (PEEP). This can result in decreased work of breathing and improved ventilation: perfusion matching. PEEP may also reduce left ventricular preload beneficially.

Mechanical Assist Devices such as an intra-aortic balloon pump may be of benefit by reducing left ventricular work and increasing cardiac output. Left and right ventricular assist devices are becoming increasingly available.

Angiographic/Surgical Intervention including cardiac transplant, angioplasty and urgent coronary artery bypass grafts can be considered.

New Agents The B-type natriuretic peptide, nesiritide (Natrecor) shows promise as a new treatment for heart failure.

◗ Coronary Artery Revascularisation Procedures and Subsequent Non-cardiac Surgery

Topics Covered in this Section
▶ Coronary Artery Bypass Grafts (CABG)
▶ Coronary Artery Stents (CAS)
▶ Percutaneous Transluminal Coronary Angioplasty (PTCA)
▶ Brachiotherapy
▶ Does Coronary Artery Revascularisation Prior to Non-cardiac Surgery Reduce Mortality?

Coronary Artery Bypass Grafts (CABG)

Coronary artery bypass grafting may decrease mortality during subsequent non-cardiac surgery. However the overall peri-operative mortality of CABG is about 3%[72] and in high risk patients it rises to 6.5%.[73] Therefore CABG prior to non-cardiac surgery may reduce the combined risk of both procedures only in patients who are at low risk from the CABG procedure. Patients with multivessel disease and unstable angina are likely to benefit from CABG prior to high-risk procedures. Patients undergoing low-risk procedures are unlikely to derive benefit from CABG performed prior to the procedure unless there is an indication for urgent CABG. One study by Breen et al. showed an increased mortality if CABG was performed within 1 month of high risk vascular surgery.[74] There may be increased mortality associated with simultaneous CABG and vascular surgery.[75] It may be safest to delay non-cardiac surgery for at least 6 weeks and up to 6 months after CABG if possible.[76]

Coronary Artery Stents (CAS)

Coronary artery stenting carries less risk than CABG with a 30-day mortality of about 0.5%.[72] CAS are either bare metal or drug eluting. Drug eluting stents prevent neo-intimal proliferation resulting in stenosis within the stent. The commonly used substances in drug eluting stents are sirolimus or paclitaxel. Both bare metal and drug eluting stents are thrombogenic. If thrombosis does occur in the stent or embolisation occurs distally there is a 50% incidence of MI and a 20% mortality. Therefore the use of antithrombic drugs (usually aspirin + clopidogrel or ticlopidine) is mandatory until endothelialisation of the stent(s) occurs. Recommended antithrombotic treatment periods are:

1   drug eluting stents: 12 months[77]
2   bare metal: 4–6 weeks

In patients with bare metal stents, non-urgent surgery should be delayed at least 4–6 weeks. Some clinicians advise 3 months as a minimum waiting period. For patients with drug eluting stents, elective surgery should be delayed for 12 months. When elective surgery is performed consult the patient's cardiologist. Surgery should be performed in a hospital where coronary artery intervention therapy is available. If semi-urgent surgery must be performed while on clopidogrel or ticlodipine, consider the following regimen recommended by Broad et al:[78]

1   Cease clopidogrel 5 days before surgery. Maintain aspirin therapy throughout the peri-operative period if the patient is on aspirin.
2   Three days before surgery commence a tirofiban and heparin infusion in the cardiology unit aiming for full anticoagulation.
3   Cease the infusions 6 h before surgery.
4   Restart clopidogrel on the first Postoperative day with a loading dose of 300 mg plus give prophylactic subcut heparin.
5   Resume daily clopidogrel 75 mg.

Chassot et al. argue that except for surgery in which bleeding is enclosed e.g. neurosurgery/spinal surgery, the risk of ceasing clopidogrel/aspirin therapy will be greater than the risk of haemorrhage.[77]

Percutaneous Transluminal Coronary Angioplasty

Following angioplasty arterial recoil and acute thrombosis may occur in the first few hours or days after the procedure. In patients who have undergone percutaneous transluminal cardiac angioplasty (PTCA) elective surgery should be delayed for at least 4 weeks.[25] However some investigators recommend even greater caution. Posner et al. found in their study that any potential benefit from PTCA was negated if subsequent high-risk surgery was performed within 90 days.[79]

Brachiotherapy

This involves intra-coronary artery irradiation with gamma or beta emitters and is used to treat recurrent in-stent restenosis. These patients usually require dual anti-platelet therapy and are at high risk if this is stopped for non-cardiac surgery.

Does Coronary Artery Revascularisation Prior to Non-cardiac Surgery Reduce Mortality?

The Coronary Artery Revascularisation Prophylaxis (CARP) trial compared patients who received revascularisation interventions with optimal medical therapy prior to elective vascular surgery. There was no difference in the incidence of death and myocardial infarction in the short term or long term.[80] It is debatable whether coronary artery revascularisation is appropriate in high risk elderly patients requiring vascular surgery because:[81]

1 They may not survive the coronary revascularisation procedure.
2 Their vascular surgery is delayed.
3 Their life span is not increased.
4 Optimised medical therapy alone may provide the same level of protection as coronary artery revascularisation.

◖ Coronary Artery Stents

See entry above.

◖ COVER ABCD A SWIFT CHECK Crisis Management Algorithm[82]

Summarised with permission from the Australian Safety Foundation. This algorithm is an easy reference summary for the rapid identification of the aetiology of a crisis during anaesthesia. It is both systematic and comprehensive. 'COVER ABCD' applies to patients with a tracheal tube. 'AB COVER ABCD' refers to patient's receiving mask anaesthesia.

COVER ABCD Algorithm[82]

COVER ABCD covers 95% of incidents, of which 3% are cardiac arrests. The percentages quoted below in brackets are the percentage of incidents caused by or related to the corresponding letter of the algorithm.

C1 Circulation—Feel pulse (rate, rhythm and character of pulse). If pulseless (3%) start CPR, get help and complete the core algorithm as soon as possible. *See* Cardiac Arrest.

C2 Colour—Note saturation (cyanosis?). Test pulse oximetry probe on your own finger if necessary, while proceeding with *O1* and *O2* (see below).

O1 Oxygen—Check rotameter settings (hypoxic mixture?). Increase FiO_2 to 1.0 and check that only the O_2 flowmeter is operating. (2%)

O2 Oxygen Analyser—Check that the oxygen analyser shows a rising O_2 concentration distal to the common gas outlet. (0.2%)

V1 Ventilation—Ventilate the lungs by hand and assess breathing circuit integrity, airway patency, chest compliance and air entry. Observe chest movement and auscultate the chest. Also inspect the capnography trace. (20%)

V2 Vaporiser—Note settings and level of contents in the vaporiser and

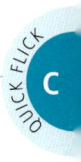

check for leaks. Consider the possibility of the wrong agent being in vaporiser. (4%)

E1 Endotracheal Tube—Check the endotracheal tube for patency, kinks and any possible obstruction. Check the capnography trace to confirm tracheal intubation. Consider the possibility of endobronchial tube placement. If necessary adjust, deflate cuff, pass a catheter through the ET tube, or remove and replace the ET tube. (14%)

E2 Elimination—Eliminate the anaesthetic machine and ventilate with a self-inflating bag using 100% O_2 (from an alternative source if necessary). Retain the gas monitor sampling tubing, but be aware of the possibility of gas sampling/monitoring problems. (15%)

R1 Review Monitors—Review all monitors in use. They should all be correctly sited, checked and calibrated. (4%)

R2 Review Equipment—Review all other equipment in contact with or relevant to the patient e.g. diathermy, humidifiers, heating blankets, endoscopes, probes, prostheses, retractors and other appliances. (2%)

A Airway—Check patency of the unintubated airway. Consider laryngospasm (6%) or the presence of a foreign body in airway (1%), or aspiration/regurgitation (5%). (Total 12%)

B Breathing—Assess pattern, adequacy and distribution of ventilation. Exclude hypoventilation (2%), bronchospasm (2%), pulmonary oedema, lobar collapse and pneumo/haemothorax (1%).

C Circulation—Evaluate peripheral perfusion, pulse, blood pressure, ECG. Exclude obstruction to venous return (e.g. supine hypotensive syndrome of pregnancy), raised intrathoracic pressure (e.g. inadvertent PEEP) or direct interference to, or tamponade of, the heart. Note any trends on records, e.g. bradycardia/ bradyarrhythmia (5%), tachycardia/tachyarrhythmia (2%), hypotension (5%), hypertension (1%) or ischaemia (1%). (Total 14%)

D Drugs—Review intended and unintended drug or substance administration (e.g. bone cement). Consider failure of drug to reach patient e.g kinked cannula. (Total 3%)

A SWIFT CHECK Algorithm
A SWIFT CHECK is a second crisis algorithm to be applied when the cause of an emergency is not revealed by the COVER ABCD algorithm. *A* covers 4% and *SWIFT CHECK covers* 1% of anaesthetic emergencies.
A Air Embolus, Anaphylaxis, Air in Pleura Awareness

S1 Surgeon/ Situation—Vagal stimulation, caval compression, bleeding, direct myocardial stimulation.

S2 Sepsis—Hypotension, desaturation, acidosis, hyperdynamic circulation.

W1 Wound—Trauma, bleeding, tamponade, pneumothorax, problems due to retractors.

W2 Water Intoxication—Electrolyte disturbance, fluid overload.

I1 Infarct—Myocardial conduction, ST or rhythm problem, hypotension or poor cardiac output.

I2 Insufflation—Vagal tone, reduced venous return, pulmonary or paradoxical arterial gas embolism.

F1 'Fat Syndrome'—Desaturation +/– hypotension especially after induction and in lithotomy position (with obese or distended abdomen), profuse bronchial secretions.

F2 Full Bladder—May cause marked haemodynamic changes +/– sympathetic stimulation.

T1 Trauma—Consider spinal injury, undiagnosed sub- or extra-dural haematoma, bronchial or diaphragmatic injury, ruptured viscus, concealed haemorrhage, myocardial contusion.

T2 Tourniquet Down—LA toxicity, unseen bleeding, failed block.

C Catheter/IV Cannula, Chest Drain Problems, Cement.

H Hyper/hypothermia, Hypoglycaemia.

E1 Embolus—Fat, thrombus, amniotic fluid.

E2 Endocrine—Hyper- or hypothyroid/adrenal medulla or cortex/ -pituitary/ diabetes/ 5-HT.

C Check—Check right patient, right operation, right body part, correct side. Check case notes, old notes for pre-operative status, diseases, drugs.

K1 K^+—Exclude potassium (and any other) electrolyte abnormality.

K2 Keep—Unless surgery can be ceased immediately, keep the patient asleep until a new anaesthetic machine can be obtained.

Note: 99.9% of incidents should have been identified by now. If the problem has not been solved, direct available resources to its solution. Get experienced help. Work from first principles. Think laterally.

❍ COX 2 Inhibitors

See Non-steroidal Anti-inflammatory Drugs (NSAIDs).

◗ Creutzfeldt-Jacob Disease (CJD)

Also called subacute spongiform encephalopathy. This illness is an infectious fatal neurological disorder. It is caused by prions which are extremely resistant to destruction by routine sterilisation and decontamination measures.

Operating Theatre Guidelines when CJD is Suspected

1 Schedule the case as last for the day.
2 Remove all unnecessary staff, equipment and supplies from the operating theatre and cover all essential exposed surfaces with plastic or impervious disposable drapes.
3 Minimise traffic through the theatre.
4 Use disposible anaesthetic and surgical equipment.
5 Air powered surgical equipment should not be used.
6 All operating theatre staff must wear appropriate disposable protective clothing and eye protection.
7 All relevant staff must be notified of CJD risk such as domestic services, pathology staff. All CJD material must be clearly labelled.
8 After the procedure surfaces are cleaned with 1–2 M sodium hydroxide.

◗ Cricoid Pressure

See *Rapid Sequence Induction (RSI)*.

◗ Cricothyroid Puncture and Cricothyrotomy

Anatomy

The cricothyroid ligament connects the cricoid cartilage to the base of the thyroid cartilage. The thyroid cartilage can be identified by feeling for the thyroid notch at the top of the laryngeal prominence (Adam's apple). Run your finger caudally down the laryngeal prominence until a gap is felt. This is the cricothyroid ligament. The next structure felt moving caudally is the cricoid cartilage which feels like a prominent hard ring shape. The cricoid cartilage lies at the level of C6 in the adult. **See** *Larynx, Anatomy and Innervation*.

Technique for Cricothyroid Puncture

1 Identify the cricothyroid ligament between the cricoid and thyroid cartilages.
2 Insert a 14 G cannula with a 10 mL syringe attached, in the midline through this membrane. Insert the cannula at an angle of 30° caudad. Pierce the trachea and confirm this position by aspirating air. Withdraw the stylet into the cannula before advancing the cannula fully into the trachea (hub of the cannula on skin).
3 Fully remove the stylet and confirm the position of the cannula again by aspirating air.

4 Ventilate through the cannula using high pressure jet ventilation (200 kPa) with a device such as a Sanders injector.

See *Transtracheal Jet Ventilation*.

Advantages
Quick and easy to perform.

Disadvantages
1 For effective ventilation a jet ventilation device is required. Low-pressure systems e.g. using an anaesthetic circuit will not work effectively.[83]
2 There must be enough patency of the upper airway for exhalation to occur (4–4.5 mm d.) otherwise O_2 entering the lungs cannot escape. Exhalation through the cannula is too slow ($\approx$ 34 sec).[84]
3 There is a risk of barotrauma and subcutaneous emphysema if jet ventilation is used.
4 One rescuer must hold the cannula in place at all times.
5 Spontaneous ventilation by the patient is impossible.
6 Temporary airway. Definitive airway control is still required.

Technique for Cricothyrotomy
This can be done either 'open' or percutaneous.

Technique for Open Cricothyrotomy
1 Identify cricothyroid membrane and make a transverse incision through the skin and lower half of the membrane with a scalpel.
2 With the handle of the scalpel, widen this incision sufficiently to enable passage of an endotracheal tube. Insert the tube through incision into the trachea. Ideally a 6 mm cuffed tracheotomy tube should be used, otherwise use any suitably sized ET tube that comes to hand.
3 Inflate the cuff of the ET tube and ventilate.

Technique for Percutaneous Cricothyrotomy
Dedicated percutaneous cricothyrotomy kits are available but are awkward to use in an emergency without prior adequate training. An example is the 5 mm Melker Cuffed Emergency Cricothyrotomy Catheter Set.
1 Insert the introducer needle into the trachea through the cricothyroid membrane in a caudad direction as described above. Advance the needle until able to aspirate air using the 5 mL syringe provided.
2 Pass the guide wire through the needle, then remove the introducer needle.
3 Use the scalpel to widen the puncture wound.
4 Insert the cuffed airway catheter containing the curved dilator over the guide wire.
5 Remove the guide wire and dilator leaving the cuffed airway catheter in the trachea.

QUICK FLICK C

Advantages
1 Easy to perform.
2 Spontaneous ventilation is possible.
3 High-pressure ventilation is not required.
4 The airway provided is 'definitive' i.e. aspiration risk is reduced and necessary surgery can be commenced.

Disadvantages
1 More 'invasive' than cricothyroid puncture and takes longer to perform.
2 Risk of haemorrhage.
3 Cricothyrotomy should not be performed on pre-pubescent children because of the risk of damaging the cricoid cartilage with subsequent airway collapse.[83] Perform needle cricothyroid puncture and jet ventilation instead.[83]

See Difficult Airway Management.

�‣ Cryoprecipitate (and Cryodepleted Plasma)

Cryoprecipitate
Cryoprecipitate is formed when fresh frozen plasma from a single unit of whole blood is thawed to between 1°C and 6°C and the resultant precipitate is collected. The precipitate is then refrozen. It is rich in factor VIII (100 units) and fibrinogen (250 mg). It also contains factor XIII, fibronectin and von Willebrand factor in a total volume of 15 mL. It is stored at −30°C, and is stable for 6 months. 1 unit of cryoprecipitate should increase fibrinogen levels by 5–10 mg/100 mL in the adult. Once thawed cryoprecipitate should be used within 6 h (or within 4 h if the unit has been opened).

Indications for Cryoprecipitate
Cryoprecipitate is indicated for the treatment of fibrinogen deficiency or dysfibrinogenaemia associated with blood loss or potential blood loss. The half-life of fibrinogen is 3–5 days. Cryoprecipitate can be used for the following conditions but only if specific therapies are not available:
1 haemophilia A (factor VIII) deficiency. Aim to increase factor VIII to > 30% of normal.
2 von Willebrand's disease.
3 factor XIII deficiency
4 fibrinonectin deficiency.
5 fibrinogen deficiency (< 80–100 mg/100 mL) due to severe blood loss and associated coagulopathy.

Cryodepleted Plasma (CDP)
This is the plasma remaining after cryoprecipitate has been removed. CDP can be used for:

1 Plasma exchange in ITP.
2 As an alternative to FFP in the treatment of warfarin overdose or reversal.
3 Coagulopathy with bleeding not requiring those factors in cryoprecipitate.

⊙ Cyanide Poisoning Treatment

See *Sodium Nitroprusside (SNP)*.

⊙ Cytotoxic Drugs

See *Immunosuppressive Drugs, Anaesthetic Implications*.

REFERENCES

1   Department of Health and Social Security. Report on: *Confidential Enquiries into Maternal deaths in the United Kingdom*, 1994–1996. London HSMO; 1999.
2   Hawkins JL, Koonin LM, Palmer SK, Gibbs CP. Anaesthesia related deaths during obstetric delivery in the United States, 1979–1990. *Anesthesiology* 1997; 86: 277–284.
3   Barnardo PD, Jenkins JG. Failed tracheal intubation in obstetrics: a 6 year review in a UK region. *Anaesthesia* 2000; 55: 685–94.
4   Preston R. Editorial: The evolving role of the laryngeal mask airway in obsterics. *Can J Anaesth* 2001; 48: 1061–5.
5   Han T-H, Brimacombe J, Lee E-J. The laryngeal mask airway is effective (and probably safe) in selected healthy patients for elective Caesarean section: a prospective study of 1067 cases. *Can J Anaesth 2001*; 48: 1117–21.
6   Dhonneur G, Ndoko S, Amathieu R et al. Tracheal intubation using the Airtraq® in morbid obese patients undergoing emergency Cesarean delivery. *Anesthesiol* 2007; 106: 629–30.
7   Morris S. Management of difficult and failed intubation in obstetrics. *Br J Anaesth CEPD Reviews* 2001; 4: 117–121.
8   Awan R, Nolan JP, Cook TM. Use of the ProSeal™ laryngeal mask airway for airway maintenance during emergency Caesarean section after failed tracheal intubation. *Br J Anaesth* 2004; 92: 144–6.
9   Kuczkowski KM, Reisner LS, Benumof JL. Airway problems and new solutions for the obstetric patient. *J Clin Anesth* 2003; 15: 552–63.
10 Levy DM. Review Article: Emergency Caesarean section: best practice. *Anaesth* 2006; 61: 786–91.
11 Dansereau J, Joshi A, Helewa ME, et al. Double-blind comparison of carbetocin versus oxytocin in prevention of uterine atony after cesarean section. *Am L Obstets Gynecol* 1999; 180: 670–6.
12 Kinney MAO, Warner ME, Nagorney DM, et al. Perianesthetic risks and outcomes of abdominal surgery for metastatic carcinoid syndromes. *Br J Anaesth* 2001; 87: 447–52.

13 Consensus on resuscitation science and treatment recommendations. Part 2: Adult basic life support. *Resuscitation* 2005; 67: 187–201.

14 Paradis NA, Martin GB, Goetting MG et al. Simultaneous aortic, jugular bulb and right atrial pressure during cardiopulmonary resuscitation in humans: insight into mechanisms. *Circulation* 1989; 80: 361–8.

15 Eftestol T, Wik L, Sunde K, Steen PA. Effects of cardiopulmonary resuscitation on predictors of ventricular fibrillation defibrillation success during out-of-hospital cardiac arrest. *Circulation* 2004; 110: 10–15.

16 Mason JJ, Owens DK, Harris RA, Cooke JP, Hlatky MA. The role of coronary angiography and coronary revascularization before noncardiac surgery. *JAMA* 1995; 273: 1919–25.

17 Soni N. *Practical Procedures in Anaesthesia and Intensive Care.* Butterworth–Heinemann, Oxford 1994; 79.

18 Cheung KW, Green RS, Magee KD. Systematic review of randomized controlled trials of therapeutic hypothermia as a neuroprotectant in post cardiac arrest patients. *J Can Assoc Emerg Physician* 2006; 8: 329–37.

19 Mallampalli A, Guy E. Cardiac arrest in pregnancy and somatic support after brain death. *Crit Care Med* 2005; 33: S325–S331.

20 Katz V, Balderston K, DeFreest M. Perimortem cesarean delivery: were our assumptions correct? *Am J Obstets Gynaecol* 2005; 192: 1916–21.

21 Younberg JA. Anesthetic considerations for major vascular surgery. Annual refresher course lecture. *American Society of Anesthesiologists* 1997; 245: 1–7.

22 Fleisher LA, Barash PG. Review article. Preoperative cardiac evaluation for noncardiac surgery: a functional approach. *Anesth Analg* 1992; 74: 586–98.

23 Poldermans D, Arnese M, Fioretti PM, Salustri A, et al. Improved cardiac risk stratification in major vascular surgery with dobutamine-atropine stress echocardiography. *J Am Coll Cardiol* 1995; 26: 648–53.

24 Palacios IF, Miller SW. Coronary arteriography and left ventriculography. In: Eagle KA, Haber E, DeSanctis RW, Austen WG, eds. *The Practice of Cardiology*, 2nd edn. Little, Brown and Company 1989; 1644–7.

25 Report of the American College of Cardiology/American Heart Association Task Force on Practice Guidelines. ACC/AHA 2007 Guidelines on perioperative cardiovascular evaluation and care for non cardiac surgery. *Circulation* 2007; 116: e418–e499.

26 Chassot P-G, Delabays A, Spahn DR. Preoperative evaluation of patients with, or at risk of, coronary artery disease undergoing non-cardiac surgery. *Br J Anaesthesia* 2002; 89: 747–59.

27 Park KW. Review Article: Perioperative cardiology consultation. *Anesthesiology* 2003; 98: 754–62.

28 Wallace AW, Galindez D, Salahieh A, et al. Effect of clonidine on cardiovascular morbidity and mortality after no cardiac surgery. *Anesthesiol* 2004; 101: 284–93.

29 Durazzo AE, Machado FS, Ikeoka DT, et al. Reduction in cardiovascular events after vascular surgery with atorvastatin: a randomized trial. *J Vasc Surg* 2004; 39: 967–75.

30 Howel SJ. Carotid endarterectomy. *Br J Anaesth* 2007; 99: 119–31.

31 McCarthy RJ, Walker R, McAteer P, Budd JS, Horrocks M. Patient and hospital benefits of local anaesthesia for carotid endarterectomy. *Eur J Vasc Endovasc Surg* 2001; 22: 13–18.

32 Stoneham MD, Knighton JD. Review article:regional anaesthesia for carotid endarterectomy. *Br J Anaesth* 1999; 82: 910–19.

33 Fox AA, Fleisher LA. Is there a difference in perioperative morbidity and mortality in patients undergoing carotid endarterectomy with local versus general anesthesia? In: Fleisher LA ed. *Evidence-Based Practice of Anesthesiology*. Philadelphia, Pennsylvania: Saunders 2004: 372–6.

34 Olympio MA. The pre-operative evaluation of symptomatic carotid endarterectomy: a debated issue. *J Neurosurgical Anesthesiol* 1996; 8: 310–13.

35 Mazer CD. Con: Combined coronary and vascular surgery is not better than separate procedures. *J Cardiothoracic Vascular Anesth* 1998; 12: 228–30.

36 Wilke HJ, Ellis JE, McKinsey JF. Carotid endarterectomy: perioperative and anaesthetic considerations. *J Cardiothoracic Vasc Anesth* 1996; 7: 928–49.

37 Lien CA, Van Poznak A. Carotid Endarterectomy. In: Yao F-S F, ed. *Yao and Artusio's Anesthesiology: Problem Orientated Patient Management*, 4th edn. Lippincott-Raven 1998; 455–81.

38 Gottlieb A, Satariano-Hayden P, Schoenwald P, Rykman J, Piedmonte M. The effects of carotid sinus nerve blockade on hemodynamic stability after carotid endarterectomy. *J Cardiothoracic Vasc Anesth* 1997; 11: 67–71.

39 Davies MJ, Dysart RH, Silbert BS, Scott DA, Cook RJ. Prevention of tachycardia with atenolol pre-treatment for carotid endarterectomy under cervical plexus blockade. *Anaesth Intensive Care* 1992; 20: 161–4.

40 Stoneham MD, Knighton JD. Review article: regional anaesthesia for carotid endarterectomy. *Br J Anaesth* 1999; 82: 910–19.

41 Lewis MP, Thomas P, Wilson LF, Mulholland RC. The 'whoosh' test. A clinical test to confirm correct needle placement in caudal epidural injections. *Anaesthesia* 1992; 47: 1002–3.

QUICK FLICK C

42 Prentiss JE. Cardiac arrest following caudal anaesthesia. *Anesthesiology* 1979; 50: 51.

43 Sinclair JC, Fox HA, Lentz JF, Fuld GL et al. Intoxication of the fetus by a local anaesthetic. A newly recognized complication of maternal caudal anaesthesia. *N Eng J Med* 1965; 273: 1173.

44 Gravlee GP. Blood conservation strategies. *Audio Digest Anesthesiology* 1996; 38: 23.

45 Brown V. Clinical strategies to avoid blood transfusion. *Anaesth Intensive Care Medicine* 2004; 5: 68–70.

46 Esler MD, Douglas MJ. Planning for hemorrhage. Steps an anesthesiologist can take to limit and treat hemorrhage in the obstetric patient. *Anesthesiol Clin North Am* 2003; 21: 127–44.

47 Al-Shari R, White PM, Davenport RJ, Lindsay KW. Subarachnoid haemorrhage. *Br Med J* 2006; 333: 235–40.

48 Greenberg MS. SAH and aneurysms. In: Greenberg MS ed. *Handbook of Neurosurgery*. 2000, 5th edn. Thiem Medical New York: 754–83.

49 Priebe H-J. Aneurysmal subarachnoid haemorrhage and the anaesthetist. *Br J Anaesth* 2007; 99: 102–18.

50 Sutcliffe AJ. Subarachnoid haemorrhage due to cerebral aneurysm. *Br J Anaesth CEPD Reviews* 2002; 2: 45–8.

51 Hunt WE, Hess RM. Surgical risk as related to time of intervention in the repair of intracranial aneurysms. *J Neurosurg* 1968; 28: 14–20.

52 Bedfort NM, Hardman JG, Nathanson MH. Cerebral hemodynamic response to the introduction of desflurane: a comparison with sevoflurane. *Anesth Analg* 2000; 91: 152–5.

53 Young WL. Cerebral aneurysms: current anaesthetic management and future horizons. *Can J Anaesth* 1998; 45: R17–R24.

54 Todd MM, Hindman BJ, Clark WR, Torner JC. The Intraoperative Hypothermia for Aneurysm Surgery Trial (IHAST) Investigators. Mild intraoperative hypothermia during surgery for intracranial aneurysm. *N Eng J Med* 2005; 352: 135–45.

55 Mack PF. Cerebral Aneurysm. In Yao F-S F, ed. *Anesthesiology Problem-Orientated Patient Management* 4th edn, Lippincott-Raven, Philadelphia 1998; 504–24.

56 Lepzig TJ, Morgan J, Horner TG, Payner T, Redelman K, Johnson CS. Analysis of intraoperative rupture in the surgical treatment of 1964 saccular aneurysms. *Neurosurgery* 2005; 56: 455–68.

57 Lai YC, Manninen PH. Anesthesia for cerebral aneurysms: a comparison between interventional neuroradiology and surgery. *Can J Anaesth* 2001; 48: 391–5.

58 Emery G, Handley G, Davies MJ, Mooney PH. Incidence of phrenic nerve block and hypercapnia in patients undergoing carotid endarterectomy under cervical plexus block. *Anaesth Intensive Care* 1998; 26: 377–81.

59 Kam AC, O'Brien M, Kam PCA. Pleural drainage systems. *Anaesthesia* 1993; 48: 154–61.

60 Eisenach J, De Kock M, Klimscha W. Alpha 2 adrenergic agonists for regional anaesthesia; a clinical review of clonidine (1984–1995). *Anesthesiology* 1996; 85: 655–74.

61 Goldsack C, Scuplak S, Smith M. A double-blind comparison of codeine and morphine for postoperative analgesia following intracranial surgery. *Anaesthesia* 1996; 51: 1029–32.

62 Hirsch N. Advances in neuroanaesthesia. *Anaesthesia* 2003; 58: 1162–203.

63 Williams DG, Hatch DJ, Howard RF. Review Article: Codeine phosphate in paediatric medicine. *Br J Anaesth* 2001; 86: 413–21.

64 Eichinger S, Schreiber W, Heinz T, et al. Airway management in a case of neck impalement: use of the oesophageal tracheal combitube airway. *Br J Anaesth* 1992; 68: 534–5.

65 Vézina M-C, Trépanier CA, Nicole PC, Lessard MR. Complications associated with the esophageal-tracheal Combitube® in the prehospital setting. *Can J Anesth* 2007; 54: 124–8.

66 Hatzakorzian R, Li Pi Shan W, Côté AV, Schricker T, Backman SB. Case Report: The management of severe emergence agitation using droperidol. *Anaesthesia* 2006; 61: 112–15.

67 Findlow D, Doyle E. Congenital heart disease in adults: Review Article. *Br J Anaesth* 1997; 78: 416–30.

68 *Cardiovascular Drug Guidelines*, 2nd edn. Victorian Medical Postgraduate Foundation Therapeutics Committee, Melbourne 1995: 133.

69 Dobb CJ. Cardiogenic shock. In: Oh TE, ed. *Intensive Care Manual*, 4th edn. Butterworth–Heinemann, Oxford 1997: 146–52.

70 Johnson MR. Congestive heart failure. In: Parrillo JE, ed. *Current Therapy in Clinical Care Medicine*, 3rd edn. Mosby, St Louis 1997; 109–15.

71 Francis GS. Congestive heart failure: Inotropic agents. In: Parrillo JE, ed. *Current Therapy in Clinical Care Medicine*, 3rd edn. Mosby, St Louis 1997: 116–21.

72 Mathens D, Stone DJ, Dent JM. Special article: preoperative cardiac risk stratification: ritual or requirement. *J Cardiothoracic Vascular Anaesthesia* 2001; 15: 626–30.

73 Kaluza GL, Joseph J, Lee JR, Raizner ME, Raizner AE. Catastrophic outcomes of noncardiac surgery soon after coronary stenting. *J Am Coll Cardiol* 2000; 35: 1288–94.

74 Breen P, Lee J-W, Pomposelli F, Park KW. Timing of high-risk vascular surgery following coronary artery bypass surgery: a 10 year experience from an academic centre. *Anaesthesia* 2004; 59: 422–7.

75 Reul GJ, Cooley DA, Duncan JM, et al. The effect of coronary artery bypass surgery on outcome of peripheral vascular operations in 1093 patients. *J Vasc Surg* 1986; 3: 788–98.

QUICK FLICK

C

76 Cruchley PM, Kaplan JA, Hug CC Jr, Nagle D, Sumpter R, Finucane D. Non-cardiac surgery in patients with prior myocardial revascularization. *Can Anaesth Soc J* 1983; 30: 629–34.

77 Chassot PG, Delabays A, Spahn DR. Perioperative anti platelet therapy: the case for continuing therapy in patients at risk of myocardial infarction. *Br J Anaesth* 2007; 99: 316–28.

78 Broad L, Lee T, Conroy M et al. Successful management of patients with a drug eluting stent presenting for elective non-cardiac surgery. *Br J Anaesth* 2007; 98: 19–22.

79 Posner KL, Van Norman GA, Chan V. Adverse cardiac outcomes after noncardiac surgery in patients with prior percutaneous transluminal coronary angioplasty. *Anesth Analg* 1999; 89: 553–60.

80 McFalls EO, Ward HB, Moritz TE, Goldman S, Krupski WC, Littooy F, et al. Coronary-artery revascularization before elective major vascular surgery. *N Engl J Med* 2004; 351: 2795–804.

81 Priebe H-J. Review article. Perioperative myocardial infarction—aetiology and prevention. *Br J Anaesth* 2005; 95: 3–19.

82 Runciman WB, Webb RK, Klepper ID et al. Crisis management—validation of an algorithm by an analysis of 2000 incident reports. *Anaesth Intensive Care* 1993; 21; 579–92.

83 Scrase I, Woollard M. Needle vs. surgical cricothyroidotomy: a short cut to effective ventilation. *Anaesthesia* 2006; 61: 962–74.

84 Dworkin R, Benumof JL, Karagianes TG. The effective tracheal diameter that causes air trapping during jet ventilation. *J Cardiothoracic Anesth* 1990; 4: 731–6.

○ Dalteparin

Dalteparin (Fragmin) is a type of low molecular weight heparin. *See Heparin (Unfractionated and Low Molecular Weight Heparins)* and *Deep Venous Thrombosis (DVT) Prophylaxis.*

○ Danaparoid

This drug is classed as a low molecular weight heparinoid and acts by inhibiting factor Xa. It is used IV or subcut for thromboprophylaxis and the dose must be reduced if there is renal impairment. It can be used in HITS patients but there is a risk of cross-reactivity with HITS antibodies. *See Heparin Induced Thrombocytopenia (HITS).*

○ Dantrolene

See Malignant Hyperthermia (MH).

○ D-dimer Test

This test detects elevated levels of fragments of fibrin and is a specific measure of fibrin degradation. *See Fibrin Degradation Products (FDPs).* Elevated D-dimers occur with disseminated intravascular coagulation (DIC) and is the most reliable lab test for DIC. *See Disseminated Intravascular Coagulation (DIC).* The normal level of D-dimer is < 500 ng/mL.

○ Decreased Level of Consciousness Postanaesthetic

See Confusion, Agitation, Decreased Level of Consciousness, Postanaesthetic.

○ Deep Venous Thrombosis (DVT) Prophylaxis

Topics Covered in this Section
▶ Risk of DVT
▶ Thrombophilia
▶ Points to Note Regarding DVT Prophylaxis
▶ Strategies for DVT Prophylaxis
▶ Postpartum Prophylaxis

For treatment of DVT *see Heparin (Unfractionated and Low Molecular Weight Heparins).*

The following guidelines are based mainly on recommendations from the Australian and New Zealand Working Party on the Management and Prevention of Venous Thromboembolism, July 2005.[1]

Risk of DVT

Many common surgical procedures are associated with a very high risk of DVT e.g. > 50% for hip replacement without thromboprophylaxis. Patients can be divided into low-, medium- and high-risk groups for DVT. Major surgery is defined as intra-abdominal surgery and other operations lasting more than 45 min. Risk factors for DVT include increasing age, obesity, cancer, previous DVT or PE, smoking, varicose veins, pregnancy, immobility, dehydration, sepsis, thrombophilia and hormone replacement therapy (HRT) or oral contraceptive pill (OCP) therapy.

Catergories of DVT Risk
Low Risk (Risk of DVT < 10%, risk of pulmonary embolus (PE) 0.01%)
1　Minor surgery lasting < 30 min in patients < 60 yrs.
2　Major surgery in a patient <40 yrs with no other risk factors.

Moderate Risk (Risk of DVT 10–40%, risk of PE 0.1–1%)
1　Major surgery in patient 40–60 yrs without other risk factors.
2　Minor surgery in patients aged 40–60 yrs with other risk factors.
3　Minor surgery in patient aged greater than 60 yrs.

High Risk (Risk of DVT 40–80%, risk of PE 1–10%)
Patients at high risk include:
1　Major surgery in patients > 60 yrs old.
2　Major orthopaedic surgery (e.g. hip fracture, hip replacement) or fracture of pelvis, hip or knee.
3　Multitrauma.
4　Abdominal or pelvic surgery for cancer.
5　Major surgery in patients aged 40–60 yrs with other risk factors.
6　Lower limb paralysis or amputation.
7　Thrombophilia.

Thrombophilia

Thrombophilia is an increased propensity to thromboembolic disease due to coagulation abnormalities. Thrombophilia can be due to acquired or congenital factors. Acquired causes include lupus anticoagulant, antiphospholipid antibodies and myeloproliferative disease. Congenital causes include activated protein C resistance (factor V Leiden), protein C deficiency and protein S deficiency and high homocysteine levels. Thrombophilia should be suspected in patients with:
1　family history of DVT/PE
2　recurrent DVT

3   unexplained DVT or PE before the age of 40.

Points to Note Regarding DVT Prophylaxis

1   Consider stopping HRT or the OCP in patients in the high- and moderate-risk categories. Cease HRT 6 weeks before surgery. The OCP should be stopped during the cycle before planned surgery.
2   Start subcut heparin 2 h before surgery unless epidural or spinal anaesthesia is planned. Continue heparin therapy until the patient is ambulant. Spinal or epidural anaesthesia reduces the incidence of DVT and PE.
3   Despite the high incidence of DVT in neurosurgery the risk of intracranial or intraspinal haemorrhage is also high with anticoagulation. Recommendations for patients having neurosurgery are:
   a) Mechanical methods of prophylaxis should be used in the peri-operative period. These include intra-operative and postoperative pneumatic compression stockings and graduated compression stockings.
   b) Five days should elapse after surgery before anticoagulant drugs are commenced.

Strategies for DVT Prophylaxis

Low-risk Group

Use intra-operative pneumatic compression stockings plus graduated compression stockings. Aim for early mobilisation post operatively.

Medium-risk Group

Use either fractionated or unfractionated heparin in the following dose:
1   *Heparin* 5000 units subcutaneously 8 h or 12 h.
2   *Dalteparin* (Fragmin) 2500 units subcutaneously as a single dose per 24 h.
3   *Enoxaparin* (Clexane) 20 mg subcutaneously as a single dose per 24 h.
4   *Nadroparin calcium* (Fraxiparin) 0.3 mL (2850 IU) subcutaneously as a single dose per 24 h.
Continue preferred drug for 7 days or until the patient is mobile. Use compression stockings on the ward plus intra-operative pneumatic compression stockings.

High-risk Group

Use one of the following recommended regimens:
1   *Dalteparin* (Fragmin) 5000 u subcutaneously on the evening before surgery and then every evening after surgery until at least 10 days postoperatively. Reduce dose to 2500 u/24 h if the patient is <50 kg or >80 yrs old.
2   *Enoxaparin* (Clexane) 40 mg subcutaneously on the evening before surgery

and then every evening after surgery until at least 10 days postoperatively. Reduce the dose to 20 mg if the patient is <50 kg or >80 yrs old. Use compression stockings on the ward plus intra-operative pneumatic compression stockings.

3 Therapy should continue for at least 10 days and up to 4–6 weeks for hip replacement surgery.

Note: If the risk of peri-operative bleeding is high, consider withholding the pre-operative dose and giving the first postoperative dose 24 h or more after surgery.

Postpartum Prophylaxis

Patients who have had CS or who are morbidly obsese (BMI>30) or vaginal deliveries with 4 or more risk factors should have clexane 40 mg daily until discharge. Risk factors include:

1 Age > 35.
2 Labour >12 h or instrumented vaginal delivery or major blood loss.
3 Parity > 4.
4 Major intercurrent illness.
5 Gross varicose veins.
6 DVT/PE in a first degree relative.
7 Heterozygous factor V (Leiden) or prothrombin gene mutation.

◐ Defibrillation

See *Cardioversion*.

◐ Defibrillators

Four different types of defibrillators are discussed:

1 Manual monophasic.
2 Manual biphasic.
3 Automated external defibrillators (AEDs) These are all biphasic.
4 Implantable (all biphasic). Also termed Automatic Implanted Cardiac Defibrillators (AICD).

Monophasic Defibrillators

These defibrillators deliver the shock (current) in a single direction from one paddle or electrode pad to the other.

Biphasic Defibrillators

These deliver a shock in two directions, from one paddle or electrode pad to the other then the current reverses direction. Biphasic waveforms decrease the threshold for successful defibrillations. This means biphasic defibrillators are more effective than monophasic defibrillators and use less electrical energy to defibrillate or cardiovert (around half the energy of monophasic defibrillators).[2] Using less electrical energy results in less post-shock myocardial dysfunction and a lower risk of skin burns.[3]

Automated External Defibrillators (AEDs)

Also called semi-automatic defibrillators. These devices are intended for use by rescuers with little or no level of CPR training from doctors to lay people. For example, emergency out of hospital defibrillation by security guards at casinos has resulted in a survival rate to hospital discharge of 74% (compared to 15% with in-hospital cardiac arrests).[4]

AEDs are indicated for use with patients who have collapsed and show no signs of life.

The steps to use these devices are:

1 Turn the machine 'on'. With some devices this will be achieved by opening the lid.
2 Voice prompts instruct the user to attach defibrillation electrodes (pads) to the chest wall in the positions illustrated on the electrode packet.
3 The voice prompt then requests that the patient not be touched and that the patient's rhythm be analysed.
4 If VF or rapid VT is diagnosed, the device will verbally advise that a shock be given and a button will 'light-up'. The machine will advise to stand clear and for the operator to push the button. After a single shock is given the device will advise that BLS be provided for 2 min and will then re-analyse the rhythm.
5 If 'no shock advised' the machine will recommend BLS measures.

Points to note with AEDs:

1 These devices can be used unmodified in children 8 years or older and/or >25 kg.
2 For patients aged 1–8 yrs use paediatric pads with an attenuator. If this is not available use the machine unmodified but do not let the pads touch each other.
3 Do not use the AED on children less than 1 year old.
4 Patients must be dried off if wet prior to using the AED.

Automatic Implanted Cardiac Defibrillators

See *Pacing, Pacemakers and Anaesthesia*.

◗ Depodur

See *Morphine, Extended Release Epidural*.

◐ Dermatomes

Table D1 Key dermatome landmarks

Dermatome	Anatomical site	Dermatome	Anatomical site
C5–T1	Upper Limb	T12–L1	Inguinal Ligament
C7	Middle finger	L3	Front of Knee
T3	Apex of Axilla	L4	Medial Side of Calf
T5	Nipple	L5	Outer Calf
T7	Tip of Xiphoid	S1	Outer Border of Foot
T10	Umbilicus	S2	Back of Knee

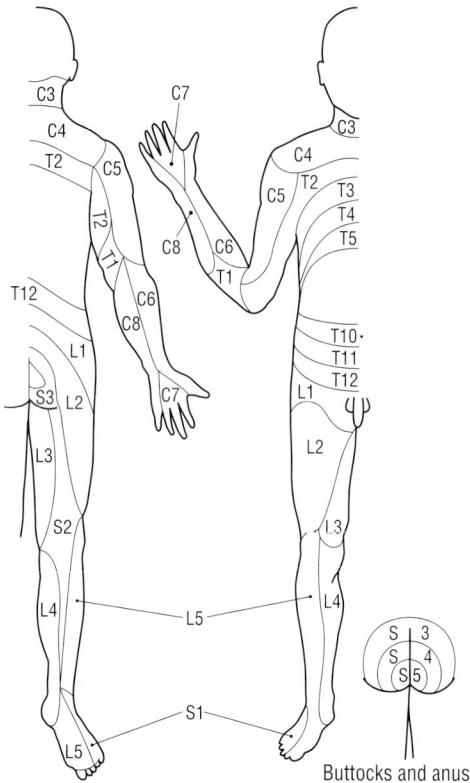

Figure D1 Dermatomes

◗ Desflurane

Methyl ethyl ether inhalational anaesthetic agent, very similar in structure to isoflurane.

Physical Properties and MAC

Blood:Gas Solubility Coefficient	0.42
Oil:Gas Solubility Coefficient	18.7
Saturated Vapour Pressure (20°C)	664 mm Hg
	(88.5 kPa)
Boiling Point	22.8°C
MAC	6.0

Comments and Dosing Guide (based on Dosing Guidelines from Baxter)

1 MAC varies with age. For children aged 1–12 years 8.1–9.1% is suggested. For elderly patients 5.2% is suggested.
2 Following IV induction of anaesthesia, a reasonable initial vaporiser setting is 4–6% with a fresh gas flow (FGF) of 3–5 L/min.
3 Gradually increase the delivered desflurane concentration by increments of 1% or less every few breaths with a FGF of 4–6 L/min, until the desired anaesthetic depth is reached. Do not attempt to increase anaesthetic depth quickly by rapidly increasing the inhaled desflurane concentration.
4 Once an adequate anaesthetic depth has been attained FGF rates can be reduced to a low flow e.g. 1 L/min.
5 Use of desflurane is associated with rapid emergence. Therefore, ensure that surgery is complete and that the timing of emergence is appropriate (e.g. turning patient from the prone position) prior to ceasing desflurane. Also ensure that muscle relaxation is reversed and the patient is adequately analgesed prior to ceasing desflurane.
6 Coughing on emergence can be attenuated with a small dose of opioid, propofol or lignocaine.

Advantages

1 Rapid onset and offset of effects due to low blood gas solubility. Desflurane has the lowest blood gas solubility of the potent inhalational anaesthetic agents.
2 Metabolised to a very small extent (0.02%). This is less than isoflurane.[5]
3 Pharmacodynamic effects are similar to isoflurane.

Disadvantages

1 Requires a unique and complex vaporiser which is electrically heated to 39°C and thermostatically controlled. Output from the vaporiser is determined by an electronically controlled pressure regulating valve. Vaporisers such as the Tec 6 weigh over 9 kg.[3]

QUICK FLICK

D

2   It has a low potency and is the least potent of the modern anaesthetic agents.
3   Its severe pungency makes it unsuitable for inhalational induction. Irritation of the airways by desflurane may be of particular concern in patients with bronchospastic disease.[6] Desflurane can cause bronchoconstriction, particularly in smokers.[7]
4   Rapidly increasing the inhaled concentration of desflurane or exceeding 1.25 MAC can result in significant sympathetic nervous system stimulation with tachycardia and hypertension.[8] Desflurane is not recommended for anaesthetic induction in patients with coronary artery disease.
5   Desflurane impairs cerebral autoregulation at concentrations greater than 0.5 MAC.[8] It is less suitable for neurosurgery and patients with raised ICP than sevoflurane.[8]
6   Interaction between desflurane and CO_2 absorbers can result in significant carbon monoxide formation. This tends to occur when the absorbent is dried e.g. flow of dry fresh gas over the absorbent for several hours between cases.[9]
7   Desflurane can cause malignant hyperthermia.
8   Desflurane has been associated with liver injury (but less commonly than with halothane or isoflurane).[10]

◐ Desmopressin (DDAVP)

An analogue of vasopressin, desmopressin may be useful for:
1   Treatment of diabetes insipidus.
2   To boost factor VIII concentration in mild-to-moderate haemophilia A.
3   To boost levels of von Willebrand factor. Although DDAVP is useful for the treatment of Type I von Willebrand's disease, it is contraindicated in Type II B disease.
4   To improve platelet function in illnesses where platelet function may be impaired e.g. renal disease.[11]
5   Situations involving heavy blood loss e.g. major orthopaedic surgery.[11]

Dose of DDAVP for Bleeding Associated with 2 to 4 Above
0.3 µg/kg/12 h. Give diluted in 50 mL N/S over 30 min. Monitor patient carefully for side effects such as vasodilatation and hypotension.

Risks
A review of desmopressin use to reduce blood loss indicated a small decrease in peri-operative haemorrhage and a 2.4-fold increase in the risk of myocardial infarction.[12]

◐ Dexamethasone

Powerful long-acting glucocorticoid drug with minimal mineralocorticoid activity, useful for the treatment of:

1 Cerebral oedema due to brain tumour.
2 Adrenal insufficiency.
3 Prevention of nausea and vomiting. A dose of 4–10 mg IV is effective in adults.[13] A dose of 0.5 mg/kg (up to 8 mg) has been found to be effective in children.[14] The combination of dexamethasone plus a 5-HT$_3$ antagonist such as ondansetron is probably the most effective drug combination to prevent postoperative nausea and vomiting.[15]

Note: If given in the awake patient dexamethasone can cause an unpleasant burning sensation in the lower pelvis due to an unknown mechanism.

◐ Dexmedetomidine

Dexmedetomidine is a potent, highly selective α2 adrenoreceptor agonist. The α2 to α1 ratio is 1600:1.

Mechanism of Action
Dexmedetomidine acts by decreasing noradrenaline release centrally and peripherally. This results in decreased sympathetic outflow from the CNS and decreases plasma noradrenaline concentrations.

Clinical Uses
It can be used in ICU by IV infusion to provide satisfactory analgesia and sedation as a single agent.[16]

Dose
Give an IV loading dose of 1 µg/kg over 10 min then an infusion of 0.2–0.7 µg/kg per h. Do not run infusion for more than 24 h.[17]

Adverse Effects
1 hypotension and bradycardia
2 hypoxia
3 atrial fibrillation,[17] sinus bradycardia[18]
4 dizziness.[19]

◐ Dextrans

Dextran is a polysaccharide derived from sucrose. Dextran 40 (10% solution) and dextran 70 (6% solution) are mixed with either 5% glucose or N/S. These solutions are used as volume expanders and in plastic surgery to reduce the risk of occlusion of microvascular anastamoses. Severe hypersensitivity reactions occur in 1 in 3300 patients. Dextran 1 (Promit) should be infused 1–2 min before the infusion of other dextran solutions. Use 20 mL for adults and 0.3 mL/kg for children.[20] This decreases the incidence of anaphylactic/anaphylactoid reactions by a factor of 35.[20]

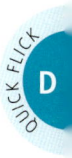

Dextran 70
Dextran 70 is used for plasma volume expansion via its osmotic effects. It has an intravascular half life of 6–12 hours.[21]

Dextran 40
Dextran 40 is used for:
1 Antithrombotic effects by inhibiting platelet adhesiveness and diluting clotting factors.[22]
2 Improves peripheral perfusion by decreasing blood viscosity, thus may be useful for graft and reimplantation procedures.
3 Dextran 40 is rapidly excreted by the kidney and if urinary flow is low, a high urinary concentration of Dextran 40 can result. This can lead to renal failure.[21] The plasma half life of Dextran 40 is 2–3 hours.[21]

Dextran and Volume Expansion
Titrate the volume infused to the desired clinical response. If more than 20 mL/kg is given within 24 h, increased bleeding may occur due to anticlotting effects. Dextran 40 is less effective than Dextran 70 for intravascular volume expansion and the effects are less long lasting. Dextrans are not the solutions of choice for volume expansion.

Dose of Dextran 40 for Thrombosis Prevention and Improving Microcirculation During Low Flow States
Give 500 mL over 4–6 h in the peri-operative period.
Repeat the dose in 24 h and, for high-risk patients, continue dextran on alternate days for up to 2 weeks.[23]

◖ Diabetes Mellitus, Preparation for Surgery

If possible, schedule the diabetic patient to be first on the morning or afternoon list, to minimise fasting times.

Topics Covered in this Section
▶ Insulin Dependent Diabetics (IDDM or Type I Diabetes)
▶ Preparing and Running an Insulin Glucose Infusion
▶ Non-insulin Dependent Diabetics (NIDDM or Type II Diabetics)
▶ Diet-controlled Diabetics

Insulin Dependent Diabetics (IDDM or Type I Diabetes)
IDDM patients can be suitable for day of surgery admission if their diabetes is well controlled and they do not require prolonged pre-operative fasting. One of several regimens may be used.

Regimen A
Morning Surgery
On the morning of surgery start 5% glucose IV at 125 mL/h and give half the

patient's usual morning insulin dose subcutaneously. Measure BSL 2 h and give subcutaneous insulin 5 units if BSL >12 mmol/ L.

Afternoon Surgery

1 If the patient is on unmixed insulin, give two-thirds of the usual morning dose of short-acting insulin and omit long-acting insulin prior to a light breakfast.
2 If the patient is on premixed insulin give half the usual insulin dose prior to breakfast.
3 Commence 5% glucose infusion at 1100 hrs.

Regimen B
Morning and Afternoon Surgery

On the morning of surgery commence an insulin/glucose infusion. Run 5% glucose at 125 mL/h and insulin at a rate dependent on patient's BSL, i.e. a sliding scale. Any values chosen for the scale need to be revised depending on the patient's response. Aim to keep BSL at ≈ 5–10 mmol/ L. If the patient is on the afternoon list allow an early light breakfast.

Patients with Insulin Pumps

Patients receiving insulin subcutaneously by a pump should have their pump switched off and be commenced on an insulin glucose infusion on the morning of surgery.[24]

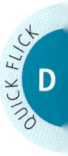

Preparing and Running an Insulin Glucose Infusion

Run 5% glucose at 80 mL/h. For renal failure patients on a fluid restriction run 10% glucose at 40 mL/h.

Insulin Infusion

Load 50 units of soluble insulin such as actrapid into a syringe with 50 mL of N/S. Flush the injection tubing with the above solution and discard the flush. This will saturate insulin binding sites on the plastic tubing. Start the infusion at 1–2 units per h.

Table D2 Example of a sliding scale for an insulin/glucose infusion

BSL (mmol/L)	Units of insulin/h
< 4	0 (call RMO)
4–8	1
8–12	2
12–16	3
> 16	4 (call RMO)

Measure BSL 2 h pre-operatively and 1 h intra- and postoperatively. If hypoglycaemia occurs (BSL <4 mmol/L) give 20–50 mL of 50% glucose and cease insulin. Notify medical staff.

Note: The half life of IV actrapid is only 5 min and with an IV infusion steady state is reached in 25–30 min.

Non-insulin Dependent Diabetics (NIDDM or Type II Diabetes)

1 Minor Surgery—Morning or Afternoon Lists
   a) No oral hypoglycaemic drugs on the day of surgery. If taking chlorpropamide, cease this for 24 h prior to surgery.
   b) Measure BSL pre-surgery, and at 6 h intervals if prolonged fasting. If BSL > 12 mmol/L consider the need for insulin/glucose infusion depending on such issues as the length of time before surgery and co-morbid conditions. If blood sugars are low (BSL <5 mmol) commence a glucose infusion. If the patient is on the afternoon list, give a light breakfast to finish 6 h before the scheduled operation time and clear fluids until 4 h before the operation. The patient should not have his/her usual morning anti-diabetic medication and an insulin/dextrose infusion commenced if patient becomes hypo/hyperglycaemic.
2 Major Surgery
   a) Cease oral agents as above.
   b) Measure BSL pre-operatively:
       i)   If BSL 6–11 mmol/L no specific preparation is required.
       ii) If BSL< 6 mmol/L start IV 5% glucose 125 mL/h.
       iii) If BSL > 11 mmol/L start insulin/glucose infusion as for IDDM (see below).
   c) If an insulin/glucose infusion is not required pre-operatively the anaesthetist may commence one intra-operatively if needed.

Diet-controlled Diabetics

Treat as for non-diabetic patients. As for all diabetics avoid lactate containing solutions (such as Hartmann's solution) as lactate is gluconeogenic. This view has been questioned in recent times. **See** *Hartmann's Solution (Ringer's Lactate)*.

◐ Diacetylmorphine/Diamorphine

Diamorphine (heroin) is a synthetic diacetylated derivative of morphine with strong analgesic properties. It is 1.5–2 × more potent than morphine. It is a prodrug which acts through its metabolites, 6-monoacetylmorphine and morphine.

Dose in Adults for Analgesia

IM 5–10 mg

IV Boluses 2.5 mg IV titrated to effect to 10 mg.

Epidural Dose a dose of 2.5 mg is appropriate for postoperative analgesia after CS.[25]

Intrathecal Dose 0.25–0.375 mg depending on the size and fitness of the patient.[26] Levy recommends a dose of 0.25 mg intrathecally for postoperative analgesia after CS.[25]

Advantages

Faster onset of action than morphine due to its higher lipid solubility. Possibly less nausea and vomiting than morphine.[27]

Disadvantages

Diamorphine produces marked euphoria and has a high addiction potential. Its medicinal use is banned in the United States but it is a popular analgesic in the United Kingdom.

◯ Diazepam

Benzodiazepine drug useful for sedation, anxiolysis, anterograde amnesia, muscle relaxation and for status epilepticus. Use of the IM route produces a suboptimal effect due to slow and erratic absorption from muscle.

Dose for Status Epilepticus

Adult IV 5–10 mg initially. May require up to 20–30 mg. ***See*** *Epilepsy, Status*.

Child 0.2 mg/kg/dose IV or 0.5 mg/kg PR.
Note: Diazepam is dissolved in propylene glycol which is very irritating to the veins and can cause pain on injection and thrombophlebitis. Give via a central line if one is available. In contrast, diazepam emulsion (diazemuls) is much better tolerated. Midazolam is an appropriate alternative.

Sedation/Anxiolysis

Adult 2–60 mg/day in divided doses PO.

Child 0.2–0.5 mg/kg/dose 8–12 h PO.

◯ Diazoxide

Diazoxide is a benzothiadiazine antihypertensive drug which is particularly useful in the treatment of pre-eclampsia/eclampsia (***see*** *Pre-eclampsia/ Eclampsia*). Acts directly on arteriolar smooth muscle causing relaxation. Also used to treat intractable hypoglycaemia. Acts by decreasing insulin secretion and inhibiting the peripheral utilisation of glucose.

Dose for Hypertensive Emergencies

Adult Give IV boluses of 30 mg up to a maximum of 150 mg as a single bolus dose. Hennessey et al. found that boluses of 15 mg of diazoxide 3 min

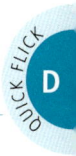

as needed were safe and effective for controlling blood pressure due to pre-eclampsia. Up to 300 mg could be given in an hour according to their protocol.[28]
Note: Single bolus doses of 300 mg have been associated with angina and with myocardial and cerebral infarction.[29]

Child 1–3 mg/kg IV repeat × 1 prn, then 2–5 mg/kg 6 h.

Diclofenac

Non-steroidal anti-inflammatory drug useful for the treatment of musculoskeletal and postoperative pain. Diclofenac is contraindicated in patients with peptic ulcer disease, gastro-intestinal bleeding and hypersensitivity to aspirin. Use with caution or avoid in asthmatic patients. ***See*** *Non-steroidal Anti-inflammatory Drugs (NSAIDS)*.

Dose
Adult 25–50 mg PO 8 h with food.

Child 1 mg/kg/dose (max 50 mg) 8 h.
Note: Diclofenac has been associated with hepatic toxicity and, rarely, acute immune haemolytic anaemia.[30]

Difficult Airway Management

All medical staff who practise intubation must have a plan for failed intubation which should be practise regularly so that it becomes second nature. Each practitioner should master some techniques and devices depending on what is available in their hospitals, and personal preference, to use when the need arises. Patients with difficult airways must be notified of this and provided with a suitable letter.

Topics Covered in this Section

- Predicting Difficult Intubation
- Management of Recognised Difficult Airway in Patients Requiring Intubation
- Management of Unrecognised Difficult Airway in Patients Requiring Intubation
- Extubation Strategy

Predicting Difficult Intubation

Failure to manage the difficult airway is the most common cause of anaesthetic death or brain damage.[31] The incidence of difficult intubation is 1–4% and the incidence of impossible intubation is 0.05–0.35%.[32] Obstetric patients have a higher incidence of failed intubation, about 1 per 250–300. ***See*** *Caesarean Section (CS)*. Up to 16% of difficult intubations can *not* be predicted from the risk assessment techniques described below.[33] Predictors of difficult intubation include the following:

1 Mallampati Test (as modified by Samsoon and Young)[34]
   The patient is asked to maximally protrude the tongue from the fully open mouth while sitting upright. Visible pharyngeal structures are used to classify the airway as follows.
   a) Class 1—soft palate, fauces, uvula and pillars all visible.
   b) Class 2—as above but pillars obscured.
   c) Class 3—only soft palate and base of uvula visible.
   d) Class 4—hard palate only visible.
   Note: The higher the class the more potentially difficult is the intubation. This test predicts only about 50% of difficult intubations and has a high incidence of false positives.[35]

2 Thyromental Distance
   This is the straight line distance between the thyroid notch and the lower border of the chin with the head extended.[36] It is predicted that:
   a) > 6.5 cm—easy laryngoscopy.
   b) 6–6.5 cm—difficult laryngoscopy.
   c) < 6 cm—very difficult/impossible laryngoscopy.[37]

3 Wilson Risk Sum Score[38]
   Evaluates 5 factors felt to be correlated with difficult intubation. These are weight, head and neck movement, mouth opening, jaw development (receding or non-receding) and prominence of upper incisors. Each factor has 3 possible scores (0, 1 or 2) and the range of scores is 0–10. A score of 2 predicts 75% of difficult intubations.[35] This scoring system has a sensitivity of ≈ 40–75%,[38,39] a specificity of ≈ 90% and a positive predictive value of ≈ 9%.[39]

Management of Recognised Difficult Airway in Patients Requiring Intubation

Cooperative Patient

The following options are to be considered.

1 Evaluate the suitability of local or regional anaesthesia for the surgery planned.

2 If local or regional anaesthesia is not a viable option (e.g. patient refusal) the next best option is to **secure the airway awake**. Intubation awake will almost always be the safest option. In borderline cases consider topicalising the oral airway with LA (+/– sedation) and performing a direct laryngoscopy. If the laryngeal view is good induce GA.

3 When securing the airway awake give supplemental oxygen therapy during the procedure e.g. by nasal prongs. Techniques that can be used include:
   a) Fibre-optic intubation (**see** *Awake Fibre-optic Intubation*).

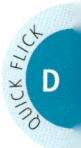

b) Use of an optical/video laryngoscope such as an Airtraq or GlideScope.

c) Use of a C-Trach™, Fastrach™ or LMA to facilitate intubation. *See Laryngeal Mask Airway (Including ProSeal™, Fastrach™ and C-Trach™)*.

e) Blind nasal intubation (*see Blind Nasal Intubation*).

f) Retrograde intubation techniques (*see Retrograde Intubation*).

g) Use of the Lightwand in the awake patient (*see Lightwand Intubation*).

h) Surgical airway under LA. *See Cricothyroid Puncture and Cricothyrotomy*.

Uncooperative Patient

This situation has the potential to result in an anaesthetic crisis situation (i.e. hypoxic brain injury/death). Options are to perform a gaseous induction/gradual IV propofol induction or a surgical airway with LA. Spontaneous ventilation must be maintained until the airway is secured. The following issues must be considered:

1 How much planning time is available? Is the patient's life immediately threatened if surgery does not proceed, or if the airway is not secured?

2 What is the intubation plan?

3 What is the 'plan B' if the intubation plan fails?

4 Is the appropriate equipment and personnel immediately available e.g. surgeon to perform emergency surgical airway? The 'intubation plan' is usually a gaseous induction followed by direct laryngoscopy. If this is not successful (as predicted) use your preferred device as described for securing the airway awake e.g. FOB, Airtraq. Plan B may be to perform surgery with a ProSeal™, formation of a surgical airway or to wake the patient up depending on circumstances. If spontaneous ventilation ceases and the patient cannot be ventilated by bag and mask, this is a crisis situation and the following steps should be taken:

a) Summon skilled assistance and notify the surgeon.

b) Insert a LMA or ProSeal™.

c) If still unable to ventilate obtain a surgical airway.

Management of Unrecognised Difficult Airway in Patients Requiring Intubation

The following discussion assumes the patient is under general anaesthesia and the first attempt at intubation is unsuccessful. Do not attempt intubation via direct laryngoscopy more than 3 times. *Oxygenation not intubation* is the overriding goal.

Optimising Intubating Conditions

1 Ensure that the patient is in the best possible position for intubation. This means with the neck slightly flexed and the head extended on the neck at the atlanto-occipital joint aligning the oral, pharyngeal and laryngeal

Patient cooperative?

Yes ◄─────────────────────────► No

Regional technique appropriate?

Yes   No

Proceed ◄── Awake intubation e.g. FOB
or surgical airway awake

Inhalational or propofol
infusion induction. Maintain
spontaneous ventilation

Direct laryngoscopy
Able to intubate?

Yes ◄─────► No

Able to Mask Oxygenate?

Yes   No

Able to intubate? ◄── Intubate using special device
e.g. FOB, Airtraq, C-Trach, Fastrach™

Insert LMA, ProSeal™
Able to oxygenate?

Yes

Yes ◄─── No

Yes

No
Options depending on circumstances
a) wake patient up
b) proceed with LMA/ProSeal™
c) surgical airway

Proceed with Definitive ◄──────────────── Surgical airway
Surgical Airway (tracheotomy, cricothyrotomy)
Or wake patient depending on circumstances

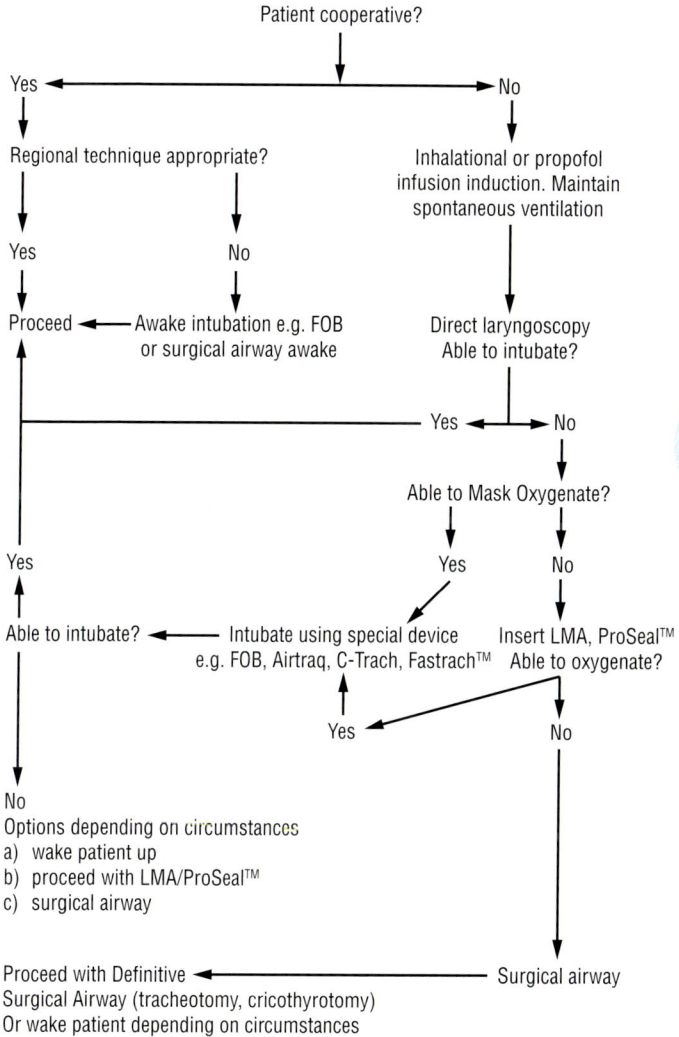

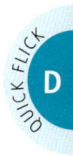

Figure D2 Management of the recognised difficult airway requiring intubation

D

QUICK FLICK

axes into a straight line. In obese patients it may be necessary to place pillows and/or blankets behind the back shoulders and head to obtain the best 'sniff' position. Placing the patient slightly sitting up by breaking the middle of the bed may help obstacles like large pendulous breasts 'flow away' from the airway rather than towards it. Lee et al. found that a 25° back-up position significantly improved laryngeal view.[40]

2 The person attempting the intubation for the second time should be the most 'experienced' anaesthetist immediately available. Optimal external laryngeal manipulation should be undertaken to improve the laryngeal view. This may be backwards, upwards and rightwards pressure—the so called BURP manoeuvre.[41] Consider the 2-anaesthetist technique in which the first anaesthetist uses the laryngoscope and laryngeal manipulation to obtain the best view and the second anaesthetist inserts the tube. Note that inexpertly applied cricoid pressure itself may make intubation difficult and this may need to be relaxed briefly to allow intubation.

3 Mandibular advancement (an assistant pulls the jaw forward) may improve the laryngeal view.[42]

4 Consider using the McCoy laryngoscope. It has a hinged distal tip activated by a lever on the handle and is particularly useful in this situation.

5 Consider using a Teflon bougie if there is any view of the epiglottis. In this technique the distal 1 cm of the bougie is formed into a slight hook shape. While an assistant gently steadies the distal end, the proximal end is positioned by the anaesthetist to scrape along the posterior surface of the epiglottis towards the larynx exactly in the midline. The distal tip of the bougie may thus enter the trachea blindly and this can be confirmed by feeling a bumping sensation on the tracheal rings. The ET tube is then railroaded over the Teflon bougie.

6 Consider using the Airtraq, an optical laryngoscope which requires minimal preparation time. **See** *Airtraq*.

7 Henderson describes a technique using a straight blade (e.g. Miller) lateral to the tongue when a McIntosh (curved blade) has failed.[43] With the head slightly turned to the left, a size 3 Miller blade is inserted through the right corner of the mouth, over the molars, and along the groove between the right tonsil and tongue. The tongue is pushed to the left and the epiglottis is lifted with the anterior pharyngeal structures. It is helpful to have an assistant retract the right corner of the mouth and to use a semi-rigid stylet in a hockey-stick shape. Alternatively a Teflon bougie can be inserted into the trachea and then the tube railroaded over this as described above.

Unable to Intubate but Able to Ventilate—Steps in Management

The priority at this stage is to maintain oxygenation and ventilation with bag-mask technique. To optimise mask ventilation:

1 Optimise the airway by providing maximal jaw thrust, adequate head tilt

and use of jaw support (opening the mouth slightly).

2 Use a 2-handed grip on the mask, while an assistant squeezes the reservoir bag (2-anaesthetist ventilation technique).

3 Insert an oral (guedel) and/or nasal airway.

If able to mask ventilate and surgery is not immediately urgent allow the patient to wake up and formulate a new plan. **See** the section above on management of the recognised difficult airway for intubation.

If surgery is immediately urgent options are:

1 Surgery under mask anaesthesia.

2 Surgery using a ProSeal™ or LMA.

3 Intubation using techniques such as the FOB, C-Trach™, Fastrach™ or Airtraq. Other techniques such as retrograde intubation or the Lightwand can be considered.

4 Obtaining a surgical airway.

Unable to Intubate and Unable to Ventilate–This is a CRISIS SITUATION

1 Summon urgent skilled assistance and notify the surgeon.

2 Insert a LMA or ProSeal™. It may be necessary to partly or fully release cricoid pressure to enable correct placement of the laryngeal mask or ProSeal™.[44] A technique of ProSeal™ insertion described by Brimacombe[45] may be ideally suited to this situation. This technique involves:

    a) The ProSeal™ is deflated and shaped in the usual way in preparation for insertion.

    b) A well-lubricated gum elastic bougie (GEB) is passed through the drain tube of the ProSeal™. Use a thin Teflon bougie if a GEB is not available.

    c) A laryngoscope is used to visualise the oesophagus and the GEB is deliberately inserted down the oesophagus.

    d) The ProSeal™ is then railroaded over the GEB into place over the larynx. This appears to be the most efficient method yet discovered for insertion of the ProSeal™ into an anatomically correct position.

3 If ventilation is adequate options are:

    a) Wake patient up and proceed with management of the recognised difficult airway for intubation as described above.

    b) If the risk of not proceeding with surgery is greater than the risk of surgery with a supraglottic airway, proceed with surgery.

    c) Intubate the patient using fibre-optic bronchoscope, Airtraq, Glidescope, C-Trach™, Fastrach™, Lightwand retrograde intubation or other suitable technique. For a method of using the LMA as a conduit for intubation **see** *Laryngeal Mask Airway (Including ProSeal™, Fastrach™ and C-Trach™)*.

4 If still unable to ventilate the patient then a surgical airway must be obtained. Options are cricothyroid puncture, cricothyrotomy or tracheostomy. **See** *Cricothyroid Puncture and Cricothyrotomy*.

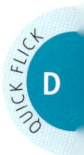

Unrecognised difficult Intubation
First attempt at intubation fails

↓

Optimise next 2 attempts (consider the use of the Airtraq
if immediately available) then cease intubation attempts

↓

Attempt mask ventilation.
Successful?

Yes ←——————————————————————→ No

Yes branch:

↓

Surgery must proceed?

Yes → Proceed path (Mask ventilation adequate for surgery?)

No → Wake patient up

Mask ventilation
adequate for
surgery?

Yes → Proceed

No ------ Consider → Intubate using e.g. Airtraq, C-Trach, Fastrach™, FOB or retrograde technique or surgical airway

No branch:

↓

Insert LMA, ProSeal™.
Ventilation successful?

Yes → Surgery must proceed?

No → Wake patient up

Yes → LMA/ProSeal™ adequate for surgery?

No → Surgical
(Definitive
Surgical Airway if
surgery must proceed
e.g. tracheostomy,
cricothyrotomy)
Otherwise wake
patient up

LMA/ProSeal™ adequate
for surgery?

No → Intubate using e.g. Airtraq, C-Trach, Fastrach™, FOB or retrograde technique or surgical airway

Yes → Proceed

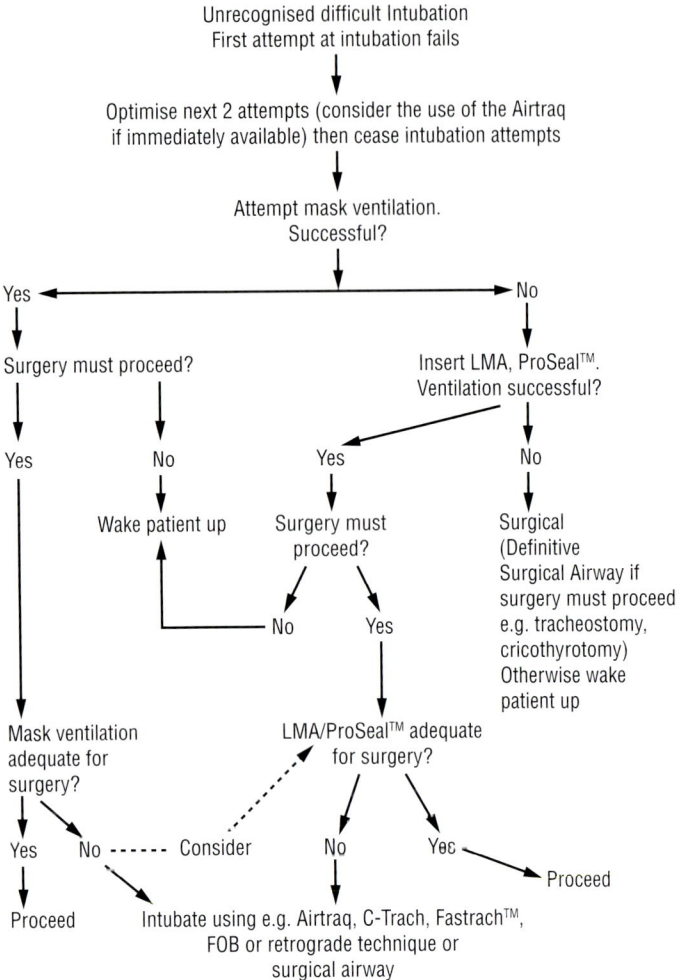

Figure D3 Management of the unrecognised difficult airway

Special Considerations

The ASA Difficult Airway Algorithm recommends that if the LMA is unsuccessful and the 'cannot intubate/cannot ventilate' scenario occurs, that consideration be given to using the Combitube (**see** *Combitube*™). If this is unsuccessful proceed to creating a surgical airway.[46]

Extubation Strategy

There must always be a contingency plan for the patient with a difficult airway in case extubation fails.

1 Extubate the patient when he/she regains consciousness. Do not attempt deep extubation.
2 Consider inserting an Airway Exchange Catheter (AEC) through the ET tube and extubating over this, leaving the AEC in the trachea. Oxygen can be provided through a connection at the proximal end of the AEC. If extubation is not tolerated an ET tube can be railroaded over the AEC into the trachea. **See** *Airway Exchange Catheters (AEC)*.
3 Obviously if a particular device such as the Airtraq was successfully used to intubate the patient then the same device may again be successful.

◖ Digital Nerve Block

Anatomy

The fingers/toes are supplied by 4 nerve branches of the digital nerve, 2 palmar/plantar and 2 dorsal.

Technique for Finger Block

1 Place the hand palm down on a flat surface.
2 Insert a 25 G needle on one side of the base of the proximal phalanx aiming to almost transfix the finger as close to the proximal phalanx as possible. Inject a total of 2 mL of 2% lignocaine on each side.

Note: Do not use Adrenaline containing solutions.

◖ Digoxin

Digoxin is a cardiac glycoside which acts by inhibiting Na^+/K^+ – ATP-ase leading to decreased Na^+/K^+ pump function. This results in increased intracellular Na^+ which in turn causes increased intracellular Ca^{2+} resulting in a positive inotropic effect on cardiac myocytes. Digoxin also decreases intracellular K^+ leading to a slowing of atrio-ventricular conduction and of depolarisation of pacemaker cells. In addition, digoxin increases vagal activity. Digoxin is useful for the treatment of:

1 Atrial fibrillation and flutter.
2 Congestive cardiac failure.

Dose

See *Atrial Fibrillation (AF), Acute and Chronic*. TR of digoxin is 1–2 ng/mL.

◖ Direct Acting Thrombin Inhibitors (DTI)[47]

These drugs are anticoagulants that act by binding directly to thrombin. They include hirudins (from leeches), bivalirudin and argatroban which are used

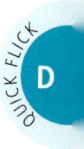

parentally and ximelagatran which is used orally. These drugs are useful anticoagulants for patients who cannot have heparin due to heparin induced thrombocytopenia (HITS) for indications such as cardiopulmonary bypass, dialysis and percutaneous coronary angiography. *See Heparin Induced Thrombocytopenia Syndrome (HITS)*. For discussion regarding individual drugs *see Fondaparinux* and *Argatroban*.

DTIs and Anaesthesia/Surgery
Most of these drugs have short half-lives and can be stopped several hours before surgery. At this stage no guidelines are available regarding these drugs and neuro-axial blockade.

Treatment of Bleeding in the Presence of DTI Drug
There is no direct acting antidote. Treatment options include:
1 prothrombim complex concentrates given with vitamin K
2 FFP
3 recombinant factor VIIa
4 dialysis with polymethyl-methyl acrylate membranes (for hirudin)
5 modified ultrafiltration (bivalirudin).

◖ Disseminated Intravascular Coagulation (DIC)

Pathophysiology
DIC is a syndrome that is always secondary to another disease process. It is characterised by massive systemic intravascular coagulation leading to deposition of fibrin in the microvasculature, thrombin generation, consumption of platelets and deficiency in clotting and anticlotting blood factors. This process leads to:
1 Haemorrhage due to consumption of platelets and clotting factors as well as the anticoagulant effect of fibrin degradation products (FDPs). *See Fibrin Degradation Products (FDPs)*.
2 Microvascular obstruction due to microclot and fibrin deposition leading to end organ damage. Features such as renal failure and ARDS may occur.
3 CVS collapse, death. Both DIC and the underlying causative disorder(s) are associated with very high mortality rates.

Aetiology
DIC can be triggered by any condition which produces damage to vascular endothelium, or that releases damaged or necrotic tissue into the blood stream. Such precipitating events include:
1 Obstetric complications including haemorrhagic shock, infection, placental abruption, pre-eclampsia/eclampsia, amniotic fluid embolus and fetal death in utero.
2 Sepsis e.g. meningococcaemia.
3 Trauma, especially brain and crush injuries and burns.

4   Transfusion reactions.
5   Malignancy.
6   Severe liver failure.
7   Severe toxic or immunological reactions e.g. snake bite, transplant rejection.
There are many other causes and the condition can be acute and fulminant
or chronic and subtle.

Clinical Manifestations of Acute DIC

These are highly variable. The effects of microvascular thrombi may
predominate initially then haemorrhagic effects may be more significant.
Clinical symptoms and signs include:

1   Delirium, coma, cerebral infarction.
2   Renal impairment/failure.
3   Skin ulceration, necrosis, gangrene.
4   Cyanosis, hypoxia, dyspnoea, pulmonary infarction.
5   Bruising, petechiae.
6   Severe haemorrhage from lungs, GIT, genitourinary tract and wounds.
    Intracranial haemorrhage may occur.

Diagnosis

DIC is characterised by:

1   Low fibrinogen levels (NR 200–400 mg/100 mL).
2   Elevated FDP levels (NR <10 µg/mL) in almost all cases. In DIC FDPs may
    be > 40 µg/mL.
3   D-dimer test confirms fibrin degradation. D-dimer is a measure of
    fragments of cross-linked fibrin. *See D-dimer Test*.
4   Reduced platelet count and reduced levels of anti-thrombin III and
    factors V and VIII.
5   Abnormal clotting studies. Total clotting time, prothrombin time (PT)
    and activated partial thromboplastin time (APTT) may all be prolonged.
    See *Prothrombin Time* and *Activated Partial Thromboplastin Time (APTT)*.
6   In many cases PT and APTT can be in or below the normal range due to
    activated factors affecting these tests.[48]

Treatment

1   Resuscitate the patient ensuring an adequate airway and ventilation.
    Maintain the patient's circulation with appropriate fluids (i.e. crystalloid/
    colloid/blood) + inotropic support. *See Blood Transfusion*.
2   Identify the pathological process triggering DIC and treat definitively if possible.
3   Attempt to reverse the coagulopathy and reduce blood loss. *Organise
    urgent consultation with a haematologist.* A combination of blood,
    platelets, fresh frozen plasma, cryoprecipitate and clotting factor
    concentrates will be required. Aim to maintain APTT in the normal range
    and platelet count > 50 × 10⁹/L. In general PT should be ignored.[49]

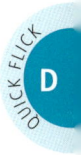

4 Cryoprecipitate infusion should be targeted towards a fibrinogen level of 100–150 mg/dL.

5 Heparin therapy is controversial. It is indicated for patients with overt thromboembolism or with severe end-organ damage due to fibrin deposition.[50] The rationale is that DIC is driven by the pathological production of thrombin and heparin inhibits thrombin. At the 'right dose' it is hypothesised that heparin will inhibit the low concentration of thrombin in the circulation without preventing appropriate haemostatic plugs forming at extravascular sites. Several heparin regimens are suggested. Horne[49] recommends heparin 20 u/kg bolus then 5 u/kg/h. Measure platelet count and fibrinogen levels which should both increase with treatment. APPT cannot be used to monitor therapy and PT may not be helpful. Increase dose by 25% every 4–6 h until the platelet and fibrinogen levels stabilise at a satisfactory level. If bleeding worsens stop heparin or decrease infusion rate.

Feinstein[51] suggests giving IV heparin at a rate of 7.5 u/kg/h. After 1–2 h give platelets to increase levels to 50 000/mL and cryoprecipitate to increase fibrinogen levels to 150 mg/100 L. Measure platelet and fibrinogen levels 30–60 min after transfusion. If adequate counts and levels are not achieved or maintained, increase the rate of heparin infusion by 2.5 u/kg/h. Repeat this sequence of evaluation.

6 Antithrombin III concentrates appear to have a beneficial effect on laboratory parameters but survival rates are not significantly increased.[50]

7 Recombinant activated Protein C administration appears to significantly reduce mortality.[50]

8 Recombinant activated factor VII (rFVIIa) has produced dramatic haemorrhage control in patients with intractable bleeding and DIC.[52] ***See** Recombinant Activated Factor VII (RFVIIA).*

◗ Dobutamine

Dobutamine is a synthetic isoprenaline derivative. Dobutamine is used for its positive inotropic effects in situations where there is low cardiac output due to such causes as myocardial infarction, cardiac surgery or cardiomyopathy.

Acts mainly on β1 adrenergic receptors, with a slight action on β2 and α adrenergic receptors. Dobutamine's main effects are to increase cardiac contractility and heart rate, with a modest decrease in systemic vascular resistance.

Dobutamine has similar properties to a combination of dopamine and sodium nitroprusside i.e. a fixed combination of inotropic drug and vasodilator.

Preparation and Administration
Mix 250 mg dobutamine with 100 mL of 5% glucose. Administer preferably via a central line, but as there is little vasoconstrictor activity, it can be given via a peripheral cannula temporarily.

Dose

Titrate to desired effect. Dose range: 0.5–40 µg/kg/min. Start with 2.5–5 µg/kg/min.

Table D3 Rate of infusion of dobutamine for a 70 kg patient

Rate of infusion	Dose
1.7 mL/h	1 µg/kg/min
4.2 mL/h	2.5 µg/kg/min
25.5 mL/h	15 µg/kg/min

Alternatively mix (3 × body wt) mg in 50 mL N/S, 1 mL/h = 1 µg/kg/min.

◖ Dolasetron Mesylate

Long-acting single daily dose anti-emetic which acts through selective 5-HT$_3$ receptor antagonism. No dosage adjustment is required in the presence of renal or hepatic impairment.

Dose

Adult For the *prevention* of nausea/vomiting (N/V) give 12.5 mg IV over 30 s or 50 mg PO daily. For the *treatment* of N/V give 12.5 mg IV over 30 s daily. Not currently approved for use in children.

◖ Dopamine

Naturally occurring catecholamine used for its positive inotropic and chronotropic actions and its effects on systemic vascular resistance, via its actions on α and β adrenergic receptors. Dopamine also has the ability to increase renal blood flow via its action on specific dopamine receptors and to increase urine output. Some researchers argue that dopamine's cardiac inotropic effect is the main mechanism for increased renal blood flow, and increased urine output may be due to a direct tubular action.[53]

Uses

1 Positive inotropic agent in low cardiac output states.
2 Impending renal failure to improve renal perfusion and urine output. There is no good scientific evidence that low dose dopamine can prevent or reverse acute renal failure.

Dose

Depends on desired effect, dose range 1–20 µg/kg/min.

Low Dose > (1–5 µg/kg/min) Stimulates mainly dopamine receptors causing renal vasodilatation and increased renal blood flow and urine output. There is no evidence of renal benefit with dopamine use.

Medium Dose > (5–10 µg/kg/min) β Adrenergic effects predominate with increased cardiac output mainly due to increased stroke volume. Blood pressure may fall due to β2 adreno-receptor mediated vasodilatation causing decreased systemic vascular resistance.

High Dose > (>15 µg/kg/min) α Adrenergic effects predominate with increased systemic vascular resistance and subsequent increased blood pressure. May get baroreceptor mediated reflex bradycardia. Renal blood flow is decreased.

Preparation and Administration
Mix 200 mg dopamine with 100 mL 5% glucose. Administer only by a central venous line.

Table D4 Rate of administration of dopamine (2 mg/mL) for 70 kg patient

µg/kg/min (mL/h)	Used for
3 (6.3 mL/h)	Improving Renal Function
8 (17 mL/h)	Mainly β Effects
16 (34 mL/h)	Mainly α Effects

Alternatively Mix (3 × body wt) mg with 50 mL N/S
1 mL/h = 1 µg/kg/min.

Other Effects of Dopamine
1 Increased Na^+ excretion by the kidney.
2 Emetic effect.
3 Increased prolactin release.
4 Tachycardia and tachydysrhythmias.
5 Depressed respiratory drive (hypoxic and central).
6 Increased intra-pulmonary shunt.
7 Gut ischaemia may occur.

▷ Dopexamine

Dobutamine analogue, agonist at Dopamine (DA) 1 and β2 adreno-receptors with lesser effect on DA2 and β1 adreno-receptors. Dopexamine has minimal α adreno-receptor effects.

Uses
Improving cardiac output (CO) in low CO states e.g. post cardiac surgery and acute heart failure.

Main Effects
Dopexamine increases CO and heart rate. It decreases systemic vascular resistance with little change in blood pressure. It causes increased renal blood flow due to its DA1 receptor stimulation effects with increased urinary output.

Dose
Given by IV infusion 0.5–6 µg/kg/min, titrate to desired clinical effect.

◗ Double Lumen Endotracheal Tubes

See One Lung Ventilation.

◗ Doxacurium

Benzylisoqninolinium type non-depolarising neuromuscular blocking drug. It is long acting and 2.5–3 × more potent than pancuronium.

Dose

For intubation, give 50–80 µg/kg. 'Top up' dose: 5–10 µg/kg. Duration of action ≈ 100 min.

Note: Doxacurium is not metabolised, it is excreted in bile and urine unchanged. The drug does not release histamine and is very cardiovascularly stable.

◗ Doxapram

Respiratory stimulant drug which acts by stimulating peripheral carotid chemoreceptors and the medullary respiratory centres. Used for:

1   Counteracting post-anaesthetic respiratory depression.
2   Treating laryngospasm.

Dose

1 mg/kg IV, acts in 20–40 s and lasts 5–12 min.

Can also be given by infusion: 1–3 mg/min (in the adult).

Note: Doxapram should not be used in patients with epilepsy, thyrotoxicosis, ischaemic heart disease or hypertension.

◗ Drixine

See Oxymetazoline.

◗ Droperidol

Butyrophenone derivative useful for its anti-emetic effects and in the treatment and prevention of postoperative agitation. Droperidol exerts its effects by dopamine 2 receptor blockade, post-synaptic GABA antagonism and some α adrenergic receptor blocking effects. It may be more effective for preventing nausea than vomiting.

Dose

Dose for Antiemesis in Adult 0.625 mg–1.25 mg IV. Its duration of action is limited by its elimination half-life of ≈ 2 h.

Dose for Antiemesis in Child 10–20 µg/kg IV.

Dose for Prevention and Treatment of Emergence Agitation in Adults 4–8 mg may be effective.[54] **See** Confusion, Agitation, Decreased Level of Consciousness, Postanaesthic.

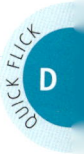

Note:

1 Droperidol causes dose-dependent sedation and drowsiness. Droperidol can cause neuroleptic malignant syndrome. ***See*** *Neuroleptic Malignant Syndrome (NMS)*.[55]

2 Droperidol increases the Q-T interval in a dose dependent fashion. This can result in dysrhythmias such as torsades de pointes and cardiac arrest. These effects are very rare at a dose of less than 2.5 mg.[56] Do not use droperidol if the QTc interval is prolonged (> 450 ms for males and >470 ms for females). ***See*** *Long QT Syndrome (LQTS)*.

3 Droperidol may be useful for morphine PCA induced PONV in adults e.g. consider adding droperidol 2.5 mg to 100 mg of morphine for PCA use.[57]

▶ Dynastat

See *Parecoxib (Dynastat)*.

▶ Dystonic Reaction, Acute

This syndrome is characterised by tonic muscular contractions such as torticollis, oculogyric crisis and opisthotonis. Exaggerated posturing of the head, neck and/or jaw and laryngo-pharyngeal spasm may also be seen. It occurs as an idiosyncratic reaction to drugs such as metoclopramide and prochlorperazine. This side effect is due to the central dopaminergic 2 receptor blockade effect of these drugs.

Treatment

Give benztropine mesylate 0.5–2 mg IV or IM *or* procyclidine 5–10 mg IV.

REFERENCES

1 *The Australian and New Zealand Working Party on the Management and Prevention of Venous Thromboembolism* (Booklet) Prevention of Venous Thromboembolism. Health Education and Management Innovations 2005.

2 Mittal S, Ayati S, Stein KM, et al. Comparison of a novel rectilinear biphasic waveform with a damped sine wave monophasic waveform for transthoracic ventricular defibrillation. *J Am Coll of Cardiol* 1999; 34: 1595–601.

3 Bardy GH, Marchlinski FE, Sharma AD, et al. Multicenter comparisons of truncated biphasic shocks and standard dampened sine wave monophasic shocks for transthoracic ventricular defibrillation. *Circulation* 1996; 94: 2507–14.

4 Valenzuela TD, Roe DJ, Nichol G, et al. Outcomes of rapid defibrillation by security officers after cardiac arrest in casinos. *N Eng J Med* 2000; 343: 1206–9.

5 Ball C, Westhorpe RN. Desflurane. *Anesth Intensive Care* 2007; 35: 657.

6   Apfelbaum JL. The new inhaled agents. Audio-Digest *Anesthesiology*
     1996; 21.

7   Goff MJ, Shahbaz RA, Ficke DJ, Uhrich TD, Ebert TJ. Absence of
     bronchodilation during desflurane anaesthesia. *Anesthesiology* 2000; 93:
     404–8.

8   Bedfort NM, Hardman JG, Nathanson MH. Cerebral hemodynamic
     response to the introduction of desflurane: a comparison with
     sevoflurane. *Anesth Analg* 2000; 91: 152–5.

9   Frink EJ. Toxicologic potential of desflurane and sevoflurane. *Acta
     Anaesthesiol Scand* 1995; 39: 120–3.

10   Anderson JS, Rose N, Martin JL et al. Desflurane hepatitis associated with
     hapten and auto antigen-specific antibodies. *Anesth Analg* 2007; 104:
     1452–3.

11   Ramsey JG. Methods of reducing blood loss and non blood substitutes.
     Can J Anaesth 1991; 3: 595–612.

12   Levy JH. Novel pharmacologic approaches to reduce bleeding. *Can J
     Anesth (Suppl)* 2003; 50: S26–S30.

13   Coloma M, Duffy LL, White P et al. Dexamethasone facilitates discharge
     after outpatient anorectal surgery. *Anesth Analg* 2001; 92: 85–8.

14   Aouad MT, Siddik SS, Rizk LB, et al. The effect of dexamethasone on
     postoperative vomiting after tonsillectomy. *Anesth Analg* 2001; 34:
     684–8.

15   Tramér MR. A rational approach to the control of postoperative nausea
     and vomiting: evidence from systemic reviews. Part 1. Efficacy and harm
     of antiemetic interventions, and methodological issues. *Acta Anaesthesiol
     Scand* 2001; 45: 4–13.

16   Hall JE, Uhrich TD, Barney JA, et al. Sedative, amnestic, and analgesic
     properties of small dose dexmedetomidine infusions. *Anesth Analg* 2000;
     90: 699–705.

17   Van Heerden PV. Sedation, Analgesia and Muscle Relaxation in the
     Intensive Care Unit. In Bersten AD, Soni N, Oh TE eds. *Oh's Intensive Care
     Manual* 5th edn. Butterworth–Heinemann, Edinburgh 2003: 833–40.

18   Aantaa R, Scheinin M. Alpha$_2$-adrenergic agents in anaesthesia. *Acta
     Anaesthesiol Scand* 1993; 37:433–48.

19   Aantaa R, Kanto J, Scheinin M. Intramuscular dexmedetomidine, a
     novel alpha$_2$-adreno receptor agonist, as premedication for minor
     gynaecological surgery. *Acta Anaesthesiol Scand* 1993; 35: 283–8.

20   Ljungström K-G. Dextran 40 made safer by pretreatment with dextran 1.
     Plastic and Reconstructive Surg 2007; 120: 337–40.

21   Pleuvry BJ. Plasma expanders. *Anaesthesia and Intensive Care Med* 2002;
     3: 228–31.

22   Miller RD. Transfusion therapy. In Miller RD, ed. *Anesthesia*. Vol 2, 3rd
     edn, Churchill Livingstone, New York 1990: 1495.

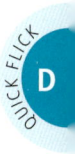

23 Sasada MP, Smith SP. *Drugs in Anaesthesia and Intensive Care*, 2nd edn. Oxford University Press, Oxford,1998: 96–7.

24 Gold BS. Anaesthetic care of patients with diabetes mellitus for ambulatory surgery. *ASA Refresher Courses in Anesthesiology* 1999; 27: 73–81.

25 Levy DM. Review Article: Emergency Caesarean section: best practice. *Anaesth* 2006; 61: 786–91.

26 Van de Velde M. What is the best way to provide analgesia after Caesarean section? *Curr Opin in Anesthesiol* 2000; 13: 267–70.

27 Wood M. Opioid agonists and antagonists. In: Wood M, Wood A, eds. *Drugs and Anesthesia: Pharmacology for Anesthesiologists*, 2nd edn. Williams and Wilkins, Baltimore 1990; 145–6.

28 Hennessey A, Thornton C, Makris A, et al. A randomized comparison of hydralazine and mini-bolus diazoxide for hypertensive emergencies in pregnancy: the PIVOT trial. *ANZJOG* 2007; 47: 279–85.

29 British National Formulary. *British Medical Association and the Pharmaceutical Press* 1991; 22: 73.

30 Tarkkila P, Rosenberg PH. Perioperative analgesia with non-steroidal analgesics. *Curr Opin Anaesthesiol* 1998; 11: 407–10.

31 Henderson JJ, Popat MT, Latto IP, Pearce AC. Difficult Airway Society guidelines for management of the unanticipated difficult intubation. *Anaesthesia* 2004; 59: 675–94.

32 Crosby ET, Cooper RM, Douglas MJ et al. The unanticipated difficult airway with recommendations for management. *Can J Anaesth* 1998; 45: 757–76.

33 Murphy GS, Vender JS. ASA Scientific Papers emphasise patient safety. *APSF Newsletter* Winter 2001; 16(4): 49–64.

34 Samsoon GLT, Young JRB. Difficult tracheal intubation: a retrospective study. *Anaesthesia* 1987; 42: 487–90.

35 Cobley M, Vaughan RS. Recognition and management of difficult airway problems. *Br J Anaesth* 1992; 68: 90–7.

36 Mathew M, Hanna LS, Aldrete JA. Pre-operative indices to anticipate difficult tracheal intubation. *Anesth Analg* 1989; 68: S187.

37 Bond A, Nussey A. Clinical prediction of a difficult intubation. *Anaesth Intensive Care* 1993; 21: 358–60.

38 Wilson ME, Spiegelhalter D, Robertson JA, Lesser P. Predicting difficult intubation. *Br J Anaesth* 1988; 61: 211–16.

39 Nath G, Sekar M. Predicting difficult intubation—a comprehensive scoring system. *Anaesth Intensive Care* 1997; 25: 482–6.

40 Lee BJ, Kang JM, Kim DO. Laryngeal exposure during laryngoscopy is better in the 25° back-up position than in the supine position. *Br J Anaesth* 2007; 99: 581–6.

41 Knill RL. Difficult laryngoscopy made easy with a 'BURP'. *Can J Anaesth* 1993; 40: 798–9.

42 Tamura M, Ishikawa T, Kato R, Isono S, Nishino T. Mandibular advancement improves the laryngeal view during direct laryngoscopy performed by inexperienced physicians. *Anesthesiology* 2004; 100: 598–601.

43 Henderson JJ. The use of a paraglossal straight blade laryngoscopy in difficult tracheal intubation. *Anaesthesia* 1997; 52: 552–60.

44 Benumof JL. Laryngeal mask airway and the ASA difficult airway algorithm. *Anesthesiology* 1996; 84: 686–99.

45 Brimacombe J, Keller C, Judd DV. Gum elastic bougie-guided insertion of the ProSeal™ laryngeal mask airway is superior to the digital and introducer tool techniques. *Anesthesiology* 2004; 100: 25–9.

46 American Society of Anesthesiologists Task Force on Difficult Airway Management. Practice guidelines for the management of the difficult airway. *Anesthesiology* 2003; 98: 1269–77.

47 Kam PCA, Kaur N, Thong CL. (Review Article) Direct thrombin inhibitors: pharmacology and clinical relevance. *Anaesthesia* 2005; 60: 565–74.

48 White M. Disseminated Intravascular Coagulation. In Parsons PE, Wiener-Kronish JP eds. *Critical Care Secrets*. Hanley & Belfus Inc, Philadelphia 1992: 267–70.

49 Horne MK. Hemorrhagic and Thrombotic Disorders. In Parrillo JE, ed. *Current Therapy in Clinical Care Medicine*, 3rd edn. Mosby, St Louis 1997; 357–8.

50 Marcel L. Current understanding of disseminated intravascular coagulation. *Br J Haem* 2004; 12: 567–76.

51 Feinstein DI. Treatment of disseminated intravascular coagulation. *Semin Thromb Hemost* 1988; 14: 351–62.

52 Franchini M, Manzato F, Salvagno GL, Lippi G. Potential role of recombinant activated factor VII for the treatment of severe bleeding associated with disseminated intravascular coagulation: a systemic review. *Blood Coagulation and Fibrinolysis* 2007; 18: 589–93.

53 Cuthbertson BH, Hunter J, Webster NR. Inotropic agents in the critically ill. *Br J Hosp Med*. 1996; 56: 386–98.

54 Hatzakorzian R, Li Pi Shan W, Côté AV, Schricker T, Backman SB. Case Report: The management of severe emergence agitation using droperidol. *Anaesthesia* 2006 ; 61: 112–15.

55 Shaw A, Matthews EE. Postoperative neuroleptic malignant syndrome. *Anaesthesia* 1995; 50: 246–7.

56 Habib AS, Gan TJ. Food and Drug Administration Black Box warning on the preoperative use of droperidol; a review of the cases. *Anesth Analg* 2003; 96: 1377–9.

57 Tramér MR. A rational approach to the control of postoperative nausea and vomiting: evidence from systemic reviews. Part II. Recommendations for prevention and treatment, and research agenda. *Acta Anaesthesiol Scand* 2001; 45: 14–19.

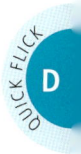

QUICK FLICK
D

E

▷ Ebstein's Anomaly

See *Tricuspid Regurgitation and Ebstein's Anomaly*.

▷ Eclampsia

See *Pre-eclampsia/Eclampsia*.

▷ ECG Monitoring

See *Electrocardiography and Myocardial Ischaemia, Peri-operative*.

▷ EDLA

Stands for an extended duration LA preparation consisting of polylactic-co-glycolic acid polymer microspheres 25–125 μm in diameter which contain bupivacaine +/– dexamethasone. These microspheres biodegrade over 7 days thus prolonging the LA effect. In 1 comparative study of LA skin infiltration, EDLA analgesia lasted 96 h compared to 24 h with plain bupivacaine.[1]

Mild indurations and pruritis were noted at the site of infiltration. The use of EDLA for nerve blocks is being investigated.

▷ Eisenmenger's Syndrome

More than a brief outline of this complicated condition is beyond the scope of this manual. Evidence from the literature is mainly anecdotal and theoretical due to the rareness of this condition.

Definition

In this syndrome, an atrial or ventricular septal defect (VSD) or other congenital cardiac abnormality causes blood to pass from the systemic to the pulmonary circulation (left-to-right shunt). This results in an increased load on the pulmonary circulation causing pulmonary hypertension and right ventricular hypertrophy. In time, the pulmonary vascular resistance increases to the point where pulmonary pressure is equal to or greater than systemic pressure (termed balanced circulation) and the shunt becomes bi-directional or reversed (right-to-left shunt). This causes cyanosis. The Eisenmenger complex is a large VSD, an over-riding aorta and right ventricular hypertrophy. Although regional and general anaesthesia are associated with considerable risk in patients with Eisenmenger's syndrome, many types of anaesthetic have been used successfully in this condition. Mortality for major non-cardiac surgery is about 24%.[2]

Clinical Effects of Eisenmenger's Syndrome

As with other types of congenital cyanotic heart disease (**see** *Congenital Heart Disease (CHD) in Adults and Non-cardiac Surgery*) these patients suffer from:[3]

1 dyspnoea, fatigue, syncope due to poor cardiac output
2 hyper-viscosity, polycythaemia, thromboembolism
3 increased bleeding tendency due to thrombocytopenia, platelet dysfunction, deficient fibrinolysis
4 congestive cardiac failure
5 haemoptysis
6 factors precipitating shunt reversal such as pregnancy can lead to rapid cardiac deterioration and death.

Management Aims

The main aim is to minimise the degree of right-to-left shunt. This shunt will be increased by factors which:

1 increase pulmonary vascular resistance (PVR)
2 decrease systemic vascular resistance (SVR).

Therefore it is important to:

1 Prevent further elevation of PVR. **See** *Pulmonary Hypertension*. Factors which increase PVR include:
   a) hypoxia
   b) hypercarbia
   c) acidosis
   d) hypothermia
   e) lung hyperinflation
   f) positive end expiratory pressure.
2 Pre-operative levels of SVR should be maintained.
3 Systemic blood pressure and cardiac output should be well maintained throughout the peri-operative period.
4 Maintain optimal intravascular fluid volume and replace fluid losses promptly. Unreplaced extracellular fluid loss is poorly tolerated.
5 In some Eisenmenger's syndrome patients, the PVR decreases with O_2 therapy and the degree of right-to-left shunt is reduced.[4] (Note that hypoxaemia due to right-to-left shunt is not usually reversible by O_2 therapy.)
6 Administration of an α adrenergic receptor agonist may increase SVR more than PVR and produce a reduction in right-to-left shunting and thus be beneficial.[4]
7 Consider the use of selective pulmonary vasodilator drugs such as nitric oxide and inhaled prostacyclin.
8 Provide antibiotic prophylaxis against bacterial endocartis. **See** *Bacterial Endocarditis (BE) Prophylaxis*.

E
QUICK FLICK

9 These patients are at increased risk of thrombo-embolic disease due to an elevated haematocrit (Hct) and require appropriate anticoagulant therapy. Venesection for polycythaemia may be required for Hct > 0.65.

10 Bradycardia and other dysrhythmias must be prevented.

Anaesthetic Management

Local infiltration or nerve blocks are preferable to GA or neuro-axial anaesthesia if appropriate. Regional anaesthesia is associated with a lower mortality than general anaesthesia but this may be more related to the type of surgery than to the anaesthetic.[2]

Pre-induction Phase

1 Ensure the patient's intravascular volume is optimal.

2 In addition to routine monitoring, insert an arterial cannula for invasive blood pressure readings.

3 Use of a pulmonary artery catheter is *not* advised because of:[4]
   a) Increased risk of pulmonary artery rupture due to pulmonary hypertension.
   b) Increased risk of dysrhythmias, thrombosis and embolism (including paradoxical embolus).
   c) Extremely difficult interpretation of PA catheter readings in the presence of a bidirectional shunt.

4 Central venous pressure (CVP) monitoring is useful to measure right ventricular (RV) filling pressure. Optimal RV filling may help minimise right-to-left shunt and an excessive elevation in CVP may indicate that the RV is failing.[4]

Induction Phase

Agents used for induction of anaesthesia include:

1 Ketamine has been used successfully and does not cause a reduction in SVR; however it may increase PVR.[5]

2 Etomidate appears appropriate for use in this condition as it has the least cardiovascular effects.[6]

3 Sammut and Paes suggest the availability of a noradrenaline infusion to maintain satisfactory SVR.[7]

Maintenance Phase

1 Several different inhalation agents have been used successfully in this syndrome, but N_2O should not be used as it can cause reduced ventricular function and pulmonary vasoconstriction, which may be detrimental.

2 Use IPPV with low inflation pressures. Plan for early extubation.

3 There is an increased risk of paradoxical embolism of gas, fat, clot or amniotic fluid. Do not allow air to enter intravenous lines.

Postoperative Phase

These patients should be monitored closely for postoperative deterioration in ICU or the high dependency ward. Many patients with this disease may survive surgery only to die soon after operation from thromboembolic disease,[8] heart failure or other complications.

Obstetric Implications

1. Pregnancy is contraindicated in this condition, and termination is frequently recommended. The mortality of termination is about 7%.[9]
2. The combination of Eisenmengers's syndrome and pregnancy is associated with a mortality of about 40–50%.[10] The fetal loss rate is about 8%.[8]
3. Caesarean section maternal mortality rate in Eisenmenger's syndrome patients is between 46 and 70%.[9]
4. It is unclear whether patients with Eisenmenger's syndrome should be allowed to labour and deliver vaginally or whether elective CS should be performed. A decision about the preferred mode of delivery must be made for each individual case well before term.
5. Well-managed epidural anaesthesia has been successfully used for labour and delivery in these patients.[11] The main concern is reduction in SVR which must be avoided. Do not use adrenaline containing solutions due to the potential for peripheral vasodilating β adrenergic receptor effects.[12]
6. Syntocinon may cause a dramatic reduction in arterial O_2 tension due to vasodilatation.[13] Cole et al. recommended uterine massage and slow syntocinon infusion rather than a syntocinon bolus.[14]

Laproscopic Surgery

Can be hazardous in these patients due to the effects of pneumoperitoneum including decreased venous return.

Other problems include:

1. PVR may be increased by elevation of airway pressure as intra-abdominal pressure rises.
2. Hypercarbia/acidosis due to CO_2 gas insufflation can also increase PVR.

It is recommended that:

1. Intra-abdominal pressure should be < 15 mm Hg.
2. Avoid the Trendelenburg position.[7]
3. Gasless laparoscopy with mechanical abdominal wall elevation may be preferable.[15]

◐ Elbow Blocks

Anatomy

Ulnar Nerve (C7, C8, T1) A branch of the medial cord of the brachial plexus passes along the posterior surface of the medial epicondyle at the elbow. It enters the forearm between the 2 heads of flexor carpi ulnaris. *Supplies:*

sensory to the dorsal and palmar aspects of the little and half the ring finger and ulnar side of hand. Motor to the medial 2 lumbricals and the interossei, adductor pollicis, flexor carpi ulnaris and the medial half of flexor digitorum profundus.

Median Nerve (C5, C6, C7, C8, T1) Arises from the medial and lateral cords of the brachial plexus. The nerve crosses the elbow in the antecubital fossa lying on the brachialis medial to the brachial artery.

Supplies: Sensory to the thenar eminence and palmar aspect of the lateral 3½ digits and the skin on the dorsal tips of the same fingers. Motor to lateral 2 lumbricals, opponens pollicis, adductor pollicis brevis, flexor pollicis brevis (LOAF).

Radial Nerve (C5, C6, C7, C8, T1) Arises from the posterior cord of the brachial plexus. The radial nerve winds around the lower end of the humerus to end in front of the lateral epicondyle. Here it divides into the superficial radial nerve and the posterior interosseous nerve. *Supplies:* Skin over posterior arm, postero-lateral lower arm and forearm, dorsal aspect of thumb base and the back of the lateral 3½ digits except for the tips. Motor to triceps, brachialis, brachioradialis and extensor carpi radialis longus.

Lateral Cutaneous Nerve of Forearm is the continuation of the musculocutaneous nerve. In the antecubital fossa it lies just lateral to the biceps tendon at the elbow crease. *Supplies*: skin on the lateral half of the forearm as far as the wrist and a variable area on the dorsum of the hand.

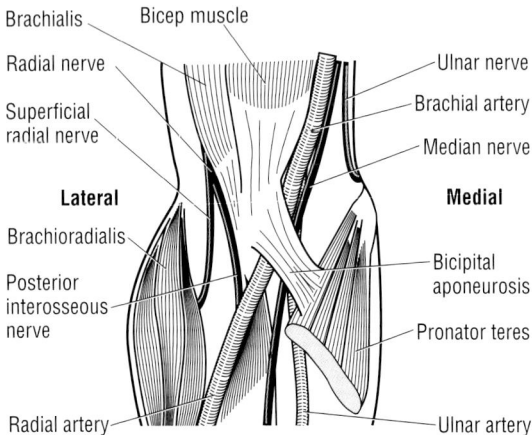

Figure E1 Nerves of the antecubital fossa

Nerve Blocks

Ulnar Nerve Block Flex the elbow to 30° and identify the ulnar nerve in the sulcus of the medial epicondyle.

Insert a 25 G 38 mm needle 1–2 cm proximal to this position and elicit paraesthesia. Inject 2 mL lignocaine 1% with adrenaline over 10–20 s.

Median Nerve Block

1 Extend the elbow and identify the medial and lateral epicondyles. Draw a line between them which should be ≈ 3–4 cm proximal to the flexion crease.
2 Palpate the brachial artery and insert a 25 G 38 mm needle on the epicondylar line about 0.5 cm medial to the brachial artery and elicit paraesthesia deep to the artery. It may be necessary to fan the needle in order to elicit paraesthesia.
3 Inject 5 mL of LA solution. If paraesthesia is not obtained inject a wall of LA alongside and deep to the brachial artery.

Radial Nerve Block

1 Identify the biceps tendon by asking the patient to flex the elbow.
2 Extend the elbow and draw a line between the medial and lateral epicondyles. Insert a 25 G 38 mm needle just lateral to biceps tendon in the groove between it and the brachioradialis muscle on the epicondylar line. Direct the needle slightly cephalad and medial to contact the lateral condyle of the humerus.
3 Inject 2–4 mL of LA while the needle is withdrawn ≈ 0.5 cm, then withdraw the needle almost to the skin. Reinsert 2 × more, each time aiming more medially, and injecting while withdrawing.

Lateral Cutaneous Nerve of the Forearm Block

This nerve, which lies superficially to the radial nerve, can be blocked by injecting 5 mL of LA subcutaneously in the groove between the biceps tendon and brachioradialis.

Using Ultrasound for Nerve Blocks Around the Elbow

The median, radial and ulnar nerves are easily visualised at the elbow with ultrasound. The median nerve will be seen medial to the brachial artery, and is hyperechoic. The radial nerve is seen as its deep and superficial branches between the brachioradialis and brachialis muscle just lateral to the insertion of the biceps tendon. The median and radial nerve can be blocked with a short axis view in the antecubital fossa (probe long axis in same plane as epicondyles). The ulnar nerve can be visualised with the arm placed flexed over the head. It can be blocked either above or below the ulnar canal. Do not block the nerve in the canal as this may lead to a pressure neuropathy. Usually only 2–2.5 mL of LA is needed as long as there is good circumferential spread. Use a 23 G needle.

QUICK FLICK **E**

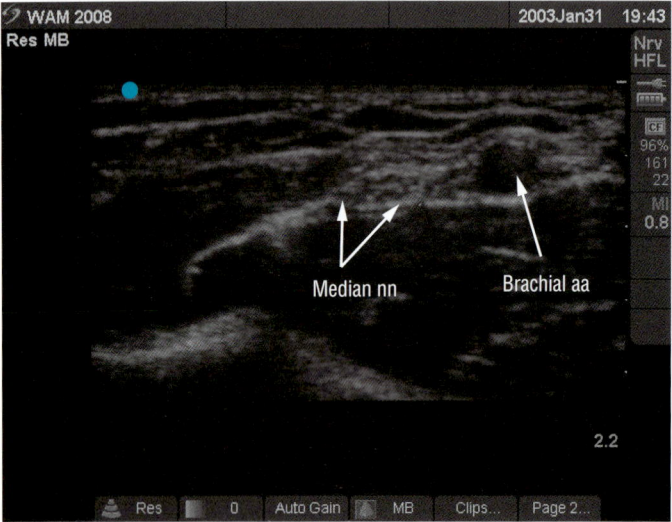

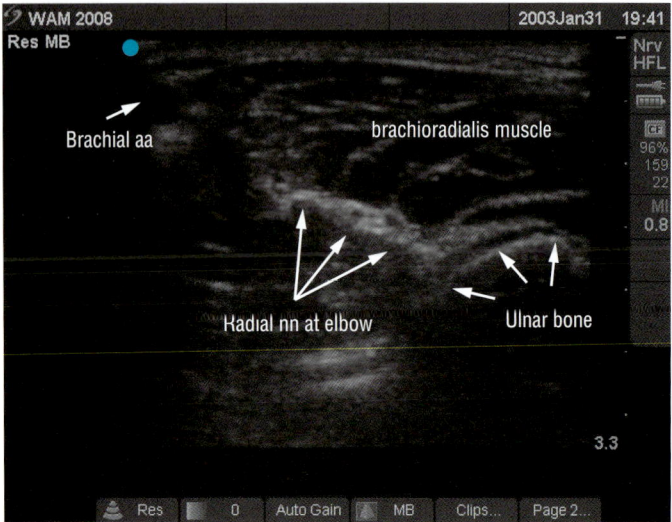

Figure E2 Image of the median, radial and ulna nerves at the level of the elbow

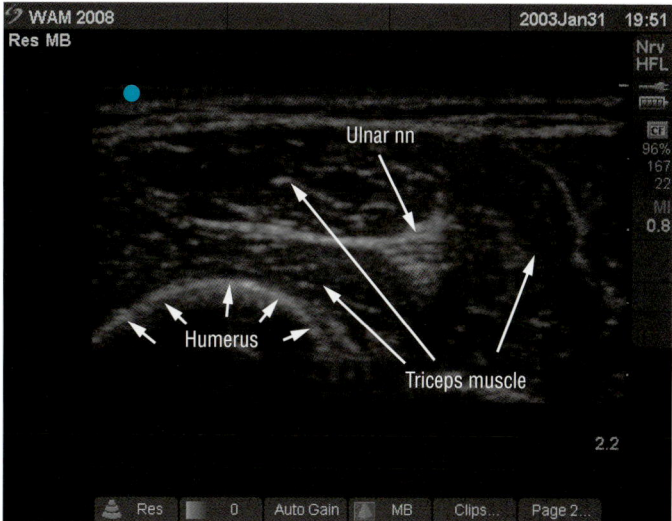

○ Electrocardiography

Topics Covered in this Section

▶ Lead Placement for Standard 12-Lead ECG Recording
▶ Lead Positions for Monitoring
▶ Normal ECG Values
▶ Some Important Diagnostic ECG Patterns

Lead Placement for Standard 12-Lead ECG Recording

There are 4 limb leads and 6 chest leads. The chest leads are positioned as follows:

1 V1 Fourth intercostal space (ICS) at the right sternal border (SB).
2 V2 Fourth ICS, left SB.
3 V3 Between V2 and V4.
4 V4 Fifth ICS in the midclavicular line (MCL).
5 V5 Fifth ICS in the anterior axillary line.
6 V6 Fifth ICS in the midaxillary line.

Lead Positions for Monitoring

Standard 3-Lead Monitoring

Right arm lead (white) on the right shoulder, left arm lead (black) on the left shoulder, left leg lead (red) on left lower chest. Usually monitor lead II

CM5 Configuration

Is a means of optimising the 3-lead system in order to detect ischaemia. This is achieved by placing the left arm electrode (black) on the V5 position and right arm lead (white) over the manubrium. The third (indifferent) lead is placed on the left shoulder. Monitor lead I (not II).

5-Lead ECG Monitoring

Place the right arm lead (white) on the right shoulder and the left arm lead (black) on the left shoulder. Place the right leg lead (green) in the mid-axillary line low on the chest. Place the left leg lead (red) in the same position on the left side. Place the chest lead (brown) in the V5 position (see above). Monitor leads II and V. **See** *ST Segment Analysis.*

Normal ECG Values

Standard recording speed 25 mm/s. Therefore 1 cm = 0.4 s and 1 mm = 0.04 s. 1 cm (2 large squares) amplitude = 1 mV.

PR Interval NR 0.12–0.2 s.

QRS NR < 0.12 s.

QT Interval Corrected QT interval $(QTc) = \dfrac{Q-T}{\sqrt{(R-R\ interval)}}$

NR QTc = 0.39 s + 0.04 s. See QT Interval Abnormalities below.

Normal Axis –30° to +120°

J Point is the end of the QRS complex.

Some Important Diagnostic ECG Patterns

1 *Axis Abnormalities*
   A significant left axis deviation is indicated by a negative QRS complex in lead II. A significant right axis deviation is indicated by a negative QRS complex in lead I.

2 *Abnormal ECG Waves*
   a) *U Wave* occurs after the T wave. An inverted U wave in leads I, II and V5 may be seen in ischaemic heart disease (IHD) and hypertension.
   b) *Delta Wave* slurred upstroke on the R wave. Classically seen in Wolff-Parkinson-White syndrome. **See** *Wolff-Parkinson-White (WPW) Syndrome.*
   c) *J Wave* rounded hump like wave on the down stroke of the R wave. Also called an Osborne wave. Seen in hypothermia.

3 *P Wave Abnormalities*
   a) *P Mitrale*—a bifid P wave is associated with left atrial hypertrophy, as can occur with mitral stenosis.
   b) *P Pulmonale*—a tall peaked P wave. This pattern is associated with right atrial enlargement as can occur with pulmonary hypertension and tricuspid valve stenosis.

4 *Strain Pattern*

Depression of the ST segment and T wave inversion. This pattern may be seen with myocardia ischaemia.

5 *QT Interval Abnormalities*

a) *Prolonged QTc Interval* **see** *Long QT Syndrome (LQTS).*

b) *Shortened QTc Interval* can occur with digoxin therapy, hyperthermia, hypercalcaemia and vagal stimulation.

6 *Electrolyte Disturbances*

a) *Hyperkalaemia*—prolonged PR interval, widened QRS, flattening of the P wave, tall and peaked T waves, deep S wave. Ultimately get a sine wave ECG pattern which precedes asystole.

b) *Hypokalaemia*—prolonged PR interval, T wave amplitude diminishes and then becomes inverted, development of U waves.

c) *Hypermagnesaemia*—prolonged PR interval and widened QRS due to a non specific intraventricular conduction system delay. Sino-atrial and atrio-ventricular node block may occur. **See** Magnesium Therapy in *Pre-eclampsia/Eclampsia* for more information.

d) *Hypomagnesaemia*—increased PR and QT interval and myocardial irritability.

e) *Hypercalcaemia*—increased PR and QRS intervals and a shortened QT interval. T wave flattening and widening and AV nodal block progressing to complete heart block.

f) *Hypocalcaemia*—prolonged QT interval, T wave inversion, heart blocks and ventricular fibrillation.

g) *Hyponatraemia*—Na < 115 mmol/L, QRS widened and ST segment elevation. Na < 100 mmol/L may cause ventricular dysrhythmias such as ventricular tachycardia or fibrillation.

7 *Bundle Branch Conduction Defects*

a) *Right Bundle Branch Block (RBBB)*—rSR pattern in V1, and a broad and slurred S wave in V5 and V6. With incomplete RBB the QRS complex duration is between 0.10 s and 0.12 s.

With complete RBBB the QRS duration is > 0.12 s.

b) *Left BBB* QRS > 0.12 s—a wide, notched M shaped QRS complex is seen in leads V5 and V6.

c) *Fascicular Blocks*—these include left anterior and left posterior hemiblocks.

   i) *Left Anterior Hemiblock*—left axis deviation, tall R wave in AVL, deep S wave in II, III and AVF. QRS widened but < 0.12 s.

   ii) *Left Posterior Hemiblock*—right axis deviation and prominent S wave in I and AVL. Tall R waves in II, III and AVF (but especially III).

d) *Bifascicular Blocks*—include combinations of RBBB and fascicular blocks.

QUICK FLICK **E**

   i) *RBBB and Left Anterior Hemiblock*—right bundle branch block
       pattern with a left axis deviation.
   ii) *RBBB and Left Posterior Hemiblock*—right bundle branch block
       pattern, right axis deviation, prominent S wave in I and AVL. Tall R
       waves in II, III and AVF.
 e) *Trifascicular Block* consists of a right bundle branch block plus a
    fascicular block and a type of atrio-ventricular conduction block (see
    below).

8 Heart Block or Atrio-ventricular Block **see** *Heart Block*.

9 *Ventricular Hypertrophy*
  a) *Right Ventricular Hypertrophy*—right axis deviation, large R wave in
     V1, V2 with initial slur. May also see inverted T wave in V2, V3 and a
     strain pattern V1–V4 with prominent S wave in I, II, III.
  b) *Left Ventricular Hypertrophy*—left axis deviation. Tall R wave in V5, V6.
     Deep S wave in V1, V2. S wave in V1+ R wave in V5 or V6 > 35 mm.

10 *Myocardial Ischaemia*
   Myocardial ischaemia is suggested by horizontal or down sloping
   depression of the ST segment (1 mm or more) with an upright T wave or
   T wave inversion. Left bundle branch block may occur with significant left
   axis deviation. Sharply pointed symmetrical T waves may occur that may
   become taller than on non ischaemic ECG.

11 *Myocardial Infarction (MI)*
   ECG changes include:
   a) ST segment elevation—occurs in minutes.
   b) Tall and widened T waves—occurs in minutes.
   c) Inversion of T waves.
   d) Appearance of pathological Q waves i.e. > 0.04 s wide and > 0.2 mV
      deep. These appear over hours to days.
   Localising the site of infarction:
   a) *Inferior*—changes in leads II, III, AVF.
   b) *Posterior*—tall R waves and tall wide asymmetrical T waves in V1–V3.
   c) *Anteroseptal*—V1–V4 changes.
   d) *High anterolateral*—I, AVL, V5, V6 changes.
   e) *Extensive anterior*—I, AVL, V1–V5 changes.

12 *Pulmonary Embolus*
   May cause an acute strain on the right ventricle with right bundle
   branch block, right axis deviation, prominent S wave in I, Q wave in III
   and inverted T wave in III. May also see non-specific ST changes and T
   inversion in anterior leads, P pulmonale and atrial dysrhythmias.

13 *Pulmonary Hypertension*
   See right axis deviation, ECG changes of right ventricular hypertrophy and
   P pulmonale. A right bundle branch block pattern is common.

◐ Electroconvulsive Therapy (ECT) and Magnetic Seizure Therapy (MST)

Electroconvulsive Therapy

This procedure requires:

1   Full pre-anaesthetic assessment.
2   Pre-oxygenate then induce anaesthesia with methohexitone 1 mg/kg or thiopentone. Propofol can also be used but lignocaine mixed with the propofol may interfere with the seizures.[16] Seizures with propofol tend to be shorter but appear to be therapeutic.
3   Give suxamethonium 0.3–0.5 mg/kg IV.
4   When the patient is paralysed insert a mouth guard if the patient has teeth. Inform the psychiatrist that the patient is ready for treatment.
5   After the seizure has stopped ventilate the patient with 100% O_2 until the patient is breathing spontaneously then transfer the patient to recovery.

Special Circumstances and ECT

1   Pacemakers including those that are rate responsive do not need to be modified for ECT.[17]
2   For patients who cannot have suxamethonium (e.g. severe sux myalgia), mivacurium is the best alternative muscle relaxant. *See Mivacurium*. Rocuronium followed by sugammadex will be a better alternative when sugammadex becomes available.
3   Remifentanil 1 µg/kg IV combined with a reduced dose of IV anaesthetic drug e.g. methohexitone 0.5 mg/kg plus suxamethonium results in longer seizure time with possibly greater efficacy.[18] A larger dose of remifentanil (500 µg) can be used with methohexitone to ablate the CVS responses to ECT (hypertension and tachycardia).[19]

Magnetic Seizure Therapy (MST)

This is a new technique in which rapidly alternating magnetic fields are used to induce seizures.[20] The peak magnetic field strength is 2 Tesla. *See Magnetic Resonance Imaging (MRI) Anaesthesia*. The seizure activity is more 'focal' and cognitive side effects such as disorientation and amnesia are reduced. As recommended by White et al. GA for MST requires smaller doses of sux (e.g. 40 mg) than ECT because of faster recovery.[20] They also recommended etomidate 0.15–2 mg/kg, glycopyrrolate 2.5 µg/kg, ketorolac 0.4 mg/kg.

Contraindications to ECT/MST

There are probably relatively few absolute contraindications to ECT but common sense must prevail. Conditions such as cervical spine instability and severe thrombocytopenia would probably preclude ECT.

Certain conditions are of great concern if ECT is contemplated.

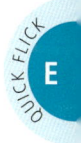

These include:

1 Cerebral pathology such as intracranial mass lesion, cerebral aneurysms and brain vascular malformations.
2 Poor CVS status.
3 Phaeochromocytoma.

�‣ Electromechanical Dissociation (EMD)

See *Cardiac Arrest*.

�‣ Emergence Agitation

See *Confusion, Agitation, Decreased Level of Consciousness, Postanaesthetic*.

�‣ EMLA

Topical anaesthetic agent useful for anaesthetising intact skin. EMLA stands for Eutectic Mixture of Local Anaesthetic Agents. A eutectic mixture is one in which the melting point is lower than the constituents of the mixture. EMLA is a mixture of equal parts lignocaine and prilocaine.

The resulting mixture has a melting point of 16°C. The LA agents are emulsified with water to give a final concentration of 25 mg lignocaine and 25 mg prilocaine per gram of EMLA.

Dose

For venepuncture, apply over a suitable vein and cover with an occlusive dressing for at least 1 h.

For superficial skin surgery such as harvesting of skin grafts, apply over the donor site and cover with an occlusive dressing for at least 2 h prior to the procedure.

Note: There is a risk of toxic blood levels if the cream is swallowed, especially by small children.

�‣ Endocarditis

See *Bacterial Endocarditis (BE) Prophylaxis*.

�‣ Endotracheal Intubation, Attenuating Hypertensive Response to

See *Hypertensive Response to Intubation (Attenuation of)*.

�‣ Endotracheal Tube Sizes

All sizes quoted are for the internal diameter of the endotracheal (ET) tube in mm.

Table E1 ET tube sizes for different ages of patient

Age	Tube size in mm
Premature neonate	2.5
Term neonate	2.5–3.0
1–3 months	3–3.5
3–6 months	3–3.5
6–9 months	3–3.5
9–14 months	3.5–4
15 mths–2 yrs	4–4.5
3–4 yrs	4.5–5
5–6 yrs	5–5.5
7–9 yrs	6–6.5
10–12 yrs	7–7.5
13–15 yrs	7–7.5 cuffed

Adult Male 8.0–8.5 **Female** 7.0–7.5.

Formula for Calculating Tube Size in the Child

$$\frac{Age}{4} + 4$$

Formula for Tube Length at Lips When Tube is in Good Position

$$\frac{Wt\ (kg)}{2} + 7\ cm \text{ or } 2 \times tube\ size + 3\ cm$$

Formula for Calculating Length of Tube at the Nares for a Nasal Tube in Good Position.

$$\frac{Age}{2} + 15\ cm$$

Some Important Lengths

Neonates Gums to vocal cords 5 cm, vocal cords to carina 5 cm.

Adults Tracheal length 10–12 cm, cords to carina 14–15 cm.

◗ Enoxaparin

Enoxaparin (Clexane) is a low molecular weight heparin drug used for its anticoagulant effect.

Dose
DVT Prophylaxis
Moderate-risk Patient 20 mg subcutaneously daily. Give the first dose 2 h before surgery.
High-risk Patient 40 mg subcutaneously on the evening before surgery then 40 mg daily (beginning with the evening after surgery) Continue for 7–10 days or until DVT risk has diminished.

DVT Treatment

1 mg/kg 12 h subcutaneously or 1.5 mg once daily subcutaneously until warfarinised.
See *Heparin (Unfractionated and Low Molecular Weight Heparins)* and *Deep Venous Thrombosis (DVT) Prophylaxis*.

◗ Enoxamine

Phosphodiesterase (PDE III) inhibitor useful for the treatment of:
1 Acute or chronic heart failure.
2 Weaning from and postcardiac bypass.
3 Patients awaiting a heart transplant.
The main actions of enoxamine are positive inotropism and peripheral vasodilatation. Cardiac output and left ventricular stroke work index are increased without an increase in myocardial O_2 consumption.

Dose by IV Infusion

90 μg/kg/min over 10–30 min, or slow bolus of 0.5 mg/kg, then infusion of 5–20 μg/kg/min.[21] Onset of effect 10–30 min, duration of effect 4–6 h.[21]

Advantages of Enoxamine Compared to Other PDEIII Drugs

1 Available as an oral agent.
2 Low incidence of associated dysrrhythmias.

◗ Entropy

Entropy is a measure of disorder in a system and has values from 0 (completely ordered) to 1 (maximum disorder). In the awake patient, EEG signals are highly irregular so the entropy value is high and under anaesthetic the EEG becomes regular and entropy values approach 0. The Datex-Ohmeda S/5™ Entropy module (M-ENTROPY) measures the level of 'disorder' (signal unpredictability) in the EEG and the frontalis electromyography (FEMG) and uses this information to calculate the level of consciousness. Two numbers are generated giving the state entropy (SE) and the response entropy (RE).

State Entropy (SE)

State entropy is computed over a frequency range of 0.8–32 Hz. As it includes the EEG-dominant part of the spectrum it primarily reflects the cortical state of the patient (level of hypnosis).[22] State entropy provides a *stable* indicator of the effects of anaesthetic/hypnotic drugs on the cortex similar to BIS monitoring. (*See* *Bispectral Index (BIS) EEG Monitor*.) The number generated is from 0 to 91 and < 60 corresponds to anaesthesia.

Response Entropy (RE)

Response entropy is calculated over a frequency range of 0.8 Hz to 47 Hz and is sensitive to activation of the facial muscles. RE is designed to have a faster response time than SE and thus gives an early warning of arousal and potential consciousness. RE indicates emergence from anaesthesia about 7 sec faster than SE.[23] RE is measured from 0–100 and again < 60 indicates anaesthesia.

Relationship between RE and SE

The system normalises RE and SE in such a way that RE becomes equal to SE when the EMG power (sum of spectral power between 32 Hz and 47 Hz) is equal to zero. The RE-SE difference then serves as an indication of EMG activation.[22]

During stable periods of anaesthesia the RE and SE values are similar. A sudden peak in RE suggests lightening of anaesthesia.

Application of the Electrodes

1 The skin on the forehead and temple is carefully wiped with an alcohol wipe and allowed to dry.
2 A disposable Entropy™ Sensor with 3 electrodes is applied to the forehead and temple.

Effects of Drugs and Electrical Interference on Entropy[22]

1 *NDNMBDs*—electrical activity in the facial muscles is very resistant to neuromuscular blocking drugs.
2 *Electrocautery*—the software of the entropy module is able in most cases to detect that electrocautery interference is occurring and reject the data.
3 *Cardiac Pacemakers*—no effect.
4 *Blinking and Eye Movement* The monitor is able to detect and reject these signals.

◑ Ephedrine

Sympathomimetic drug derived from the Ma Huang plant. Ephedrine stimulates α and β adrenergic receptors directly, and also causes endogenous release of noradrenaline. It is useful for the treatment of:

1 Hypotension associated with regional and GA.
2 Nasal decongestion.

Dose

Adult 3–6 mg IV boluses titrated to the desired clinical effect. Onset of effect is rapid and effects last for about 1 h. Can also be given as 15 mg IM when a sustained effect on blood pressure is required.

Note: Ephedrine has a long duration of action due to its resistance to metabolism by COMT and MAO. Tachyphylaxis occurs with prolonged use.

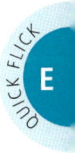

QUICK FLICK

E

◐ Epidural Abscess

The incidence of epidural abscess associated with epidural anaesthesia is estimated to be about 1 per 110 000–145 000.[24] The rate of *spontaneous* epidural abscess in the general hospital population is calculated to be in the range of 1–2 per 10 000 hospital admissions.[25] The mean time of onset of symptoms and signs is about 5 days after epidural insertion.

Clinical Presentation

Symptoms and signs of epidural abscess include:

1 Back pain, nerve root pain radiating from the involved spinal area.
2 Spinal tenderness, swelling and erythema.
3 Fever (absent in 30–40%).
4 Sphincter incontinence, sensory deficit and paresis/paralysis (late signs).

Investigations

1 The definitive investigation for epidural abscess is a MRI scan with gadolinium contrast. Myelography followed by CT scan is also highly sensitive for diagnosis.[25]
2 ESR and WBC are usually raised.
3 Positive blood cultures are helpful but only obtained in about 25% of cases.[26] In the majority of cases the causative organism is *Staphylococcus aureus* or *Staphylococcus epidermidis*. Gram negative bacilli and anaerobic bacteria may also be causative agents.
4 Send pus obtained from the abscess site for gram stain and culture.
5 Remove the epidural catheter if it is still in-situ and send the tip for culture.
6 Lumbar puncture should not be done as it may cause meningitis or neurological deterioration.

Treatment

1 Urgent neurosurgical consultation. Emergency surgical decompression and drainage of pus is usually required if neurological signs are present.
2 IV antibiotics depending on gram stain and sensitivities. For urgent antibiotic treatment while awaiting sensitivities a reasonable choice of agents would be ceftazidime and vancomycin.[25]

Prognosis

Mortality is about 7%.[27] Development of paralysis is irreversible in up to 50% of cases, and this is especially likely to occur if paralysis is present for more than 48 h.[28]

◐ Epidural Anaesthesia

Topics Covered in this Section

▶ Anatomy of the Epidural Space
▶ Contraindications to Epidural Anaesthesia

▶ Technique for Lumbar Epidural Insertion and Epidural Analgesia for Labour Pain

▶ Epidural Anaesthesia for Caesarean section

▶ Technique for Thoracic Epidural Insertion and Dosage Recommendations

▶ Epidural Anaesthesia for Postoperative Pain Relief

▶ Troubleshooting Problems with Epidural Infusions

▶ Dural Puncture (Spinal) Headache and Blood Patching

▶ Intravenous Injection of Bupivacaine/Ropivacaine

▶ Unintentional Extensive Subarachnoid Blockade ('Total Spinal')

▶ Anticoagulant Therapy and Epidurals

▶ Thrombocytopenia and Epidurals

▶ Combined Spinal Epidural Anaesthesia

▶ Complications of Epidural Anaesthesia

Anatomy of the Epidural Space

The epidural space extends from the foramen magnum to the sacral hiatus and surrounds the dura. It is bounded anteriorly by the posterior longitudinal ligaments of the spinal column. Laterally the epidural space is bounded by the intervertebral foramina and pedicles and posteriorly by the ligamentum flavum. The epidural space contains nerve roots, fat, lymphatic and blood vessels, and areolar tissue. The structures encountered when inserting a Tuohy needle into the epidural space, using a midline approach, are: skin, supraspinous ligament, interspinous ligament and ligamentum flavum.

QUICK FLICK

E

Contraindications to Epidural Anaesthesia

The absolute contraindications to epidural anaesthesia are:

1 patient refusal
2 coagulopathy
3 infection at the site of insertion.

Technique for Lumbar Epidural Insertion and Epidural Analgesia for Labour Pain

Technique for Lumbar Epidural Insertion

1 Assess the patient adequately and identify possible contraindications to the procedure.
2 Ensure that the patient gives informed consent and is cooperative.
3 Insert 16–18 G IV cannula and commence IV N/S or Hartmann's solution. Adjust rate of IV fluid infusion to maintain normovolaemia.
4 Ask the patient to fully flex the lumbar spine in the sitting or lateral position. Identify a suitable intervertebral space, usually L3–4 (**see** *Spinal Anatomy*). Sterilise and drape the site using a strict aseptic technique.

5 Inject 1% lignocaine into the skin and deeper structures of the chosen intervertebral space, using 38 mm 23 G needle.

6 Insert the Tuohy needle into interspinous ligament, remove the trocar, and attach a low resistance syringe filled with either saline or air. Air use does carry the risk of pneumocephalus and subsequent headache.[29] Other potential risks of using air (identified from published reports) include spinal cord and nerve root compression, venous air embolus and inadequate analgesia.[30] Air related complications could be potentially worsened by subsequent use of N_2O.

7 Identify the epidural space by the sudden loss of resistance as the syringe and Tuohy needle are slowly and carefully advanced with pressure on the syringe plunger. Resistance to needle advancement will increase just prior to entering the epidural space because of the ligamentum flavum. Do not advance needle during a uterine contraction in a labouring patient. In 80% of cases the space will be at a depth of between 4 and 6.5 cm.[31]

8 Insert the epidural catheter through the Tuohy needle and remove the needle over the catheter. Pull the catheter back so that only about 3–4 cm remains in the epidural space. Do not insert the catheter during a uterine contraction. *Note:* Never pull the catheter out through the needle as this may shear the catheter.

9 Attach the filter connector to the catheter and use a syringe to attempt to aspirate CSF or blood. If neither of these fluids is aspirated, flush the filter with LA agent and attach it to the filter connector. Secure the epidural catheter to the patient with sterile adhesive dressings.

Epidural Analgesia for Labour Pain

Epidural anaesthesia in labour does not increase the rate of Caesarean section.[32] It does not increase the duration of labour, but does increase the likelihood of an instrumental delivery.[33] Discontinuing the epidural late in labour does not appear to decrease the incidence of instrumental delivery.[34] Epidural anaesthesia does not increase the risk of long-term backache.[33]

Test Dose

Inject a test dose through either the Tuohy needle or the catheter. Use 3 mL of 2% lignocaine. Addition of adrenaline to the test dose may or may not result in a tachycardia and is not reliable for detecting intravascular injection in the obstetric patient.[35]

Establishing the Block for Patient in Labour

1 Give 500 mL to 1 L of Hartmann's solution or N/S prior to initiating epidural blockade.

2 Inject 15–20 mL of bupivacaine 0.125% with 1:400 000 adrenaline and fentanyl 5 µg/mL. Inject slowly and incrementally. Ask the patient to report any ill effects such as tinnitus, tingling in lips and tongue or

dysphoria (suggesting IV injection). Alternatively use ropivacaine 0.2% (2 mg/mL) with fentanyl 2 μg/ml in similiar volumes to bupivacaine 0.125%.

3 Ensure ephedrine and/or aramine is available at all times to treat hypotension.

'Top Up' Doses

Give 15–20 mL of the same mixture used to establish the block up to every 1–2 h as required to treat the patient's distress. Another option is to use an infusion of bupivacaine 0.125% with fentanyl 2.5 μg/mL run at an initial rate of 10 mL/h (7–15 mL/h) with 10 mL boluses as required up to each h. Alternatively use a ropivacaine 0.2% with fentanyl 2 μg/mL at 10 mL/h (6–14 mL/h). Patient controlled epidural top ups can also be used, for example bupivacaine 0.125% 5 mL/h infusion plus 5 mL boluses with a 20 min lockout (max dose per h 20 mL).[36]

Epidural Anaesthesia and Chorioamnionitis

With covering antibiotic therapy the risk of epidural abscess associated with chorioamnionitis appears to be very low.[37]

Epidural Anaesthesia for Caesarean Section

See Caesarean Section (CS).

Technique for Thoracic Epidural Insertion and Dosage Recommendations

Thoracic epidural anaesthesia can provide excellent analgesia following abdominal or chest surgery, rib fractures, pancreatitis and unstable angina. It is a considerably more difficult technique to perform than lumbar epidural placement and there is a increased risk of spinal cord injury.

1 Site of Thoracic Epidural Insertion

The epidural space for insertion of the catheter should correspond to the mid-dermatomal innervation of the surgical incision. Some examples are:

a) Abdominal aortic aneurysm surgery—T7–T8 or T8–T9.

b) Upper abdominal surgery—T6–T7 or T7–T8.

c) Lower abdominal surgery—T9–10.

2 Anatomical Considerations

The vertebral prominence at the base of the neck corresponds to the C7 level and the inferior angle of the scapula corresponds with T7 level. The thoracic dorsal spines are angulated and this angulation is maximal in the mid thoracic region (T5–T8). A paramedian approach may thus be more successful than a midline approach in this region.

The ligamentum flavum in the thoracic region is thinner than in the lumbar region and may also be softer.

The epidural space is much thinner in the thoracic region compared with the lumbar region. See the following table.

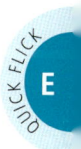

Table E2 Width of the epidural space at various spinal levels

C5	1.0–1.5 mm
T6	1.5–3 mm
L3	5–6 mm

There is a significant risk of spinal cord damage if the needle passes through the epidural space. The spinal cord becomes the cauda equina at the L1–L2 disc space in the adult and at the L3 vertebra in the newborn.

3　Midline Approach to Thoracic Epidural Placement

　a) Position the patient either sitting or laterally with maximal spinal flexion. Little flexion of the thoracic spine is possible because the intervertebral joints allow mainly for rotational movements.

　b) Sterilise and drape the site of entry as for lumbar epidural insertion. Anaesthetise the skin and deeper structures with a 32 mm 23 G needle. While infiltrating, use this needle to evaluate the correct angle of epidural needle insertion to pass it between the spinous processes.

　c) Insert the epidural needle and use a 'loss of resistance' technique to identify the epidural space.

　d) When the epidural space is identified insert the epidural catheter. Aim to leave about 3–4 cm of the epidural catheter in the epidural space. Remove the needle and secure the catheter.

4　Paramedian Approach to Thoracic Epidural Placement

　a) Prepare the patient as described above.

　b) At the selected vertebral level palpate the spinous process. The insertion point is ≈ 1.5 cm lateral to the spinous process.

　c) Use a 32 mm 23 G needle to anaesthetise the skin and deeper structures. Insert the needle perpendicularly to the skin and attempt to contact the vertebral lamina.

　d) Insert the Tuohy needle through the initial puncture wound, then 'walk' the needle aiming for ≈ 10–45° medial angulation and ≈ 45–55° of cephalad angulation (in the mid-thoracic region). These angles will vary greatly from patient to patient and between thoracic levels. The aim is to identify the cephalad medial edge of the lamina. At this site bone will not be encountered at the expected depth.

　e) The Tuohy needle is then advanced with extreme care through the thin ligamentum flavum and into the epidural space.

　f) Once the epidural space is identified proceed as described above.

5　Thoracic Epidural Dose

　a) Give a test dose of 3 mL of lignocaine 2%. Subsequent doses depend on the type and duration of surgery and the patient's size and cardiovascular stability. As a rough guide thoracic epidural dosages are generally 30–50% lower than lumbar dosages to block the same number of dermatomes. For example, for a large bowel resection give ≈ 0.1 mL/kg bolus of bupivacaine 0.25% with fentanyl 5–10 μg/mL prior to surgical incision. Alternatively give 0.1 mL/kg ropivacaine 7.5 mg/mL with fentanyl 5–10 μg/mL.

b) Give a further 2.5–5 mL boluses intra-operatively depending on the patient's physiological responses to surgery and the epidural itself, to a total of ≈ 15 mL.

Epidural Anaesthesia for Postoperative Pain Management

1 Epidural Infusions of LA + Opioid

a) *Bupivacaine and Fentanyl*
Use a solution of bupivacaine 0.125% + fentanyl 2.5 μg/mL.
Adults Run the infusion at 6–20 mL/h for a lumbar catheter and 4–12 mL/h for a thoracic catheter.
Children The maximum theoretical infusion rate for children is 0.3–0.4 mL/kg/h of this solution.

b) *Bupivacaine and Morphine*
Mix 4 mg of morphine with 200 mL of bupivacaine 0.125%.
Adults Run the infusion at 4–12 mL/h. This type of epidural infusion is particularly useful for abdominal wounds extending over many dermatomes e.g. from xiphisternum to pubis.

c) *Ropivacaine and Fentanyl*
Use a solution of ropivacaine 2 mg/mL with fentanyl 2–4 μg/mL.
Adults run the infusion at 6–14 mL/h for a lumbar or thoracic epidural.

2 Pethidine Epidural Patient Controlled Anaesthesia (PCA)
Adults Give 50 mg pethidine loading dose epidurally. Use a solution containing 300 mg pethidine in 60 mL N/S. Set the PCA pump to give 20 mg boluses (4 mL) with a 10 min lockout and a background infusion of 5 mg/h (1 mL).

3 Epidural Morphine Boluses
These provide excellent analgesia lasting about 16 h.
Dose Adult 1–5 mg depending on the size and fitness of patient (average dose 3 mg).

4 Morphine Epidural Infusion
Give morphine at a rate of 0.2–0.6 mg/h. A morphine infusion may be safer than intermittent bolusing.[38]
Note: Epidural morphine use is associated with an increased risk of late respiratory depression.

Trouble Shooting Problems with Epidural Infusions

1 Inadequate Epidural Anaesthesia

a) Check the dermatomal level of the block with ice. Identify which dermatomes are analgesed and whether the epidural blockade is partially or fully unilateral. Give the patient a bolus of the usual hourly rate of the infusion and assess the response. If there does not appear to be any significant epidural blockade, check that the catheter has not fallen out and that the infusion pump is working.

b) If the catheter is in place and a dermatomal level cannot be identified, give a bolus of 5–10 mL of lignocaine 2% (the dose depending on the site of the epidural catheter) to re-establish the block. If an epidural block cannot be re-established abandon the epidural and substitute with an alternative analgesia regimen or resite the epidural catheter.

c) If the lignocaine bolus is effective, increase the epidural infusion rate by 2–3 mL/h and reassess the patient in 2–3 h or sooner if the patient becomes uncomfortable.

d) If analgesia is still inadequate despite demonstrating that some epidural blockade is occurring, treatment options include:

i) Increase the fentanyl in the epidural solution to 5 μg/mL.

ii) Continue the epidural infusion with opioid free bupivacaine or ropivacaine solution and provide the patient with IV opioid PCA or a pethidine epidural PCA.

iii) Change the patient over to epidural PCA pethidine and cease the epidural LA agent (see above).

iv) Give an epidural bolus dose of morphine (or infusion). This will take ≈ 1 h to provide effective analgesia. During this time analgese the patient with an appropriate dose of IV opioid.

v) If the pain problem is due to a 'missed segment' or asymmetrical dermatomal blockade, pulling back the catheter slightly using an aseptic technique may help improve the quality of the block.

2 Blocked Epidural Catheter

Flush the epidural catheter with 1 mL N/S or LA solution. Check that connection between the filter and filter connector is not too tight.

3 Hypotension

a) Establish the clinical urgency of situation i.e. is patient symptomatic, is there evidence of a 'high block'? (See Total Spinal below.)

b) Elevate the patient's legs.

c) Give a vasopressor drug such as ephedrine, or metaraminol. **See** *Ephedrine* and *Metaraminol (Aramine).*

d) IV fluid loading with colloid such as gelofusine 250–1000 mL rapidly depending on the urgency of the situation.

e) Cease the epidural infusion if the level of epidural blockade is excessive.

f) Exclude/diagnose/treat other causes of hypotension e.g. haemorrhage, sepsis.

Dural Puncture (Spinal) Headache and Blood Patching

CSF can be distinguished from saline used to find the epidural space. CSF feels warm on the gloved hand, and is positive for glucose and protein on using urine test sticks.[39] The pH of CSF is 7.5 or greater whereas the pH of saline is usually less than 7.5.[39] The incidence of post dural puncture headache (PDPH) using an 18 G Tuohy needle is approximately 75–85%.[40]

Initial Management of Dural Puncture

If dural puncture occurs, inform the patient and discuss the implications fully and frankly. There are various options of management. For patients in labour one approach is to reattempt epidural insertion one intervertebral space higher. Once the epidural catheter is sited:

1   Give a test dose as described above, then give the full epidural dose slowly and incrementally looking for any evidence of subarachnoid block.
2   Subsequent 'top up' bolus doses for labour pain should be given by the anaesthetist and any evidence of subarachnoid block sought.

Another approach is suggested by Kuczkowski and Benumof.[41] These authors aimed at maintaining CSF volume by the following steps:

1   Reinjection of CSF seen in a loss of resistance syringe attached to the Tuohy needle.
2   Injection of 3–5 mL of preservative-free normal saline intrathecally.
3   Insert the epidural catheter through the Tuohy needle into the subarachnoid space.
4   Establish SAB anaesthesia for labour with 1 mL of bupivacaine 0.25% plus 10 µg fentanyl.
5   To maintain analgesia, an intrathecal infusion of bupivacaine 0.0625% with fentanyl 2 µg/mL is run at 2 mL/h.[42]
6   The intrathecal catheter is left in situ for 8–12 h post delivery.

This approach resulted in an incidence of PDPH of only 14%.

Prevention of PDPH

There is no evidence that bed rest or keeping the patient excessively hydrated will prevent the development or reduce the severity of headache.[43] Prophylactic blood patching through an epidural catheter placed just after the dural tap does not reduce the incidence of PDPH but it may shorten the duration of PDPH symptoms.[44]

If headache occurs:

1   Treat the headache initially with simple oral analgesics such as paracetamol and oxycodone. Use IM morphine if oral analgesics are inadequate. Consider giving stool softener therapy (e.g. lactulose) if opioids are used, to reduce the risk of constipation and straining.
2   Caffeine 300 mg PO or theophylline 300 mg PO are reported to be effective in some patients.[43] Sumatriptan has also been used successfully

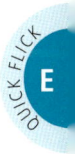

to treat post dural puncture headache.[45] The dose is 6 mg subcutaneously, with repeat dose given in 24 h if the headache reoccurs. Relief occurred in 30 min in one series.

3   If severe headache persists after 24–48 h perform an epidural blood patch (EDBP) unless there is a contraindication e.g. the patient is anticoagulated or septic. The success rate for epidural blood patching is estimated to be ≈ 90% and a further 8% are successfully treated by a second EDBP.[46] This high rate of success is reduced if the procedure is undertaken in the first 24 h after dural puncture or if < 10 ml of blood is used.[47] The following technique is suggested:

   a) After preparing and anaesthetising the same intervertebral level as the site of dural puncture, insert a Tuohy needle into the epidural space. If unable to identify the epidural space at this level reattempt 1 space caudad rather than more cephalad. This is because blood in the epidural space tends to spread in a cephalad direction.[48]

   b) An assistant aseptically withdraws 20 mL of blood and this is injected slowly into the epidural space. 15–20 mL of blood is injected. Discontinue the injection if the patient complains of discomfort such as back or leg pressure.

   c) The patient should lie flat for 2 h after the procedure.[43]

   d) The patient should avoid straining or lifting for 4–5 days and seek medical attention if headache re-occurs.

   e) Patients should be followed up in the out-patient clinic until full recovery has occurred.

Note: PDPH has been treated successfully in patients using an epidural patch with substances other than blood. For example a modified fluid gelatin called Plasmion® was used in a patient with sickle cell disease.[49] ***See*** *Sickle Cell Disease*.

Intravenous Injection of Bupivacaine/Ropivacaine

Prevention

Evron et al. recommend that to prevent the epidural catheter entering an epidural vein, the following be done.[50]

1   Identify the epidural space with a 'loss of resistance' technique.

2   Inject 5 mL N/S into the Tuohy needle and keep the plunger depressed on the syringe for 20 sec.

3   Insert the epidural catheter.

The researchers claimed that the incidence of epidural catheter cannulation of an epidural vein was decreased by 14% and there was a lower incidence of unblocked segments.

Diagnosis

The patient may notice tingling in the lips or tongue or tinnitus. Seizures and CVS collapse can occur.

Treatment

Mild reactions can be treated with reassurance. For the treatment of more severe reactions ***see*** *Bupivacaine* and *Intralipid for the Treatment of Bupivacaine/Ropivacaine Toxicity.*

Unintentional Extensive Subarachnoid Blockade ('Total Spinal')

May result in ascending sensation loss and weakness leading to respiratory compromise. The patient may lose consciousness. Cardiovascular effects include hypotension, bradycardia and cardiac arrest.

Treatment

1 *Airway* Optimise the airway. If the patient loses consciousness and there is a risk of aspiration (e.g. pregnant), apply cricoid pressure, give IV suxamethonium and intubate the trachea. If the patient is conscious, but unable to self ventilate, perform a rapid sequence induction with thiopentone, cricoid pressure and suxamethonium.
2 *Breathing* Ventilate with 100% O_2.
3 *Circulation* Support blood pressure aggressively with IV fluid loading and vasopressor agents such as ephedrine, metaraminol and, if necessary, adrenaline. Treat bradycardia with atropine. *Maintain left lateral tilt if the patient is pregnant.*
4 If a patient with an epidural in situ is progressing to total spinal anaesthesia, aspiration of CSF from the epidural catheter (20–30 mL) may prevent 'total spinal' from occurring, or reduce its effects.[51] In addition after aspirating CSF, consider injecting 20 mL of N/S or a combination of N/S and Hartmann's solution through the epidural catheter. This may be of further benefit by diluting the remaining intrathecal LA.[52]

Anticoagulant Therapy and Epidurals

1 *Heparin* Do not attempt epidural anaesthesia if the patient is fully heparinised. If the patient is receiving subcutaneous heparin in prophylactic doses, do not attempt epidural anaesthesia within 6 h of the last dose. In addition, do not remove the epidural catheter within 6 h of the last heparin dose. Do not give the next dose of heparin for at least 2 h after catheter removal. If patients are on heparin for 4 days or more prior to epidural catheter removal, check the platelet count. ***See*** *Heparin Induced Thrombocytopenia Syndrome (HITS).* If the patient is to be fully heparinised intraoperatively or postoperatively, defer heparinisation for at least 1 h after the epidural is inserted.[53]
2 *Low Molecular Weight (LMW) Heparin* For patients on prophylactic single daily dose LMW heparin therapy e.g. clexane 40 mg, do not insert or remove an epidural catheter within 12 h of the last dose. Delay the next dose for at least 2 h after epidural catheter insertion or removal. If blood is seen in the epidural catheter resite and delay the next dose of

E

LMW heparin for 24 h.[54] If patients are on therapeutic LMW heparin e.g. clexane 1 mg/kg, do not insert or remove an epidural catheter within 24 h of the last dose. Delay the next therapeutic dose for at least 6–8 h after epidural catheter insertion. Additional antiplatelet drugs such as aspirin or non selective NSAIDs should be avoided in patients receiving LMW heparin and regional anaesthesia.

3 *Aspirin* Probably safe to proceed if there is no clinical evidence of increased bleeding tendency.[55]

4 *NSAIDs* Probably safe to proceed unless other complicating factors are present.[56]

5 *Platelet Adenosine Diphosphate (ADP) Receptor Antagonists* e.g. ticlopidine and clopidogrel. These drugs inhibit the binding of platelets to fibrinogen and platelet–platelet interaction. The risk of epidural haematoma in the presence of these drugs is unknown. It is advisable to delay regional anaesthesia until drug effects have dissipated (clopidogrel 7 days, ticlopidine 14 days). *See Platelet Adenosine Diphosphate (ADP) Receptor Antagonists*.

6 *Platelet Glycoprotein IIb/IIIa Receptor Antagonists* e.g. abciximab (RePro), eptifibatide and tirofiban. The risk of epidural haematoma in the presence of these drugs is unclear from the literature. Do not use epidural anaesthesia until the effects of the following drugs have fully dissipated:

   a) abciximab 12–24 h

   b) eptifibatide 4–8 h

   c) tirofiban 4–8 h.

   See Platelet Glycoprotein IIb/IIIa Receptor Antagonists.

7 *Direct Acting Thrombin Inhibitors* Due to a lack of relevant information neuro-axial blockade should not be used in the presence of these drugs.

8 *Fondaparinux* There is little information published on the use of fondaparinux and regional anaesthesia. If neuro-axial blockade is used a pre-operative dose should not be given. The first dose should be given 6 h postoperatively.[57]

9 *Warfarin* Do not insert or remove an epidural catheter unless the INR is 1.3 or less.

Thrombocytopenia and Epidurals

If the platelet count is > 80 000/mm^3 and platelet function is normal it is probably safe to insert an epidural block. If the platelet count is < 50 000/mm^3 epidural block is absolutely contraindicated.

Combined Spinal Epidural Anaesthesia

See Subarachnoid Block (SAB).

Complications of Epidural Anaesthesia

1 Headache (see above). The overall risk of dural puncture followed by headache is about 1:200 epidurals.
2 Epidural haematoma (see below)
3 Epidural abscess (**see** *Epidural Abscess*)
4 Cranial nerve palsies. These occur in 1–3.7 per 100 000 obstetric epidurals and the abducens nerve is the most commonly affected causing diploplia.[58]
5 Persistent/permanent neurological injury. The risk of this occurring for obstetric epidurals is between about 1:20 000[59] and 1:100 000.[58]

◯ Epidural Haematoma

Epidural haematoma is a rare complication of epidural or spinal anaesthesia. The incidence of epidural haematoma associated with epidural anaesthesia is estimated to be about 1 in 150 000–190 000.[53,54] The risk of an epidural haematoma associated with an obsteric epidural is about 1:500 000.[58] Predisposing factors include:

1 Anticoagulant therapy. **See** *Epidural Anaesthesia (Anticoagulant Therapy and Epidurals).*
2 Haemostatic abnormalities such as thrombocytopenia.
3 Elderly patients.

Presentation and Diagnosis

Typically patients present with:

1 Neurological deficit such as paralysis of the lower limbs, decreased leg sensation.
2 Back pain.
3 MRI is the diagnostic test of choice.

Treatment

Epidural haematoma with neurological deficit is a neurosurgical emergency requiring urgent decompression. A relatively good outcome is expected if decompression laminectomy is performed within 8 h of the onset of neurological symptoms.[60]

◯ Epiglottitis

This disease is typically seen in children 2–6 yrs but can occur at any age. The usual causative organism is *Haemophilus influenzae* type b (Hib). The disease is much less common in children since the introduction of Hib vaccination and presentations are now more frequent in adults than children.[61]

Presentation in Children

The usual presentation is:

1 Drooling, sitting up.

2   Tachypnoea, stridor and suprasternal recession.
3   Cough is absent.
4   Complete airway obstruction may occur at any time.
5   Fever, tachycardia.

Treatment in Children

1   Stay with the child until the airway is secure. Do not examine the pharynx. Do not insert an IV cannula or upset the child in any way.
2   Notify the on-call ENT surgeon and paediatrician.
3   Before induction of anaesthesia, ensure a surgeon is available who is competent to perform an urgent tracheostomy.
4   Perform a gaseous induction with O_2 and sevoflurane. When the patient is deeply anaesthetised obtain IV access and give atropine 10 µg/kg. If the airway is difficult to maintain, try pulling the tongue forward to disimpact the epiglottis. Typically the epiglottis is swollen and 'cherry red'.
5   Intubate the patient orally with an endotracheal tube that is 0.5 mm smaller than normal. Inspect epiglottitis to make the diagnosis, and obtain throat swab and take blood for blood culture and full blood count. Post obstructive pulmonary oedema may occur requiring intermittent positive pressure ventilation.
6   Give cefotaxime 50 mg/kg/12 h IV.
7   When the situation is completely controlled change the oral endotracheal tube to a nasal tube under direct vision.
8   Secure the patient's arms with splints to prevent self extubation and transfer the patient to ICU.
9   Give rifampicin antibiotic prophylaxis to all family members and other close contacts.

Presentation in Adults

Adult epiglottitis has a slower onset than in the child, and there is less risk of acute airway occlusion.[61] Causative organisms include *Strep pneumoniae*, beta-hemolytic strep and *Staph aureus*. Hib is a rare cause of adult epiglottitis.

1   Diabetes mellitus is frequently associated with this condition in adults.[62]
2   Fevere, sore throat, difficulty breathing.
3   Inflammation extending into the supraglottic structures is more common than in children.
4   Drooling, muffled voice.

Treatment in Adults

1   Obtain urgent ENT review. The ENT specialist may perform nasendoscopy to confirm the diagnosis and assess severity.
2   Nebulised adrenaline can be considered.
3   The need for airway intervention (intubation/tracheotomy) is based on

the severity of symptoms. Of special concern are the need to sit upright, drooling, muffled voice, dyspnoea and exhaustion.

4 Options for airway intervention are gaseous induction and direct laryngoscopy and intubation when 'deep', awake fibre-optic intubation[63] (***see*** Awake Fibre-optic Intubation) or tracheotomy under LA.
5 Antibiotic treatment with cefotaxime and metronidazole.
6 If the patient is not intubated monitor in a high dependency area.

◗ Epilepsy, Status

Status epilepticus is defined as a seizure lasting more than 30 min or 2 or more sequential seizures without recovery of full consciousness between seizures.[64] It is a *medical emergency* with a mortality of up to 30% in adults and 8% in children especially with convulsive seizures (limb stiffness and jerking).[65] Complications of prolonged seizures may include:[66]

1 permanent brain damage
2 lactic acidosis
3 hypoglycaemia
4 myoglobinuria, renal failure
5 cardiac arrest.

Aetiology

Possible causes include:

1 *Intracerebral Disorders*
    a) epilepsy, especially if anticonvulsant withdrawal is occurring.
    b) cerebral tumour, haemorrhage, infection, trauma.
    c) hypoxic brain damage.
2 *Metabolic Causes*
    a) electrolyte disturbances such as hyponatraemia.
    b) alcohol withdrawal.
    c) hypoglycaemia.
3 *Systemic Illness*
    a) eclampsia. ***See*** Pre-eclampsia/Eclampsia.
    b) severe sepsis.

Treatment

1 *Airway* Ensure adequate airway, intubate the patient if required.
2 *Breathing* Ensure adequate ventilation and consider hypoxia/hypercarbia in the differential diagnosis of seizure aetiology.
3 *Circulation* Provide adequate circulatory support. Consider a cardiovascular cause for the seizure e.g. dysrhythmia.
4 Check BSL, FBC, UEC, calcium, magnesium, phosphate, ABG and, if relevant, anticonvulsant levels, blood alcohol and drug screen.

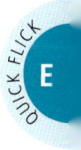

QUICK FLICK

E

5 If hypoglycaemia is the possible cause of seizures, give IV thiamine 100 mg IV then 50 mL of 50% glucose. Thiamine should be given before glucose to avoid precipitating Wernicke's encephalopathy.

6 *Benzodiazepines:* Diazepam *Adult* 5–10 mg IV increments to a maximum dose of 20–30 mg. *Child* 0.2 mg/kg IV—repeat as necessary. If unable to site IV give 0.5 mg/kg PR. Alternatively lorazepam 0.1 mg/kg IV can be used and may be superior to diazepam.[64]

7 *Paraldehyde:* Should be considered in children with status epilepticus (100 μg/mL) 0.2 mL/kg IM (maximum 10 mL). Use a glass syringe.

8 *Phenytoin: Adult/Child* 15–20 mg/kg IV in N/S no faster than 50 mg/min. May cause hypotension or heart block—slow Infusion rate if these occur. Use ECG monitoring during infusion. If seizures persist give an additional phenytoin dose of 5 mg/kg.

9 For ongoing seizures give phenobarbitone 20 mg/kg IV at 100 mg/min.

10 If seizures continue perform a rapid sequence induction with thiopentone 3–5 mg/kg, cricoid pressure, suxamethonium 1.5 mg/kg and intubation. *See Rapid Sequence Induction (RSI)*.

11 Consider an infusion of thiopentone 1–5 mg/kg/h[67] and a muscle relaxant infusion e.g. cisatracurium.

12 Seek urgent ICU/neurologist consultation. Search for a precipitating cause through history, physical examination and relevant investigation.

◔ Epsilon-aminocaproic Acid

Lysine analogue antifibrinolytic drug useful for reducing blood loss in surgery typically associated with massive blood loss such as liver transplant. This drug acts by binding to the plasminogen molecule. It is cheap and eliminated renally.

◔ Eptacog Alpha (Activated)

See Recombinant Activated Factor VII (RFVIIA).

◔ Eptifibatide

See Platelet IIb/IIIa Receptor Antagonists.

◔ Ergometrine Maleate

Contains ergonovine, an ergot alkaloid, which causes uterine contractions superimposed on tonic contraction and peripheral vasoconstriction. Used to prevent/treat postpartum haemorrhage (*see Postpartum Haemorrhage*) and haemorrhage associated with incomplete abortion. Ergometrine can cause hypertension.

Dose

200–500 μg IM. Onset of action takes 5–7 min and effects last ≈ 45 min.

Dose for Emergency Control of Haemorrhage 100–500 µg IV.
Note: IV ergometrine can cause vasoconstriction and severe hypertension especially in the pre-eclamptic patient.

Syntometrine is a combination of ergometrine 500 µg and oxytocin 5 units in a volume of 1 mL.

◐ Esmolol

Relatively selective β1 adreno-receptor blocker particularly useful for its rapid onset and offset of effects (elimination half-life 10 min). Metabolised by hydrolysis via plasma esterases.

Uses
1   Acute supraventricular dysrhythmias including atrial fibrillation and flutter.
2   Control of peri-operative hypertension.
3   Treatment of myocardial infarction.
4   Reducing the hypertensive response to intubation.

Dose
Give 500 µg/kg over 1 min then an infusion of 50–150 µg/kg/min, titrated to response. Given in a concentration of 10 mg/mL, preferably via a peripheral line. In 70 kg man give 20–60 mL/h. Onset of effect occurs in 5–10 min, effects cease after ≈ 20 min.

Bolus Dose (to Blunt the Response to Intubation) 2–3 mg/kg 2 min prior to intubation or 1–2 mg/kg + opioid 4 min before intubation.[68]

Esmolol and Pregnancy
Esmolol may not be effective for treating pregnancy induced hypertension.[69] Esmolol also causes persistent β blockade in the fetus and severe bradycardia may occur.[70]

◐ Etomidate

Carboxylated imidazole IV anaesthetic drug.

Dose for Induction of Anaesthesia
0.3 mg/kg.

Advantages
1   Excellent cardiovascular stability. Etomidate is indicated for IV induction in patients with unstable CVS status e.g. shocked patients, and patients with known cardiovascular disease.
2   Etomidate causes a reduction in ICP and intraocular pressure (IOP).

Disadvantages
1   May get pain on injection (25–50%). This is reduced by the addition of lignocaine.

QUICK FLICK

E

2 Involuntary movement.
3 Causes adreno-cortical suppression and is not suitable for prolonged use by IV infusion because of this effect.
4 Etomidate is contraindicated in patients with porphyria. **See** *Porphyria*.
5 Causes nausea and vomiting (more than thiopentone).
6 Dissolved in propylene glycol which causes a high incidence of thrombophlebitis.
7 Etomidate should be avoided in patients with known seizure disorders.

○ Ex-utero Intrapartum Treatment (EXIT) Procedure

This technique is used during Caesarean section surgery for the management of a fetus with potentially life-threatening airway obstruction. The aim of this technique is to maintain utero-placental circulation (maternal-fetal bypass) while securing the compromised fetal airway prior to full delivery. This procedure has also been termed operation on placental support (OOPS) and airway management on placental support (AMPS). A large number of additional staff are required including a paediatric anaesthetist, paediatric airway surgeon, a neonatologist and appropriate nurse support. A second anaesthetic machine and appropriate monitors for the neonate are also required.

Anaesthetic Technique
The aims of the technique are:
1 Adequate safe anaesthesia for the mother.
2 Full uterine relaxation (usually by deep volatile anaesthesia).
3 Maintenance of uterine volume i.e. only the head and neck and upper torso are delivered through the uterine incision until the fetal airway is secured.
4 Maintenance of adequate uteroplacental blood-flow.
5 Appropriate anaesthesia and muscle relaxation of the fetus.

Pre-induction Phase
1 Ensure adequate staff and expertise are present as described above.
2 Ensure blood is available for maternal transfusion.

Maternal Anaesthesia
Although this procedure can be done under regional anaesthesia, general anaesthesia is usually preferred.
1 Consider establishing a lumbar epidural block for intra-operative and postoperative analgesia.
2 Induce general anaesthesia as described in *Caesarean Section (CS)*. Placing the mother in the lithotomy position enables the fetal airway anaesthetist/surgeon to stand between the mother's legs and provides good access to the fetal head.

3 Uterine relaxation can be attained by high dose inspired volatile anaesthetic (about 2–3 × MAC) in 100% oxygen e.g. sevoflurane 2.8–4.5%[71] or isoflurane 1.8–2.2%.[72] It may take 20 minutes or longer to achieve adequate uterine relaxation.

4 Some authors advocate maintaining uterine volume by infusing warm saline (aminioinfusion).[73]

5 If uterine relaxation is inadequate with volatile anaesthetic alone, consider adding a glyceryl trinitrate (GTN) infusion. Boluses of 50–100 μg plus an infusion of 15–20 μg/kg/min are usually effective. Cease the infusion when the cord is clamped.

6 Blood loss from the uterus can be reduced by a continuous suture around the uterine incision or by uterine staples.[74]

7 Once the fetal airway is secured and the fetus delivered reduce the concentration of inhaled volatile anaesthetic and administer oxytocin 10 units IV then an infusion of 40 units of oxytocin in 1000 mL of Hartmann's solution over 6 h. If the uterus will not contract **see** *Postpartum Haemorrhage*.

8 Treat maternal hypotension in the usual way with appropriate IV fluids and boluses of ephedrine and/or metariminol or other vasoconstrictor.

Fetal/Neonatal Anaesthesia

In addition to the inhalational agent administered to the mother, Bui et al. recommended the following drugs IM for fetal anaesthesia:[72]

1 fentanyl 10 μg/kg
2 vecuronium 0.2 mg/kg
3 atropine 10 μg/kg.

Monitor the fetus with pulse oximetry. Mean fetal preductal oxygen saturation is only about 50%.[75] The mean value for SpO_2 during EXIT procedures is about 71%.[73] Do not let fetal SpO_2 fall below this value. A fetal scalp electrode can also be placed to measure the heart rate. Prevent/treat fetal bradycardia (HR < 110). An IV cannula in the fetal hand is useful if surgery is necessary.

◗ Extracorporeal Membrane Oxygenation (ECMO)

More than a brief description of this complex treatment modality is beyond the scope of this manual. ECMO is a technique of respiratory support used for extremely hypoxic patients especially newborns with a reversible cause e.g. meconium aspiration. Basically blood is oxygenated and CO_2 is removed outside the body using hollow fibre oxygenators. The lungs are 'rested' and the harmful effects of ventilating the severely diseased lung are reduced. ECMO is very successful in newborns but results in adults are less encouraging.

There are several forms of ECMO including:

1 Veno–venous—blood is drained from the venous system, oxygenated and then returned to the venous system. No cardiac support is required.

2 Veno–arterial—blood is drawn from the venous system, oxygenated and then returned to the arterial system with a biopump providing cardiac support. The blood must be anticogulated, usually with heparin.

In neonates the right internal jugular (RIJ) vein is used for veno–venous bypass and veno–arterial bypass utilises the RIJ and the right common carotid artery. In the adult, veno–arterial ECMO involves accessing the right atrium or IVC for venous blood drainage to the oxygenator and then pumped infusion of the oxygenated blood into the femoral artery.

○ Eye Blocks

These are used for procedures such as cataract surgery.

Innervation of the Eye

Afferent fibres from the cornea and conjunctiva pass through the ciliary ganglion in the retrobulbar space and thence to the ophthalmic division of the trigeminal nerve. The lateral rectus muscle is supplied by the abducent (VI cranial nerve), the superior oblique by the trochlear nerve (IV cranial nerve) and the remainder by the oculomotor nerve (III cranial nerve). Remember $LR_6SO_4R_3$. Two types of block are described. With each type first establish IV access.

Topics Covered in this Section

▶ Peribulbar Eye Blocks
▶ Sub-Tenon's Block

Peribulbar Eye Blocks

Two-injection Site Technique

1 Use a mixture of bupivacaine 0.5%, 4 mL + lignocaine 2% and hyaluronidase 150–300 units. Alternatively, use ropivacaine 10 mg/mL with hyaluronidase. Use a 25 G 33 mm orbital block needle. Although adrenaline containing solutions are frequently used,[76] they are not without risk. Adrenaline does not prolong the effects of bupivacaine and results in a reduction in ophthalmic artery pressure.[77] Adrenaline should not be used if orbital vascular pathology is suspected.[76,77]

2 Surgically prep the skin with a suitable antiseptic. Ask the patient to fix the eye on an object on the ceiling so that the eye does not move and is in the neutral position. Anaesthetise the conjunctiva with amethocaine 1%. Consider sedating the patient prior to LA injection with a small dose of propofol e.g. 10–30 mg IV.

3 *First Injection* Insert percutaneously into the lower outer quadrant of the orbit at the junction of the lateral third and medial two-thirds of the

inferior orbital rim. Direct the needle posteriorly. Once past the equator of the eye, angle the needle superomedially so that the tip lies near the apex of the orbital cone, at a depth of about 2.5 cm. Ensure that the eye moves freely, and that it has not been penetrated. If aspiration is negative, inject 4–6 mL of LA. The upper eyelid should droop almost immediately. Inject another 1 mL while withdrawing the needle.

4   *Alternatively for First Injection—Inject Transconjunctivally* Retract the lower eyelid, and insert the needle into the inferior fornix at the 7:30 clock position in the right eye and 4:30 clock position for the left eye, 2 mm lateral to the limbus.[76] Advance the needle tangentially between the rim of the orbit and the globe. When the needle tip is past the equator, angle the tip medially and cephalad and insert to a depth of 2.5 cm. Inject as above.

5   *Second Injection* Insert needle percutaneously 2 mm inferior and 2 mm medial to the supraorbital notch. Direct the needle posteriorly and slightly superiorly to a depth of 2 cm, then 0.5 cm medially.[78] Inject 2–3 mL of LA.

6   After the above injections, tape the eye closed, and apply pressure via a Honan balloon or similar mercury filled device. Aim to apply 20–30 mm Hg pressure for 5–10 min.[76] Do not apply for more than 20 min.[76]

7   If the block is inadequate after 10 min, 'top up' the block with 2–5 mL of 2% lignocaine via the first injection site.

Peribulbar Block Single Injection Technique

In this variation a relatively large volume of ropivacaine plus hyaluronidase is used.

The site of injection is identical to the first injection site described above.

For the average sized orbit inject 8 mL of ropivacaine 10 mg/mL plus hyaluronidase 750 units over 30–45 s.[79] Inject an additional 2–4 mL if a 'top-up' injection is required 10 min after the initial injection.[79]

Sub-Tenon's Block

This block is less likely to injure the eye than peribulbar or retrobulbar techniques.

Anatomy

Tenon's capsule is a dense layer of white connective tissue surrounding the globe and the extraocular muscles at the front of the orbit. It lies directly under the conjunctiva and is superficial to the sclera. Tenon's capsule merges with the conjunctiva about 1 mm from the limbus and extends posteriorly to attach to the fibrous ring around the optic nerve. Sub-Tenon's space is a potential space between the sclera and Tenon's capsule.

Technique

1   The patient is directed to look upwards and outwards, and amethocaine 1% is instilled onto the medial portion of the bulbar conjunctiva.

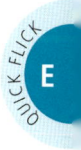

QUICK FLICK **E**

2 Instil 1–2 drops of 5% povidone to sterilise the conjunctiva.

3 Position the eyelid speculum to keep the eye open. Ask the patient to look upwards and outwards relative to the eye to be anaesthetised.

4 Using small, sterile (e.g. Moorfield's) forceps, pick up the conjunctiva and anterior Tenon's capsule at the infer-nasal point at least 5 mm from the limbus (7:30 clock position for the left eye). Take care to avoid conjunctival vessels.

5 With a curved pair of spring scissors (e.g. Wescott) make a small cut 1–2 mm long through the conjunctiva and Tenon's capsule so that bare white sclera is visible. The closed scissors are gently advanced to create a space between the sclera and Tenon's capsule.

6 Still holding the conjunctiva and Tenon's capsule with the forceps insert a sterile lacrimal cannula through the incision. Gently advance the lacrimal cannula (Southampton needle) along sub-Tenon's space and following the curvature of the globe, to the posterior part at the back of the eye. The direction of insertion is between the attachments of the media and inferior rectus muscles. Hydrodissection (used gently) can be applied to clear adhesions between the sclera and the Tenon's capsule as the cannula is passed beyond the equator of the eye. Fully insert the cannula.

7 Inject 3–4 mL of LA solution over 15–30 s. Use a 1:1 mixture of 2% lignocaine and 0.5% bupivacaine, or 1% ropivacaine. Add hyaluronidase to the LA to give a concentration of 15–60 u/mL. Consider changing the cannula tip position slightly after each mL to make injection easier.

8 Remove the eyelid speculum and apply a Honan balloon or gentle digital pressure for 5 min.

9 Consider a facial nerve block achieved by infiltration with 1.5 mL of LA into the lateral aspect of each eyelid deep to orbicularis oculi.

Problems

1 Subconjunctival haemorrhage may occur.

2 Subconjunctival fluid accumulation can occur if the cannula is too superficial.

Contraindications to sub-Tenon's Block

Anatomical features of the eye which may preclude a sub-Tenon's block include a large pterygium or the presence of a retinal band.[80]

○ Eye Injury, Penetrating

If the patient is *not fasted* and surgery is urgent and the eye is salvageable, the first priority is to prevent aspiration of gastric contents. The second priority is to prevent loss of intraocular contents. The most appropriate technique in the 'open eye, full stomach' scenario is controversial, as discussed below:

1 Consider the following drugs to reduce the risk and effects of aspiration:
   a) Ranitidine 50 mg IV.
   b) Metoclopramide 10 mg IV.
   c) Sodium citrate 0.3 M 30 mL PO.

2 Pre-oxygenate for 5 minutes, and consider the following drugs to attenuate the effects of laryngoscopy and intubation on intraocular pressure (IOP):
   a) Lignocaine 1.5 mg/kg IV.
   b) Fentanyl 2 µg/kg.
   Give both drugs 3–4 min prior to intubation.
   c) Thiopentone 3–5 mg/kg or propofol 2–2.5 mg/kg. Both of these drugs cause a reduction in intraocular pressure. Khosravi et al. reported that rises in IOP due to sux and laryngoscopy were less with propofol than with thiopentone.[81]

3 Apply cricoid pressure with the onset of anaesthesia.

4 Suxamethonium 1.5 mg/kg (immediately after thiopentone or propofol). Suxamethonium is known to increase IOP in the normal eye and theoretically could cause further damage to the open eye. However, despite its widespread use in this situation there have been *no* reports of additional eye damage.[82] In contrast, if the patient coughs, loss of intraocular contents is likely.

5 Intubate, ventilate and maintain anaesthesia with O_2, N_2O and volatile agent + nondepolarising muscle relaxant.

6 Extubate in the lateral position only when the patient is able to protect their own airway.

Alternatively

If suxamethonium is contraindicated or considered unsuitable, a modified rapid sequence technique can be used, utilising rocuronium 0.6–0.9 mg/kg. However suxamethonium remains the muscle relaxant of choice in this situation. ***See*** *Rapid Sequence Induction (RSI)*.

Regional Anaesthesia

Anaesthesia for a penetrating eye injury is normally done under GA because it is felt that eye blocks may aggravate the injury. However there are reports in the literature of eye surgery for penetrating injury being performed successfully under retrobulbar and peri bulbar blocks.[83] This approach should not therefore be automatically dismissed.

REFERENCES

1 Pederson JL, Lilles JD, Hammer NA, et al. Bupivacaine in micro spheres prolongs analgesia after subcutaneous infiltration in humans: a dose-finding study. *Anesth Analg* 2004; 99: 912–18.

2   Martin JT, Tautz TJ, Antognini JF. Safety of regional anaesthesia in Eisenmenger's syndrome. *Regional Anaesthesia and Pain Medicine* 2002; 27: 509–13.

3   Jones HG, Stoneham MD. Continuous cervical plexus block for carotid body tumour excision in a patient with Eisenmenger's syndrome. *Anaesthesia* 2006; 61: 1214–18.

4   Pollack KL, Chestnut DH, Wenstrom KD. Anesthetic management of a patient with Eisenmenger's syndrome. *Anesth Analg* 1990; 70: 212–15.

5   Morray JP, Lynn AM, Stamm SJ et al. Hemodynamic effects of ketamine in chidren with congenital heart disease. *Anesth Analg* 1984; 62: 895–9.

6   Jones P, Patel A. Anaesthetic dilemma: Eisenmenger's syndrome and problems with anaesthesia. *Br J Hosp Med* 1995; 54: 214.

7   Sammut MS, Paes ML. Anaesthesia for laparoscopic cholecystectomy in a patient with Eisenmenger's syndrome. *Br J Anaesth* 1997; 79: 810–12.

8   Hytens L, Alexander JP. Maternal and neonatal death associated with Eisenmenger's syndrome. *Acta Anaesthesiologica Belgica* 1986; 37: 45–51.

9   Smedstad KG, Morison DH. Pulmonary hypertension and pregnancy: a series of eight cases. *Can J Anaesth* 1994; 41:6: 502–12.

10 Yentis SM, Steer PJ, Plaat F. Eisenmenger's syndrome in pregnancy: maternal and fetal mortality in the 1990s. *Br J Obstet Gynaecol* 1998; 105: 921–2.

11 Spinnato JA, Kraynack BJ, Cooper MW. Eisenmenger's syndrome in pregnancy: epidural anaesthesia for elective Caesarean section. *N Eng J Med* 1981; 20: 1215–17.

12 Stoelting RK, Dierdorf SF. *Anesthesia and Co-existing Disease*. 4th edn. Churchill-Livingstone, Philadelphia 2002: 58.

13 Mason R. *Anaesthesia Data Book—A Perioperative and Peripartum Manual*, 3rd edn. Greenwich Medical Media Limited, London 2001; 166.

14 Cole PJ, Cross MH, Dresner M. Incremental spinal anaesthesia for elective Caesarean section in a patient with Eisenmenger's syndrome. *Br J Aneasth* 2001; 86: 723–6.

15 Temelcos C, Kuhn R, Stribley C. Sterilisation of women with Eisenmenger's syndrome: report of 4 cases. *Aust NZ Obstet Gynaecol* 1997; 37: 121–3.

16 Ding Z, White P. Anesthesia for electroconvulsive therapy. *Anesth Analg* 2002; 94: 1351–64.

17 McPherson RD, Barrett N. Electroconvulsive therapy in patients with cardiac pacemakers. *Anaesth Intensive Care* 2006; 34: 470–4.

18 Anderson FA, Arsland D, Holst-Larsen H. Effects of combined methohexitone-remifentanil anaesthesia in electroconvulsive therapy. *Acta Anaethesiol Scand* 2001; 45: 830–3.

19 Locala J, Irefin S, Malone D et al. The comparative hemodynamic effects of methohexital and remifentanil in electroconvulsive therapy. *J of ECT* 2005; 21: 12–15.

20 White P, Amos Q, Zhang Y et al. Anesthetic considerations of magnetic seizure therapy. *Anesth Analg* 2006; 103: 76–80.

21 Sasada MP, Smith SP. *Drugs in Anaesthesia and Intensive Care*, 3rd edn. Oxford University Press, Oxford,1998: 138–9.

22 Viertiö-Oja H, Maja V, Särkela M et al. Description of the Entropy™ algorithm as applied in the Datex-Ohmeda S/5™ Entropy Module. *Acta Anaesthesiol Scand* 2004; 48: 154–61.

23 Vakkuri A, Yli-Hankala A, Talija P. Time-frequency balanced spectral entropy as a measure of anesthetic drug effect in central nervous system during sevoflurane, propofol, and thiopental anesthesia. *Acta Anaesthesiol Scand* 2004; 48: 145–53.

24 Ruppen W, Derry S, McQuay H, Moore A. Incidence of epidural hematoma, infection and neurological injury in obstetric patients with epidural analgesia/anesthesia. *Anesthesiol* 2006; 105: 394–9.

25 Darouchi RO. Spinal epidural abscess. *N Eng J Med* 2006; 355: 2012–20.

26 Kindler CH, Seeberger MD, Staender SE. Epidural abscess complicating epidural anaesthesia and analgesia. *Acta Anaesthesiol Scand* 1998; 42: 614–20.

27 Del Curling O, Gower DJ, McWhorter JM. Changing concepts in spinal epidural abscess: a report of 29 cases. *Neurosurgery* 1990; 27: 185–92.

28 Danner RL, Hartman BJ. Update of spinal epidural abscesses: 35 cases and review of the literature. *Reviews of Infectious Diseases* 1987; 9: 477–94.

29 Smarkusky L, DeCarvalho H, Bermudez A et al. Acute onset headache complicating labour epidural caused by intrapartum pneumocephalus. *Obstets and Gynecol* 2006; 108: 795–8.

30 Saberski LR, Kondamuri S, Osinubi OYO. Identification of the epidural space: Is loss of resistance to air a safe technique? A review of the complications related to the use of air. *Regional Anaesth and Pain Med* 1997; 22: 3–15.

31 Brown DL, Wedel DJ. Spinal, epidural and caudal anaesthesia. In: Miller RD, ed. *Anaesthesia*, 3rd edn, Churchill Livingstone, New York 1990: 1397.

32 Wong CA, Scavone BM, Peaceman AM et al. The risk of cesarean delivery with neuraxial analgesia given early versus late in labour [see comment]. *N Engl J Med* 2005; 352: 655–65.

33 Anim-Somuah M, Smyth R, Howell C. Epidural versus non-epidural or no analgesia in labour. *Cochrane Database Systematic Reviews* (4: CD000331), 2005.

QUICK FLICK E

34 Torvaldsen S, Roberts CL, Bell JC, Raynes-Greenow CH. Discontinuation of epidural analgesia late in labour for reducing the adverse delivery outcomes associated with epidural anaesthesia. Cochrane Database Systematic Reviews (4: CD004457), 2004.

35 Blomberg RG, Lofstrom JB. The test dose in regional anaesthesia. *Acta Anaesthesiol Scand* 1991; 35: 465–8.

36 Evron S, Glezerman M, Sadan O et al. Patient-controlled epidural anaesthesia for labour pain: effect on labour, delivery and neonatal outcome of 0.125% bupivacaine vs. 0.2% ropivacaine. *Internat J Obstet Anesth* 2004; 13: 5–10.

37 Goodman EJ, Dehorta E, Taguiam JM. Safety of spinal and epidural anaesthesia in patients with chorioamnionitis. *Reg Anesth* 1996; 21: 436–41.

38 De Lem-Casasola OA, Lema MJ. Postoperative epidural opioid analgesia: What are the choices? *Anesth Analg* 1996; 83: 867–75.

39 El-Behesy, JD, Koh KF et al. Distinguishing cerebrospinal fluid from saline used to identify the extradural space. *BJA* 1996; 77: 784–5.

40 Collier CB. Complications of regional anaesthesia. In: Birnbach DJ, Gatt S, eds. *Textbook of Obstetric Anesthesia*. New York: Churchill Livingstone, 2000: 504–23.

41 Kuczkowski KM, Benumof JL. Decrease in the incidence of post-dural puncture headache: maintaining CSF volume. *Acta Anaesthesiol Scand* 2003; 47: 98–100.

42 Kuczkowski KM. Decreasing the incidence of post-dural puncture headache: an update. (Letter) *Acta Anaesthesiol Scand* 2005; 49: 594.

43 Gielen MJM. Post dural puncture headache: a review. *Regional Anaesthesia* 1989; 14: 101–6.

44 Scavone B, Wong C, Sullivan J, et al. Efficacy of a prophylactic epidural blood patch in preventing post dural puncture headache in patients after inadvertent dural puncture. *Anesthesiol* 2004; 101: 1422–7.

45 Carp H, Sing PJ, Vadhera R, Jayaram A. Effects of serotonin-receptor agonist sumatriptan on postdural headache: report of 6 cases. *Anesth Analg* 1994; 79: 180–2.

46 Morgan P. Review article: Spinal anaesthesia in obstetrics. *Can J Anaesth* 1995; 42: 1145–63.

47 Rivindran RS. Epidural autologous blood patch on an outpatient basis. *Anesth Analg* 1984; 63: 962.

48 Beards SC, Jackson A, Griffiths AG, Horsman EL. Magnetic resonance imaging of extradural blood patches: appearances from 30 min to 18 h. *BJA* 1993; 71: 182–8.

49 Chiron B, Laffon M, Ferrandière M, Pitter J-F. Postdural puncture

headache in a patient with sickle cell disease: use of an epidural colloid patch. *Can J Anesth* 2003; 50: 812–14.

50 Evron S, Gladkov V, Sessler D, et al. Predistension of the epidural space before catheter insertion reduces the incidence of intravascular epidural catheter insertion. *Anesth Analg* 2007; 105: 460–4.

51 Southorn P, Vasdev GM, Chantigin RC, Lawson GM. Reducing the potential morbidity of an unintentional spinal anaesthesia by aspirating cerebrospinal fluid. *Br J Anaesth* 1996; 76: 467–9.

52 Tsui BCH, Malherbe S, Koller J, Aronyk K. Reversal of an unintentional spinal anaesthetic by cerebrospinal lavage. *Anesth Analg* 2004; 98: 434–6.

53 Haljamoe H. Thromboprophylaxis, coagulation disorders and regional anaesthesia. *Acta Anaesthesiol Scand* 1996; 40: 1024–40.

54 Horlocker TT. Low molecular weight heparin and neuraxial blockade. *Thrombosis Research* 2001; 101: V141–V154.

55 Sage DJ. Epidurals, spinals and bleeding disorders in pregnancy: A review. *Anaesth Intensive Care* 1990; 18: 319–26.

56 Horlocker TT, Wedel D, Schroeder D et al. Perioperative antiplatelet therapy does not increase the risk of spinal haematoma associated with regional anaesthesia. *Anesth Analg* 1995; 80: 303–9.

57 Motte S, Samama CM, Guay J et al. Prevention of postoperative venous thromboembolism. Risk assessment and methods of prophylaxis. *Can J Anesth* 2006; 53: S68–S79.

58 Scott DB, Hibbard BM. Serious non-fatal complications associated with extradural block in obstetric practice. *Br J Anaesth* 1990; 64: 537–41.

59 Aromaa U, Lahdensuu M, Cozanitis DA. Severe complications associated with epidural and spinal anaesthesia in Finland 1987–1993. A study based on patient insurance claims. *Acta Anaesthesiol Scand* 1997; 41: 445–52.

60 Schmidt A, Nolte H. Subdural and epidural haematomas following epidural anaesthesia. A literature review. *Anaesthetist* 1992; 41: 276–84.

61 Wood N, Menzies R, McIntyre P. Epiglottitis in Sydney before and after the introduction of vaccination against *Haemophilus influenzae* type b disease. *Internal Medicine J* 2005; 35: 530–5.

62 Chang YL, Lo SH, Wang PC, Shu YH. Adult acute epiglottitis: experience in a Taiwanese setting. *Otology—Head and Neck Surgery* 2005; 132: 689–93.

63 Neligan PJ. Infectious Diseases and Bioterrorism. In: Fleisher LA, ed. *Anesthesia and Uncommon Diseases*, 5th edn. Philadelphia Pennsylvannia, Saunders Elsevier 2006: 377–411.

64 Prasad K, Krishnan P, Al-Roomi K, Sequeira R. Anticonvulsant therapy for status epilepticus. *Br J Clin Pharmacol* 2007; 63: 640–7.

QUICK FLICK

E

65 Treatment of convulsive status epilepticus. Recommendations of the Epilepsy Foundation of America's Working Group on Status Epilepticus. *JAMA* 1993; 270: 854–9.

66 Kelly BJ. Status Epilepticus. In Parsons PE, Weiner-Kronish, eds. JP. *Critical Care Secrets*, Hanley & Belfus, Philadelphia, 1992: 284–7.

67 Opdam H. Status Epilepticus. In Bersten AD, Soni N, Oh TE eds. *Oh's Intensive Care Manual* 5th edn. Butterworth–Heinemann, Edinburgh 2003: 485–93.

68 Hall RI. Editorial. Esmolol—just another beta blocker? *Can J Anaesth* 1992; 39: 757–64.

69 Malinow AM. Anaesthetic considerations for pre-eclamptic patient. *Audio Digest, Anesthesiology* 1995; 37: 21.

70 Ramanathan J, Bennett K. Pre-eclampsia: fluids, drugs and anaesthetic management. *Anesthesiol Clin North Am* 2003; 21: 145–63.

71 Dahlgren G, Törnberg HDC, Pregner K, Irestedt L. Four cases of the ex utero intrapartum treatment (EXIT) procedure: anaesthetic implications. *International J Obstet Anesth* 2004; 13: 178–82.

72 Bui TH, Grunewald C, Frenckner B et al. Successful EXIT (ex utero intrapartum treatment) procedure in a fetus diagnosed with congenital high obstruction syndrome due to laryngeal atresia. *Eur J Pediatric Surg* 2000; 10: 328–33.

73 Bouchard S, Johnson MP, Flake AW, et al. The EXIT procedure: experience and outcome in 31 cases. *J Pediatric Surg* 2002; 37: 418–26.

74 Hirose S, Farmer DL, Lee H et al. The ex utero intrapartum treatment procedure: looking back at the EXIT. *J Pediatric Surg* 2004; 39: 375–80.

75 Dildy GA, Clark SL, Loukas CA. Intrapartum fetal pulse oximetry: past, present and future. *Am J Obstet Gynecol* 1996; 175: 1–9.

76 Anathanam JJK, Francis RI. How to do a peri-bulbar block: the transconjunctival approach modified for the anxious patient. *Br J Hosp Med* 1994; 52: 295–8.

77 Wong DHW. Regional anaesthesia for intraocular surgery. *Can J Anaesth* 1993; 40: 635–57.

78 Berry CB, Murphy PM. Regional anaesthesia for cataract surgery. *Br J Hosp Med* 1993; 49: 10: 689–701.

79 Corke PJ, Baker J, Cammack R. Comparison of 1% ropivacaine and a mixture of 2% lignocaine and 0.5% bupivacaine peribulbar anaesthesia in cataract surgery. *Anesth Intensive Care* 1999; 27: 248–52.

80 Koh JWM, Cammack R. Sub-Tenon's block in cataract surgery—a comparison of 1% ropivacaine and a mixture of 2% lignocaine and 0.5% bupivacaine. *Anaesth Intensive Care* 2005; 33: 597–600.

81 Khosravi MB, Lahasee M, Azemati S, Eghbal MH. Intraocular pressure

changes after succinylcholine and end tracheal intubation. (Letter) *Indian J Ophthalmology* 2007; 55: 164.

82 Ferrari LR. The injured eye. *Anesthesiol Clin N Am* 1996 March; 14(1): 125–50.

83 Niemi-Murola L, Immonen I, Kallio H, Maunuksela EL. Preliminary experience of combined peri- and retro bulbar block in surgery for penetrating eye injuries. *Eur J Anaesthesiol* 2003; 20: 478–81.

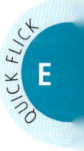

QUICK FLICK

E

F

◖ Failed Intubation

See *Difficult Airway Management*.

◖ Failure to Regain Consciousness after General Anaesthesia

See *Confusion, Agitation, Decreased Level of Consciousness, Postanaesthetic*.

◖ Fasting Pre-operatively

These guidelines relate to elective surgery. **See also** *Aspiration, Prevention and Treatment*.

Adult Fast for solid food for 6 h, and for clear fluids for 4 h preoperatively. Clear fluids more than 2 h before anaesthesia are probably acceptable.[1] Alcoholic beverages delay gastric emptying and are not acceptable as clear fluids.[2] Gum chewing before surgery probably does not increase the risk of aspiration.[2]

Child Fast for solid food and formula milk for 6 h preoperatively. Clear fluids and breast milk can be given up to 4 h preoperatively. Clear fluids more than 2 h before anaesthesia are probably acceptable.[3]

◖ Fastrach™ Device

A laryngeal mask type device used as an aid to intubation.
See *Laryngeal Mask Airway (Including ProSeal™, Fastrach™ and C-Trach™)*.

◖ Fat Embolism Syndrome and Bone Cement Implantation Syndrome

Topics Covered in this Section
▶ Fat Embolism
▶ Bone Cement Implantation Syndrome

Fat Embolism

In this condition fat globules and bone marrow elements cause potentially life threatening clinical effects on the lungs and brain. The source of the fat emboli can be:

1 Long bone fractures.
2 Surgery on bones e.g. joint replacement, intramedullary nailing.
3 Bone marrow transplant.
4 Liposuction.[4]

The presence of intravascular fat globules is probably very common with long bone fractures or instrumentation but only a small percentage of such patients develop the syndrome.[5] These fat globules cause acute lung and brain injury through as yet unexplained mechanisms. Fat may enter the systemic circulation and travel to the brain via a patent foramen ovale, or by traversing the pulmonary circulation and entering the systemic circulation.[6] It is not known how or why the fat causes organ injury. This could be due to mechanical obstruction by the fat or pulmonary vasoconstriction.

Clinical Manifestations

1 Hypoxia, bilateral pulmonary infiltrates, ventilation-perfusion mismatch and shunting. Florid pulmonary oedema may occur.
2 Pyrexia.
3 Confusion and restlessness, coma.
4 Petechial rash particularly affecting the upper half of the body, conjunctiva and mucous membranes of the mouth.
5 Retinal examination may reveal exudates and haemorrhages. Fat droplets may be seen traversing the retinal vessels.
6 Coagulopathy and thrombocytopenia may occur.

Diagnosis

1 The diagnosis can be made from the clinical picture with manifestations occurring within 48 h of a relevant procedure or injury.[7]
2 CXR may show poorly defined diffuse pulmonary infiltrates.
3 ECG may show a right ventricular strain pattern with right bundle branch block, right axis deviation, prominent S wave in I, Q wave in III and inverted T wave in III.
4 ABG may show a severe alveolar-arterial oxygen tension gradient of greater than 100 mm Hg.
5 Examination of urine and sputum may reveal the presence of fat globules.
6 A fall in $ETCO_2$ during surgery may indicate that fat embolisation is occurring.
7 Cerebral MRI may be diagnostic for brain fat embolism.

Treatment

1 Treatment is largely supportive and predominantly aimed at improving oxygenation. Death is usually due to respiratory complications. Consider high concentration O_2 therapy, CPAP, or intubation and IPPV + PEEP. Massive severe fat embolism has been successfully treated with veno-arterial ECMO.[8]
2 Neurological damage may be considerable and cause long-term disability.
3 The mortality is between 10 and 45% in florid cases.[7]

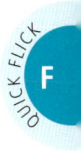

Bone Cement Implantation Syndrome

Description and Pathophysiology[9]

This syndrome occurs in association with cemented total hip replacement surgery during the procedure. The cause of the syndrome is unclear. It does not appear that the bone cement actually enters the circulation but other material such as fat and other bone marrow contents do embolise and effects are similar to fat embolism. Hayakawa et al. hypothesised that some of the embolised material might be bone powder from the reaming process.[10]

Clinical Manifestations[7]

Clinical features include:

1 hypotension
2 hypoxaemia
3 pulmonary hypertension
4 cardiac dysrhythmias, pulseless electrical activity
5 cardiac arrest and death.

Treatment

The syndrome may last seconds to minutes particularly in patients with healthy hearts. Treatment is supportive. Cardiac output and blood pressure must be maintained with:

1 IV fluid loading.
2 Vasoactive drugs such as metaraminol.
3 Inotropes such as adrenaline may be required.
4 Maintained oxygenation.

◗ Fatty Liver of Pregnancy, Acute

This very rare condition is of unknown aetiology and occurs in the third trimester of pregnancy. Its incidence is about 1:13 000–16 000 pregnancies.[11] The liver abnormalities may be confused with, or overlap with, pre-eclampsia. Mortality is between 10 and 20% and liver transplantation may be required.[12]

Clinical Picture

The main symptoms, signs and biochemical abnormalities are:

1 nausea, vomiting, heartburn, oesophagitis, gastric erosions and haematemesis.
2 upper right abdominal pain.
3 jaundice which is often mild.
4 coagulopathy, DIC.
5 elevated liver transaminase values.
6 leucocytosis, hyperuricaemia, hypoglycaemia.
7 renal failure.
8 fulminant hepatic failure with encephalopathy/hepatic coma.

Diagnosis

Definitive diagnosis is by liver biopsy or typical findings on CT scan. There is microvascular fatty infiltration of the liver.

Treatment

1 Delivery provides the only definitive treatment resulting in reversal of the condition unless liver damage is very severe.[12]
2 Monitor BSL frequently. A continuous infusion of 10% glucose to prevent/treat hypoglycaemia may be required.
3 Correct clotting abnormalities, if present, with FFP, vitamin K, platelets.
4 Optimise intravascular volume.
5 Epidural anaesthesia is probably preferable to GA for Caesarean section but is contraindicated if a significant coagulopathy is present.

◯ Femoral Nerve Block and 3 in 1 (Triple Nerve) Block

The 3 in 1 block aims to block the femoral and obturator nerves and the lateral cutaneous nerve of thigh.

Anatomy

Femoral Nerve (L2, L3, L4) arises from the lumbar plexus and is sensory to the anterior thigh. Through the saphenous nerve branch it also supplies sensation to the medial leg, ankle and foot. The motor supply of the femoral nerve is to the muscles of the anterior thigh including the quadriceps. The nerve enters the thigh beneath the inguinal ligament just lateral to the femoral artery.

Obturator Nerve (L2, L3, L4) also arising from the lumbar plexus, this nerve innervates the skin on the medial side of the thigh and the knee and hip joint.

Lateral Cutaneous Nerve of Thigh (L2, L3) supplies the skin over the antero-lateral thigh to the knee.

Technique for Femoral Nerve Block

Secure IV access, sterilise the skin at the injection site.

1 Insert a short bevelled 22 G block needle in a 30° cephalad direction just lateral to the femoral artery and just below the inguinal ligament.
2 Feel for 2 'pops' as the needle passes first through the fascia lata and then the fascia iliaca. The tip of the needle should lie just lateral to, and slightly deeper than, the femoral artery and preferably the needle should be seen to pulsate slightly. A nerve stimulator can also be used, looking for contractions of the quadriceps, with a stimulating current of ≈ 0.4–0.6 mA.

QUICK FLICK

F

3   Inject 15 mL of bupivacaine 0.5% incrementally ensuring negative
    aspiration prior to and during injection. Ropivacaine 20 mL of 1% can also
    be used.

Technique for 3 in 1 Block

The site of injection is identical to above but a greater volume of LA is used.
Inject 30 mL (2–2.5 mg/kg) of bupivacaine 0.5% while applying pressure
distal to the injection site to encourage LA spread towards the lumbar plexus.

Ultrasound Guided Femoral Nerve Block

1   Secure IV access and use strict sterile technique at all times.
2   Place the ultrasound probe just below the inguinal ligament (short axis
    view-probe placed parallel to ligament).
3   The femoral artery is the main landmark. It is round, usually smaller than
    the femoral vein and is pulsatile. If a second artery is seen, the femoral
    artery has given off its profunda femoris branch.
4   The femoral vein is medial to the artery and is compressible.
5   The femoral nerve is lateral to the artery and is triangular or oval in shape.
    The nerve gives off branches laterally hence the medial side appears
    thicker than the lateral side.

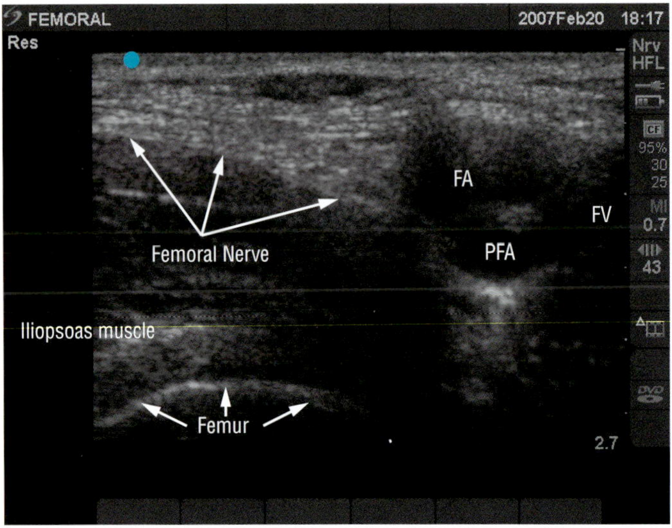

Figure F1 Ultrasound image of femoral nerve

FA = Femoral artery   PFA = Profunda femoris artery
FV = Femoral vein

6 One can imagine a figure wearing a dunce's hat, the vein is the body, the artery the head and the nerve the hat.

7 The injection needle should be positioned at least twice, once medially close to the artery and once laterally towards the apex of the triangle.

8 The injection of the anaesthetic should give the appearance of a doughnut with the nerve at the centre.

Continuous Femoral Nerve Blockade

This can be achieved using a kit such as Pajunk Plexalong and a stimulating catheter. The steps are as for femoral nerve block as described above to locate the nerve. Then:

1 Insert the guide wire through the catheter.

2 Remove the stimulating catheter and insert the infusion catheter over the guide wire.

3 Establish femoral nerve blockade with 20 mL of ropivacaine 0.75%.

4 Commence infusion of ropivacaine 0.2% 10–12 mL/hr.

Comments

The femoral nerve block provides analgesia for femoral shaft and neck fractures and surgery involving the anterior thigh. Three in 1 (triple nerve) block has been used for hip replacement surgery combined with sedation and an additional separate block of the lateral cutaneous nerve of thigh.[13]
See *Lateral Cutaneous Nerve of Thigh Block*.

◐ Fenoldopam

Fenoldopam is a selective dopamine 1 receptor agonist. Its effects include renovascular vasodilatation ($3.5 \times$ more potent than dopamine) and natriuresis. It is thought that this drug may provide some protection against renal failure in at-risk patients having procedures associated with renal insult. Rannuci et al. found that fenoldopam reduced the incidence of renal failure in patients having CABG who were deemed at high risk for this complication.[14]

Dose

0.1 µg/kg/min by IV infusion.

◐ Fentanyl

Synthetic phenylpiperidine derivative (like pethidine) with opioid-type analgesic properties. $60–80 \times$ more potent than morphine, with a more rapid onset of action. Fentanyl has a high margin of safety producing little cardiovascular depression but may cause bradycardia. Also has a short duration of action at low dose (< 10 µg/kg) but becomes a long acting drug at high dose (50–100 µg/kg). Elimination half-life 1.5–6 h.

Dose

Non-cardiac Surgery Dose depends on the duration and nature of surgery.
Adult Dose For minor surgery 50–100 µg is a reasonable dose in the adult with effects lasting 30–60 min. Higher doses will cause more prolonged effects.
Child Dose 1–2 µg/kg.

Cardiac Surgery 50–100 µg/kg IV. Effects last ≈ 6 h.

IV Infusion (for Postoperative Analgesia) 50 µg/kg in 50 mL N/S run at 1–4 mL/h (equivalent to 1–4 µg/kg/h).

Epidural 50–100 µg. **See** *Epidural Anaesthesia* and *Patient Controlled Epidural Analgesia (PCEA)*.

Intrathecal 25 µg is effective and safe to supplement LA used for SAB.

Topical Fentanyl Applied in the form of fentanyl patches which are currently available in 4 different strengths; 25, 50, 75 and 100 µg/h delivered to the systemic circulation. The patches are applied for 72 h and are used in the treatment of chronic cancer pain. Fentanyl 50 µg/h is ≈ 135–244 mg/day of oral morphine (transdermal fentanyl product information).

Intranasal Fentanyl Intranasal fentanyl is about 70% as effective as IV fentanyl.[15]

Fentanyl Buccal Tablets These are rapidly effective providing analgesia in 10–15 min.

❍ Fetal Death in Utero

See *Intrauterine Fetal Death*.

❍ Fetal Resuscitation in Utero

The following steps are recommended by Levy for patients with a non-reassuring fetal cardiotocograph trace, to optimise fetal condition while an urgent Caesarean section is organised:[16]

1 Cease syntocinon infusion.
2 Position the patient fully left lateral.
3 Supplementary oxygen by face mask.
4 Infuse 1 L of crystalloid.
5 If blood pressure is low give ephedrine or metaraminol.
6 Consider tocolysis with terbutaline 250 µg subcut or glyceryltrinitrate 400 µg sublingually.

❍ Fibre-optic Intubation

See *Awake Fibre-optic Intubation*.

◗ Fibrin Degradation Products (FDPs)

NR < 10 µg/mL. Plasmin causes the breakdown of fibrin into FDPs. FDP levels therefore reflect fibrinolysis. The effects of FDPs include:[17]

1 Possibly inhibiting clot formation by competing with fibrin polymerisation sites.
2 Interfering with platelet function and inhibit thrombin.
3 Possibly damaging vascular endothelium.

FDPs thus inhibit coagulation and FDP levels are increased by syndromes involving increased fibrinolysis and defibrination such as disseminated intravascular coagulation (DIC), in which FDP levels increase to >40 µg/ml.

◗ Fibrinogen

NR 200–400 mg/100 mL. Low levels occur in conditions such as disseminated intravascular coagulation. **See** *Cryoprecipitate (and Cryodepleted Plasma)*.

◗ Fist Pacing

See *Pacing, Pacemakers and Anaesthesia*.

◗ Fitting

See *Epilepsy, Status*.

◗ Fluid Replacement Therapy

Paediatric Patient: Maintenance Fluid Requirement per Hour

4 mL/kg first 10 kg + 2 mL/kg for next 10 kg + 1 mL/kg for rest of weight. For example a 32 kg child requires 40 + 20 + 12 mL/h = 72 mL/h maintenance. Standard fluid in child up to 1 year: N/4 saline + 5–10% glucose. Older child: N/4 saline + 3.75% glucose.

Potassium requirements are 3 mmol/kg/day. Add 10 mmol KCl per 500 mL bag of fluid. Ensure urine output established before giving potassium.

Adult Maintenance Fluid Requirements

A healthy 70 kg patient requires ≈ 125 mL/h maintenance fluid.

Table F1 Insensible losses occurring intra-operatively in adults

Surgery type	Insensible loss/ third space loss
GA alone	1–2 mL/kg/h
Small incision	3–4 mL/kg/h
Large incision	5–6 mL/kg/h
Bowel drawn out of wound	7–8 mL/kg/h
Major viscus or vascular surgery	9–10 mL/kg/h[18]

QUICK FLICK F

Note: Blood loss (up to the point of requiring transfusion) should be replaced in the following ratios: with colloid 1 mL blood:1 mL colloid, with crystalloid 1 mL blood:3–5 mL crystalloid.

Flumazenil

An imidazobenzodiazepine used as a competitive antagonist of benzodiazepine drugs.

Dose

Adult 200 µg IV over 15 s then 100 µg at 60 s intervals, titrate to response. Max total dose in adult 1 mg (2 mg in ICU). Effects last 15–140 min and resedation may therefore occur. IV Infusion 100–400 µg/h.

Child 5 µg/kg bolus, repeat dose at 60 s intervals to max 40 µg/kg total dose. *IV Infusion* 2–10 µg/kg/h

Fondaparinux

This is a new pentasaccharide selective factor Xa inhibitor, useful for the prevention and treatment of venous thromboembolism (DVT and PE). It has a long half-life of about 17 h.

Dose in Adults

2.5 mg subcut daily.

Advantages

1. This drug may be a useful alternative to heparin in patients with HITS. **See** *Heparin Induced Thrombocytopenia Syndrome (HITS)*.
2. Appears to be more effective than fractionated heparin in reducing the incidence of DVT.[19]

Disadvantages

1. Renally excreted. Not suitable for use in patients with renal failure.
2. Relatively long half-life with activity up to 48 h or longer after last dose. Can probably be reversed by recombinant activated factor VII in an emergency.[20]

Fontan Procedure

Only a brief discussion of this complex topic is possible in this manual. The Fontan procedure, also called single ventricle repair, is used for conditions such as tricuspid atresia and severe Ebstein's anomaly. The aim is to connect the systemic venous return directly to the pulmonary artery bypassing the congenital cardiac lesion that was the indication for the procedure. This approach excludes one ventricle creating a single ventricle systemic pump. CVP becomes the driving pressure for the pulmonary circulation. Originally the Fontan procedure involved anastamosis of the right atrium and pulmonary artery with interposition of a homograft valve. This operation was improved and now involves anastomosis of the right atrial appendage directly to the main pulmonary artery avoiding the use of any prosthetic material. In further modifications of the procedure total cavo-pulmonary connections are being used with a cavo–caval baffle directing IVC blood to the SVC orifice and anastomosing the SVC to the pulmonary artery. A small fenestration is made to the baffle to create a right-to-left shunt to the left atrium to reduce systemic venous pressure.

High systemic venous pressures can lead to:

1 Peripheral oedema.
2 Hepatomegaly, ascites and cirrhosis.
3 Pleural and pericardial effusions.
4 Protein losing enteropathy.
5 Pulmonary arteriovenous fistulae.
6 Progressive right atrial dilatation if the right atrium is included in the circulation. This can lead to atrial dysrhythmias such as SVT/atrial flutter/atrial fibrillation.

Other manifestations include:

1 Conduction disturbances such as the bradycardia/tachycardia syndrome.
2 Poor exercise tolerance.
3 Increased thrombosis/stroke risk.

Anaesthesia and the Fontan Procedure

The aims of anaesthesia are to:

1 Maintain blood flow through the lungs.
2 Maintain CO.

Towards these aims:

1 Careful patient evaluation in discussion with the patient's cardiologist is essential. **See** *Cardiac Investigations*.
2 Usually after successful repair no murmur is audible and oxygen saturation should be around 95%.
3 Invasive monitoring should be carefully considered depending on the patient's condition and type of surgery.
4 Maintain or slightly increase pre-load which is the driving pressure for the pulmonary circulation.
5 Afterload reduction is generally well tolerated if blood pressure, HR and preload are maintained.
6 Increased intrathoracic pressure may cause cardiac output to fall due to decreased venous return and decreased pulmonary blood flow therefore keep ventilation pressures low and do not use PEEP above 5 cm H_2O.[21]
7 Avoid factors that may increase pulmonary vascular resistance such as hypercarbia, acidosis, hypoxia and catecholamines.
8 Regional anaesthesia can usually be used successfully in these patients.

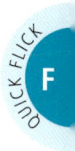

QUICK FLICK

F

9 Any technique used should be titrated slowly and carefully.

10 Endocarditis prophylaxis should be considered for at-risk procedures.

11 Treat hypotension with Trendelenburg/anti-Trendelenburg positioning and IV fluids.[22] Metaraminol may be preferable to ephedrine if a vasoconstrictor is required.

Pregnancy

Patients with a Fontan circulation tend to tolerate pregnancy poorly due to low or fixed cardiac output.

Epidural for Labour

1 Use ECG monitoring to detect dysrhythmia.

2 Do not use a loss of resistance to air technique for identifying the epidural space. Use saline instead.

3 Epidural LA must be given slowly in order to allow the patient time to physiologically adapt.

4 Maintain normovolaemia.

CS

1 Maintenance of left lateral tilt is particularly important.

2 Either GA or epidural block can be used depending on the preference and experience of the anaesthetist. Do not use SAB.

3 Epidural anaesthesia should be titrated slowly to effect to avoid rapid CVS changes.

◯ Forehead Block

Requires the blocking of the supraorbital nerve, which supplies the upper eyelid medially and the forehead and scalp to the vertex, and the supratrochlear nerve which supplies the conjunctiva and the skin of the medial upper eyelid and skin of the medial orbit and the root of nose.

Technique

Raise a wheal of LA just above the orbital ridge (5 mL). Also inject 2 mL of LA just above the supraorbital notch. Extend the wheal to the midline to block the supratrochlear nerve.

◯ Fresh Frozen Plasma (FFP)

Description and Storage

A unit of FFP is collected from a single unit of whole blood. It contains all the coagulation factors found in plasma including 200 units of factor VIII, 200 units factor IX and 400 mg of fibrinogen. The FFP bag also contains citrate. The total volume is 150–300 mL which is stored at –25°C. FFP is considered expired 1 year after the collection date. If thawed FFP can be stored at 2–6°C for up to 24 h (or up to 5 days if treating a condition other than factor VIII deficiency).[23]

Compatibility

Compatibility tests prior to transfusion are not required. Give ABO group compatible FFP but in an emergency non-goup compatible FFP can be used. Only group O FFP should be given to group O blood type recipients.

Indications

1 Coagulopathic patients with blood loss. In adults 4–8 units of FFP is required for a significant clinical effect. **See** *Blood Transfusion*. In children give 10–20 mL/kg over 1 h.
2 Reversal of warfarin. Sufficient FFP (depending on the degree of warfarinisation) will reverse the effects of warfarin for ≈ 6–8 h.[24]
3 DIC. **See** *Disseminated Intravascular Coagulation (DIC)*.
4 Severe liver disease and bleeding.
5 Thrombotic thrombocytopenic purpura often with plasma exchange.

FFP Reactions

FFP transfusion can result in rash, itchiness, tachycardia and hypotension. Mild reactions can be treated with:

1 Promethazine 25 mg IM; and
2 Hydrocortisone 100 mg IV.

For more severe reactions **see** *Anaphylaxis/Anaphylactoid Reactions*.

○ Frozen Storage, Red Cells

These are prepared by adding glycerol to RBC before freezing. The glycerol must be removed before transfusion by washing the thawed cells in N/S. Frozen blood can be stored for 10 years and is useful for:

1 Special situations e.g. battle-field hospitals.
2 Private blood banks.
3 Patients with very rare red cell phenotypes.

REFERENCES

1 Stoelting RK. 'NPO' and aspiration: new perspectives. *American Society of Anesthesiologists refresher course lectures* 1997; 111: 1–7.
2 Stoelting RK. NPO: Fact and fiction. *Audio-Digest Anesthesiology* 1995; 37: 15.
3 Phillips S, Daborn AK, Hatch DJ. Preoperative fasting and paediatric anaesthesia. *Br J Anaesth* 1994; 73: 529–36.
4 Fourme TC, Vieillard-Baron A, Loubieres Y et al. Early fat embolism after liposuction. *Anesthesiology* 1988; 89: 782–4.
5 Lafont ND, Kalonjii MK, Barre J et al. Clinical features and echocardiography of embolism during cemented hip arthroplasty. *Can J Anaesth* 1997; 44: 112–17.

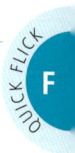

6 Colonna DM, Kilgus D, Brown W et al. Acute brain fat embolization occurring after total hip arthroplasty in the absence of a patent foramen ovale. *Anesthesiol* 2002; 96: 1027–9.

7 Mason R. *Anaesthesia Data Book—A Perioperative and Peripartum Manual*, 3rd edn. Greenwich Medical Media Limited, London 2001: 194.

8 Igarashi M, Kita A, Nishikawa K et al. Use of percutaneous cardiopulmonary support in catastrophic massive pulmonary fat embolism (Case report). *Br J Anaesth* 2006; 96: 213–15.

9 Byrick RJ. Cement implantation syndrome: a time limited embolic phenomenon (Editorial). *Can J Anaesth* 1997; 44: 107–11.

10 Hayakawa M, Fujioka Y, Morimoto Y. Pathological evaluation of venous emboli during total hip arthroplasty. *Anaesthesia* 2001; 56: 571–5.

11 Corke PJ. Anaesthesia for Caesarean section on a patient with acute fatty liver of pregnancy. *Anaesth Intensive Care* 1995; 23: 215–18.

12 Long CJ. Hepatic Disease. In Birnbach DJ, Gatt SP, Datta S, eds: *Textbook of Obstetric Anesthesia*. Churchill Livingstone, Philadelphia, 2000: 607–16.

13 Lim W, Kennedy N. Hemiarthroplasty of the hip under triple nerve block. *Anaesth Intensive Care* 1994; 22: 722–3.

14 Ranucci M, Soro G, Barzaghi N, et al. Fenoldopam prophylaxis of postoperative acute renal failure in high-risk cardiac surgery patients. *Ann Thoracic Surg* 2004; 78: 1332–7.

15 Striebel HW, Krämer J, Lubmann I et al. Pharmacokinectics of intranasal fentanyl (German). *Der Schmerz* 1993; 7: 122–5.

16 Levy DM. Review Article: Emergency Caesarean section: best practice. *Anaesth* 2006; 61: 786–91.

17 Yentis SM, Hirsch NP, Smith GB. *Anaesthesia and Intensive Care A–Z*, 2nd edn. Butterworth–Heineman, Oxford 2000: 216.

18 Mazzei WJ. Cardiovascular monitoring. *Audio-Digest Anesthesiology* 1996; 38: 5.

19 Turpie AGG. The design of venous thromboembolism trials: fondaparinux is definitely more effective than enoxaparin in orthopaedic surgery. *Int J Clin Practice* 2004 May; 58: 483–93.

20 Roberts HR, Monroe DM, Escobar MA. Current concepts of hemostasis. *Anesthesiol* 2004; 100: 722–30.

21 Baum V. The adult paient with congenital heart disease. *J Cadiothoracic and Vasc Surg* 1996; 10: 261–82.

22 Ioscovich A, Briskin A, Fadeev A et al. Emergency cesarean section in a patient with Fontan circulation using an indwelling epidural catheter (Case report). *J Clin Anaesth* 2006; 18: 631–4.

23 Downes KA, Yomtovian R, Sarode R. Serial measurements of clotting factors in thawed plasma stored for 5 days. *Transfusion* 2001; 41: 570.

24 Hardy J, Belisle S, Robitaille D. Blood Products: when to use them and how to avoid them. *Can J Anaesth* 1994; 41: 5: R52–R61.

○ Gabapentin and Pregabalin

Gabapentin is an anticonvulsant drug that is useful in the treatment of chronic neuropathic pain and acute and chronic postoperative pain. It acts possibly by blocking calcium channels and reducing excitability of dorsal horn neurones to afferent nerve nocioception signals. Gabapentin is used orally and has dose limited absorption due to saturation of absorption pathways. Pregabalin acts in the same way as gabapentin but absorption is not limited. Both drugs are excreted renally entirely so caution must be used in renally impaired patients.

Suggested Doses for Acute Pain
Give 300 mg 8 h of gabapentin[1] or 600 mg/day of pregabalin.

○ Gas Embolism, Venous

Gas embolism is due to venous entrainment of air or other gas e.g. CO_2 or N_2O used for laparoscopy. The physiological disturbance from CO_2 insufflation is 6.5 times less than air due to the higher blood solubility of CO_2.[2] In the adult 100–300 mL of air embolised rapidly can be fatal.[3] The effect of intravenous air embolism is greater in the child than the adult on a mL/kg basis.[2] Larger volumes of air can be tolerated if it is infused slowly.

Clinical Effects
1 Gasping respiration, coughing.
2 Dyspnoea.
3 Light-headedness.
4 Chest pain.
5 Altered mental state, coma. Cerebral air embolism can occur through a patent foramen ovale (present in about 20% of the population).

Diagnosis
1 Decrease in end-tidal CO_2 concentration (by >2 mm Hg) unless CO_2 is the causative gas.
    Increased end-tidal N_2 concentration by 2–3% with air embolus.[4]
2 Fall in O_2 saturation measured by pulse oximetry.
3 Loud, coarse continuous 'millwheel' heart murmur.
4 Rales, wheezing on chest auscultation.
5 Hypotension, bradycardia, tachyarrhythmia, shock.
6 CVP rises.

7 ECG changes—peaked p waves, RV strain pattern (RBBB, RAD), prominent S wave in I, Q wave in III and T wave in point 3 (see above), may also see myocardial ischaemia changes—***see*** *Electrocardiography*.

8 Changes in sound detected by a precordial doppler (described as an irregular roaring noise).

9 Bubbles of gas are easily detected by TOE.

Treatment

1 Notify the surgeon immediately, cease the cause of gas embolus e.g. egress of laparoscopic gas.

2 If the source of gas entry is a wound, flood the surgical field with saline. Providing a Valsalva manoeuvre by squeezing the reservoir bag may reveal the vascular entry site of air. In neurosurgical cases, compress the jugular veins bilaterally to reveal the site of bleeding and reduce the degree of air entrainment.

3 Cease administration of N_2O, give 100% O_2.

4 Check that central venous access lines are not entraining air.

5 If cardiac arrest, resuscitate as per section on *Cardiac Arrest*. ECC may help force air into the smaller pulmonary vessels.

6 Position the patient so that the surgical site is *below* the heart level, and preferably place the patient in the left lateral position, tilted head down 15°. This manoeuvre may reduce the amount of air entering the heart. There is little evidence for efficacy with this strategy.[5]

7 Attempt to aspirate air from a central venous line. The optimal site for the tip of the catheter for this purpose is in the right atrium 2 cm below the junction of the right atrium and the SVC.[2] Possibly the best available device for this purpose is the Bunegin-Albin multi-orifice catheter by Cook with a success rate of up to 60%.[5]

8 Cardiopulmonary bypass may be lifesaving in extreme cases if available. Thoracotomy and direct aspiration of air from the heart and great vessels may be needed.

9 Inotropic support may be required.

10 Add positive end-expiratory pressure of 5 cm H_2O, to reduce the pressure gradient favouring air entrainment. This may cause a further decline in cardiac output.

11 Consider using hyperbaric oxygen if available. This is helpful for venous embolism but not arterial embolism.[5]

12 Experimental therapies include the use of fluorocarbon derivatives to enhance the solubility of gases into blood e.g. FP-43.[5] ***See*** *Blood Substitutes*.

◗ Gelofusin

Description and Composition

Gelofusin is a synthetic colloid solution with an average molecular weight of 35 000 Daltons and contains 4% succinylated bovine gelatin in saline. Gelatin is obtained through the hydrolysis of collagen creating a purified protein.

Gelofusin contains:

Sodium	154 mmol/L
Chloride	120 mmol/L
pH of	7.4 +/− 0.3
Osmolarity	274 mOsm/L.

There are minimal amounts of potassium and calcium. It has a shelf-life of 3 years.

Uses

Gelofusin is used to treat hypovolaemia and for isovolaemic haemodilution. The plasma half life is less than 4 h. It is recommended in the product information to give the first 20–30 mL slowly as anaphylaxis can occur with this solution.

Problems

1 In patients on angiotensin converting enzyme inhibitors under anaesthesia who are hypotensive, the hypotension may be worsened by gelofusin.[6]
2 The emergence of bovine spongioform encephalomyopathy (Mad Cow Disease) has raised concerns regarding the use of bovine gelatin and the risk of prion contamination.

◗ Glasgow Coma Scale (GCS)

Originally developed for grading severity and outcome for head injury.[7]

	SCORE
EYES OPEN	
Spontaneously	4
To speech	3
To pain	2
Nil	1
BEST MOTOR RESPONSE	
Obey commands	6
Localise pain	5
Withdraw to pain	4
Abnormal flexion	3
Extensor response	2
Nil	1
VERBAL RESPONSE	
Orientated	5
Confused	4

QUICK FLICK

G

Inappropriate words	3
Sounds other than words	2
Nil	1

▷ Glenn Shunt

This is a caval-pulmonary shunt procedure in which blood from the SVC is diverted into the right pulmonary artery. This procedure is done for conditions such as Ebstein's anomaly. Because IVC blood still undergoes right-to-left shunting hypoxia continues and is progressive. This is due to decreased flow to the contralateral lung and increasing communication channels between the SVC and IVC. Pulmonary arterio-venous shunts may also develop. A bi-directional Glenn shunt involves anastomosis of the SVC to the main pulmonary artery allowing perfusion of both lungs. Pulmonary hypertension may result from this procedure.

▷ GlideScope Video Laryngoscope (GVL)

This device has a small camera mounted at the tip of the 50–60° angled laryngoscope blade. The camera images are illuminated by a LED light source and relayed to a colour screen by a cable attached to the laryngoscope handle. The GVL is intended to aid intubation in patients who can open their mouth wide enough to admit the GVL (≈ 18 mm) and:
1 Are suspected or known to be difficult to intubate.
2 Fail attempted conventional direct laryngoscopy after GA is induced.
3 Patients requiring cervical spine immobilisation during intubation.

Technique for Using the GlideScope
1 Insert the GVL in the midline without the normal positioning for direct laryngoscopy.
2 Visualise the larynx on the video screen.
3 Insert the ET tube with a semi-rigid stylet with a hockey stick angulation on the tip into the pharynx.
4 Under vision from the GVL camera intubate the larynx and trachea.
The GlideScope requires sterilisation between uses. The GlideScope Cobolt works in the same way as the GVL but uses a disposable clear plastic blade over a slim video 'baton' housing the camera light source and antifogging mechanism. The video screen is more compact than on the standard GVL. A specially designed GlideScope rigid stylet is also marketed to make shaping of the ET tube easier and a GlideRite tube which has a flexible tip is suggested.

Advantages
1 Consistently provides an excellent view of the larynx.
2 The device is easy to use and requires little training.[8]
3 It is available in adult (>15 kg) and paediatric (10–15 kg) sizes.

Disadvantages

1. The GVL is expensive retailing at about $AUS15 000 at the time of printing.
2. There is no guiding channel on the GVL for the ET tube. This means that the ET tube must be inserted blindly into the oropharynx with a stylet in situ, and manipulated into the field of view of the camera. This manoeuvre has been associated with oropharyngeal injuries. Chin et al. describe a 1.5 cm laceration to the soft palate due to ET tube manipulation while using the GlideScope.[9] Cooper described 2 patients who suffered perforation of the paltopharyngeal arch during GVL intubations.[10]
3. It can be difficult to advance the ET tube off the stylet and into the trachea. The tip of the ET tube tends to impinge onto the anterior commissure or impact into a cartilaginous ring on the anterior wall of the trachea.[11]
4. Oropharyngeal tissue can tent into the field of vision[9]
5. There may be suboptimal space between the GlideScope and the patient's teeth or other structures when manipulating the ET tube into the larynx.[9]

◗ Glucose-6-Phosphate Dehydrogenase (G6PD) Deficiency

G6PD deficiency results in episodic haemolytic anaemia due to accumulation of methaemoglobin and deficiency of reduced glutathione in red blood cells.[12] These episodes can be precipitated by certain drugs including: primaquine and chloroquine, quinidine, sulphonamides, nalidixic acid, nitrofurantoin, penicillins and probenicid.[13] Also avoid streptomycin, chloramphenicol, sulphonamides, isoniazid, nitrates, aspirin in high doses, phenacetin, vitamins K and C (very high doses) and methylene blue. It occurs most commonly in males of negroid origin and people of Mediterranean origin (X linked disorder). Paracetamol should be used with caution or in reduced dosage due to increased risk of liver injury from metabolites. *See* Paracetamol.

Anaesthetic Implications[12]

Do not exceed the maximum safe doses of drugs such as prilocaine and sodium nitroprusside which can result in haemolysis due to concurrent production of oxidising subtances.[12] If methaemoglobinaemia occurs, methylene blue is ineffective in treatment and may cause haemolysis.

◗ Glyceryl Trinitrate

Organic nitrate which produces venodilation at low doses and arterial vasodilatation at higher doses. Acts by increasing production of nitric oxide in vascular smooth muscle cells causing relaxation. Results in redistribution of coronary blood flow to ischaemic myocardium and is less likely to produce coronary steal than sodium nitroprusside.[14]

Uses

1 Myocardial ischaemia.
2 Left ventricular failure associated with myocardial infarction.
3 Treatment of hypertension.
4 Induction of hypotension.
5 For producing uterine relaxation for situations such as retained placenta and uterine inversion. *See Uterine Relaxation for Retained Placenta*.

Dose for IV Infusion

1 Add 250 mg glyceryl trinitrate to 500 mL 5% glucose in a glass container.
2 Administer via an approved administration set (to reduce absorption into plastics).
3 Usual dose range 0.5–6 µg/kg/min, equals 4–50 mL/h of the above solution.

Dose for Uterine Relaxation

IV Dose Remove 1 mL from an ampoule containing 50 mg of glyceryl trinitrate in 10 mL (5 mg) and dilute to 10 mL with N/S. Take 1 mL (500 µg) from this solution and dilute to 10 mL resulting in a final concentration of 50 µg/ml. Give 1 mL boluses as required. The dose required is variable but 100–200 µg is usually effective.[15]

Sublingual Dose 2 sprays of sublingual glyceryl trinitrate (800 µg) has been reported as effective and well tolerated.[16]

❍ Glycopyrronium (Glycopyrrolate)

Quaternary ammonium anticholinergic compound with similar actions to atropine, but does not cross the blood–brain barrier and thus has no central actions. Glycopyrronium causes less tachycardia than atropine.

Uses

Antisialogogue, treatment of bradycardia, and for protection against the muscarinic effects of anticholinesterase drugs such as neostigmine.

Dose

10 µg/kg IV.

❍ Granisetron

Potent, long-acting and highly selective $5-HT_3$ receptor antagonist that also decreases serotonin release. Granisetron is useful for the treatment and prevention of postoperative nausea and vomiting. Effects last for 24 h.

Dose

Adult 1 mg IV. Up to 3 mg can be given in 24 h for postoperative nausea and vomiting.

Child 20–40 µg/kg IV has been used for chemotherapy nausea prophylaxis.

Advantages
1　Does not decrease the effects of tramadol (**see** *Ondansetron*).
2　Long acting.

REFERENCES

1　Gray P. Successful use of gabapentin in acute pain management following burn injury: a case series. *Pain Medicine* 2008; 9: 371–6.

2　Chiu PT, Gin T, Oh TE. Anaesthesia for laparoscopic general surgery. *Anaesth Intensive Care* 1993; 21: 163–71.

3　Webber S, Andrzejowski J, Francis G. Gas embolism in anaesthesia. *Br J Anaesth CEPD Reviews* 2002; 2: 53–7.

4　Gabba DM, Fish JF, Howard SK. *Crisis Management in Anesthesiology*. Churchill Livingstone, New York 1994: 116–19.

5　Waltier DC. Diagnosis and treatment of vascular air embolism (Review Article). *Anesthesiol* 2007; 106: 164–77.

6　Powell CG, Unsworth DJ, McVey FK. Severe hypotension associated with angiotensin-converting enzyme inhibition in anaesthesia. *Anaesth Intensive Care* 1998; 26: 107–9.

7　Teasdale G, Jennett B. Assessment of coma and impaired consciousness: a practical scale. *Lancet* 1974; 2: 81–3.

8　Cooper RM, Pacey JA, Bishop MJ, McCluskey SA. Early clinical experience with a new video laryngoscope (GlideScope) in 728 patients. *Can J Anaesth* 2005; 52: 191–8.

9　Chin KJ, Arango MF, Paez AF, Turkstra TP. Palatal injury associated with the GlideScope®. *Anaesth Intensive Care* 2007; 35: 449–50.

10　Cooper RM. Complications associated with the use of the GlideScope® video laryngoscope. *Can J Anesth* 2007; 54: 54–7.

11　Dow WA, Parsons DG. 'Reverse loading' to facilitate GlideScope® intubation. *Can J Anesth* 2007; 54: 161–2.

12　Mason RA. *Anaesthesia Databook: A Perioperative and Peripartum Manual*. Greenwich Medical Books Limited, London 2001: 208–9.

13　Stoelting RK, Dierdorf SF. *Anaesthesia and Co-existing Disease*, 3rd edn. Churchill Livingstone, New York 1993; 399–40.

14　Klein L. Cardiogenic shock. In: Parrillo JE, ed. *Current Therapy in Critical Care Medicine*, 3rd edn. Mosby, St Louis 1997: 72–8.

15　Axemo P, Fu X, Lindberg B et al. Intravenous nitroglycerine for rapid uterine relaxation. *Acta Obstet Gynecol Scand* 1998; 77: 50–3.

16　Dawson NJ, Gabbott DA. Use of sublingual glyceryl trinitrate as a supplement to volatile inhalational anaesthesia in a case of uterine inversion. *Internat J Obstet Anaesth* 1997; 6: 135–7.

QUICK FLICK G

H

○ Haemaccel

Contains polygeline, a polypeptide manufactured from urea linked bovine gelatin, with an average molecular weight of 30 000. Gelatin is obtained through the hydrolysis of collagen from animals creating a purified protein.

Haemaccel also contains:

Sodium	145 mmol/L
Potassium	5.1 mmol/L
Calcium	6.25 mmol/L
Chloride	145 mmol/L
pH	7.4 +/− 3
Osmolarity	301 mOsm/L.

Uses

Colloid plasma volume expander. Stays in the intravascular space longer than crystalloid solutions but for a shorter time than dextrans.[1] Plasma half-life of haemaccel ≈ 4h.[1]

Problems

1   May cause clotting of citrated blood used for transfusion if mixed in the same IV giving set, due to haemaccel's calcium content.
2   Reactions to haemaccel occur in 0.04% of administrations ranging from minor to severe allergic responses.[2]
3   Haemaccel administration can result in increased bradykinin production resulting in hypotension. Bradykinin production is inhibited by angiotensin converting enzyme (ACE). Patients on ACE inhibitors appear to be more susceptible to haemaccel induced hypotension for this reason.
4   The emergence of bovine spongioform encephalomyopathy (Mad Cow Disease) has raised concerns regarding the use of bovine gelatin.

○ Haematoma Block

This simple block is useful for the closed reduction of wrist, forearm, ankle and femur fractures. It is used mainly for wrist fractures. The block can be supplemented by IV analgesia (fentanyl/ketamine), inhaled N_2O and/or sedation (e.g. midazolam).

The procedure involves the following steps:

1   Site a cannula in the non-fractured arm.
2   Sterilise the skin overlying the fracture and use aseptic technique.

3 Insert a 20 gauge needle into the fracture site and aspirate blood to confirm that the needle is in the fracture haematoma.

4 Inject LA e.g. 10 mL of 2% lignocaine for adults. A further 5 mL of LA can be injected around the fracture site.

5 Lignocaine 2.5 mg/kg is suggested as an appropriate dose in children.[3]

6 Wait 10 min before manipulating the fracture.

◐ Haemoglobin

Table H1: Normal Hb levels for age

Age in months/years	Hb g/100 mL
Birth	13.6–19.6
3 months	10–11
1 yr	11.2
10 yrs	12.9
Adult male	13.5–18
Adult female	11.5–16.4

◐ Haemoptysis, Massive

Massive haemorrhage into the airway is an anaesthetic and surgical emergency with a mortality of between 30 and 85% in non-trauma cases.[4] It can be defined as > 600 mL in 24 h.[5] Death usually results from asphyxiation due to alveolar blood rather than exsanguination. Emergency thoracic surgical consultation should be sought. A respiratory physician skilled in bronchial procedures will also be helpful.

Causes

These are many and include:

1 Tuberculosis is the leading cause in developing countries, and cancer in the lung (primary or secondary) is the leading cause in developed countries.[5]

2 Aspergilloma, necrotising pneumonia, hydatid cyst.

3 Bronchiectasis/sarcoma.

4 Iatrogenic e.g. due to pulmonary artery catheter complications.

5 Trauma.

6 Vascular abnormalities e.g. arteriobronchial fistula.

7 Wegener's granulomatosis, Goodpasture's disease.

Management

1 *Airway* Place the patient in a left lateral head down position and suction the airway. If the side of bleeding is known e.g. known right lung cancer, place the bleeding side down. If the patient is in danger of asphyxiation obtain IV access and secure the airway with an ET tube using a rapid

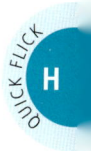

sequence induction (**see** *Rapid Sequence Induction*) with the patient supine if necessary. Ideally a double lumen tube (DLT) should be used to isolate the bleeding side but a single lumen tube will suffice until a DLT is available.

2   *Ventilation* Provide 100% O_2. Use IPPV but avoid high airway pressures which may cause gas embolus. Do not use jet ventilation because this may cause blood in the airway to dry and solidify.

3   *Identify the Site of Bleeding* This may be achieved by suctioning of the ET tube and trachea, then insertion of a FOB. It may be possible to see the site of bleeding. Direct the FOB into bronchus that is not bleeding then railroad the tube over this to ventilate the non-bleeding lung and protect it from further soiling. Additionally a Fogarty size 14 catheter can be passed through the cords next to the ET tube. The ET tube can be withdrawn into the trachea and a FOB through the ET tube used to direct the catheter into the bronchus on the side of bleeding.[6] Inflate the balloon on the catheter. An ET tube with a bronchial blocker can be used in a similar way.

   A double lumen tube (DLT) if available can provide rapid isolation of the bleeding lung and a channel for Fogarty catheter insertion.

   Once the side of bleeding is known place the patient lateral with the bleeding side down.

4   *Circulation* Resuscitate the patient's intravascular volume. Urgent blood transfusion may be required. Check the patient's coagulation status and reverse any abnormality.

5   *Non-surgical Bleeding Control* Strategies include rigid and or fibre-optic bronchoscopy to identify the site of bleeding. Iced saline + adrenaline lavage, adrenaline injected into the site of bleeding, and placement of balloon catheters may control or reduce bleeding. Topical application of thrombin and thrombin-fibrinogen solutions has also been used successfully.[5] CXR and CT scanning may help elucidate the site and cause of bleeding. Pulmonary/bronchial angiography may also identify the site of bleeding, and enable control of bleeding by selective bronchial artery embolisation using e.g. polyvinyl alcohol foam granules.

6   *Surgery* May be required immediately e.g. rupture of a thoracic aneurysm into a bronchus.[4]

7   *Other Treatments* For immunological mediated diffuse alveolar haemorrhage consider steroid and cytotoxic therapy + plasmaphoresis.[6]

○ Haemorrhage

See *Blood Loss Assessment and Initial Management* and *Blood Transfusion.*

◐ Halothane

Halogenated hydrocarbon volatile inhalational anaesthetic agent.

Physical Properties and MAC

Blood: Gas Solubility Coefficient	2.3
Oil: Gas Solubility Coefficient	224
Saturated Vapour Pressure at 20°C	244 mm Hg (32 kPa)
Boiling Point	50.2°C
MAC	0.75

Advantages

Sweet, non-irritating odour suitable for inhalational induction. Potent agent.

Disadvantages

1 Requires preservative, 0.01% thymol, accumulation of which can interfere with vaporiser function.
2 Risk of halothane hepatitis.
3 Sensitises myocardium to catecholamines more than other modern inhalational agents.
4 Causes prolongation of the Q-T interval predisposing the patient to ventricular tachycardias such as torsade de pointes.
5 Produces vagal stimulation which can result in marked bradycardia.
6 Halothane is a potent trigger for malignant hyperpyrexia.

Recommendations

1 Avoid repeated exposure. Do not use halothane within 6 months of previous halothane anaesthetic unless there is an overriding clinical indication.
2 A history of unexplained jaundice or pyrexia after previous halothane anaesthetic is an *absolute contraindication* to repeat halothane exposure.
3 Caution with adrenaline because of the risk of cardiac dysrhythmia such as ventricular ectopic beats and ventricular tachycardia. Avoid using concentrations of adrenaline > 1:100 000 and volumes of this concentration > 10 mL in 10 min or > 30 mL/h.
4 Do not use halothane in patients with a prolonged Q-T interval or patients taking drugs known to prolong the Q-T interval. **See** *Long QT Syndrome (LQTS)*.

◐ Hartmann's Solution

Hartmann's solution (Ringer's Lactate) is a crystalloid solution containing:

Sodium	131 mmol/L
Potassium	5 mmol/L
Calcium	2 mmol/L
Chloride	111 mmol/L

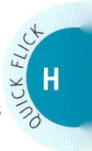

Lactate   29 mmol/L
Osmolarity 274 mOsm/L (hypotonic)
pH   5–7.

Lactate is metabolised by both gluconeogenesis and oxidation (mainly in the liver) to bicarbonate and glucose. Hirsch states that Hartmann's solution should not be given to diabetic patients as it may increase glucose levels and cause elevated ketone levels.[7] In contrast, Robertshaw and Hall state that Hartmann's can be used safely in diabetic patients.[8]

◗ Heart Block (HB)

HB (atrioventricular block) can be divided into 3 main types:

1 *First Degree HB* P-R interval > 0.20 s (5 mm).
2 *Second Degree HB* Subdivided into:
   a) Wenckebach or Morbitz Type I—Gradual lengthening of P-R interval until a dropped beat occurs then the cycle repeats.
   b) Morbitz Type II—Fixed ratio of P waves to QRS complexes e.g. 2:1, 3:1.
3 *Third Degree HB* No relationship between P waves and QRS complexes.

Treatment

First degree and Morbitz type 1 second degree HB usually require no treatment. Morbitz type 2 and third degree HB require treatment if cardiovascular compromise is present. For emergency management of adult:

1 Isoprenaline 2 mg in 50 mL 5% glucose, start at 5 mL/h. Infusion range. Can give boluses of 10–20 µg (0.25–0.5 mL of the above diluted solution).[8]
2 Use an adrenaline infusion if isoprenaline is not available.
   See *Adrenaline*.
3 External transcutaneous pacing.
4 Temporary transvenous pacing wire.
5 Permanent pacemaker. ***See*** *Pacing, Pacemakers and Anaesthesia*.

◗ Heart Failure

See *Congestive Cardiac Failure (CCF)*.

◗ Heart Transplant Patients, Anaesthetic Considerations for Non-cardiac Surgery

Physiological Considerations

1 The transplanted heart is denervated and is paced by the donor atrium at a resting rate of 90–100 beats per minute. Systemic vascular resistance is increased in these patients and ventricular hypertrophy is usual.[9]
2 The donor heart is responsive to volume loading by increasing stroke volume via the Frank-Starling mechanism.[10] In addition, heart rate increases over 5–6 minutes in response to the release of endogenous catecholamines.[10] The transplanted heart is preload dependent and

responds poorly to hypovolaemia and decreased systemic vascular resistance. It is very important to maintain pre-load peri-operatively.

3 The donor heart does not respond to Valsalva manoeuvres and carotid sinus massage.

Pathophysiological Considerations

1 There is accelerated coronary artery atheromatous disease.[11] However the patient will not experience chest pain due to myocardial ischaemia.

2 There is an increased incidence of dysrhythmias such as ventricular ectopic beats. First degree atrioventricular block, right bundle branch block and bradyarrhythmias are common.[9] Episodes of dysrhythmia may indicate rejection. Note that the ECG often contains 2 P waves due to the presence of residual recipient atrial tissue. About 10% of recipients require a permanent pacemaker.

3 Immunosuppressive drugs result in an increased susceptibility to infection and can have other side effects. About 75% of patients develop hypertension secondary to cyclosporin A therapy. **See** *Immunosuppressive Drugs, Anaesthetic Implications.*

Pharmacology and the Transplanted Heart

1 The donor heart rate will have no response to drugs with autonomic activity such as anticholinergics (atropine, glycopyrrolate) and anticholinesterases (neostigmine) but heart rate will increase with sympathomimetic amines such as adrenaline, isoprenaline, ephedrine, dobutamine and dopamine.

2 Reflex tachycardia with vasodilators such as sodium nitroprusside is absent and the hypotensive effects of these drugs may be exaggerated.

3 The transplanted heart is usually exquisitely sensitive to adenosine and this drug should be used with extreme caution. Use a starting dose of 1 mg.[12]

4 Digoxin is ineffective in the transplanted heart for AV nodal slowing but does still provide positive inotropy.[12]

5 Atropine can cause AV block and sinus arrest.[13]

Pre-operative Assessment and Preparation

1 Liaise with the patient's cardiologist and the transplant team if possible.

2 Look for any evidence of rejection such as increasing symptoms of heart failure, dysrhythmias, low voltage ECG and deteriorating ventricular function on echocardiography.[9]

3 If possible avoid procedures which may result in infection such as nasal intubation and invasive monitoring. Use strict asepsis when performing invasive procedures.

4 Use appropriate antibiotic prophylaxis including anti-staphylococcal cover (e.g. flucloxacillin).

5 Continue immunosuppressive therapy throughout the peri-operative

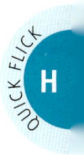

period. Azathioprine can be given IV at the same dose as PO. Patients will require peri-operative steroid coverage.

6   Establish monitoring as appropriate for the procedure and the patient's physiological condition. If central venous pressure monitoring is required do not use the right internal jugular vein. This is because this vein is used for cardiac biopsies.[11] TOE monitoring may be preferable to invasive central pressure monitoring.

7   Ensure adequate fluid preload prior to the induction of anaesthesia and at all other times.

8   Ensure isoprenaline and/or transcutaneous pacing is readily available to treat bradycardia. *See* *Isoprenaline*.

Intra-operative Care

1   General and/or regional anaesthesia has been used successfully in heart transplant patients.

2   Significant hypotension may occur with epidural or spinal anaesthesia if preload is not maintained.[9] Therefore, maintain adequate preload at all times.

3   Avoid myocardial depressant drugs.

4   Hypotension can be treated with ensuring adequate preload and vasoconstrictors such as metaraminol or phenylephrine.

5   For bradycardia consider isoprenaline or pacing.

6   Use adrenaline if severe cardiac decompensation occurs.

7   Use atropine or glycopyrrolate with neostigmine to reverse residual neuromuscular blockade. This is because unopposed neostigmine may cause cholinergic side effects such as bronchospasm (but not bradycardia).

Postoperative Care

1   Liaise with the patient's cardiologist and transplant team regarding postoperative management including immunosuppressive therapy while the patient is nil by mouth.

2   Remove all unnecessary intravascular lines, drains and other invasive equipment to reduce the risk of infection.

○ HELLP Syndrome

This term describes a form of severe pre-eclampsia/eclampsia with **H**aemolysis, **E**levated **L**iver **E**nzymes and **L**ow **P**latelets. *See* *Pre-eclampsia/ Eclampsia*.

○ Hemoglobin Raffimer

This is a purified, cross-linked human Hb solution manufactured from expired donated blood units. The purified Hb is bound to o-raffinose and presented as a solution containing 10 g/100 mL Hb tetramer 9 (2 α chains and 2 β chains) with a molecular size of 64 kDa. It is stored in a deoxygenated state and currently undergoing trials as a substitute for RBC transfusion. The intravascular half life is 15–18 h.

Advantages

1 May be acceptable to Jehovah's Witness patients.[14]
2 Minimal renal toxicity due to high molecular weight.

Disadvantages

1 There is an increased incidence of myocardial infarction in cardiac surgical patients given Hemoglobin Raffimer during CABG.[14]
2 Hemoglobin Raffimer binds nitric oxide which can lead to arterial vasoconstriction and hypertension.

○ Heparin Induced Thrombocytopenia Syndrome (HITS)

This condition is due to the production of IgG antibodies to heparin/platelet factor 4 complexes resulting in thrombocytopenia and venous and/or arterial thrombosis. The incidence is about 1% of heparin treated patients and about 0.1% of patients treated with fractionated heparin.[15] In patients who develop HITS, fractionated heparin also results in antibody production in 90% of cases and is thus also contraindicated. HITS usually develops 4–10 days after commencement of heparin or sooner if the patient has been given heparin in the last 100 days.

Diagnosis

Thrombocytopenia with thrombosis are the main features. Deep venous thrombosis and/or pulmonary embolus occur in about 50% of patients.[15] The detection of HITS antibodies may aid diagnosis.

Treatment

1 Discontinue heparin or fractionated heparin.
2 Perform APTT, do not initiate alternative anticoagulant therapy until APTT <90 sec.
3 Use alternative anticoagulant treatment such as lepirudin or other direct thrombin inhibitors. Give lepirudin 0.4 mg/kg IV over 20 s then IV infusion 0.15 mg/kg/h. Adjust infusion rate to keep APTT between 50 and 90 s. Note that about 50% of patients will have thrombotic complications after heparin withdrawal without anticoagulant intervention.[15] *See Direct Acting Thrombin Inhibitors (DTI).*
4 Fondaparinux, a new pentasaccharide anticoagulant, may be a suitable alternative. *See Fondaparinux.*

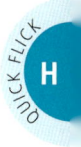

QUICK FLICK H

Thromboprophylaxis in Patients with a History of HITS
Use danaparoid 750 units subcut 12 h.

○ Heparin (Unfractionated and Low Molecular Weight Heparins)

Topics Covered in this Section
▶ Unfractionated Heparin
▶ Low Molecular Weight (LMW) Heparins

Unfractionated Heparin

Heparin is an anticoagulant drug that acts by binding reversibly to antithrombin III causing its activation. Antithrombin III in turn inactivates thrombin, factors XII, XI, X, IX and other proteases involved in blood clotting. Heparin also inhibits platelet aggregation by fibrin. This drug is used for:

1 Prevention and treatment of venous and arterial thrombo-embolic disease.
2 Anticoagulation for cardiac bypass surgery.
3 Priming dialysis and cardiopulmonary bypass machines to prevent extra-corporeal clot formation.

Dose in Adults

1 *Prevention of Deep Venous Thrombosis (DVT) and Pulmonary Embolus (PE)* 5000 u subcutaneously 8–12 h.
2 *Treatment of DVT* 5000 u IV loading dose then IV infusion 1250 u/h. Check APTT after 4 h. Aim for therapeutic APTT range of 60–85 s. Increase or decrease the infusion rate accordingly.
3 *Treatment of PE* **see** *Pulmonary Embolism (PE).*
4 *Reversal of Heparin* **see** *Protamine.*

Low Molecular Weight (LMW) Heparins

These anticoagulant drugs act by catalysing the inhibition of activated factors IX, X, XI and XII by antithrombin III.

Advantages of LMW Heparins

1 Inhibit platelets less than heparin and may produce less intra-operative bleeding.[16]
2 They have a longer duration of action than heparin making administration easier.
3 LMW heparins have less risk of producing heparin-induced thrombocytopenia.
4 LMW heparins are more effective in reducing mortality from pulmonary embolus than heparin.[16]
5 Less monitoring of the anticoagulant effect of LMW heparin is required compared with heparin.

Disadvantages of LMW Heparins

1 Measuring the anticoagulant effects of LMW heparin is more difficult. This is done by measuring anti-Xa activity. The therapeutic range for treatment of established DVT/PE is 0.3–0.8 anti–Xa units/mL at 3–5 h after the dose.

2 In cases of bleeding LMW heparin is more difficult to reverse than heparin. See below.

3 Patients who are susceptible to heparin-induced thrombocytopenia cannot receive LMW heparin due to 90% cross-reactivity.

Dose in Adults

1 *Prevention of DVT and PE* **See** *Deep Venous Thrombosis (DVT) Prophylaxis.*

2 *Treatment of DVT and PE*
    a) Dalteparin (Fragmin) 100 u/kg/12 h subcutaneously or 200 u/kg/day.
    b) Enoxaparin (Clexane) 1 mg/kg/12 h subcutaneously or 1.5 mg/kg/day.
    Therapy with LMW heparin should be continued for at least 5 days overlapping with oral warfarin therapy from day 1. INR must be in the therapeutic range (2.0–3.0) for at least 2 days before ceasing LMW heparin. This is because initiation of warfarin causes a prothrombotic state by inhibition of protein C and protein S.

3 *Reversal of LMW Heparin Activity* LMW heparin can be ≈ 60% neutralised by protamine and fresh frozen plasma is also effective. **See** *Protamine.* Give 1 mg protamine per mg of enoxaparin or per 100 u of dalteparin.

◖ Hepatitis B and C

See *Needle-stick Injury.*

◖ Hepatorenal Syndrome (HRS)

This term describes the development of renal failure in the presence of severe liver disease (usually advanced cirrhosis) without another identifiable cause. The mechanism of renal injury is thought to be:

1 Extreme splanchnic vasodilation. There can be vasoconstriction of liver and brain vascular beds.[17]

2 Arterial under-filling.

3 Renal intra-arteriolar vasoconstriction.[17]

The most common precipitating factor for this condition is spontaneous bacterial peritonitis.[17] Other causes are blood loss and large volume paracentesis without albumin replacement fluid. HRS is divided into:

1 Type 1—rapidly progressive form over days in patients with severe hepatic impairment.

2 Type 2—slowly progressive form in patients with less severe chronic liver impairment.

Mortality for this condition is high. However, modern treatments can

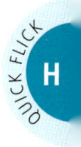

QUICK FLICK

H

prolong survival until liver transplant—the only curative treatment—can be undertaken.[18]

Measures to Prevent Hepatorenal Syndrome Developing Peri-operatively

1 Adequate hydration, with IV fluids for at least 12 h pre-operatively.
2 Mannitol 20% 100 mL immediately pre-operatively. Give a second dose postoperatively if urine output < 50 mL/h.[19]
3 Consider sodium taurocholate 1 g PO 8 h for 48 h.[20]
4 Albumin infusions reduce the incidence of HRS developing in patients with spontaneous bacterial peritonitis[21] and may have a role in pre-operative prevention although this hypothesis is yet to be tested.
5 Long-term norfloxacin therapy was found in one trial to reduce the incidence of HRS by decreasing the incidence of spontaneous bacterial peritonitis.[22] This may also have implications for peri-operative HRS prevention.

Treatment of Hepatorenal Syndrome

This condition is usually fatal. Treatments include:

1 Liver transplant.
2 Vasopressin therapy with drugs such as terlipressin, ornipressin, omipressin, noradrenaline, dopamine, midodrine.
3 Volume expansion with albumin solution.[17,18] Albumin appears to enhance the effects of terlipressin.[17]
4 Trans jugular intrahepatic portosystemic stent (TIPS) to restore effective blood volume has been successful in some patients.
5 Extracorporeal liver support such as extracorporeal albumin dialysis.

◐ Herbal Medicines and Anaesthesia

It is advisable to ask all patients if they are taking herbal or other non-prescribed medication. Although most herbal medicines are probably harmless it may be prudent to ask the patient to cease all herbal remedies for at least 2 weeks prior to surgery.[23] Adverse effects of specific herbal medicines include:

1 *Echinacea* This herb is contraindicated in patients taking immunosuppressive drugs, or with autoimmune disease and human immunodeficiency virus infection.[24]
2 *Ephedra* Use of this drug has been associated with hypertension, tachycardia, seizures, intracranial haemorrhage, myocardial infarction and psychosis.[24] Its use has been banned in the US since April 2004.
3 *Feverfew (Tancacetum parthenium)* Can cause platelet dysfunction.
4 *Garlic (Allium sativum)* Anecdotal reports suggest heavy garlic intake can cause an increased bleeding tendency with unexpected surgical bleeding and a report of a spontaneous epidural haematoma.[25,26] Garlic should not

be taken with warfarin, aspirin or other NSAIDs.[27] The effects of garlic last about 7 days.

5 *Ginger (Zingeber officinale)* May potentiate the effects of warfarin and decrease platelet aggregation.

6 *Ginkgo biloba* has also been associated anecdotally with bleeding tendencies. As for garlic, ginkgo should not be taken with warfarin, aspirin or other NSAIDs. Ginkgo effects last about 36 h.

7 *Ginseng* Can induce tachycardia and hypertension and decrease blood sugar. Ginseng can also interfere with warfarin decreasing its effect. This herb inhibits platelets and the risk of bleeding is increased in patients on anti-platelet therapies. Patients on antidepressants may develop mania if given ginseng.

8 *Goldenseal (Hydrastis canadensis)* Can cause hypertension, oedema or hypokalaemia due to its mineralocorticoid effects.

9 *Kava* Interacts with levodopa and can potentiate Parkinson's disease. It also causes sedation and an increased risk of suicide in patients with depression. Kava use has resulted in liver failure and its use is banned in Europe.

10 *St John's Wort* Increases uterine tone and should be avoided in pregnancy. St John's Wort decreases the efficacy of warfarin, digoxin and anti-convulsants. This herb can potentially interact with tramadol and SSRIs to cause serotonin syndrome. *See Serotonin Syndrome*. St John's Wort can also decrease the efficacy of HIV protease inhibitor drugs.

11 *Licorice (Glycyrrhiza glabra)* can cause hypertension, low potassium levels or oedema.

12 *Valerian* Causes sedation and thus may enhance the effects of sedative drugs such as benzodiazepines. It can prolong barbiturate induced sleep.

Heroin

See Diacetylmorphine/Diamorphine.

Human Immunodeficiency Virus (HIV)

See Needle-stick Injury.

Hydralazine

A pthalazine derivative which acts directly on vascular smooth muscle causing arteriolar vasodilation. Used for the treatment of moderate to severe hypertension, and severe heart failure.

Treatment of Hypertension

Dose IV Adult 5–10 mg IV boluses every 20 min to a max dose of 20–40 mg. Duration of action 2 6 h.

QUICK FLICK

H

◐ Hydromorphone (Dilaudid)

This analgesic drug is a semi-synthetic modification of morphine. 2 mg of hydromorphone is equivalent to morphine 10 mg.

Dose

Adult PO 1–8 mg 4 h. *IM/Subcut* 1–2 mg 4–6 h. IV 0.5 mg 4–6 h.

Child[28] *PO* 0.05–0.1 mg/kg/dose. *IM/Subcut* 0.02–0.05 mg/kg/dose. *Slow IV* 0.01–0.02 mg/kg/dose 4–6 h.

Advantages

1   Hydromorphone may have a lower incidence of side effects such as nausea and vomiting, sedation and pruritis compared to morphine.[29] For patients who suffer intolerable side effects with morphine, hydromorphone is therefore a good alternative to consider.[30]
2   Hydromorphone is as effective for analgesia as morphine at equivalent doses.
3   Epidural hydromorphone may produce less respiratory depression, itch and urinary retention than epidural morphine.[31]

Disadvantages

1   Hydromorphone may have a higher incidence of mood and sleep disturbances than morphine when both are used by the PCA route.[32] Psychomimetic effects of hydromorphone may be due to accumulation of the 3-glucuronide metabolite.
2   Hydromorphone and its metabolites are excreted renally. Caution must therefore be used in patients with renal impairment.
3   Like morphine, hydromorphone causes histamine release. Hydromorphone is therefore contraindicated in conditions where histamine release is undesirable such as phaeochromocytoma. **See** *Phaeochromocytoma*.

◐ Hydroxyethylated Starch (Hydroxyethyl Starch, HES)

These solutions are manufactured by treating starch from maize or sorghum with ethylene chlorohydrin and pyrimidine. Hydroxyethylated starch contains 90% amylopectin. Hetastarch, with an average molecular weight of 450 000 Daltons, is the most common form used. It is primarily excreted by the kidneys.

Uses

Hydroxyethylated starch is used for plasma expansion and hetastarch has a half-life in the plasma of less than 24 h.[33] It is the most commonly used colloid in the United States. The maximum recommended dose is 33 mL/kg/day.[34]

Advantages

There is no concern about transmission of animal diseases such as bovine spongiform encephalomyelitis as with gelofusin.

Disadvantages

High molecular weight HES solutions can cause a coagulopathy by reducing levels of factor VIII and von Willebrand factor.

▶ Hyper/Hypocalcaemia

See Calcium.

▶ Hyper/Hypokalaemia

See Potassium.

▶ Hypercapnia

The normal range of arterial $PaCO_2$ is 35–45 mm Hg.
Hypercapnia can result from respiratory and non-respiratory causes.

Respiratory Causes of Hypercapnia

1 Hypoventilation.
2 Increased anatomical or non anatomical dead space.
3 Increased ventilation/perfusion (V/Q) mismatch.

Non-respiratory Causes of Hypercapnia

1 Rebreathing of CO_2 e.g. failure of the CO_2 absorber.
2 Exogenous CO_2 e.g. during laparoscopy.
3 Sodium bicarbonate administration.
4 Hypermetabolic state e.g. fever, sepsis and malignant hyperpyrexia.

▶ Hyperperfusion Syndrome

This condition can occur after carotid endarterectomy surgery and is due to increased cerebral perfusion. *See Carotid Endarterectomy (CEA)*.

▶ Hypertension

QUICK FLICK

H

Definition

Defined as a systolic > 139 mm Hg and diastolic > 89 mm Hg. Severe hypertension is systolic > 179 mm Hg and diastolic > 109 mm Hg.[35] Malignant hypertension is a blood pressure of >200/140 and is a medical emergency.

Significance of Pre-existing Hypertension

Controlled hypertension is not an independent risk factor for peri-operative morbidity. Uncontrolled hypertension is a minor predictor of peri-operative cardiac morbidity/mortality. ***See*** *Cardiovascular Peri-operative Risk Prediction for Non-cardiac Surgery*. If a patient has severe hypertension SBP > 180 mm Hg, DBP > 110 mm Hg and has not been investigated or treated, then elective surgery should probably be postponed. Patients who have been investigated and treated can probably proceed with surgery with control of their hypertension with IV agents. Antihypertensive medication should be taken up to the day of surgery with the exception of ACE inhibitors and angiotensin receptor antagonists. ***See*** *Angiotensin Related Antihypertensive Drugs and Anaesthesia*.

Hypertension during Anaesthesia

Causes of hypertension during anaesthesia include:

1 Physiological, e.g. nociceptive stimulation, awareness, laryngoscopy/intubation, volume overload, hypoxia, hypercarbia.
2 Pathological, e.g. raised intracranial pressure, phaeochromocytoma, pre-eclampsia, renovascular and essential hypertension.
3 Pharmacological, e.g. acute withdrawal of antihypertensive medication, vasopressor drugs.

Treatment

Depends on cause. ***See*** *COVER ABCD A SWIFT CHECK Crisis Management Algorithm*.

Must exclude hypoxia, ensure that the depth of anaesthesia is adequate and that the blood pressure reading is not artifactual. Consider:

1 *Deepening Anaesthesia.* Increase inspiratory concentration of inhalational agent, and/or bolus of IV anaesthetic agent e.g. thiopentone, propofol.
2 *Supplementing Analgesia.* Give opioid drug IV or additional LA + opioid via the epidural catheter.
3 *Antihypertensive Drugs.* Suitable agents include:
   a) β blocker. Especially useful if there is an associated tachycardia or a tachycardia is undesirable. For example, give metoprolol 1–2 mg IV boluses minutely to a maximum total dose of 15–20 mg. Do not use a β blocker if phaeochromocytoma suspected.
   b) Hydralazine 5–10 mg IV boluses.
   c) Phentolamine 0.5 mg boluses IV.
   d) Glyceryl trinitrate infusion 250 mg in 500 mL 5% glucose 0.1–6 µg/kg/min (10–400 µg/min).
   e) Sodium nitroprusside infusion 50 mg in 100 mL 5% glucose, run at 0.5–6 µg/kg/min.

See entry for each drug.

◑ Hypertensive Response to Intubation (Attenuation of)

Attenuation of the hypertensive responsive to intubation is particularly desirable in conditions such as:

1. phaeochromocytoma **see** *Phaeochromocytoma*.
2. cerebral aneurysm **see** *Cerebral Aneurysm Surgery*.
3. pre-eclampsia/eclampsia **see** *Pre-eclampsia/Eclampsia*.

Techniques

The following dosages are, in general, quoted for situations in which a single agent is used. If using multiple agents together lower doses should be used to avoid significant hypotension:

1. Ensure that the patient is well anaesthetised prior to intubation with a judicious dose of IV induction agent or inhalational drug.
2. Opioids: Consider fentanyl 5–10 μg/kg IV or sufentanil 0.5–1.0 μg/kg IV, 3–5 min before intubation.[36] Alfentanil 25–50 μg/kg IV is also effective. Remifentanil 2 μg/kg with a propofol induction will ablate the haemodynamic response to intubation.[37] However a bolus of this magnitude may result in severe bradycardia and hypotension before intubation.[38] Alternatively use a remifentanil infusion of 1–1.5 μg/kg/min run for 60–90 s prior to induction.[39]
3. Lignocaine 1.5–2 mg/kg IV 90 s before induction.
4. β blocker: e.g. Esmolol 2–3 mg/kg[40] or labetalol 0.15–0.45 mg/kg IV.[41]
5. Hydralazine 5–10 mg IV 15 min before induction of anaesthesia.[42]
6. Glyceryl trinitrate infusion 5–50 μg/kg/min just prior to laryngoscopy.[42]
7. Sodium nitroprusside 1–2 μg/kg.[41]
8. Magnesium sulfate 40 mg/kg given immediately after induction of anaesthesia appears to be effective in reducing the hypertensive response to intubation in pre-eclamptic patients. **See** *Pre-eclampsia/Eclampsia*.
9. Using a nerve stimulator, ensure that the patient is completely paralysed prior to intubation.

◑ Hypertrophic Cardiomyopathy (HCM)

This condition is defined as hypertrophy of the left ventricle, without dilation, in the absence of an identifiable cause.[43] Over 70% of cases are familial with autosomal dominant inheritance and variable penetrance. There is a 2–3% annual death risk.[44] It is the most common cause of sudden cardiac death in the young and the incidence is about 0.2%.[45]

Pathophysiology and Investigations

1. Hypertrophy of the anterior ventricular septum, although the site of hypertrophy can be highly variable.
2. Abnormal diastolic relaxation and excessive contractility in systole.

QUICK FLICK **H**

3 Decreased LV compliance, high diastolic filling pressures and decreased end-diastolic ventricular volume (i.e. a low capacity stiff ventricle).

4 Structural and functional abnormalities of the mitral valve.

5 Dynamic LV outflow obstruction may be present and is due to abnormal forward motion of the mitral valve with impaction of the anterior leaflet against the hypertrophied septum. This occurs in about 60% of patients. The previous term for this condition was hypertrophic obstructive cardiomyopathy or idiopathic hypertrophic subaortic stenosis.

6 If LV outflow obstruction occurs it is worsened by factors that increase contractility or which increase ventricular emptying (decreased preload or afterload). Mitral valve regurgitation can occur during periods of obstruction due to increased LV cavity pressure.

7 Relevant investigations include:
   a) *ECG* may indicate left ventricular hypertrophy, ST segment depression and T wave changes.
   b) *Echocardiography* typically shows left ventricular wall thickening. If the ratio of intraventricular septal thickness to left ventricular free wall thickness is >1.3:1 the diagnosis of HCM must be considered.[46]

Clinical Features

1 Ventricular dysrhythmias, supraventricular tachycardia and atrial fibrillation may occur and can be fatal.

2 Patients may experience dyspnoea, angina, syncope, heart failure and sudden death.

3 A systolic ejection murmur may be present.

Treatment

HCM patients are frequently treated with β blockers which relieve angina and dyspnoea. Calcium channel blockers may improve diastolic relaxation and increase exercise tolerance. These patients may also be on antiarrhythmic therapy e.g. amiodarone, sotalol, antiocoagulants (for atrial fibrillation) and have implanted defibrillators. Other treatments include dual chamber pacemakers, septal myotomy-myomectomy, catheter based alcohol septal ablation, and cardiac transplant.

Anaesthetic Management

It is imperative to avoid factors which increase myocardial contractility, decrease ventricular filling or increase ventricular emptying. Aim for strict haemodynamic stability and modest bradycardia. Consult directly with the patient's cardiologist or obtain cardiology review if the patient is newly diagnosed.

Anaesthesia Aims

1 Maintain preload. Ensure the patient is well hydrated (but not over hydrated) with IV fluids pre-operatively and maintain intravascular volume

throughout the peri-operative period. Do not use vasodilators such as sodium nitroprusside.

2   Maintain afterload, as a fall in systemic vascular resistance can result in increased ventricular emptying with increased outflow tract obstruction. Epidural/spinal anaesthesia may be extremely hazardous in the presence of HCM and these procedures have been associated with severe bradycardia, hypotension, myocardial infarction and death.[47] However, epidural anaesthesia has been used successfully in labouring patients.[48]

3   Consider invasive monitoring including intra-arterial BP, CVP line, PAC and transoesophageal echocardiography. Pulmonary capillary wedge pressure (PCWP) measurements can help predict optimal fluid loading of the left ventricle. Cardiac output monitoring can also help assess the response to therapeutic measures. Also the PCWP waveform can be observed for evidence of mitral valve regurgitant flow (giant V waves) indicating increased outflow obstruction.[49]

4   Avoid tachycardia which can increase outflow obstruction and decrease cardiac output. Bradycardia can be beneficial by increasing preload. Do not use ephedrine, atropine, ketamine or pancuronium which may increase heart rate.

5   Avoid increases in myocardial contractility. Do not give inotropic drugs such as digoxin and dobutamine.

6   Bacterial endocarditis prophylaxis should be 'considered' for relevant procedures.[43] *See Bacterial Endocarditis (BE) Prophylaxis.*

7   Maintain sinus rhythm as atrial contraction is extremely important for ventricular filling. Consider immediate cardioversion if a dysrhythmia occurs.

8   Avoid morphine which can produce venodilation. Use fentanyl instead.

Induction Phase

1   Propofol or thiopentone are suitable induction agents. Do not use ketamine, which may cause a tachycardia and increase contractility.[46]

2   Use rocuronium or cisatracurium for muscle relaxation. Do not use pancuronium which may produce a tachycardia.

Maintenance Phase

1   If the patient needs to be ventilated, avoid high airway pressures, PEEP and the Valsalva manoeuvre. This is to avoid decreases in preload. Small tidal volumes and higher respiratory rates are preferable during ventilation.

2   Sevoflurane or halothane are the inhalational anaesthetic agents of choice and are preferable to isoflurane and desflurane (both of which can increase HR and BP).[45] N_2O should not be used.

3   Hypotension should be treated with intravascular volume loading.

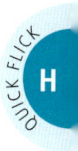

QUICK FLICK

H

If this is ineffective administer an α_1 adreno-receptor agonist such as phenylephrine (50–100 µg increments) or methoxamine (1 mg IV boluses).[50] Do not use ephedrine as it will increase HR.

4 Hypertension should be treated with increased concentration of inhalational anaesthetic agent. If this is inadequate use esmolol (*see Esmolol*). Do not use vasodilators such as GTN or SNP.

5 If AF develops intraoperatively treat with cardio version rather than pharmacologically.

Recovery Phase

In addition to the principles outlined above, ensure the patient is warm and well analgesed.

Treatment of Heart Failure

If heart failure occurs in a patient with HCM treatment principles include:

1 Optimise preload with IV fluids.

2 Optimise afterload with an α adreno-receptor agonist such as metaraminol.

3 Decrease heart rate and contractility with a β adreno-receptor blocker drug.

4 Give frusemide if pulmonary oedema occurs.[51]

HCM and Obstetric Anaesthesia

Pre-term Labour

If there is LV outflow obstruction betamimetic tocolytic agents for premature labour are absolutely contraindicated.[44] Magnesium sulfate would probably be safer.[44]

Epidural Analgesia for Labour

Epidural anaesthesia has been used successfully in HCM patients in labour.[48, 52] Recommendations include:

1 Consider starting an epidural infusion early in labour.

2 Use low concentrations of LA agent e.g. bupivacaine 0.125%. Titrate dose gradually.

3 Do not use adrenaline containing solutions in order to avoid any adrenaline induced increase in myocardial contractility or heart rate.

4 Consider an arterial line to monitor blood BP closely.

5 ECG monitoring.

6 Oxytocin may cause adverse effects due to relaxation of vascular smooth muscle. It must be administered slowly and carefully. Boccio et al. recommend ergonovine as an alternative.[53]

Anaesthesia for CS

Opinion regarding optimal anaesthesia for CS in HCM patients favours GA.[53, 54] Minnich et al. argue that for patients with HCM with an epidural for labour pain already present, it would be reasonable to gradually and carefully 'top-up' the epidural for CS.[53] Their recommendation is to revert to GA if significant CVS deterioration occurs that is not responsive to fluids and vasopressors. Autore reported 3 cases of successful epidural anaesthesia for CS.[55]

◯ Hyperviscosity Syndrome

This syndrome is due to polycythaemia, which may be primary or secondary to causes such as congenital cyanotic heart disease. It consists of headache, dizziness and visual disturbance and the treatment is venesection if the Hct is > 0.65. *See Congenital Heart Disease (CHD) in Adults and Non-cardiac Surgery*.

◯ Hypocapnia

Hypocapnia is defined as $PaCO_2 < 35$ mm Hg. It can result from:

1 hyperventilation
2 reduced CO_2 production.

◯ Hypotension

Specific treatment depends on cause. Causes can be divided into:

1 *Inadequate Preload* Hypovolaemia e.g. blood loss, venodilator drugs, supine hypotensive syndrome (*see Supine Hypotensive Syndrome*).
2 *Cardiac Impairment* E.g. tamponade, tension pneumothorax, dysrhythmia, ischaemia.
3 *Reduced Afterload* E.g. sepsis, neuro axial anaesthesia, arterial vasodilators, anaphylaxis.

Treatment

Urgency and aggressiveness of treatment depends on severity of hypotension and cause. Principles of management are:

1 *Optimise Preload* Give IV fluids of appropriate type and volume (crystalloid, colloid, blood).
2 *Correct Cardiac Impairment* E.g. reduce/cease administration of volatile anaesthetic agent. If no palpable pulse, commence immediate external or internal cardiac massage. *See Cardiac Arrest*.
3 *Optimise Afterload* Give vasoconstrictor drug e.g. ephedrine 3–6 mg boluses IV, metaraminol 0.5–1 mg IV boluses, adrenaline 10 µg–1 mg IV depending on severity of situation + IV infusion (*see Adrenaline*).

QUICK FLICK

H

Diagnosis of Hypotension Using COVER ABCD Algorithm (Search for Cause Simultaneously with Treatment)

- *C (Circulation & Colour)* Feel pulse for rate, rhythm and character. Pulse quality may indicate that the blood pressure measurement is artifactual, or a dysrhythmia is present. Assess the patient's colour looking especially for cyanosis, or erythema suggesting an anaphylaxis. Look at the ECG tracing and treat significant dysrhythmias if present.

- *O (Oxygen supply, Oxygen analyser)* Ensure that the patient is adequately oxygenated. Ventilate with 100% O_2 if severe hypotension is present. Look at the pulse oximetry trace. The presence of a pulse waveform is suggestive that some output is present.

- *V (Ventilation & Vaporiser)* Assess ventilation. Examine the chest for tension pneumothorax/bronchospasm. Listen to the heart sounds. May hear muffled valve sounds in tamponade or 'mill wheel murmur' with gas embolus. Check the capnograph trace. The presence of expired CO_2 indicates some cardiac output is present. Check the vaporiser setting. An overdose of volatile anaesthetic agent may be the cause of the hypotension. Reduce delivered concentration or cease volatile administration.

- *E (Endotracheal Tube & Elimination)*

- *R (Review Monitors and Equipment)* Recheck pulse oximetry, capnography, ECG and any other monitors in use such as CVP. Check equipment such as drug infusion pumps e.g. is inotropic drug failing to reach patient due to infusion pump or IV line problems? Check surgeon's positioning of instruments as this may be causing decreased venous return. Assess degree of blood loss (check suction bottles). Excessive insufflation of gas during laparoscopy may also be a cause.

- *A (Reassess Airway)*

- *B (Reassess Ventilation)*

- *C (Reassess Circulation)* i.e. Preload (blood loss?) cardiac function (myocardial ischaemia?) and afterload (total spinal?). Optimise the above.

- *D (Drug effects)* Review intended, possible/actual unintended drug administration or substance administration e.g. bone cement, accidental rapid infusion of vancomycin. Reconsider failure of a drug to reach patient e.g. kinked cannula. If the cause of hypotension still not apparent move onto A SWIFT CHECK algorithm.

See COVER ABCD A SWIFT CHECK Crisis Management Algorithm.

◗ Hypoxia/Hypoxaemia

Hypoxaemia can be defined as a $PaO_2 < 60$ mm Hg or O_2 Saturation $< 90\%$. Hypoxia is an anaesthetic emergency requiring immediate treatment. Causes include the following:

1 Pre-airway Issues:
   a) Inadequate inspired FiO_2.
   b) Inadequate ventilation e.g. ventilator failure or switched off.
   c) Disconnection.
   d) Blocked filter.
   e) Blocked anaesthetic gas tubing.
2 Airway Problems:
   a) Oesophageal intubation.
   b) Blocked ET tube.
   c) Laryngospasm.
   d) Laryngeal swelling (e.g. anaphylaxis) or compression (e.g. haematoma).
   e) Tracheal/bronchial obstruction e.g. bronchial intubation or compression e.g. mediastinal mass.
   f) Material in the airway such as blood or vomitus.
   g) Bronchospasm (**see** *Brochospasm*).
3 Problems Distal to the Airways:
   a) Ventilation-perfusion mismatch.
   b) Shunt.
   c) Diffusion block i.e. impaired transfer of O_2 across alveolar wall to pulmonary capillary as can occur with pulmonary oedema.
   d) Inadequate cardiac output.
   e) Decreased O_2 carrying capacity of blood e.g. anaemia, carbon monoxide poisoning.

Hypoxia Management 'Drill'

1 Most cases of hypoxia are detected by the pulse oximeter reading. Check that the pulse oximeter is properly attached to the patient. Always assume the pulse oximeter reading is correct until proven otherwise.
2 Check the oxygen analyser and flow meters and ensure that O_2 is being delivered to the patient. Look at the other monitors especialy capnography, ECG and blood pressure for any abnormalities.
3 Perform a rapid screen of the anaesthetic circuit from the wall oxygen outlet to the patient, looking for obvious causes of inadequate ventilation such as disconnections.
4 Eliminate the ventilator. Hand ventilate the patient with the reservoir bag. Increase the inspired O_2 concentration of the delivered gas to 100% and ensure the oxygen analyser shows a rising O_2 concentration in the inspired gas. Feel lung compliance and look at the capnography trace and other monitors. Get help early if situation is not resolving rapidly. If there is any doubt about the oxygen supply quality, or the integrity of the anaesthetic circuit, use a self inflating bag and separate oxygen cylinder supply. If this equipment is unavailable use expired air ventilation (mouth to mouth/LMA/tube).

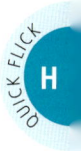

QUICK FLICK

H

5 Examine the patient. Check for:
   a) Presence of adequate pulse and blood pressure.
   b) Rash, swelling of the lips and eyelids suggesting anaphylaxis.
   c) Evidence of aspiration such as secretions in the LMA.
   d) Equal chest expansion on inspiration.
   e) Subcutaneous emphysema.
   f) Auscultate the chest for abnormalities such as wheezes, absent breath sounds unilaterally.

6 Consider airway causes such as patient biting the LMA, bronchial intubation, blocked or kinked ET tube or blocked filter. If there is any doubt about the ET tube, change the tube. The filter can be checked by disconnecting it from the tube and squeezing the reservoir bag, ensuring that gases pass easily through the filter.

7 If no apparent airway, lung pathology or anaesthetic circuit causes are identified consider rarer causes such as methaemoglobinaemia.

8 Obtain an urgent chest X-ray and consider other investigations such as fibre-optic bronchoscopy.

Diagnosis of Hypoxia Using the COVER ABCD Crisis Management Algorithm

The COVER ABCD A SWIFT CHECK crisis management algorithm should be immediately applied with simultaneous diagnosis and treatment. If patient is undergoing mask anaesthesia, begin with A B.

- *A (Ensure Patent Airway).*
- *B (Ensure Patient is Breathing)* If not ventilate, with 100% O_2
- *C (Circulation and Colour)* Feel pulse, ensure circulation is adequate, if not treat as per *Hypotension* above. Check patient's colour for cyanosis or erythema (suggesting allergic reaction).
- *O (Oxygen Supply and Oxygen Analyser)* Increase FiO_2 (to 100% if hypoxia severe) and ensure O_2 analyser shows a rising concentration of O_2 distal to the common gas outlet. Always consider a contaminated O_2 supply. If contamination is suspected, use cylinder O_2. If no cylinder O_2 use your own expired O_2.
- *V (Ventilation and Vaporiser)* Ventilate lungs by hand to assess lung compliance, circuit integrity, and airway patency. Look at chest expansion and perform auscultation to detect wheezing/asymmetrical breath sounds. If unilateral chest expansion consider endobronchial intubation, pneumothorax or sputum plugging of bronchus. Consider urgent chest X-ray/fibre-optic bronchoscopy. **See** *Pneumothorax*. Check capnography trace. If expired CO_2 low consider pulmonary embolus + decreased cardiac output (**see** *Hypercapnia*). Check vaporiser setting.
- *E (Endotracheal Tube and 'Eliminate')* Check ET tube for patency/kinks. Pass suction tubing down the ET tube and suck out secretions.

Consider ET tube cuff herniation (deflate cuff), bronchial/oesophageal intubation, tracheal tear (tube passes through cords but tip of tube lies outside trachea). 'When in doubt take it out' i.e. replace tube. 'Eliminate' the anaesthetic machine if contaminated O_2 supply suspected, or undiagnosed equipment problem is occurring. Use self inflating bag and cylinder O_2 to ventilate patient. For example a near fatal tension pneumothorax occurred at Westmead Hospital due to kinked expiratory limb tubing (personal communication).

- *R (Review Monitors and Equipment)* Review all monitors especially pulse oximetry, capnography ECG, BP. Check for hyperthermia and exclude malignant hyperpyrexia. Review all equipment including surgical equipment e.g. gas insufflation for laparoscopy may be causing embolus.
- *A (Reassess Airway)*
- *B (Reassess Ventilation)*
- *C (Reassess Circulation)* Must ensure adequate pulse and blood pressure.
- *D (Drug Effect)* For example formation of methaemoglobin by drugs such as prilocaine. If the cause of hypoxia is still not apparent move onto A SWIFT CHECK algorithm. ***See*** *COVER ABCD A SWIFT CHECK Crisis Management Algorithm*.

REFERENCES

1 Pleuvry BJ. Plasma expanders. *Anaesthesia and Intensive Care Med* 2002; 3: 228–31.

2 Forbes AM. Colloids and blood products. In Oh TE, ed. *Intensive Care Manual*. 4th edn. Butterworth–Heinemann, Oxford, 1997; 754–9.

3 Luhmann JD, Schootman M, Scott JL, Kennedy RM. A randomised comparison of nitrous oxide plus hematoma block versus ketamine plus midazolam for emergency department forearm fracture reduction in children. *Pediatrics* 2006; 118: e1078–e1086.

4 Håkanson E, Konstantinov IE, Fransson S-G, Svedjeholm R. Management of life-threatening haemoptysis. *Br J Anaesth* 2002; 88: 291–5.

5 Harrison BA, Vasdev G. Anesthesia for Bronchoscopy. In Faust RJ, Cucchiara RF, Rose SH, et al (eds). *Anesthesiology Review,* 3rd edn. Churchill Livingstone, Philadelphia, 2002: 513.

6 Lordan JL, Gascoigne A, Corris PA. The pulmonary physician in critical care: Illustrative case 7: Assessment and management of massive haemoptysis. *Thorax* 2003; 58: 814–19.

7 Hirsch IB, McGill JB, Cryer PE, White PF. Perioperative management of surgical patients with diabetes mellitus. *Anesthesiology* 1991; 74: 346–59.

8 Robertshaw HJ, Hall GM. Diabetes mellitus: anaesthetic management. *Anaesthesia* 2006; 61: 1187–90.

9 Broomhead C. Management of patients with a cardiac transplant. *Br J Hosp Med* 1995; 54: 571–3.

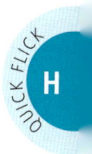

10 Cheng DCH, Ong DD. Anaesthesia for non-cardiac surgery in heart-transplanted patients. *Can J Anaesth* 1993; 40: 981–6.

11 Shaw IH, Kirk AJB, Conacher ID. Anaesthesia for patients with transplanted hearts and lungs undergoing non-cardiac surgery. *Br J Anaesth* 1991; 67: 772–8.

12 Morgan-Hughes NJ, Hood G. Anaesthesia for a patient with a cardiac transplant. *Br J Anaesth CEPD Reviews* 2002; 2: 74–8.

13 Bernheim A, Fatio R, Kiowski W et al. Atropine often results in complete atrioventricular block or sinus arrest after cardiac transplantation: An unpredictable and dose-independent phenomenon. *Transplantation* 2004; 77: 1181–5.

14 Lanzinger MJ, Niklason LE, Shannon M, Hill SE. Use of hemoglobin raffimer for postoperative life-threatening anemia in a Jehovah's Witness. *Can J Anesth* 2005; 52: 369–73.

15 de Maistre E, Gruel Y, Lasne D. Diagnosis and management of heparin induced thrombocytopenia. *Can J Anesth* 2006; 53: S123–S124.

16 Bullingham A, Strunin L. Prevention of postoperative venous thromboembolism. *Br J Anaesth* 1995; 75: 622–30.

17 Salerno F, Gerbes A, Ginés P et al. Diagnosis, prevention and treatment of hepatorenal syndrome in cirrhosis. *Gut* 2007; 56: 1310–18.

18 Witzke O, Gerken G, Kribben A, Philipp T. Das hepatorenale Syndrom: Wo stehen wir im Jahr 2007? [Hepatorenal syndrome: What's new in 2007?]. *Medizinische Klinic* 2007; 102: 203–8.

19 Grant IS. Intercurrent disease and anaesthesia. In Aitkenhead AR, Smith G, eds. *Textbook of Anaesthesia,* 2nd edn. Churchill Livingstone, New York 1990: 645–76.

20 Mason RA. Anaesthesia Databook. *A Clinical Practice Compendium.* Churchill Livingstone, New York, 1990: 136.

21 Brinch K, Moller S, Bendsten F et al. Plasma volume expansion by albumin in cirrhosis. Relation to blood volume distribution, arterial compliance and severity of disease. *J Hepatol* 2003; 39: 24–31.

22 Fernandez J, Navasa M, Planas R et al. Primary prophylaxis of spontaneous bacterial peritonitis delays hepatorenal syndrome and improves survival in cirrhosis. *Gastroenterology* 2007; 133: 1029–31.

23 Hodges PJ, Kam PCA. Review article: the peri-operative implications of herbal medicines. *Anaesthesia* 2002; 57: 889–99.

24 Gunning K. Echinacea in the treatment and prevention of upper respiratory tract infections. *Western Journal of Medicine* 1999; 171: 198–200.

25 Rose KD, Croissant PD, Parliament CF. Spontaneous spinal epidural haematoma with associated platelet dysfunction from excessive garlic ingestion: a case report. *Neurosurgery* 1990; 26: 880–2.

26 Burnham BE. Garlic as a possible risk for postoperative bleeding. *Plastic and Reconstructive Surgery* 1995; 95: 213.

27 Miller LG. Herbal medicines. Selected clinical considerations focusing on known or potential drug-herb interactions. *Archives of Internal Medicine* 1999; 159: 1857–8.

28 Shann F. *Drug Doses,* 11th edn. Collective Pty Ltd 2001: 34.

29 Sarhill N, Walsh D, Nelson KA. Hydromorphone: pharmacology and clinical applications in cancer patients. *Support Care Cancer* 2001; 9: 84–96.

30 Latta KS, Ginsberg B, Barkin RL. Meperidine: a clinical review. *American J Therapeutics* 2002; 9: 53–68.

31 Goodarzi M. Comparison of epidural morphine, hydromorphone and fentanyl for postoperative pain control in children undergoing orthopaedic surgery. *Paed Anaesth* 1999; 9: 419–22.

32 Coda BA, O'Sullivan B, Donaldson G et al. Comparative efficacy of patient-controlled administration of morphine, hydromorphone, or sufentanil for the treatment of oral mucositis pain following bone marrow transplantation. *Pain* 1997; 72: 333–46.

33 Pleuvry BJ. Plasma expanders. *Anaesthesia and Intensive Care Med* 2002; 3: 228–31.

34 Thornberry EA. Perioperative fluids. *Anaesthesia and Intensive Care Medicine* 2002: 3; 414–17.

35 Marcucci C, Fleisher LA. Hypertension: implications for anesthetic management. *Curr Opin Anaesthesiol* 1997; 10: 229–33.

36 Mack PF. Cerebral Aneurysm. In Yao F-S F, ed. *Anesthesiology Problem-Orientated Patient Management,* 4th edn, Lippincott-Raven, Philadelphia 1998; 504–24.

37 Barclay K, Kluger MT. Effect of bolus dose of remifentanil on haemodynamic response to tracheal intubation. *Anaesth Intensive Care* 2000; 28: 403–7.

38 Elliott P, O'Hare R, Bill KM et al. Severe cardiovascular depression with remifentanil. *Anesth Analg* 2000; 91: 58–61.

39 Richa F, Yaziga A, Nasser E et al. General anaesthesia with remifentanil for Cesarean section in a patient with HELLP syndrome (case report). *ACTA Anaesthesiol Scand* 2005; 49: 418–20.

40 Hall RI. Editorial: Esmolol—just another beta blocker? *Can J Anaesth* 1992; 39: 757–64.

41 Yao F-S F. Hypertension. In Yao F-S F, ed. *Anesthesiology Problem-Orientated Patient Management*, 4th edn, Lippincott-Raven, Philadelphia 1998; 316–33.

42 Sia-Kho E. Pregnancy-Induced Hypertension. In Yao F-S F, ed. *Anesthesiology Problem-Orientated Patient Management,* 4th edn, Lippincott-Raven, Philadelphia 1998; 681–703.

QUICK FLICK

H

43 Elliott PM, McKenna WJ. Management of hypertrophic cardiomyopathy. *Br J Hosp Med* 1996; 55: 419–23.

44 Shah DM, Sunderji SG. Hypertrophic cardiomyopathy and pregnancy: report of a maternal mortality and review of the literature. *Obstetrical and Gynecological Survey* 1985; 40: 444–8.

45 Poliac LC, Barron ME, Maron BJ. Hypertrophic cardiomyopathy. *Anesthesiology* 2006; 104: 183–92.

46 Stoelting RK, Dierdorf S. *Anaesthesia and Co-existing Disease,* 4th edn. Churchill Livingstone, Philadelphia 2002: 120–5.

47 Baraka A, Jabbour S, Itani I. Severe bradycardia following epidural anaesthesia in a patient with idiopathic hypertrophic subaortic stenosis. *Anesth Analg* 1987; 66: 1337–8.

48 Paix B, Cyna A, Belperio P, Simmons S. Epidural analgesia for labour and delivery in a patient with congenital hypertrophic obstructive cardiomyopathy (Case report). *Anaesth Intensive Care* 1999; 27: 59–62.

49 Edmends S, Ghosh S. Hypertrophic obstructive cardiomyopathy complicating surgery for cerebral aneurysm clipping. *Anaesthesia* 1994; 49: 608–9.

50 Loubser P, Suh K, Cohen S. Adverse effects of spinal anesthesia in a patient with idiopathic hypertrophic subaortic stenosis. *Anesthesiology* 1984; 60: 228–30.

51 Tessler MJ, Hudson R, Naugler-Colville MA et al. Pulmonary oedema in two patients with hypertrophic obstructive cardiomyopathy (HOCM). *Can J Anaesth* 1990; 37: 469–73.

52 Minnich ME, Quirk JG, Clark RB. Epidural anaesthesia for vaginal delivery in a patient with idiopathic hypertrophic subaortic stenosis. *Anesthesiology* 1987; 67: 590–2.

53 Boccio RV, Chung JH, Harrison DM. Anesthetic management of Caesarean section in a patient with idiopathic hypertrophic subaortic stenosis. *Anesthesiology* 1986; 65: 663–5.

54 Oakley GDG, McGarry K, Limb DG et al. Management of pregnancy in patients with hypertrophic cardiomyopathy. *Br Med J* 1979; 1: 1749–59.

55 Autore C, Brauneis S, Apponi F et al. Epidural anaesthesia for Caesarean section in patients with hypertrophic cardiomyopathy: a report of three cases. *Anesthesiology* 1999; 90: 1205–7.

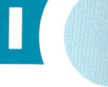

⊳ Immunosuppressive Drugs, Anaesthetic Implications

Topics Covered in this Section
▶ Bleomycin
▶ Cyclosporin
▶ Tacrolimus
▶ Azathioprine
▶ Steroids

These drugs increase the patient's susceptibility to infection and malignancy. Some specific drugs with complications are listed below.

Bleomycin
Anthracycline antibiotic type anti-cancer drug used for the treatment of malignancies such as testicular cancer and Hodgkin's disease. BLM can cause pulmonary toxicity and acute severe lung toxicity in the presence of hyperoxia.

Pre-operative Evaluation
1. Assess the patient for evidence of pulmonary and/or renal toxicity (which can result in delayed clearance of BLM).
2. Possibly increased risk if:
   a) exposure to BLM within 1–2 months.[1]
   b) > 450 mg total dose received.
3. Consider corticosteroid pretreatment.[1]

Intra-operative Management
Avoid an inspired O_2 concentration > 30%. Use the minimum inspired O_2 concentration required to maintain an O_2 saturation > 90%

Cyclosporin
Can cause renal and hepatic insufficiency, hypertension and neurotoxicity such as a reduced seizure threshold. It can also cause biliary stasis. Cyclosporin may augment neuromuscular blockade.

Tacrolimus
Can cause diabetes and be nephrotoxic. It can also cause hypertension.

Azathioprine

Haematological toxicity with thrombocytopenia and anaemia. Can also cause hepatic insufficiency and biliary stasis.

Steroids

Can cause adrenal insufficiency (**see** *Steroid 'Cover' for Surgery/Anaesthesia*), hypertension, diabetes mellitus, peptic ulcer disease, pancreatitis and psychiatric illnesses. They can also cause cataracts and aseptic bone necrosis.

◗ Infraorbital Nerve Block

Anatomy

Supplies sensory innervation to the lower eyelid, cheek, upper lip and side of nose. Emerges from the infra-orbital foramen 1.5 cm below the inferior orbital rim. This foramen lies ≈ 2 cm from the lateral border of the nose and is in line with the pupil when the eye is in the neutral position.

Technique

The nerve can be blocked by passing a 23 G needle through the skin 0.5 cm below the foramen and injecting at the orifice. Alternatively the needle can be inserted through the mucosa adjacent to the upper gum and aimed towards the palpating finger of the opposite hand held over the foramen. Inject 2 mL of LA solution (e.g. lignocaine 2% solution).

◗ Inguinal Field Block

Used for inguinal hernia repair. The inguinal region is supplied by:

1 *Iliohypogastric Nerve (L1)* Innervates the suprapubic skin and the skin immediately above the inguinal ligament.
2 *Ilioinguinal Nerve (L1)* Supplies the skin over the root of the penis and upper part of the scrotum (or labium).
3 *Genitofemoral Nerve (L1, 2)* The genital branch supplies the skin over scrotum (or labium) and adjacent thigh. The *Femoral branch* supplies the skin over the upper part of the femoral triangle.

Technique (as described by Dr C. Sparkes et al.)[2]

1 Draw a line between the anterior superior iliac spine (ASIS) and the umbilicus.
2 2 cm from the ASIS along this line sterilise and anaesthetise the skin and puncture the skin with a 19 G needle.
3 Insert a 22 G short bevelled (SB) needle at this point 90° to skin. After ≈ 1 cm, a pop is felt.
4 Inject 7 mL of lignocaine 1% + 1:200 000 adrenaline (to anaesthetise iliohypogastric nerve). Insert the needle another 0.5 cm. A second pop is felt and there is 'loss of resistance' (LOR) to injection. Inject 8 mL of LA (to anaesthetise the Ilioinguinal nerve).

5 Next identify the mid-inguinal point, anaesthetise the skin 1 cm cephalad to this point, and make a hole in the skin as above. Insert the SB needle until 2 pops are felt and there is again LOR to injection (at a depth of ≈ 4 cm). Inject 25 mL of LA solution (to block genitofemoral nerve).

6 Ask the surgeon to mark the line of incision on the patient's skin and infiltrate along this line with 20 mL of 0.5% lignocaine + adrenaline using a 9 cm 22 G spinal needle. At the lateral end of the incision line inject a further 3 mL of LA subcutaneously in the direction of umbilicus.

7 The surgeon may need to supplement the block with additional LA intra-operatively.

8 Consider an additional 5–10 mL of LA injection around the pubic tubercle percutaneosly.

▶ Insulin/Glucose Infusion

See *Diabetes Mellitus, Preparation for Surgery*.

▶ Intercostal Drain

See *Chest Drain*.

▶ Intercostal Nerve Block

Anatomy

The intercostal nerve lies in the intercostal groove at the lower edge of each rib. T2–T6 supply the chest and T7–T11 the abdomen (sensory and motor innervation).

Technique

The best access to the intercostal nerve is behind the mid-axillary line.

1 Using a sterile technique, pull the skin cephalad over the rib and insert a 23 G sharp-bevelled needle at 90° to the skin. Anaesthetise the skin, then walk the needle off the lower border of the rib.

2 At edge of the rib, angle the needle cephalad and insert the needle no more than 2 mm so that the point is in the intercostal groove.

3 If aspiration is negative inject 3–5 mL of bupivacaine 0.5% + adrenaline 1:200 000. The block will last 6–10 h.

Note: The blocks are done more easily with the patient prone or sitting.

Complications

1 Pneumothorax.

2 Inadequate ventilation due to muscle paralysis of the intercostals.

3 Systemic LA toxicity due to intravascular injection.

4 Inadvertant subdural or epidural injection producing hypotension and/or extensive blockade.

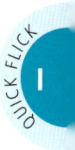

QUICK FLICK

I

Multi-level Intercostal Blockade with a Single Injection

Extensive intercostals blockade can be achieved with a single injection with a similar effect to intrapleural blockade. In a technique described by Murphy local anaesthetic is deposited in a tissue plane between the internal intercostalis aponeurosis and the deeper intercostalis intimus muscles.[3]

Technique

1   Identify the intercostal site appropriate for the surgical incision.
2   Insert a 23 G sharp bevelled needle at the angle of the rib (≈ 6 cm from the midline posteriorally).
3   Contact the rib, then walk the needle off the lower border. Insert the needle a further 3–5 mm under the rib. The needle should have pierced the aponeurosis of the internal intercostal muscle.
4   Inject 10–15 mL of LA e.g. ropivacaine 10 mg/mL.

◐ Internal Jugular Vein (IJV) Catheterisation

Anatomy

The internal jugular vein (IJV) originates from the jugular foramen at the base of the skull and terminates between and behind the clavicular and sternal heads of the sternomastoid muscle, where it joins the subclavian vein. At its origin, the IJV lies posterior to the internal carotid artery but as it descends it becomes lateral to the common carotid artery (CCA). The vagus nerve lies between and posterior to the 2 vessels.

Technique

Position the patient supine without a pillow and with the head turned slightly to the contralateral side with the bed tilted 10–20° Trendelenburg. There are 2 main approaches. Use strict aseptic technique + LA infiltration in the awake patient.

High Approach

1   Identify the midpoint between the mastoid process and the ipsilateral sternoclavicular joint. Palpate the carotid artery at this level. The IJV should lie just lateral to this pulsation.
2   Use a 23 G 'seeker' needle to identify the IJV. Be careful not to compress the vein while palpating the carotid pulse. Aim in the direction of the ipsilateral nipple. If the first pass is unsuccessful, direct the needle slightly more laterally.
3   After identifying the IJV with the seeker needle, leave this needle in place and insert an 18 G cannula or a needle suitable for insertion of the guide wire. Insert this cannula/needle parallel and alongside the seeker needle.
4   Insert the guide wire through cannula/needle and remove the latter.

5 After using a scalpel to nick the skin insert the dilator over the wire and dilate the tract to the IJV. Remove the dilator and then insert the central venous catheter over the wire.
   Note: Never lose sight of the distal end of the wire and never insert the catheter without holding the distal end of the wire.
6 Ensure blood can be aspirated from each lumen and flush each lumen with heparinised saline, then close off each lumen.
7 Suture the catheter into position. For an adult this will be at ≈ 15 cm for a right IJ line and ≈ 17 cm for a left IJ line. Apply a sterile dressing.
8 Perform a post-procedure chest X-ray to check the position of the catheter tip. The tip of the catheter should be outside the right atrium. Schuster et al. recommend that the CVC tip be located in the SVC above the level of the carina.[4]

Low Approach
1 Position the patient as above and identify the sternal and clavicular heads of the sternomastoid muscle.
2 Insert the 23 G seeker needle at 30–45° to the coronal plane aiming for the ipsilateral nipple, parallel with the long axis of the body, at the apex of the triangle formed by these 2 muscle heads. Use a stabbing motion to penetrate the IJV which normally lies in this gap closer to the clavicular than sternal head. The IJV usually lies at a depth of 0.5–2 cm.
3 Once the vein is identified, leave the seeker needle in place. Insert an 18 G cannula or a needle suitable for insertion of the guide wire parallel and alongside the seeker needle. Then proceed as above.

Aids to Success
The diameter of the internal jugular vein can be increased by a Valsalva manoeuvre, IPPV, PEEP and increasing head down tilt.[5]

Ultrasound Guided Internal Jugular Vein Catheterisation
Portable ultrasound machines such as the Sonosite are enabling visualisation of the internal jugular vein. This technology is reducing the incidence of complications[6] and is rapidly becoming a standard of care. The technique involves:
1 Prep, drape and position the patient as described above.
2 Using a sterile sheath and strict aseptic technique, use the ultrasound probe to image the carotid artery (pulsatile) and the internal jugular vein (compressible). The vein can be made more obvious by Trendelenburg positioning or a Valsalva manoeuvre. Orientate the probe in the transverse plane (at right angles to the long axis of the vein). Avoid pressing down too hard with the probe as this may make the vein hard to see.
3 Position the probe so that the vein is in the centre of the screen.

QUICK FLICK

I

4 Insert the 18 G Seldinger needle into the skin at the centre of the probe at a steep angle. It may help, while learning this technique, to have a second operator hold the probe.

5 Once the Seldinger needle enters the vein, put the probe down and pass the wire.

6 Use the probe to confirm that the wire is in the vein, then complete the procedure as described above.

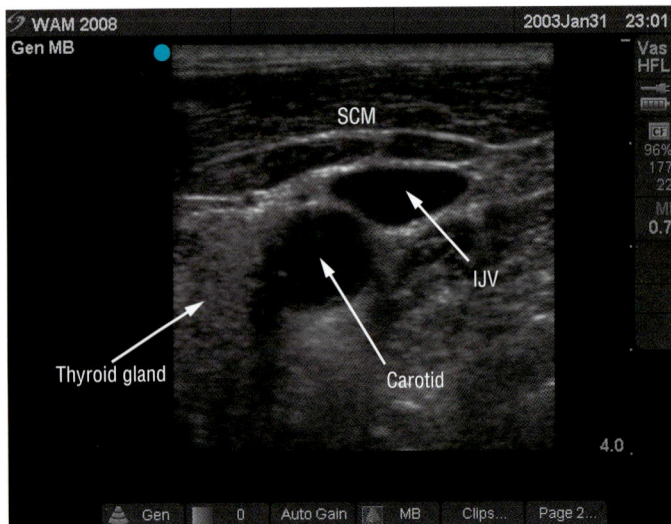

Figure I1 Ultrasound image of internal jugular vein

Complications of Internal Jugular Vein Catheterisation

1 If the tip of the central venous catheter lies within the pericardium, cardiac tamponade may occur.[7]

2 Carotid artery puncture. The incidence of this is 2–17%,[8] unless an ultrasound guided technique is used.

3 Haemorrhage with possible airway compromise.

4 Infection.

5 Pleural puncture.

◗ International Normalised Ratio (INR)

The INR was developed to improve comparability of measures of prothrombin time (PT) between laboratories. INR thus correlates with PT which measures the effectiveness of the extrinsic clotting pathway. Normal range (NR) for PT is 10–12 s, NR for INR is 0.8–1.2. Both INR and PT are elevated by deficiencies or abnormalities of clotting factors II, V, VII, X such as in the presence of warfarin therapy. The recommended INR for standard and high-dose anticoagulant therapies are 2.0–3.0 and 2.5–3.5 respectively. *See* *Warfarin*.

⭕ Intra-arterial Injection

Effects of Intra-arterial Drug Injection

The effect of intra-arterial drug injection depends on the type of drug involved. Examples from the literature include:

1 *Buprenorphine* Intra-arterial injection produced peripheral cyanosis.[9]
2 *Diazepam* Intra-arterial diazepam has resulted in effects similar to thiopentone with ischaemia and tissue necrosis.
3 *Etomidate* No significant effects from intra-arterial injection.[10]
4 *Flucloxacillin* Intra-arterial flucloxacillin can produce severe reactions with arterial vasospasm and peripheral gangrene.[11]
5 *Midazolam* Does not appear to be hazardous.[12,13]
6 *Morphine* Does not appear to be hazardous.
7 *Propofol* Intra-arterial propofol has resulted in pain, local blanching and a transient decrease (5 min) in blood flow to the distal limb. Significant limb morbidity appears less likely than with thiopentone.[14]
8 *Thiopentone* Can also cause severe vasospasm and gangrene.

Treatment of Intra-arterial Drug Injection Producing Sequelae

1 Remove any residual drug from the line, leave the arterial cannula in situ and flush with saline.
2 Look for any evidence of vascular spasm. If this does occur, consider the following vasodilators:[12]
   a) Papaverine 40–80 mg in 20 mL N/S intra-arterially.
   b) Tolazoline 25–50 mg intra-arterially.
   c) Reserpine 1.25 mg IV.
   d) Phenoxybenzamine 0.5 mg IV.
3 Intra-arterial guanethidine has been used effectively. The dose is 5 mg in 5 mL N/S.[13]
4 Iloprost, a thromboxane inhibitor. This was used to treat a buprenorphine arterial injection (combined with a Dextran 40 infusion).[9]
5 Dextran 40 infusion to improve microcirculation in the ischaemic area.[9] *See* *Dextrans*.
6 Consider urokinase intra-arterially.
7 Stellate ganglion block, brachial plexus block.
8 Flushing the cannula with procaine, phentolamine or heparinised saline is not of proven benefit.[15]

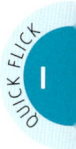

QUICK FLICK

I

⟡ Intracranial Pressure (ICP) and Treatment of Raised ICP

ICP is defined as the pressure in the lateral ventricle or in the subarachnoid space over the convexity of the cerebral cortex. Normal ICP is ≈ 13 cm H_2O or 10 mm Hg. 20–25 cm H_2O ICP is equivocal while > 25 cm H_2O (18 mm Hg) is 'raised'.

Methods of Reducing Raised ICP

1 Exclude hypoxia and hypercarbia and ensure optimal patient oxygenation.
2 Elevate the head 15–30°. Keep the head in the neutral position. Ensure that there is no venous obstruction at the neck due to e.g. tight ties around the neck for the ET tube.
3 Ensure adequate muscle relaxation, as increased thoracic and abdominal muscle tone may increase ICP.
4 Hyperventilate the patient to an end tidal expired CO_2 concentration of 30 mm Hg. Check $PaCO_2$ on arterial blood gas analysis. Excessive hyperventilation may lead to cerebral ischaemia.[16]
5 Mannitol 20% 0.25–2 g/kg IV. The usual dose is 0.5–1 g/kg. The dose given depends on the severity of the situation. Give Mannitol over 20 min, as it may cause hypotension if given faster.[17] Its effects start within 10 min and peak at about 45 min. If ICP remains persistently raised, give 0.25–0.5 g/kg every 6 h. Effects of mannitol are enhanced by the addition of frusemide 0.3 mg/kg IV.[16] Frusemide can also be used instead of mannitol in a dose of 1 mg/kg.
6 Give steroids if raised ICP is due to a brain tumour. Give dexamethasone 16 g IV LD then 4 mg 6 h.
7 Cease N_2O and volatile anaesthetic agent as these drugs may contribute to raised ICP.[18] Substitute with a propofol infusion for maintenance of anaesthesia.
8 Consider boluses of thiopentone 2–3 mg/kg. If this is helpful, consider a thiopentone infusion (4–5 mg/kg/h).[17] Blood pressure support may be required.
9 Removal of CSF may produce a marked improvement.
10 Decompressive craniotomy.

⟡ Intracranial Venous Thrombosis (ICVT)

Although this condition can occur outside of pregnancy the incidence is increased during pregnancy especially in women with a previous history of venous thrombosis. ICVT occurs about once per 5000–10 000 pregnancies.[19] This condition may be mistaken for post dural puncture headache (PDPH) and dural puncture may increase the risk of this condition. Fifty per cent of cases are associated with haemorrhagic cerebral infarcts. The onset is usually acute and often occurs post-partum. It may be related to intracranial venous congestion and endothelial injury due to labour and delivery exertion coupled with the hypercoagulable state of pregnancy. The peri-partum mortality is about 10%. Most peri-partum patients make a good recovery.

Presentation
The main symptoms are:
1 headache, dizziness, blurred vision
2 nausea and vomiting
3 lethargy
4 seizures
5 hemiparesis
6 coma and death.

Differentiation between PDPH and ICVT
1 History of previous venous thrombosis favours ICVT.
2 Presence of focal deficits and/or mental state changes and seizures are suggestive of ICVT and warrant urgent MRI examination.
3 Consider ICVT in patients at low risk for PDPH i.e. no evidence of dural puncture at time of epidural insertion and the use of small calibre spinal needles.
4 The headache with ICVT tends to change over time while PDPH headache tends to be more consistent.
5 Little headache relief with blood patching in ICVT patients.

Investigations
1 Cerebral CT scanning—this will pick up only about 30% of cases.
2 MRI + venography is the standard test for diagnosis.

Treatment
1 supportive measures
2 anticoagulation
3 endovascular thrombolysis
4 surgical thrombectomy.

▶ Intralipid for the Treatment of Bupivacaine/Ropivacaine Toxicity

In the event of cardiac arrest due to bupivacaine or ropivacaine injected intravenously, treat as per the section on *Cardiac Arrest*. If the patient is unresponsive to standard treatment, do the following while continuing CPR:[20]
1 Give intralipid 20% solution 1.5 mL/kg IV bolus (70 kg = 100 mL).
2 Infuse intralipid 20% at 0.25 mL/kg/min (70 kg = 1000 mL/hr).
3 Repeat bolus dose × 2 if needed 3 minutely.

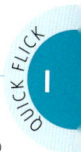

4 Continue infusion until adequate haemodynamic stability is achieved. Increase infusion rate up to 0.5 mL/kg/min if needed.

5 A suggested maximum total dose of intralipid is 8 mL/kg.

See *Bupivacaine* and *Ropivacaine*.

○ Intraoperative Myocardial Ischaemia

See *Myocardial Ischaemia, Peri-operative*.

○ Intraosseous Puncture

Useful for obtaining rapid access to intravascular space when venous cannulation has failed. This procedure can be performed in any age group. A 16 G bone marrow biopsy needle or a Cook™ interosseous needle is required.

Technique for Insertion

1 Surgically prep the insertion area e.g. the anteromedial surface of the tibia ≈ 2–3 cm below the tibial tuberosity. Other sites of insertion that have been utilised include the distal tibia, distal femur, iliac crest and sternum.

2 Use LA to anaesthetise skin and deeper structures if the patient is conscious.

3 Insert the needle with a screwing motion through the bony cortex, angling away from the joint and epyphyseal plate. There is a sensation of 'loss of resistance' as the marrow cavity is entered.

4 Aspiration of bone marrow confirms proper placement. Inject a 10 mL test dose of saline.This should inject freely. Injection of certain drugs such as sodium bicarbonate via the interosseous route is controversial because of the increased risk of tissue necrosis and osteomyelitis associated with hypertonic solutions.[21]

5 Newer IO devices for adults include the FAST1 designed for insertion into the adult manubrium 1.6 cm caudal to the sternal notch.[22]

○ Intrapleural Anaesthesia

This technique involves repeated injection of LA into the pleural space via a catheter, and can be used for postoperative analgesia and for the treatment of pain associated with chest drains.

Technique

1 Place the patient lateral with the side to be anaesthetised uppermost.

2 Aseptically prep the skin around the point of insertion, which is 10 cm lateral to the spinous processes at the sixth, seventh or eighth ribs.

3 Anaesthetise the skin and deeper tissues if the patient is awake, then insert an 18 G Tuohy needle to contact the superior surface of the rib. Remove the stylet and attach a 10 mL syringe (without the piston) filled with sterile saline.

4 Advance needle slowly over the superior surface of the rib. When the pleural space is penetrated the saline will be sucked into the pleural space. Usually a 'pop' sensation is felt.[23]

5 Insert an epidural catheter 5–6 cm into the pleural space and secure.

6 Check post-procedure chest X-ray for pneumothorax.

7 There are kits available for pleural anaesthesia such as the Arrow™ Intrapleural Set.

Dose

Adult Inject 20 mL of 0.5% bupivacaine with adrenaline 1:200 000 every 4–6 h. Inject with the patient in the supine position for 30 min.

For Patients Requiring a Chest Drain for Pneumothorax[24]

1 Insert an epidural catheter 5–10 cm into the pleural space dorsal to, and in the same intercostal space as, the chest drain.

2 Use the Tuohy needle for insertion as described above.

3 Inject bupivacaine through the pleural catheter as above, with the patient in supine position for 30 min and the chest drain clamped for 10 min if on suction.

Intrapleural Catheter

See Chest Drain.

Intrathecal Anaesthesia

See Subarachnoid Block (SAB).

Intrauterine Fetal Death

Intrauterine fetal death can be associated with disseminated intravascular coagulopathy (DIC) probably due to the release of fetal thromboplastin. DIC rarely occurs unless the dead fetus has been retained for days or weeks. Delivery soon after fetal death will usually prevent DIC occurring.[25]

Intravenous Regional Anaesthesia

See Bier Block.

Intubating Laryngeal Mask

See Laryngeal Mask Airway (Including ProSeal™, Fastrach™ and C-Trach™).

Intubation, Hypertensive Response

See Hypertensive Response to Intubation (Attenuation of).

Isoflurane

Halogenated methyl ether inhalational anaesthetic agent.

QUICK FLICK

I

Physical Properties and MAC

Blood:Gas Solubility Coefficient	1.4
Oil:Gas Solubility Coefficient	91
Saturated Vapour Pressure at 20°C	239 mm Hg (32 kPa)
Boiling Point	48.5°C
MAC	1.15

Advantages

Potent anaesthetic agent suitable for virtually all types of surgery.

Disadvantages

1 May have a 'coronary steal' effect, but the clinical significance of this is unclear.

2 Pungent odour makes isoflurane unsuitable for gaseous induction.

3 Isoflurane, like sevoflurane, significantly prolongs the Q-T heart rate corrected (Q-Tc) interval.[26] It should not be used in patients presenting with a prolonged Q-Tc interval due to the risk of precipitating torsades de pointes. *See* Long QT Syndrome (LQTS).

◖ Isoprenaline

Synthetic catecholamine used for the treatment of complete heart block until transvenous pacing can be arranged. Acts on β adreno-receptors thus causing positive cardiac inotropy and chronotropy. There are no significant α adreno-receptor effects.

Preparation

Mix 2 mg of isoprenaline with 50 ml of 5% glucose resulting in a concentration of 40 μg/mL.

Dose

Adult 10–20 μg then infusion of 0.5–8 μg/min (1 mL/h–12 mL/h).

Child 0.05 μg/kg/min.

REFERENCES

1 Mathes DD. Bleomycin and hyperoxia exposure in the operating room. *Anesth Analg* 1995; 81: 624–9.

2 Sparkes CJ, Rudkin GE, Agiomea K, Fa'arondo JR. Inguinal field block for adult inguinal hernia repair using a short bevelled needle. *Anaesth Intensive Care* 1995; 23:143–8.

3 Murphy DF. Intrapleural analgesia. *Br J Anaesth* 1993; 3: 426–34.

4 Schuster M, Nave H, Pipenbrock S et al. The carina as a landmark in central venous catheter placement. *Br J Anaesth* 2000; 85: 192–4.

5 Waldmann C, Barnes R. Cannulation of central veins. *Anaesthesia and Intensive Care Medicine*. 2004; 5: 6–9.

6   Wigmore TJ, Smythe JF, Hacking MB et al. Effect of the NICE guidelines for ultrasound guidance on the complication rates associated with central venous catheter placement in patients presenting for routine surgery in a tertiary referral centre. *Br J Anaesth* 2007; 99: 662–5.

7   Collier PE, Blocker SH, Graff DM, Doyle P. Cardiac tamponade from central venous catheters. *Am J Surg* 1998; 176: 212–14.

8   Bailey PL, Whitaker EE, Palmer LS, Glance LG. The accuracy of the central landmark used for central venous catheterization of the internal jugular vein. *Anesth Analg* 2006; 102: 1327–32.

9   Gouny P, Gaitz JP, Vayssairat M. Acute hand ischaemia secondary to intraarterial buprenorphine injection: treatment with iloprost and dextran-40. *Angiology* 1999; 50: 605–6.

10 Glass PS, Leiman BC, Reves JG. Etomidate: what is its present role in anesthesia? *Seminars in Anaesthesia* 1988; 7: 143–51.

11 McGrath P. Accidental intra-arterial flucloxacillin: management using guanethidine. *Anaesth Intensive Care* 1992; 20: 518–19.

12 Iatrou C, Robinson S, Rosewarne F. Inadvertent intra-arterial midazolam (letter). *Anaesth Intensive Care* 1997; 25: 431.

13 Sivalingam P. Inadvertent cannulation of an aberrant radial artery and intra-arterial injection of midazolam (letter). *Anaesth Intensive Care* 1999; 27: 424–5.

14 Brimacombe J. Gandin D, Bashford L. Transient decrease in arm blood flow following accidental intra-arterial injection of propofol into the left brachial artery. *Anaesth Intensive Care* 1994; 22: 291–2.

15 Evans JM, Latto IP, Ng WS. Accidental intra-arterial injection of drugs: a hazard of arterial cannulation. *Br J Anaesth* 1974: 460–3.

16 Trail R. Acute head injuries: anaesthetic considerations. In: Keneally J, ed. *Australasian Anaesthesia*. A.N.Z.C.A., Melbourne 1996: 145–50.

17 Priebe H-J. Aneurysmal subarachnoid haemorrhage and the anaesthetist. *Br J Anaesth* 2007; 99: 102–18.

18 Craen RA, Gelb AW. The anaesthetic management of neurosurgical emergencies. *Can J Anaesth* 1992; 39: 5: R29–R34.

19 Lockhart E, Baysinger CL. Intracranial venous thrombosis in the parturient (Review Article). *Anesthesiology* 2007; 107: 652–8.

20 Lipid Rescue: resuscitation for cardiac toxicity website: http://lipidrescue. squarespace.com/ (accessed July 2008).

21 Harte FA, Chalmers PC, Walsh RF, Danker PR, Shiekh FM. Intraosseous infusions: a parenteral alternative in pediatric resuscitation. *Anesth Analg* 1987; 66: 687–9.

22 Day M. Act FAST with intraosseous infusion. *Nurs* 2003; 33: 50–2.

23 Frenette L, Bourdreault D, Guay J. Interpleural analgesia improves pulmonary function after cholecystectomy. *Can J Anaesth* 1991; 38: 171–4.

QUICK FLICK

I

24 Engdahl O, Boe J, Sandstedt S. Intrapleural bupivacaine for analgesia during chest drainage treatment of pneumothorax. *Acta Anaesthesiol Scand* 1993; 37: 149–53.

25 Weiner C. The obstetric patient and disseminated intravascular coagulation. *Clin Perinatol* 1986; 13: 705.

26 Kleinsasser A, Kuenszberg E, Loekinger A et al. Sevoflurane, but not propofol, significantly prolongs the Q-T interval. *Anesth Analg* 2000; 90: 25–7.

○ Jehovah's Witnesses (JW)[1]

'Therefore I say, unto the children of Israel, ye shall eat the blood of no manner of flesh: for the life of all flesh is the blood thereof: whoever eateth it shall be cut off' (Levictus; 17: 10–16). Due to their religious beliefs, Jehovah's Witness (JW) patients may absolutely refuse blood transfusion and transfusion of some blood derivatives. The JW patient believes that a blood transfusion may result in eternal damnation. There are over 60 000 JWs in Australia plus another 50 000 associates. Associates are people who are participating in JW activities, but who have not yet fully decided to adopt all JW beliefs. Studies of extreme anaemia indicate that severe physiological decompensation tends to occur at Hb< 4.5 g/100 mL and death at Hb< 3 g/100 mL.[2]

Jehovah's Witness Hospital Liaison Committees
These committees exist in most major cities and there are over 1400 worldwide. Representatives from these committees can provide useful mediation between JW patients and medical care providers.

What is Allowed and Not Allowed
The JW church specifically bans so-called 'primary products' i.e. red cells, white cells, plasma and platelets. Pre-donation of the patient's own blood is not allowed. Individual JW patients are permitted as a matter of conscience to decide for themselves whether fractions of the 'primary products' are acceptable. These fractions include albumin, cryoprecipitate, immunoglobulins and blood factors. Systems involving extracorporeal circulation (e.g. cardiac bypass, haemodialysis) are usually acceptable but there 'must' be a continuous connection between the patient and the blood. Organ transplants and artificial blood such as Hemoglobin Raffimer[3] are usually acceptable as are cell saver devices.

JW and Epidural Blood Patch
An epidural blood patch can be done provided that there is a connection between the venous blood and the epidural needle by tubing.[4] There are reports in the literature of epidural colloid injections successfully treating post-dural puncture headache. Chiron et al. reported the epidural injection of 30 mL of Plasmion, a modified gelatine solution warmed to 35.7°C.[5] This successfully treated a PDPH in a patient with sickle cell disease.

JW Adults and the Law

Competent adult patients have an absolute right to refuse any aspect of medical treatment. The reasons for this refusal are irrelevant. If a competent adult is treated against their will, then the tort (civil wrong) of battery is committed.[2] For an elective case, the anaesthetist can refuse to be involved. In an emergency case the anaesthetist is bound ethically, medicolegally and contractually to treat the JW (or any other) patient. The anaesthetist should discuss with the JW patient alone exactly what he/she will or will not accept related to blood and blood products and the possible consequences of such refusal, including death. This discussion should be clearly documented in the medical record, signed by the patient and this should be witnessed by another doctor.

In an emergency, if the specific wishes of the unconscious patient are not known, then the patient must be treated according to the clinical judgement of the doctors involved and the defence of medical necessity applies.[2] Under these circumstances a life saving blood transfusion could be given. If the patient is semiconscious and refuses blood, the attending doctor must decide whether the patient is competent. If the decision is made that the patient is not competent then emergency treatment including life saving blood transfusion is defensible.

JW Children

In broad terms, medicolegally in Australia, a child is defined as being under the age of 18 years. For JW parents, it is extremely distressing and disturbing to their religious values for their child to have a blood transfusion or receive blood products. If blood transfusion or blood products (or any other treatment) are required for a life threatening indication for a JW child, then such treatment should be instituted and there should not be a negative medico-legal result. Such actions are covered by the *Children and Young Persons (Care and Protection) Act 1998*. The medical superintendent should be involved in this type of situation.

If blood or blood fractions are required but the treatment is not 'necessary as a matter of urgency' such treatment cannot be administered without parental consent or an order of the court. Again, the Jehovah's Witness Hospital Liaison Committee representative can be an invaluable mediator in these situations.

◗ Jet Ventilation

See *Transtracheal Jet Ventilation.*

◗ Junctional Tachycardias

See *Supraventricular Tachycardias (SVT).*

REFERENCES

1 *Jehovah's Witnesses Guidelines for their non-blood medical management*. Prepared by the Jehovah's Witnesses Hospital Liaison Services, Sydney 2000 (used with permission).

2 Cox M, Lumley J. Editorial: No blood or blood products. *Anaesthesia* 1995; 50: 583–5.

3 Lanzinger MJ, Niklason LE, Shannon M, Hill SE. Use of hemoglobin raffimer for postoperative life-threatening anemia in a Jehovah's Witness. *Can J Anesth* 2005; 52: 369–73.

4 McIlveney F, Pace NA. Jehovah's Witnesses. *Anaesthesia and Intensive Care Medicine* 2004; 5: 57–9.

5 Chiron B, Laffon M, Ferrandière M, Pitter J-F. Postdural puncture headache in a patient with sickle cell disease: use of an epidural colloid patch. *Can J Anesth* 2003; 50: 812–14.

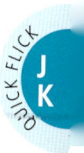

K

○ Ketamine

Phencyclidine derivative, used as an intravenous, intramuscular or oral anaesthetic agent and for its analgesic effects. Acts mainly as a non-competitive antagonist of the NMDA receptor and probably has agonist effects at opioid receptors.[1] It is particularly useful:

1   for induction of anaesthesia in patients with compromised CVS function e.g. shocked and elderly patients.
2   as a sole anaesthetic agent for brief procedures, such as change of burns dressings.
3   for anaesthesia in developing countries with limited resources.
4   for analgesia.
5   as an oral or IM premedication drug.

Advantages

1   Causes CVS stimulation via the sympathetic nervous system (increased HR and BP). Baroreceptor function is well maintained.
2   Causes bronchodilation and has been used successfully in the treatment of asthma. Mild respiratory stimulation occurs and airway reflexes are relatively preserved, compared to other IV anaesthetic agents.
3   Ketamine has potent analgesic properties even at sub-anaesthetic doses.
4   Can be given IM which is particularly useful for situations such as the uncooperative patient.

Disadvantages

1   Ketamine has a slow onset of action, and pain may occur on injection (IV and IM).
2   Sudden jerky movements or hypertonus may occur.
3   Disturbing emergence reactions may be experienced, such as unpleasant dreams and hallucinations.
4   Excessive salivation may occur (alleviated by antisialogogue premedication) and postoperative nausea and vomiting are common.
5   Causes increased intraocular pressure and intracranial pressure.
6   Subject to abuse.

Dose

Dose for Anaesthesia 1.5–2 mg/kg IV. Onset of action takes about 30 s and lasts 5–10 min. IM dose is 10 mg/kg. Onset of action 2–8 min, effects last 10–20 min. For brief painful procedures in adults, such as movement of a fractured limb, 10–20 mg IV boluses can be given, titrated to effect.

IV Infusion for Anaesthesia Ketamine can be used to maintain anaesthesia in a dose of 10–30 μg/kg/min. However other agents such as propofol will usually be more appropriate.[2]

Use by Continuous Infusion for Analgesia (IV or Subcut) Give ketamine 0.25–0.5 mg/kg as a bolus IV then an infusion of 2–10 μg/kg/min. An example of a subcut infusion regimen is 150 mg in 24 mL run at 1 mL/h.

Oral Dose as a Premedication Drug 6–7 mg/kg is an effective pre-operative sedative in children taking effect in 15–30 min.[3] Ketamine should be mixed with a sweet liquid due to its awful taste. It is claimed that emergence problems with ketamine are less frequent in children.[4] Oral secretions may be excessive and an antisialogogue is recommended.[5] In children having upper airway procedures, there may also be an increased incidence of stridor and laryngospasm in the recovery room.[5]

Epidural Ketamine Preservative-free ketamine added to opioids used epidurally improves pain relief.

PCA Ketamine Do not mix ketamine with morphine in the same PCA syringe. This does not improve analgesia.

○ Ketorolac

Non-steroidal anti-inflammatory drug with strong analgesic activity.

Dose

Over 65 yrs old 10–15 mg IM then 10–15 mg IM 4–6 h, maximum daily dose 60 mg.

Under 65 yrs old 10–30 mg IM then 10–30 mg IM 4–6 h. Maximum daily dose 90 mg.

Advantages
Potent analgesic drug in a parenteral form.

Disadvantages
1 Non selective COX inhibitor. ***See*** *Non-steroidal Anti-inflammatory Drugs (NSAIDs)*.
2 There have been several reports of renal failure associated with its use, even in young patients without other risk factors.[6]
3 There is an increased risk of peptic ulcer disease and GIT haemorrhage particularly in older patients on prolonged therapy.
4 High dose ketorolac (>120 mg/day) inhibits bone healing, but not lower dosages used for brief periods.[7]

Precautions
Do not use for more than 5 days. Do not use in patients with:

1 dehydration
2 hypovolaemia
3 moderate-to-severe renal dysfunction
4 bleeding diatheses
5 anticoagulant therapy
6 hypersensitivity to ketorolac.

REFERENCES

1 Gurnani A, Sharma PK, Rautela RS, Bhattacharya A. Analgesia for acute musculo-skeletal trauma: low dose subcutaneous infusion of ketamine. *Anesth Intensive Care* 1996; 22: 34–6.

2 White PF, Way WL, Trevor AJ. Ketamine—its pharmacology and therapeutic uses. *Anesthesiology* 1982; 56: 119–36.

3 Rainey L, Van Der Walt JH. The anaesthetic management of autistic children. *Anaesth Intensive Care* 1998; 26: 682–6.

4 Gutstein HB, Johnson KL, Heard MB, Gregory GA. Oral ketamine preanaesthetic medication in children. *Anesthesiology* 1992; 76: 28–33.

5 Filatov SM, Baer GA, Rorarius MG, Oikkonen M. Efficacy and safety of premedication with oral ketamine for day-case adenoidectomy compared with rectal diazepam/diclofenac and EMLA. *Acta Anaesthesiol Scand* 2000; 44 (1): 118–24.

6 Smith K. Halliwell RMT, Lawrence S et al. Acute renal failure associated with intramuscular ketorolac. *Anaesth Intensive Care* 1993; 21: 700–3.

7 Reuben S, Ablett D, Kaye R. High dose non-steroidal anti-inflammatory drugs compromise spinal fusion. *Can J Anesth* 2005; 52: 506–12.

Labetalol

Selective antagonist at β1and β2 adreno-receptors and to a lesser extent α1 receptors. It is used for the treatment of all grades of hypertension and hypertension associated with pre-eclampsia. Can be given IV or PO.

Dose

Adult 5–20 mg boluses IV injected over 2 min, up to a total dose of 200 mg. Acts in 5–30 min and is effective for about 50 min. Can also be given by infusion (in glucose or glucose/saline) at a rate of 20–160 mg/h IV.
Child 1–2 mg/kg IV dose (max 100 mg). ***See*** *Hypertensive Response to Intubation (Attenuation of).*

Lactate

NR 0.3–1.3 mmol/L. Elevated serum lactate levels can occur with tissue hypoxia. Serum lactate correlates well with the degree of hypovolaemic shock due to haemorrhage. A level of over 9 mmol/L is associated with a 75% mortality in ruptured abdominal aortic aneurysm patients.[1]

Laparoscopic Surgery

Laparoscopic cholecystectomy was first described in 1989.[2] A growing multitude of abdominal and pelvic laparoscopic techniques are being developed such as nephrectomy and bowel resection. With increasing frequency laparoscopic surgery is being combined with open surgery to greatly reduce the size of surgical wounds.
The main issues in laparoscopic surgery are:

1. The physiological effects of pneumoperitoneum.
2. Complications associated with the insertion of a Verres needle blindly into the peritoneal cavity.
3. Complications due to gas insufflation into the tissues or a blood vessel.

Induction Phase—To Intubate or Not Intubate

There is an increased risk of regurgitation with pneumoperitoneum.[3] Most patients should be intubated. However, brief laparoscopic surgery can be undertaken with a ProSeal™ or laryngeal tube suction in patients who are not at risk of aspiration.[4] ***See*** *Aspiration, Prevention and Treatment*. For patients having laparoscopic cholecystectomy, insert a gastric tube to deflate the stomach.

Gas Insufflation Phase

For abdominal surgery, gas is insufflated into the peritoneal cavity to provide physical and visual access. Insertion of the Verres needle may cause trauma to blood vessels or other structures. Gas insufflation is provided by high-flow insufflators with gas flows of 4–6 L/min. Complications that can occur at this stage include:

1   Gas embolism due to placement of the Verres needle into a blood vessel. **See** *Gas Embolism*.
2   Subcutaneous emphysema, pneumothorax and/or pneumomediastinum may occur. The surgeon must cease insufflation immediately. Subcutaneous emphysema can result in increased end tidal CO_2 measurements, but without increased airway pressure, unless a pneumothorax is also present. Management of subcutaneous emphysema includes increasing minute ventilation to maintain acceptable end tidal/$PaCO_2$ levels, ceasing N_2O in the inhaled gas mixture and reassuring the patient after surgery.
3   A vagally mediated bradycardia may occur as the peritoneum is stretched. This can be severe enough to produce asystole.[5] In this situation tell the surgeon to stop insufflation and let out all the gas. Give atropine 0.6 mg. If asystole persists **see** *Cardiac Arrest*.

Intra-operative Phase

1   There is a potential risk of the tip of the endotracheal tube migrating into a bronchus with pneumoperitoneum, especially with Trendelenburg positioning.[6]
2   Avoid high pressure IPPV and PEEP as this can result in a marked reduction in cardiac output in the presence of pneumoperitoneum.[7]
3   Do not allow intra-abdominal pressure (IAP) to rise above 20 mm Hg. This can result in a severe reduction in venous return causing reduced cardiac output. Renal function may also be impaired with decreased renal blood flow and glomerular filtration rate.[7] A IAP of 15 mm Hg is sufficient for most procedures.[7]
4   Functional residual capacity and pulmonary compliance are reduced by the pneumoperitoneum.[6] Airway resistance is increased.[7] Hypercarbia may occur due to absorption of insufflated CO_2. The effects of hypercarbia include tachycardia, dysrhythmias and reduced systemic vascular resistance. Treat with increased ventilation rate.
5   There is an increased risk of embolisation to the cerebral circulation during gynaecological laparoscopic procedures through a patent foramen ovale.[8] A patent foramen ovale is present in about 27% of the population.[9] This predisposition to cerebral embolisation is due to the interaction of pneumoperitoneum, head down tilt and IPPV resulting in relatively higher pressures in the right atrium than the left atrium.[10] This risk can be reduced by IV fluid loading e.g. with 500 mL of colloid.[10]

6 Concealed intra-operative haemorrhage can occur at any stage. Have a low index of suspicion for haemorrhage and always have adequate IV access.

7 If N_2O is used for pneumoperitoneum, fire or explosion can occur in the peritoneal cavity with diathermy or laser. CO_2 does not support combustion.

8 If the light cable is disconnected from laparoscope, do not allow the distal end to burn patient.

9 Do not use N_2O in the inhaled gas mixture due to increased risk of nausea and vomiting and possibly increased bowel distension.

Postoperative Phase

Nausea and vomiting are very common after laparoscopic surgery (e.g. > 60% after laparoscopic cholecystectomy).[11] **See** *Nausea and Vomiting, Prevention and Treatment*.

○ Laryngeal Anatomy

See *Larynx, Anatomy and Innervation*.

○ Laryngeal Mask Airway (Including ProSeal™, Fastrach™ and C-Trach™)

Topics Covered in this Section

▶ LMA-Classic
▶ LMA-ProSeal™
▶ Fastrach™ Intubating Laryngeal Mask
▶ LMA C-Trach™

The LMA-Classic

The LMA-Classic is a cuffed mask designed to fit over the laryngeal inlet and provide an airway for anaesthesia and resuscitation. It does not protect the trachea from aspiration of gastric contents and is usually used for spontaneously breathing patients.

Table L1: Appropriate LMA size for different sized patients

Size	Inflate with	Wt of patient
1	up to 4 mL	Neonate to 6.5 kg
1.5	up to 7 mL	5–10 kg
2	up to 10 mL	10–20 kg
2.5	up to 14 mL	20–30 kg
3	up to 20 mL	30–50 kg
4	up to 30 mL	50–70 kg
5	up to 40 mL	70–100 kg
6	up to 50 mL	100+ kg

QUICK FLICK **L**

LMA and Failed Intubation

The LMA can be lifesaving in the situation of 'can't intubate, can't ventilate' i.e. intubation fails and bag mask ventilation is unsuccessful. Inserting an LMA will often result in a satisfactory supraglottic airway and enable patient ventilation. *See Difficult Airway Management*. The LMA can also be used to provide a conduit for intubation, by passing an endotracheal tube through it. The vocal cords will lie about 3 cm from the mask aperture. Use of an extra long size 6.0 ET tube (such as a Mallinckrodt™ microlaryngoscopy tube) in adults will enable deeper insertion of the tip of the ET tube into the trachea. The LMA is left in position until extubation. In a variation of this technique, a Teflon introducer can be passed through the LMA and into the trachea. The tube is then railroaded over the introducer either with or without the LMA left in position. Another variation involves passing a fibre-optic bronchoscope (FOB) loaded with a tube through the LMA and into the trachea. Once in the trachea with the FOB, railroad the tube over the FOB.

Table L2: Maximum sized ET tube that can be passed through the various LMA sizes[12]

LMA size	Maximum size ET tube that will pass through
1	3.5
2	4.5
2.5	5.0
3	6.0 cuffed
4	6.0 cuffed
5	7.0 cuffed

LMA-ProSeal™

This device is similar to the classic laryngeal mask airway but features a modified cuff, a drainage tube and an integral bite block. The modified double cuff enables an improved seal over the laryngeal inlet to a pressure of ≈ 40–50 cm H_2O.[13] This is about twice the seal pressure of the LMA-Classic. The drainage tube runs from the distal tip of the cuff to the proximal end of the wire-reinforced airway tube. This acts as a channel for gastric fluid and gases, and also facilitates gastric tube placement. This device is designed for positive pressure ventilation. A dedicated introducer tool can be used to aid in correct placement of the ProSeal™.

Table L3: Appropriate ProSeal™ size for different sized patients

Size	Maximum inflation volume	Wt of patient	Max diameter of orogastric tube
1.5	7 mL	5–10 kg	10 fr
2	10 mL	10–20 kg	10 fr
2.5	14 mL	20–30 kg	10 fr
3	20 mL	30–50 kg	16 fr
4	30 mL	50–70 kg	16 fr
5	40 mL	70–100 kg	18 fr

Half the maximum inflation volumes quoted are usually sufficient.

Insertion of the ProSeal™ with the Introducer Tool[14]

1 Prepare the device by tightly deflating it. Lubricate the posterior tip of the deflated cuff with a water soluble lubricant such as K-Y Jelly.
2 Insert the ProSeal™ introducer. Place the tip of the introducer into the retaining strap at the rear of the cuff. Fold the ProSeal™ along the outer curve of the introducer and place the drain tube and airway tube into the appropriate slots.
3 Position the patient's head as for intubation (head extended on the neck, neck slightly flexed).
4 Press the tip of the ProSeal™ against the palate and slide the cuff in a rotational movement following the curve of the palate. Advance the device into the hypopharynx until a definite resistance is felt. The cuff must press against the palate during the insertion manoeuvre.
5 Stabilise the device with one hand while removing the introducer with the other.
6 Inflate the cuff without holding the device using about half the maximum volumes described in the table above. Do not exceed 60 cm H_2O inflation pressure.

Insertion over a Gum Elastic Bougie (GEB)

This technique is very effective and prevents the tip of the Proseal™ from rolling up. Successful insertion on the first attempt with this technique was 100% in one study.[15] This technique has obvious application to failed intubation management. *See Difficult Airway Management.*

1 The ProSeal™ is deflated tightly and the GEB is passed through the drain tube.
2 Using gentle laryngoscopy, the distal end of the GEB is placed well into the oesophagus.
3 The ProSeal™ is then railroaded into position over the GEB. There is a sensation of moderate resistance when the the ProSeal™ is correctly positioned.
4 Inflate the ProSeal™ cuff and test ventilate.

Other Points

1 If an orogastric tube is used, it must not be stiffened by refrigeration due to the potential for trauma.

2 If regurgitated fluid is expelled through the drain tube and the patient remains well oxygenated, it is advised to leave the ProSeal™ in place.[14] This is the intended function of the drain tube. Pass an orogastric tube through the drain tube into the stomach so that it can be emptied.

3 Leave the taping on the device undisturbed until the patient is awake enough to have purposeful movements.

4 The manufacturer recommends deflating the ProSeal™ prior to removal although some practitioners remove the device while still inflated.

5 Nitrous oxide can diffuse into the cuff of the ProSeal™ during long procedures increasing cuff volume and pressure. It is recommended to feel the tension in the inflation indicator balloon periodically and reduce pressure in the cuff if it becomes excessive (greater than 60 cm H_2O). Higher pressures than this may cause a sore throat.

6 The role of the ProSeal™ continues to evolve. The device appears to be a satisfactory alternative to intubation for laparoscopic cholecystectomy in selected patients.[16] The ProSeal™ does not protect against aspiration to the same degree as an ET tube and should not be used in patients at significant risk of aspiration e.g. patients with acute appendicitis. Incredibly, this has been tried with disastrous consequences.[17]

7 The LMA Supreme is a disposable form of the ProSeal™.

Fastrach™ Intubating LMA

This device is a type of laryngeal mask airway (LMA) specifically designed as a ventilation device and a guide to tracheal intubation. The Fastrach™ consists of:

1 An anatomically curved, short wide bore, stainless steel tube sheathed in silicone.

2 The steel tube is bonded to a laryngeal mask with a single, moveable aperture bar.

3 The Fastrach™ comes in sizes 3, 4 & 5 (see Table L4).

4 The stainless steel tube is also bonded to a metal guiding bar.

5 Specially designed silicone ET tubes are used. These are available in sizes 6, 6.5, 7, 7.5 and 8 mm.

Table L4: Inflation volumes for various sizes of Fastrach™

Fastrach™ size	Patient's weight	Maximum inflation volume
3	30–50 kg	20 mL
4	50–70 kg	30 mL
5	70–100 kg	40 mL

Technique for Using the Fastrach™

1 The head and neck are placed in the neutral position, not the classic sniffing position.

2 The Fastrach™ is fully deflated and a bolus of water soluble lubricant (e.g. K-Y jelly) is applied to the posterior saucer shaped tip of the device.

3 The patient should be deeply anaesthetised or the airway adequately anaesthetised in the awake patient. In most studies of Fastrach™ efficacy muscle relaxants were used.[18]

4 While holding the metal guiding bar (handle), the flattened tip of the Fastrach™ is placed against the hard palate and then inserted into the oropharynx by using a rotational movement in the sagittal plane.

5 Do not insert Fastrach™ to the 'hilt'. Observe for caudal displacement of the prominence of the thyroid cartilage.

6 Inflate the cuff (see inflation volumes in the table on page 296). About half these volumes is usually sufficient. An intracuff pressure of 60 cm H_2O is recommended.

7 The success rate of the Fastrach™ as a ventilation device on the first insertion attempt is almost 100%.[19]

8 The well-lubricated silicone ET tube is then passed through the LMA-Fastrach™ into the trachea. The longitudinal line on the ET tube should be facing the handle.

9 Intubation through the LMA-Fastrach™ is successful on the first attempt in about 80% of patients.[20] With 1–4 adjustment manoeuvres the successful intubation rate is greater than 99%.[19]

10 Adjustment manoeuvres include:
   a) Pulling the LMA-Fastrach out 6 cm without deflating the cuff then re-inserting the device (up-down manoeuvre).[19]
   b) Using the Chandy manoeuvre, which is a 2-step process. First slightly rotate the device in the sagittal plane, using the metal handle, while squeezing the 'bag' to find the best position for ventilation. Second lift the Fastrach™ away from the posterior pharyngeal wall.
   c) Rotating the ET tube.
   d) Adjusting the head-neck position.
   e) Using a smaller or larger Fastrach™.

11 Once the patient is intubated, the Fastrach™ can be deflated and left in place. Alternatively the ET connector can be removed and the Fastrach™ carefully pulled over the tube using the purpose-made 'pusher' device to keep the ET tube in place.

12 Once the Fastrach™ is removed, reattach the connector to the ET and ventilate.

Points to Note

1 The patient must be able to open their mouth at least 2.5 cm.

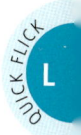

2 For patients requiring in-line head and neck stabilisation in the neutral position it is easier to place the Fastrach™ than the LMA-Classic.[21] However the LMA-Fastrach™ causes significant segmental cervical spine movement and in patients with cervical spine injury this technique may be inappropriate.[22]

   a) Intubation through the LMA-Fastrach™ is more likely to succeed on the first attempt in patients with predicted or known airway problems.[19]

   b) If cricoid pressure is applied the success rate is reduced and cricoid pressure may have to be removed temporarily to allow intubation.

Fibre-optic Intubation and the LMA-Fastrach™

If using a fibre-optic bronchoscope through the LMA-Fastrach™, note that the FOB is not stiff enough to push the epiglottic elevation bar out of the way and the tip of the FOB will be deflected to the left or right. Therefore:

1 Pass the specially designed silicone endotracheal tube to just beyond the distal epiglottic elevation bar.

2 Then pass the FOB through the ET tube to visualise the vocal cords and proceed as described above.

The LMA C-Trach™

This device is similar to the Fastrach™ but includes a fibre-optic bundle that transmits an image to a clip-on viewer on the proximal end of the device. This enables visualisation of the larynx through the device during intubation. The steps in intubation and manoeuvres for optimising position are the same as with the Fastrach™. Intubation on the first attempt is more likely with the C-Trach™ compared to the Fastrach™ and has a success rate of about 96%.[23] The C-Trach™ is available in sizes 3 (30–50 kg), 4 (55–75 kg) and 5 (>75 kg). *See Difficult Airway Management*.

▷ Laryngeal Tube (LT)

Reuseable ventilatory device for use as an alternative to mask or endotracheal intubation provided that protection of the airway against regurgitation is not required. This concept is quite similar to the Combitube™ airway. The LT consists of a blind-ended S-shaped tube with a proximal pharyngeal cuff and a distal oesophageal cuff, and a laryngeal ventilation hole. The pharyngeal cuff stabilises the tube and blocks off the naso- and oropharynx. The distal oesophageal tube blocks off the oesophagus. To insert:

1 Fully deflate and lubricate both cuffs.

2 Insert the tube centrally into the mouth until the middle horizontal 'teeth' line of the tube is aligned with the teeth, or until a distinct resistance is felt.[24]

3 Inflate the cuffs to a pressure of 80 cm H_2O, through the single pilot tube, using the cuff pressure gauge provided.

4   When the tube position has settled, press the red deflate valve to adjust to the desired pressure (60–70 cm H_2O).
5   Ventilate the patient. A ventilation pressure of 30 cm H_2O or greater is possible with this device.[25]
6   To remove the LT, deflate both cuffs and remove.

Table L5: Appropriate size of LT

Patient	LT size
Newborn–6 kg	0
Infant 6–15 kg	1
Child 15–40 kg	2
Child/small adult 30–60 kg	3
Medium adult 50–90 kg	4
Large adult >90 kg	5

Laryngeal Tube-Suction
This is a new type of laryngeal tube. It incorporates a separate channel from the proximal to distal end of the device to enable the passage of a gastric tube. This can be used to deflate the stomach and for aspiration of any gastric fluid.

◯ Laryngoscopy

See Difficult Airway Management.

◯ Laryngoscopy Grading

Table L6: Cormack and Lehane classification of the view obtained at laryngoscopy[26]

Grade	View obtained
1	Full view of cords
2	Partial view of cords
3	Epiglottis only
4	Epiglottis not visible

◯ Laryngospasm

Laryngospasm can be defined as an involuntary occlusion of the glottis and laryngeal inlet by contraction of the laryngeal muscles closing the true and/or false vocal cords. It is most likely to occur during induction and emergence from anaesthesia, when anaesthesia is light. It can result from oral secretions or regurgitated fluid stimulating the larynx.

Prevention
Strategies to prevent laryngospasm include:
1   Ensure that the patient is adequately anaesthetised prior to airway manipulation and surgical stimulation.

2 Suck away oral secretions prior to extubation and extubate 'deep' or when the patient is 'fully awake' without residual muscle relaxant effects.

Clinical Effects

1 Stridor.

2 Respiratory distress with tachypnoea, chest retraction.

3 Hypoxia.

4 Negative pressure pulmonary oedema may occur.

5 Cardiac arrest may occur due to extreme hypoxia.

Management

1 Cease or remove the stimulus causing laryngospasm if possible e.g. suck away oral secretions.

2 Decide whether you are able to 'break' the laryngospasm. This involves providing 100% oxygen with CPAP using the anaesthetic bag and mask and providing low tidal volume ventilation with short sharp squeezes on the bag. The CPAP reduces the pressure gradient across the obstruction and may stent the pharyngeal and laryngeal muscles.[27] At the same time optimise the airway with jaw thrust, head tilt and jaw support (slightly open the mouth).

3 Consider deepening anaesthesia with small incremental doses of propofol e.g. 30–50 mg.

4 If the laryngospasm does not 'break' and significant hypoxia begins to occur, give suxamethonium IV and intubate the trachea. Extubate only when the patient is fully awake and able to control their airway reflexes.

5 For the management of negative pressure pulmonary oedema *see Negative Pressure Pulmonary Oedema*.

◗ Larynx, Anatomy and Innervation

Laryngeal Cartilages (See Figure L1)

The laryngeal cartilages are the:

1 *thyroid cartilage* which has the thyroid notch anteriorly.

2 *cricoid cartilage* which is shaped like a signet ring with the narrowest part facing anteriorly. Between the thyroid and cricoid cartilages is the cricothyroid membrane.

3 *arytenoid cartilages*, which are pyramidal in shape and articulate with the supero-lateral aspects of the cricoid cartilage.

4 *epiglottis* is a leaf shaped cartilage attached at its lower end to the thyroid cartilage. The vocal cords run from the arytenoid cartilages to the posterior surface of the thyroid cartilage.

5 *corniculate cartilages* are small nodules sitting on the arytenoid cartilages.

6 *cuneiform cartilages* are flakes of cartilage within the aryepiglottic folds.

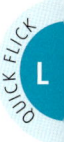

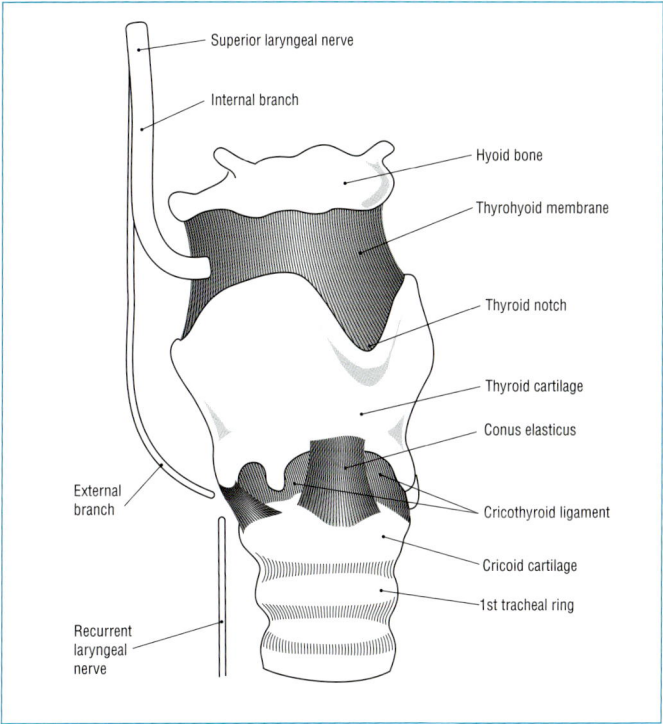

Figure L1 Laryngeal cartilages

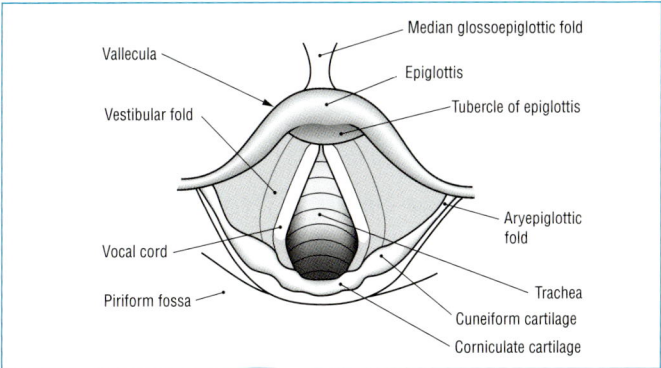

Figure L2 The laryngeal inlet

Innervation of the Larynx

1   The larynx is innervated by the vagus nerve via the superior laryngeal nerve and the recurrent laryngeal nerve.
2   The superior laryngeal nerve supplies the interior of the larynx as far as the vocal cords (via its internal branch).
3   The recurrent laryngeal nerve supplies the motor supply to the intrinsic muscles of the larynx (apart from the cricothyroid) and sensory supply to the laryngeal mucosa inferior to the vocal cords.

▷ Laser Surgery

Laser stands for Light Amplification by Stimulated Emission of Radiation.

Examples of Lasers Used Medically

1   CO_2 (wavelength 10 600 nm): used for coagulation and precision cutting.
2   Argon or Krypton (wavelength 400–700 nm): used for photocoagulation in eye and skin surgery. Neodymium yttrium-aluminium-garnet (Nd-YAG) (wavelength 1060 nm): used for tumour destruction and photocoagulation.

Precautions for Laser Surgery[28]

1   Protective glasses for staff with appropriate tint for the type of laser used. CO_2 lasers are more likely to damage the cornea while Nd-YAG lasers are more likely to damage the retina.
2   Moist gauze protection for patient's eyes.
3   If airway laser is required, use a laser resistant endotracheal tube (e.g. wrapping the tube with aluminium foil tape), with methylene blue stained saline filling the cuff. Commercially available laser resistant tubes include the Mallinckrodt™ Laser-Flex.
4   Use gas mixtures that least support combustion e.g. <30% O_2 in N_2. Alternatively use jet ventilation.
5   Sterile water/saline should be immediately available in a bucket to extinguish fire. **See** *Tracheostomy, Elective* for management of airway fire.
6   Adequate evacuation of laser plume.
7   All windows should be covered and warning signs displayed. Theatre traffic should be minimal.

▷ Lateral Cutaneous Nerve of Thigh Block

Anatomy

The lateral cutaneous nerve of thigh (L2, L3) arises from the lumbar plexus and divides into anterior and posterior branches.

Anterior branch supplies sensation to the skin over the anterolateral aspect of the thigh to the knee.

Posterior branch supplies the skin on the lateral side of the thigh just below the greater trochanter to the mid-thigh level.

Technique

1 Identify the anterior superior iliac spine and then identify the point 2.5 cm medial and 2.5 cm caudal to this landmark. The nerve lies below this point immediately beneath the fascia lata.
2 Sterilise and anaesthetise the skin, then insert a 23 G short bevelled needle in a 45° lateral direction. As the needle pierces the fascia lata a popping sensation is felt.
3 Inject 3–5 mL of LA (e.g. lignocaine 2%) as the needle is slowly withdrawn, then another 3–5 mL is injected as the needle is reinserted more medially.
4 Repeat until 15–20 mL of LA is injected from lateral to medial, above and below the fascia lata in a wall extending for about 5 cm.

◗ Latex Allergy

Latex and Anaphylaxis

Latex accounts for about 15% of anaphylaxis under anaesthesia.
See *Anaphylaxis/Anaphylactoid Reactions*.

Identifying Predisposed Patients

Attempt to identify patients who may be latex allergic and inquire specifically about latex allergy. Predisposed patients include:[29,30]

1 patients with a medical history suggesting latex allergy such as contact dermatitis due to washing-up gloves, tingling and swelling of lips when blowing up balloons and wheeze and rhinitis in the presence of airborne rubber particles.
2 healthcare workers who routinely wear latex gloves.
3 atopic patients and patients with hand eczema.
4 patients with spina bifida.
5 patients with chronic urological illness requiring repeated catheterisation.
6 spinal cord injury patients.
7 patients allergic to exotic fruit such as avocados and papaya.
8 patients with myelodysplasia.[31]
9 workers in the rubber industry.

Preventing Latex-induced Allergic Reactions

General Measures

1 Remove all latex-containing products from the operating theatre and make this case the first for the day. If emergency surgery, operate in a theatre that has not been in use for some hours.

2   Have latex allergy warning signs on the operating theatre doors and inside the operating theatre. Traffic through the theatre should be minimal.

Gloves
All gloves used by staff must be of non-latex material. The use of non-latex gloves (e.g. neoprene) by the surgeon is the most important preventative measure.[32]

Drug and Fluid Administration
1   Inject drugs via reflux valves and not through latex bungs on IV giving sets. Drugs such as antibiotics should not be drawn up through the rubber bung on the drug ampoule. Use glass syringes rather than rubber tipped plunger syringes.[30] Braun® make a 2-part non-latex containing syringe[32] and Terumo syringes are latex-free.
2   Haemaccel containers include a rubber bung and there has been a report of anaphylaxis.[33]

Anaesthetic Circuits and Airways
Non-latex containing anaesthetic circuits should be used e.g. a plastic Banes circuit with a silicone bag and mask. Laryngeal mask airways, PVC endotracheal tubes and plastic guedel airways are all safe.

Ventilators
If a silicone ventilator bellows is not available use a well used set of latex ones.[29] Washing the bellows may improve safety.

Monitoring Issues
The blood pressure cuff should be placed over a soft cotton wrapping on the patient's skin. As Datex® pulse oximeter probes contain latex, cover the finger with Tegaderm (3M®) prior to application. [32] Use Baxter® or 3M® ECG electrodes (latex-free).[29]

Tapes
Non-latex containing tapes include Micropore®, Blenderm® and Steri-strips®.[30] *Note:* There is no evidence that allergy prophylaxis with drugs such as steroids and ranitidine is effective.[31]

Treatment of Latex Allergy
In addition to measures outlined in the section on *Anaphylaxis/Anaphylactoid Reactions*, remove all latex contact from the patient.

Investigation of Suspected Latex Allergy
1   Mast cell tryptase levels will often be acutely elevated (normal level 2 µg/L).[30]
2   Skin prick testing by pricking the patient's skin through a latex glove or a suspension of latex glove particles. If the patient is allergic a wheal develops.[30]
3   Radio-allergosorbent testing for latex specific IgE antibodies is available but is not as accurate as skin prick testing.[31]

◐ Left Ventricular Ejection Fraction

See *Cardiac Investigations.*

◐ Left Ventricular Failure, Acute

See *Pulmonary Oedema.*

◐ Lepuridin

Direct thrombin inhibitor similar to hirudin from leeches but made through recombinant technology. It can be used in HITS patients for treatment of DVT/PE but there is a risk of anaphylaxis on re-exposure. *See* *Heparin Induced Thrombocytopenia Syndrome (HITS)*. It is only used intravenously and the dose must be reduced with renal impairment.

◐ Levobupivacaine

This LA agent is the levo stereoisomer of bupivacaine.

Dose
Equivalent to bupivacaine[34] (*see* *Bupivacaine*). The maximum recommended doses in adults are 150 mg acutely and 400 mg over 24 h.[34]

Advantages
About 30–50% less cardiotoxicity and CNS toxicity than racemic bupivacaine.

◐ Levosimendan

Cardiotonic drug that causes increased cardiac contractility by enhancing the sensitivity of heart muscle to calcium. This improved myocardial performance occurs without increased myocardial oxygen consumption or effects on heart rhythm. Levosimendan also acts as a vasodilator by stimulating ATPIII dependent potassium channels.

Indications
Levosimendan is useful for treating acutely decompensated severe heart failure resistant to conventional therapy (diuretics, ACE-inhibitors, digoxin and inotropes).

Contraindications
1   Renal and liver failure.
2   Severe hypotension and tachycardia.
3   History of torsades de pointes.

Dose
1   Mix 10 mL of levosimendan (2.5 mg/mL) with 500 mL of 5% glucose making a solution of 0.05 mg/mL.
2   Give a loading dose of 12–24 µg/kg infused over 10 min–1 h then an infusion of 0.1 µg/kg/min. If after 30–60 min there is evidence of

excessive hypotension or tachycardia, decrease infusion rate to 0.05 µg/kg/min. If initial infusion rate well tolerated consider increasing infusion rate to 0.2 µg/kg/min.

⊙ Lightwand Intubation

The Trachlight™ type of lightwand is used as an example of this technique.

Description of the Trachlight™
The device consists of 3 parts:
1 a reusable handle. A locking clamp is located on the front of the handle that secures the ET tube connector.
2 a flexible wand with a bright light bulb at the distal end. This wand can be shortened or lengthened by a connecting/locking device located on the handle.
3 a stiff retractable stylet encased within the wand. This allows the wand to be shaped.

Steps in Lightwand Oral Intubation
1 Prepare the device by inserting the well-lubricated lightwand into the chosen ET tube so that the light bulb is positioned at the cuff end but not protruding from it. Lock the ET tube connector to the handle. Ensure that the stylet which is inserted into the lightwand is also well lubricated.
2 The distal end of the lightwand and tube are bent to 90° (the stylet keeps this shape).
3 The patient's head and neck are positioned in the neutral position or slightly head extended position, not the classic sniffing position used for direct laryngoscopy.[35]
4 The patient must be adequately anaesthetised or have received adequate airway topical anaesthesia, prior to insertion of the device.
5 Use ambient light conditions unless the patient has a very thick neck.
6 The patient's jaw is lifted forward and the device is inserted exactly in the midline, with a rocking, arcing motion in the sagittal plane aiming to place the tip at the thyroid prominence.
7 On entering the glottic opening there is a feeling of 'loss of resistance' and a well-defined glow just below the thyroid prominence should be seen. At this point pull the stylet back 10 cm and advance the wand and ET tube into the trachea. The glow should be seen to travel down the trachea and disappear below the sternal notch.
8 Release the ET tube from the connector and remove the wand from the ET tube.

Techniques for Improving Success[36]
1 Using a smaller than usual ET tube (e.g. size 6 mm for an adult female and a size 7 mm for an adult male) may help successful placement.

2 The length of the ET tube beyond the bend should approximate the distance from the pharynx and the cords.

3 The lightwand and ET tube are inserted into the mouth with the right hand starting on the right side of the mouth (with the angled tip pointing left) and then rotating the wand medially.

4 Recently there has been some research into the use of the Lightwand combined with a Fastrach™ to assist in tracheal intubation through the Fastrach™.[37]

◐ Lignocaine

Amino-amide type LA agent and anti-arrhythmic drug. Presented in strengths of 0.5%–2% for local and regional anaesthesia and IV injection. In addition there are topical preparations including a 10% spray, 4% aqueous solution and a 1–2% jelly preparation. *See* EMLA.

Uses

1 As a local anaesthetic
2 Anti-arrhythmic drug
3 Reducing the stimulating effects of intubation and extubation (e.g. coughing, bronchospasm, hypertension)
4 Reducing the pain of propofol IV.

Local Anaesthetic Use

Lignocaine is suitable for all types of regional anaesthesia including IV limb anaesthesia (*see* Bier Block) with the exception of subarachnoid block. Lignocaine 5% (+ 7.5% dextrose) when used for subarachnoid block has been associated with transient radicular irritation.[38] It is less cardiotoxic than bupivacaine or ropivacaine. The maximum lignocaine dose for LA is 4–5 mg/kg, or 7–8 mg/kg if adrenaline is added. Lignocaine is shorter acting than bupivacaine or ropivacaine and is unsuitable for use as an infusion for regional anaesthesia.

Table L7: Effects of lignocaine toxicity at various plasma concentrations[39]

Clinical effects	Plasma concentration
Light headedness, tongue numbness	4 µg/mL
Visual and hearing disturbances, muscle twitching	8 µg/mL
Loss of consciousness	10 µg/mL
Convulsions	12 µg/mL
Respiratory arrest	20 µg/mL
Cardiac arrest	24 µg/mL

Anti-arrhythmic Use

Lignocaine is a Class 1b anti-arrhythmic drug that slows conduction through ischaemic areas of the heart. Lignocaine is indicated for shock-resistant ventricular fibrillation and pulseless ventricular tachycardia, but it is less effective than amiodarone. **See** *Cardiac Arrest*. Give 1 mg/kg initially then 0.5 mg/kg if a second dose is required.

Reducing the Stimulating Effects of Intubation and Extubation

1 1.5 mg/kg IV 1.5–3 min before intubating reduces the hypertensive response and rise in intracranial pressure due to intubation.[40] IV lignocaine reduces the incidence of reflex bronchospasm to intubation (but not bronchospasm due to allergic reaction).[41]

2 1.5 mg/kg IV 2–3 min before extubation reduces coughing post extubation and intracranial pressure.[42]

Reducing the Pain of IV Propofol

Lignocaine IV reduces the pain associated with IV propofol administration. Picard et al. found the most effective way to administer lignocaine for this purpose in adults was to inject 40 mg with a tourniquet at the forearm (50–70 mm Hg) released after 30–120 sec.[43] In children use 0.5 mg/kg.[43] This reduced the incidence of pain from 70% to 40%.

◐ Lipid Lowering Drugs

See *Statin Therapy*.

◐ Lipid Treatment for Local Anaesthetic Toxicity

See *Intralipid for the Treatment of Bupivacaine/Ropivacaine Toxicity*.

◐ Liquid Plasma

Liquid plasma is plasma removed from a unit of donated blood and refrigerated but not frozen like FFP. It is preserved in citrate-phosphate-dextrose and has a 26-day storage life. Liquid plasma has the advantage of not requiring thawing in an emergency.[44]

◐ Long QT Syndrome (LQTS)

In this condition a spectrum genetic mutations affecting cardiac ion channels results in prolonged ventricular repolarisation. This defect results in Q-T interval prolongation and predisposition to episodes of torsades de pointes. These ventricular tachydysrhythmias typically cause syncope, seizure-like episodes and ventricular fibrillation which may be fatal. **See** *Torsades de Pointes*. The incidence of this condition is between 1:1100 and 1:3000, and the disease usually presents in children and young adults.[45] The syndrome can be congenital or acquired but many patients with the acquired form probably still have an underlying previously silent genetic disorder.

Diagnosis

The QT interval varies with heart rate so a corrected value is used for Q-Tc. Q-Tc = Measured QT divided by the √ RR interval and is measured in seconds. The normal Q-Tc is 0.39 s +/– 0.04 s. Q-Tc > 0.44 s is prolonged although in 6% of patients with LQTS the Q-Tc is normal.[45] T and U wave abnormalities are common e.g. large biphasic P waves may be seen.

Prognosis

Without treatment mortality is about 50% within 10 years of diagnosis. With treatment the 10-year mortality is less than 4%.

Acquired LQTS

Some drugs prolong the Q-Tc interval and torsades de pointes may be precipitated in some patients. It is hypothesised that many of these patients have a subclinical form of congenital LQTS. These drugs include:

1 class Ia, IIc, III anti-arrhythmic drugs e.g. quinidine.
2 butyrophenones e.g. droperidol, haloperidol.
3 several antipsychotic drugs e.g. thioridizine.
4 selective 5-HT$_3$ (serotonin) re-uptake inhibitors e.g. fluoxetine.
5 5-HT$_1$ agonist drugs e.g. zolmitriptan.
6 some antibiotics e.g. erythromycin.
7 antimalarials, antihistamines.
8 prokinetic drugs e.g. cisapride.
9 volatile anaesthetic agents.

Acquired LQTS can be due to electrolyte abnormalities e.g. hypocalcaemia, hypomagnesaemia, hypokalaemia. It can also result from heart disease such as myocarditis, and sick sinus syndrome. Non-heart conditions that can cause LQTS include hypothyroidism, subarachnoid haemorrhage and right-sided neck dissection.

Treatment for Congenital LQTS

1 Beta-blocking drugs reduce the incidence of attacks and the risk of sudden death.
2 Anti-bradycardia pacing to prevent bradycardia and pauses that can induce attacks.
3 An automatic implantable cardiac defibrillator (AICD) is indicated if syncope, torsades de pointes and/or cardiac arrest occurs despite the above treatments. AICD therapy is also indicated if Q-Tc is very prolonged (>0.55–0.6 s).
4 Left cervico-thoracic sympathectomy in patients refractory to all other treatments.
5 The patient's relatives must be screened. This may be lifesaving for undiagnosed patients.

Anaesthetic Implications for Patients with Diagnosed LQTS
General Aspects of Management
Liaise with the patient's cardiologist if possible prior to surgery.
1   maintain β blocker therapy peri-operatively.
2   ensure electrolytes are normal.
3   ensure implanted pacemaker is functioning appropriately. **See** Pacemakers and Anaesthesia.
4   prevent hypothermia which prolongs QT interval.
5   ensure an external defibrillator is available.
6   avoid bradycardia and tachycardia.
7   consider invasive arterial pressure monitoring and central venous access to facilitate access for transvenous pacing.

Specific Anaesthetic Drugs
1   All volatile anaesthetic drugs probably have some effect on the Q-T interval—propofol induction and maintenance is preferable.[45]
2   Midazolam and vecuronium are probably safe.
3   Succinylcholine, pancuronium and ketamine should probably be avoided.
4   Avoid reversal of neuromuscular blockade with atropine/glycopyrrolate if possible.

Treatment of Torsades de Pointes
See Torsades de Pointes.

LQTS and Pregnancy
LQTS may be inherited by the fetus and can result in fetal perinatal death.

◑ Lorazepam

Benzodiazepine is useful for pre-operative alleviation of anxiety. Lorazepam results in sedation and profound anterograde amnesia lasting up to 6 h. Also useful for treatment of status epilepticus (IV). **See** Epilepsy, Status. It has a slow onset of action orally, taking up to 2–4 h.

Dose
1   For premedication give 50 µg/kg up to a maximum dose of 4 mg PO.
2   For seizures give 0.1 mg/kg IV.

◑ Lower Segment Caesarean Section

See Caesarean Section.

◑ Low Molecular Weight Heparins

See Heparin (Unfractionated and Low Molecular Weight Heparins).

Ⓓ Ludwig's Angina: Anaesthetic Management

Ludwig's angina is a soft tissue cellulitis of the floor of the mouth and neck resulting in progressive airway compromise due to massive swelling. The infection source is usually the lower molar teeth. Aspiration of pus into the airways can also occur.

QUICK FLICK L

Presentation

The main symptoms and signs are:

1 trismus, pain, dysphagia
2 fever, septicaemia
3 upper airway obstruction with dyspnoea, stridor, cyanosis and asphyxiation.

Anaesthetic Management

The anaesthetic management for securing the airway and surgical drainage involves the following.[46]

Pre-anaesthetic Stage

1 Antibiotic therapy. The usual organism(s) are streptococci, staphylococci, *Escherichia coli* (*E. coli*), pseudomonas or mixed infections.
   Recommended antibiotics (until the organism is known) are: clindamycin + penicillin (or ciprofloxacin) and metronidazole.[47]
2 Dexamethasone therapy.
3 Consider a drying agent such as glycopyrrolate.
4 Consider nebulised adrenaline to reduce airway swelling.
5 ENT surgeon should be available for immediate tracheostomy.
6 Nasal fibre-optic laryngoscopy can be used to assess airway oedema and predict the difficulty of intubation.

Anaesthetic Phase

Options for securing the airway are:

1 Awake tracheostomy using local anaesthesia. This is the favoured management but can be extremely difficult. A surgical airway also risks spreading the infection to deep cervical and mediastinal tissues.
2 Awake fibre-optic nasal oral intubation. **See** *Awake Fibre-optic Intubation*.
3 Gaseous induction using sevoflurane and oxygen. With the patient deep, direct laryngoscopy can be attempted. Failed intubation with the requirement for emergency tracheotomy often occurs with this technique (55% of attempts in one study).[48]
4 Use an armoured (reinforced) tube as the submandibular swelling may compress an ordinary PVC tube.[47]

5 Blind nasal intubation should not be attempted due to the risk of bleeding, and abscess perforation with lung soiling and airway obstruction.

◗ Lumbosacral Plexus (Psoas Compartment) Block

This block is useful for post-operative analgesia after surgery on the leg.

Anatomy of the Lumbar Plexus

The lumbar plexus is made up of the anterior primary rami of L1, L2, L3 and part of L4 with a contribution from T12 in 50% of cases. The branches of the lumbar plexus are:

1 Iliohypogastric and ilioinguinal nerves (L1 + T12).
2 Genitofemoral nerve (L1, L2).
3 Lateral cutaneous nerve of thigh (L2, L3).
4 Femoral nerve (L2, L3, L4).
5 Obturator nerve (L2, L3, L4)
6 Accessory obturator nerve (L3, L4).

Anatomy of the Sacral Plexus

The sacral plexus is made up of the anterior primary rami of L5, S1, S2 and S3 with contributions from L4 and S4. This plexus then gives rise to the following nerves:

1 Sciatic nerve (L4, L5 & S1, S2, S3).
2 Pudendal nerve (S2, S3, S4).
3 Pelvic sphlanchnic nerves.

Technique

1 Position the patient sitting or in the lateral position.
2 Identify the spinous process of L3, then locate the transverse process 3–5 cm laterally using a 22 G spinal needle.
3 Walk the needle off either the upper or the lower border of the transverse process. Feel for a 'pop' sensation heralding the passage of the needle through the quadratus fascia into the psoas compartment, or attempt to elicit paraesthesia. A nerve stimulator can also be used. The correct depth is about 7–10 cm.
4 Inject 20 mL of bupivacaine 0.5% with adrenaline. There should be little resistance to injection. Although anaesthesia of the femoral, obturator and lateral cutaneous nerve of thigh is expected, the sciatic nerve usually escapes.[49]

◗ Lung Function Tests

See *Respiratory Function Tests*.

◑ Lung Volumes

Table L8: Lung volumes

Lung volume	mL/ kg	For 70 kg patient
Vital capacity	70 mL/kg	5 L
Functional residual cap.	34 mL/kg	2.4 L
Residual volume	14 mL/kg	1 L
Tidal volume	7 mL/kg	500 mL

REFERENCES

1 Brimacombe J, Berry A. A review of anaesthesia for ruptured abdominal aortic aneurysm with special emphasis on preclamping fluid resuscitation. *Anaesth Intensive Care* 1993; 21: 311–23.

2 Dubois F, Berthelot G, Levard H. Cholecystectomie par coelioscopie. *Presse Med* 1989; 18: 980–2.

3 Duffy BL. Regurgitation during pelvic laparoscopy. *Br J Anaesth* 1979; 51: 1089–90.

4 Roth H, Genzwuerker HV, Rothhaas A et al. The ProSeal™ laryngeal mask airway and the laryngeal tube suction for ventilation in gynecological patients undergoing laparoscopic surgery. *Europ J Anaesthesiol* 2005; 22: 117–22.

5 Biswas TK, Pembroke A. Asystolic cardiac arrest during laparoscopic cholecystectomy. *Anaesth Intensive Care* 1994; 22: 289–92.

6 Inada T, Uesugi F, Kawachi S, Takubo K. Changes in tracheal tube position during laparoscopic cholecystectomy. *Anaesthesia* 1996; 51: 823–6.

7 Chui PT, Gin T, Oh TE. Anaesthesia for laparoscopic general surgery. *Anaesth Intensive Care* 1993; 21: 163–71.

8 Salonen M, Mäkinen J, Saraste M, Parkkola R. Is laparoscopic hysterectomy bad for the brain? *Gynaecol Endoscopy* 1999; 8: 161–4.

9 Hagen P, Scholz D, Edwards W. Incidence and size of patent foramen ovale during the first 10 decades of life. *Mayo Clin Proc* 1984; 59: 17–20.

10 Tuppurainen T, Mäkinen J, Salonen M. Reducing the risk of systemic embolization during gynecologic laparoscopy—effect of volume preload. *Acta Anaesthesiol Scand* 2002; 46: 37–42.

11 Koivusalo AM, Lindgren L. Effects of carbon dioxide pneumoperitoneum for laparoscopic cholecystectomy. *Acta Anaesthesiol Scand* 2000; 44: 834–41.

12 Benumof JL. Laryngeal mask airway and the ASA difficult airway algorithm. *Anesthesiology* 1996; 84: 686–99.

13 Keller C, Brimacombe J, Raedler C, Puehringer F. Do laryngeal mask airway devices attenuate liquid flow between the oesophagus and the

pharynx? A randomized, controlled cadaver study. *Anesth Analg* 1999; 88: 904–7.

14 *LMA-ProSeal Instruction Manual*. The Laryngeal Mask Company Limited, 2000 (with permission).

15 Brimacombe J, Keller C, Judd DV. Gum elastic bougie-guided insertion of the ProSeal™ laryngeal mask airway is superior to the digital and introducer tool techniques. *Anesthesiology* 2004; 1: 25–9.

16 Maltby JR, Beriault MT, Watson NC et al. The LMA-ProSeal is an effective alternative to tracheal intubation for laparoscopic cholecystectomy. *Can J Anaesth* 2002; 49: 857–62.

17 Putzke C, Max M, Geldner G, Wulf H. Severe ARDS following perioperative aspiration of gastric content associated with the use of a 'ProSeal' laryngeal mask airway (German). *Anasthesiology, Intensivmedizin, Notfallmedizin, Schmerztherapie* 2005; 40: 487–9.

18 van Vlymen JM, Coloma M, Tongier WK. Use of the intubating laryngeal mask airway: are muscle relaxants necessary? *Anesthesiology* 2000; 93: 340–5.

19 Brain AIJ, Verghese C, Addy EV et al. The intubating laryngeal mask II: a preliminary clinical report of a new means of intubating the trachea. *Br J Anaesth* 1997; 79: 704–9.

20 Baskett PJ, Parr MJ, Nolan JP. The intubating laryngeal mask. Results of a multicentered trial with experience of 500 cases. *Anaesthesia* 1998; 53: 1174–9.

21 Asai T, Wagle AU, Stacey M. Placement of the intubating laryngeal mask is easier than the laryngeal mask during manual in-line neck stabilization. *Br J Anaesth* 1999; 82: 712–14.

22 Kihara S, Watanabe S, Brimacombe J et al. Segmental cervical spine movement with the intubating laryngeal mask during manual in-line stabilization in patients with cervical pathology undergoing cervical spine surgery. *Anesth Analg* 2000; 91: 195–200.

23 Liu EHI, Goy RWL, Chen FG. The LMA C-Trach™, a new laryngeal mask airway for endotracheal intubation under vision: evaluation of 100 patients. *Br J Anaesth* 2006; 96: 396–400.

24 Ocker H, Wenzel V, Schmucker P et al. A comparison of the laryngeal tube with the laryngeal mask airway during routine surgical procedures. *Anesth Analg* 2002; 95: 1094–7.

25 Gabbott DA. Recent advances in airway technology. *Br J Anaesthiol CEPD Reviews* 2001; 1: 76–80.

26 Cormack RS, Lehane J. Difficult tracheal intubation in obstetrics. *Anaesthesia* 1984; 39: 1105–11.

27 Gaba DM, Fish KJ, Howard SK. *Crisis Management in Anesthesiology*. Churchill Livingstone, New York 1994: 277–9.

28 Rampil IJ. Anesthetic considerations for laser surgery. *Anesth Analg* 1992; 74: 424–35.

29 Protocol for the management of latex allergy, Flinders Medical Centre, Adelaide. In Keneally J, Jones M, eds. *Australasian Anaesthesia 1996*, Australian and New Zealand College of Anaesthetists 1996: 130–4.

30 Fisher M McD. Latex allergy during anaesthesia: cautionary tales. *Anaesth Intensive Care* 1997; 25: 302–3.

31 Holzman RS. Latex allergy: an emerging operating room problem. *Anesth Analg* 1993; 76: 635–41.

32 McAleer P, Barker D. Latex Allergy: a review. In Keneally J, Jones M, eds. *Australasian Anaesthesia 1996*, Australian and New Zealand College of Anaesthetists 1996: 123–34.

33 Schwartz HA, Zurowski D. Anaphylaxis to latex in intravenous fluids. *J Allergy Clin Immunol* 1993; 92: 358–9.

34 McLeod GA, Burke D. Review article: Levobupivacaine. *Anaesthesia* 2001; 56: 331–41.

35 Hung RO, Stewart RD. Lightwand intubation: 1—a new lightwand device. *Can J Anaesth* 1995; 42: 820–5.

36 Djordjevic D. Trachlight™—learning tips (letter). *Can J Anaesth* 1999; 46: 615–17.

37 Dimitriou V, Voyagis GS, Grosomanidis V, Brimacombe J. Feasibility of flexible light-wand guided tracheal intubation with the intubating laryngeal mask during out-of-hospital cardiopulmonary resuscitation by an emergency physician. *Europ J Anaesthesiol* 2006; 23: 76–9.

38 Albrecht A, Hogg M, Robinson S. Transient radicular irritation as a complication of spinal anaesthesia with hyperbaric 5% lignocaine. *Anaesth Intensive Care* 1996; 24: 508–10.

39 Covino BG. Clinical Pharmacology of Local Anesthetic Agents. In: Cousins MJ, Bridenbaugh PO eds. *Neural Blockade in Clinical Anesthesia and Management of Pain*, 2nd edn, Philadelphia, Pennsylvania: JB Lippincott Company 1988: 111–44.

40 Priebe H-J. Aneurysmal subarachnoid haemorrhage and the anaesthetist. *Br J Anaesth* 2007; 99: 102–18.

41 Venkatesan T, Korula G. A comparative study between the effects of 4% end tracheal tube cuff lignocaine and 1.5 mg/kg intravenous lignocaine on coughing and hemodynamics during extubation in neurosurgical patients: a randomized controlled double blind trial. *J Neurosurg Anesthesiol* 2006; 18: 230–4.

42 Downes H, Gerber N, Hirshman CA. IV lignocaine in reflex and allergic bronchoconstriction. *Br J Anaesth* 1980; 83: 873–8.

43 Picard P, Tramér M. Prevention of pain on injection with propofol: a quantitative systemic review. *Anesth Analg* 2000; 90: 963–9.

44 Burtelow M, Riley E, Druzin M et al. How we treat: management of life threatening primary postpartum hemorrhage with a standardized massive transfusion protocol. *Transfusion* 2007; 47: 1564–72.

45 Booker PD, Whyte SD, Ladusans EJ. Long QT syndrome and anaesthesia. *Br J Anaesth* 2003; 90: 349–66.

46 Neff SP, Merry AF, Anderson B. Airway management in Ludwig's angina. *Anaesth Intensive Care* 1999; 27: 659–61.

47 Gray H, Pead M. Ludwig's angina. *Anaesthesia and Intensive Care Medicine* 2002; 3: 250–2.

48 Ovassapian A, Tuncbilek M, Weitzel E, Joshi C. Airway management in adult patients with deep neck infections: a case series and review of the literature. *Anesth Analg* 2005; 100: 585–9.

49 Mulroy MF. *Regional Anesthesia; an Illustrated Procedural Guide*, 2nd edn. Little, Brown and Company, Boston 1996: 199–200.

○ Magnesium

Most abundant cation in the body after potassium. The normal blood level of Mg^{2+} is 0.75–1.0 mmol/L (1.5–2 mEq/L). Total body depletion of Mg^{2+} may not be reflected by serum Mg^{2+} levels.[1]

Effects of Hypomagnesaemia

1 Ventricular dysrhythmias.
2 Increased cardiovascular mortality.[1]
3 May lead to intracellular potassium depletion.[2]
4 Neuromuscular excitability and, rarely, convulsions.[3]

Effects of Hypermagnesaemia

See Pre-eclampsia/Eclampsia.

○ Magnesium Sulfate

Mg^{2+} has anti-dysrhythmic effects including prolongation of AV nodal conduction and suppression of conduction in accessory pathways.[1] Magnesium reduces catecholamine release, and is an antagonist at alpha-adrenergic receptors. It is also an arteriolar dilator. A 5 mL ampoule of 50% strength magnesium sulphate contains 2.465 g of magnesium sulfate (equating to 10 mmol or 20 mEq of magnesium ions).

Indications and Dosages in Adults

1 Pre-eclampsia/eclampsia. Magnesium therapy is used to prevent seizures and also may assist in lowering blood pressure by reducing systemic vascular resistance. For details of magnesium therapy in pre-eclampsia and the toxic effects of magnesium **see** *Pre-eclampsia/ Eclampsia*.
2 Torsade de Pointes. Give 2 g IV over 10 min followed by an infusion of 0.5–0.75 g/h for 12–24 h. **See** *Torsade de Pointes*.
3 Magnesium deficiency.
4 Ventricular dysrhythmias associated with digoxin toxicity.
5 To control pre-term labour.[4]
6 May reduce post acute myocardial infarction mortality, especially in the elderly and high-risk patients.[1] Give 2 g IV over 5–15 min then 18 g over 24 h.[1]
7 May be useful for atrial fibrillation with a rapid ventricular rate, supraventricular tachycardia, ventricular dysrhythmias during acute

myocardial infarction, refractory ventricular tachycardia or ventricular fibrillation and multifocal atrial tachycardia.[1]

8 Phaeochromocytoma surgery. **See** *Phaeochromocytoma*.
9 Asthma resistant to more conventional therapy.[5]

Magnetic Resonance Imaging (MRI) Anaesthesia

Basic Principles of the MRI Scanner

MRI scanning involves the use of high strength magnetic fields to provide digitalised, tomographic high resolution images of tissues and organs. The device consists of:

1 Cryogenic magnetic. Formed by a liquid nitrogen cooled superconductor in an environment of liquid helium at a temperature of 4.22°K. This magnet produces a magnetic field which can be > 6 Tesla (1.5–3.0 Tesla is usual). It takes ≈ 72 h to establish this field. 1 Tesla (T) = 1000 gauss (G). The earth's magnetic field is 5×10^{-5} T (≈ 0.5 G).
2 Gradient coils. These are loops of wire that have gradient currents induced in them during the production of radiofrequency pulses. Torque in these wires results in the audible noise of the scanning process.[6]

How an Image is Obtained

1 Atoms with net electrical charges due to an odd number of protons and/or neutrons produce a randomly orientated magnetic field. These magnetic fields are aligned by the static magnetic field of the MRI scanner.
2 A radiofrequency pulse produces a second magnetic field which deflects the orientation of these atoms. When the pulses cease the atoms return to their aligned state in the static magnetic field (termed relaxation) releasing energy.
3 These 'relaxation' rates vary between tissues and enable differentiation of structure. The 'energy' released by realignment is detected by the receiver coil and used to create the MRI image.
4 Hydrogen atoms are the most commonly used for imaging.

Contraindications to MRI Scanning or Close Exposure to MRI Equipment

1 Cardiac pacemakers, implantable defibrillators.
2 Ferromagnetic intracerebral aneurysmal clips.
3 Intra-ocular metallic foreign body.
4 Other ferromagnetic devices that can be displaced by the magnetic field such as cochlear implants, stents and coils. Heart valves may be safe but require specific clearance for each type of valve. If an implanted device is not ferromagnetic (e.g. stainless steel, nickel, titanium) then it does not present a risk.
5 A metal object in the patient that is well fixed, and the function of the object is not affected by a magnetic field (e.g. sternal wires), is not a risk to the patient. However such objects may affect image quality.

6 MRI is relatively contraindicated in pregnancy. There is no direct evidence that MRI is harmful to the fetus. If MRI is done in pregnancy it is preferable to perform MRI after organogenesis is completed (> 12 weeks gestation). The gadolinium-based contrast agents do enter the fetal circulation and could pose a potential risk.[7] Note also that in advanced pregnancy the patient cannot lie flat in the scanner (**see** *Supine Hypotensive Syndrome*), and may not fit into the narrow scanning tunnel. The fetus may suffer ear damage due to the loudness of the scanner.

7 If the patient is breast feeding and gadolinium is used breast milk must be expressed and discarded for 48 h after the scan and the baby fed with infant formula.

QUICK FLICK M

Hazards in the MRI Scanning Room

1 Patients or staff can be injured by ferromagnetic objects becoming missiles.

2 Electronically encoded information on objects such as credit cards may be destroyed by the magnetic field.

3 Patients may experience discomfort due to iron containing pigments in tattoos or makeup. The patient must be warned to inform staff if the tattoo becomes uncomfortably hot and the MRI scanning process can then be slowed down.

4 Asphyxiation may result from 'quenching' in which liquid helium leaks into the MRI room and rapidly expands. Frostbite can also occur due to the coldness of the helium. O_2 sensors must be installed and functional to warn of this hazard.[8]

5 Acoustic noise can be a risk to hearing and ear protection should be worn.

6 Do not allow cables and wires to form loops as these can be heated up by the MRI process and cause burns.

Approach to the Patient Requiring MRI Anaesthesia

Many MRI suites routinely scan anaesthetised patients and have well established MRI compatible monitors and anaesthetic machines. For a detailed description of problems with monitors in the MRI suite see Rosewarne's book.[9]

In addition to the hazards and difficulties described above other issues are:

1 Remoteness from the patient.

2 Difficulty observing the patient.

3 Inadequate space in the scanner for resuscitation. Patients may need to be removed from the MRI scanning room if resuscitation is required.

4 Infusions pumps should not be used unless placed remotely with long infusion lines.

5 The metal spring in the LMA pilot balloon valve may cause image degradation.[10]

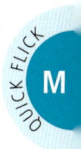

○ Malignant Hyperthermia (MH)

Topics Covered in this Section

▶ Description and Clinical Features
▶ Incidence
▶ Triggering Factors for Malignant Hyperthermia (MH)
▶ Diagnosis of MH
▶ Patients Susceptible to MH
▶ Treatment of the Acute Phase of MH
▶ Treatment of the Postacute Phase of MH
▶ Anaesthetic Management of the MH-susceptible Patient
▶ Obstetrics and MH Susceptibility
▶ Caffeine/Halothane Contraction Test and Genetic Testing

Description and Clinical Features

MH is due to a genetic condition with an autonomic dominant inheritance pattern. In this syndrome a triggering agent results in a markedly accelerated metabolic state. The triggering agent causes release of calcium ions from skeletal muscle sarcoplasmic reticulum causing hyperactive muscle fibre shortening. The genetic mutation causing MH is on the RYR1 gene on chromosome 19 and relates to the ryanodine calcium gate on skeletal muscle fibres. Two types of clinical reaction are recognised. In the first one there is muscle rigidity (75% of cases) and in the second there is absence of muscle rigidity.[11] Mortality without specific treatment is about 80%. With appropriate treatment the current mortality rate is about 8%.[12]

The main signs are:

1　Rigidity in skeletal muscle (but see above). Masseter spasm may occur (**See** *Masseter Spasm*.)
2　Fever, profuse sweating. Above 43°C proteins begin to denature and irreversible cerebral damage may occur.[13]
3　Tachypnoea and cyanosis.
4　Increased O_2 consumption and CO_2 production.
5　Tachycardia, unstable blood pressure, arrhythmias.
6　Hyperkalaemia, acidosis.
7　Dysfunction in many other organ systems.
8　Renal failure and DIC may occur.
9　MH can present with sudden cardiac arrest.

Incidence

The incidence of MH in the general adult population is about 1:40 000 and about 1:15 000 in children.[12] MH occurs in about 1:4200 anaesthetics involving suxamethonium and a volatile anaesthetic agent.

Triggering Factors for Malignant Hyperthermia (MH)

This syndrome is known to be triggered by certain drugs including:

1 All volatile anaesthetic agents.
2 Suxamethonium, decamethonium and carbachol. Curare is probably also a trigger.
3 Caffeine, xanthines, cocaine, phenothiazines.
4 Sympathomimetics are now thought to be safe.

Diagnosis of MH

The diagnosis of MH is based on clinical presentation. Supporting biochemical evidence includes elevated serum creatine kinase, myoglobinaemia and myoglobinuria. **See** *Masseter Spasm*.

Patients Susceptible to MH

People who are, or may be, susceptible to MH include:

1 Patients diagnosed as MH susceptible from muscle biopsy testing. This test is very sensitive and specific.
2 Patients who are diagnosed MH susceptible from genetic testing. Genetic testing is useful if positive but a negative test does not exclude MH susceptibility. Only about 30% of MH susceptible patients test positive with genetic testing.
3 A positive family history of MH or a suspicious episode of reaction to an anaesthetic in a family member. In one report 75% of cases did not have a known positive family history.[14]
4 Patients with musculoskeletal disorders such as strabismus, kyphoscoliosis and clubfoot.
5 Central-core disease is almost certainly related to MH. Patients with osteogenesis imperfecta, King-Denborough syndrome and other myopathies may also be susceptible. There is probably NO association between MH and neuroleptic malignant syndrome. **See** *Neuroleptic Malignant Syndrome (NMS)*.
6 Patients who experience heatstroke or rhabdomyolysis may be at increased risk.

Note: A previous exposure to a triggering anaesthetic does not guarantee a lack of susceptibility to MH. About 33% of cases of MH occur in patients who have been previously exposed to a triggering agent without MH occurring.

Treatment of Acute Phase of MH[15]

1 Declare that a crisis is occurring and summon skilled assistance. Alert the surgeon and immediately cease all possible triggering agents such as inhalational anaesthetic drugs. Hyperventilate with 100% O_2 at a gas flow of at least 10 L/min. Do not turn off the CO_2 absorber as production of CO_2 is greatly increased. Do not change the anaesthetic machine or circuit. This is not a priority.

2 Keep the patient anaesthetised with a propofol infusion until the surgery is (urgently) completed or abandoned.

3 Administer dantrolene sodium 2.5 mg/kg IV boluses until signs of MH are controlled or up to 10 mg/kg is given. Occasionally a total dose of up to 30 mg/kg will be required. Each vial of dantrolene contains 20 mg of active drug, sodium hydroxide and 3 g of mannitol and needs to be mixed with 60 mL of sterile H_2O. This task alone will entirely occupy one of the resuscitating staff. Prewarming the sterile water to no greater than 38°C will speed up the solubilisation of the dantrolene.

4 Administer sodium bicarbonate 1–2 mEq/kg or as guided by arterial blood gas analysis.

5 Actively cool the patient with a core temperature > 39°C. Use IV iced saline 15 mL/kg over 15 min × 3. Also surface cool patient with ice and consider lavage of stomach, bladder, rectum and open cavities with iced saline. Stop cooling when the patient's temperature falls below 38°. Do not induce hypothermia.

6 Hyperkalaemia is common. Treat with hyperventilation, sodium bicarbonate, Actrapid 10 units + 50 mL of 50% glucose. Calcium chloride 5–10 mL of 10% solution may also be useful. ***See*** *Potassium*.

7 Treat cardiac dysrhythmias with reversal of hyperkalaemia and acidosis + antiarrhythmic drugs appropriate for the particular dysrhythmia. Do not use calcium channel blockers. These can cause hyperkalaemia and cardiovascular collapse due to their interaction with dantrolene.

8 Monitor serum K^+, Ca^{2+}, clotting studies and urine output. Aim for at least 2 mL/kg/h urine output.

9 Do not transfer patient to the intensive care unit (ICU) until a satisfactory response to treatment has occurred as a worsening of the condition may ensue if the patient is transferred prematurely.

10 Ongoing management includes checking for rising CK and/or potassium levels or falling urine output suggesting myoglobin induced renal failure. Urine may turn cola coloured. Aim for a urine output > 1 mL/kg/h.

Treatment of Postacute Phase of MH

1 Observe the patient in the ICU for a minimum of 36 h. Give dantrolene 1 mg/kg IV 6 h for 24–48 h, then oral dantrolene 1 mg/kg 6 h for another 3 days.

2 Counsel the patient and family regarding MH and ensure that the patient understands the implications of their condition. Arrange for follow up muscle biopsy testing of the patient and relevant family members. Currently in Australia and New Zealand there are only 4 centres for testing (Sydney, Melbourne, Perth and Palmerston North, NZ).

Anaesthetic Management of the MH-susceptible Patient

1 Prepare the anaesthetic machine by removing all vaporisers. Also replace the CO_2 absorbent, anaesthetic tubing and fresh gas outlet tubing with fresh equipment. Flush the anaesthetic machine and breathing system with O_2 at 10 L/min for at least 10 min (20 min if the fresh gas outlet tubing cannot be replaced). A 'volatile anaesthetic free' anaesthetic machine can also be used but this is probably not necessary.

2 Use a 'non-triggering' anaesthetic technique. Non-triggering drugs include:
   a) Intravenous anaesthetic drugs such as barbiturates, propofol, ketamine and benzodiazepines.
   b) Opioids, N_2O, all local anaesthetic drugs (with or without adrenaline).
   c) Non-depolarising neuromuscular blocking drugs including rocuronium, vecuronium, atracurium and pancuronium. Curare is not safe.
   d) Atropine and neostigmine.
   e) Droperidol is safe.

3 Make sure that 36 vials of dantrolene are immediately available. Prophylactic dantrolene is not recommended for most MH susceptible patients.[15]

4 In addition to routine monitoring, monitor the patient's temperature carefully intraoperatively.

5 Postoperatively patients should be monitored in recovery for at least 1 h and in a phase 2 area for at least 1.5 h.

Obstetrics and MH Susceptibility

1 Monitor temperature and heart rate during labour.

2 An epidural or spinal anaesthetic is preferred for Caesarean section. LA with or without adrenaline can be used. If GA is required, use a non-triggering technique as described above.

3 Be aware of the possibility of a MH-susceptible fetus in a non-MH susceptible mother, if the father is MH susceptible.

4 Ephedrine is probably safe, as is oxytocin.

Caffeine/Halothane Contraction Test and Genetic Testing

MH is initially a clinical diagnosis. Elevated serum creatine kinase, myoglobinaemia and myoglobinuria are biochemical evidence of a possible MH reaction. Muscle biopsy testing or a positive genetic test are the only definitive diagnostic tests for MH. For muscle biopsy testing a long section of vastus lateralis muscle is removed from the patient and these muscle fibres are exposed to caffeine and halothane and contractions are measured.

A DNA test is available for detection of 1 of the 15 known abnormalities of the RYR1 gene. The role of this test is to help identify relatives that are MH-susceptible of patients that:

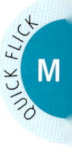

QUICK FLICK **M**

1 have a positive caffeine/halothane contraction test; and
2 are positive for genetic testing. Only 30% of patients who have a positive contraction test are also positive on genetic testing.

If a relative has a positive genetic test they are MH susceptible and do not need muscle biopsy testing. If a relative has a negative genetic test this does not exclude MH susceptibility.

Mallampati Score

See *Difficult Airway Management.*

Mannitol

An alcohol used for osmotic diuresis, mannitol is useful in the treatment of:

1 Raised intracranial pressure. **See** *Intracranial Pressure (ICP) and Treatment of Raised ICP*.
2 Preservation of renal function during procedures such as repair of abdominal aortic aneurysm. **See** *Abdominal Aortic Aneurysm (AAA) Surgery*.
3 Prevention of hepatorenal syndrome. **See** *Hepatorenal Syndrome (HRS)*.
4 Short-term management of acute glaucoma.

Dose

Depends on the indication, see relevant cross references listed above.

Masseter Spasm

Masseter spasm is defined as jaw tightness that interferes with intubation after a dose of suxamethonium. This reaction is most common in children but is occasionally noted in adults. The incidence of this reaction in children is about 0.1–0.5%.[16] It may be so severe as to prevent jaw opening (jaws of steel). It is hypothesised that a percentage of these patients are susceptible to malignant hyperthermia (up to 50%).[16] Masseter spasm may also be the first sign of MH. Some patients who develop masseter spasm have an underlying muscle abnormality.

Treatment

1 Maintain oxygenation. Relaxation of the jaw usually occurs after a few minutes at most.
2 Abandon elective surgery if the masseter spasm is marked and allow the patient to awaken. If malignant hyperthermia develops treat as above.
3 If surgery is urgent continue anaesthesia with a technique that is non-triggering for MH. See above.
4 Check CK levels immediately and at 6 h intervals until this level is in the NR (25–200 u/L). Watch for cola-coloured urine and if this develops check for urinary myoglobin.
5 Observe the patient in hospital for at least 12 h.

◑ Massive Blood Transfusion

See *Blood Transfusion*.

◑ MAST Suite

MAST stands for military anti-shock trousers. This device can be used to aid in the management of hypovolaemic shock due to severe blood loss. The mechanisms of actions are:

1 Mechanically increases peripheral resistance.
2 Compresses the IVC and lower limb vessels promoting venous return.
3 Causes redistribution of blood from the legs and splanchnic circulation to the brain and heart.
4 The suite has 2 leg components and one abdominal component. The components can be inflated with air to compress the legs and or abdomen up to a maximum pressure of 100 mm Hg. The usual pressure range is 20–40 mm Hg. This device is probably seldom used in actual clinical practice.

◑ Mediastinal Mass and Anaesthesia

Mediastinal masses can occur in any age group and have a wide variety of aetiologies. The most common causes (in order of decreasing frequency):[17]

1 lymphoma (Hodgkin's and Non-Hodgkin's)
2 thymomas, thyroid masses
3 germ cell tumours and granulomas
4 lung cancers, bronchogenic cysts
5 vascular tumours.

The most important effects of these masses is compression of vital structures including:

1 Superior vena cava. These are usually malignant masses on the right side. *See* *Superior Vena Cava Syndrome*.
2 Heart and pericardium. The heart may be directly involved by tumours and cause effects such as dysrhythmias.[18]
3 Trachea and bronchi leading to respiratory compromise.
4 Pulmonary arteries.

The major concerns therefore are that a mediastinal mass can cause catastrophic obstruction to major airways or the heart, SVC or pulmonary arteries especially under anaesthesia. Most deaths due to mediastinal mass and anaesthesia are in children.[17]

Anaesthetic Assessment, Investigation and Preparation

1 Look for any evidence of superior vena cava syndrome (*see* *Superior Vena Cava Syndrome*).
2 Evaluate for signs of pericardial tamponade such as pulsus paradoxus and consider echocardiography.

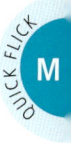

3   Look for pulmonary artery obstruction which can result in right ventricular outflow obstruction and greatly diminished pulmonary venous return to the left side of the heart. One simple test is to ask the patient to perform a Valsalva manoeuvre which may produce syncope or presyncope.[19] Pre-operative CT and MRI scans should be carefully scrutinised for this complication.

4   Look for any evidence of bronchial or tracheal obstruction. Symptoms and signs include:
    a) wheezing, stridor, decreased breath sounds.
    b) recurrent infections.

5   Appropriate investigations include:
    a) CXR.
    b) CT/MRI of chest.
    c) Mass effects on major vessels can be elucidated by echocardiography in the erect and supine position.[20]
    d) Upright and supine pulmonary function tests looking at peak expiratory flow rate and flow volume loops. Slinger and Karsli argue that these tests do not offer any useful extra information to the imaging tests described above.[17]

6   If practical and appropriate, consider pre-operative radiotherapy and/or chemotherapy to shrink the mediastinal mass prior to anaesthesia and surgery.

7   Ascertain if compression symptoms are less lying on one side or the other. If needed turn the patient to the less symptomatic side during anaesthesia.

Anaesthesia for Patients with Mediastinal Mass

A rigid bronchoscope and a doctor skilled in rigid bronchoscopy should be present in the operating theatre or other area where a GA is given to these patients.

The basic principles of anaesthesia for mediastinal mass surgery are:

1   If at all possible perform the procedure under LA e.g. CT guided needle biopsy, mediastinoscopy and biopsy. Thoracic epidural anaesthesia in the awake patient may be possible.

2   Consider awake fibre-optic intubation to ensure the tube is passed beyond an area of compressed trachea if possible, prior to GA.[21]

3   If GA is required use a gaseous or gradual propofol IV induction maintaining spontaneous ventilation preferably for the whole case but especially until the airway is definitively secured.

4   If muscle relaxants are required test ventilate the patient prior to administration and if successful use only short-acting agents.

5   Planned rigid bronchoscopy and/or cardiopulmonary bypass may be required in extreme cases. Patients with evidence of severe cardiac,

vascular or tracheobronchial obstruction cannot safely be given GA without planned cardiopulmonary bypass or ECMO.[17] *See Extracorporeal Membrane Oxygenation (ECMO).*

Unanticipated Airway Obstruction in the Patient with Mediastinal Mass
In this scenario tracheal intubation is successful but ventilation is difficult or ineffective.
1   Wake the patient up if this is appropriate.
2   Try repositioning the patient (lateral, prone) to shift the mass off the trachea/bronchus.[22]
3   Rigid bronchoscopy and ventilation distal to the site of obstruction. Life-threatening cardiovascular compression that does not respond to lightening of the anaesthesia should be treated with:
  a) Median sternotomy and elevation of the mass.
  b) Consider emergency cardiopulmonary bypass.

○ Mental Nerve Block

Anatomy
The mental nerve arises in the mandibular canal and arises from the inferior alveolar nerve. It exits the mandible through the mental foramen to supply sensation to the skin of the lower lip and chin and mucous membrane lining the lower lip.

Technique
1   Anaesthetise the mucous membrane of lower lip adjacent to the second premolar tooth (in line with the pupil, with the eyes in the neutral position) using gauze soaked in 4% topical lignocaine.
2   Insert a 25 G needle about 1 cm deep towards the mental foramen and inject 2 mL of LA (e.g. 2% lignocaine).

○ M-Entropy

See Entropy.

○ Metabolic Equivalent

See Cardiovascular Peri-operative Risk Prediction for Non-cardiac Surgery.

○ Metaraminol

Metaraminol (aramine) is a synthetic sympathomimetic amine used as a vasoconstrictor agent for the treatment of hypotension. Acts by a direct agonist effect on α receptors with lesser stimulation of β receptors. There is some uptake of metaraminol into adrenergic nerve endings from where it is released as a weak neurotransmitter.

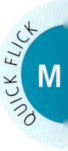

QUICK FLICK M

Dose

Adult Give 0.5–1 mg IV, titrate to desired effect. Effects begin within 1–2 min with a maximum effect in 10 min. Effects last 20–60 min.

IV Infusion Load 50 mg into 100 mL N/S and run at 1–10 mL/h.

Child 0.01 mg/kg IV boluses.

IV Infusion in Child 0.1–1 µg/kg/min, titrate against blood pressure.

◖ Methadone

Synthetic opioid agonist with efficient oral absorption and long duration of action. Less sedating than morphine. Used for:
1 analgesia for chronic pain.
2 treatment of heroin addiction.
3 cough suppression in terminal disease.

Dose

For *heroin addiction* give methadone in a dosage that is about 25% of the heroin dosage in mg.

For *analgesia* give 5–10 mg PO or subcutaneously or IM every 6–8 h as required.

Anaesthetic Implications of Long-term Methadone Therapy
1 Involve and consult the Drug and Alcohol Service at an early stage for patients on methadone for heroin addiction.
2 Methadone therapy should be continued up to the time of surgery.
3 High doses of methadone may prolong the Q-T interval and increase susceptability to torsades de pointes. This risk is increased if other drugs that increase the Q-T interval are used such as amiodarone, erythromycin and haloperidol.[23] ***See*** *Long QT Syndrome (LQTS)*.
4 Post-operatively restart methadone therapy as soon as practically possible.
5 Use PCA opioid analgesia with a background infusion if methadone cannot be restarted within 48 h and the patient has significant pain.
6 Consider supplementary ketamine by a subcut infusion. ***See*** *Ketamine*.

◖ Methaemoglobin

Methaemoglobin (MetHb) is haemoglobin in which ferrous iron in the molecule has been oxidised to the ferric state. Methaemoglobinaemia occurs when MetHb exceeds 1% of total Hb. Patients are not usually symptomatic until MetHb levels reach 8% or greater. Methaemoglobinaemia can be due to drugs such as:
1 Prilocaine in doses > 600 mg, due to the metabolite o-toluidine.
2 EMLA cream, topical benzocaine and tetracaine.

3 Nitrates, nitrites and sodium nitroprusside.
4 Dapsone.
5 Diaspirin—a purified human haemoglobin product.

Effects of Methaemoglobin[24]

1 Cyanosis may occur when MetHb levels exceed 8–12%.
2 At 20–30% MetHb may see headache, confusion and increased respiratory rate. At higher levels (> 50%) there may be decreased level of consciousness, seizures and CVS collapse and death.
3 Oxyhaemoglobin dissociation curve is shifted to the left.
4 As MetHb level increases, pulse oximetry will read 80–85% regardless of the true saturation.
5 MetHb is brownish in appearance and produces a slate grey colour in the patient. The brownish blood does not redden on exposure to oxygen. This feature can be used as a bedside test.
6 Arterial pO_2 is normal despite the cyanosis.
7 Diagnosis is by co-oximeter calculation of MetHb levels.

Treatment

1 Cease the offending agent. Treatment is not required unless the patient is symptomatic.
2 Give methylene blue 1–2 mg/kg IV (use the 1% solution) over 5 min. The dose can be repeated after 1 h. Methylene blue should not be administered to patients with G6PD deficiency. ***See*** *Glucose-6-phosphate Dehydrogenase Deficiency*.
3 Blood transfusion or exchange transfusion may be required for patients with cardiovascular collapse.
4 Hyperbaric oxygen.

Methohexitone

Intravenous methylated oxybarbiturate anaesthetic agent.

Advantages

1 Faster recovery from anaesthesia than thiopentone, hence this drug is favoured for ultra short procedures e.g. electroconvulsive therapy.
2 It is less of an irritant than thiopentone if extravasation occurs.

Methohexitone may be preferable for use in the asthmatic patient compared with thiopentone.[25]

Disadvantages

1 There is an increased incidence of excitatory effects compared with thiopentone.
2 Methohexitone may also cause an epileptiform pattern on the EEG.
3 Pain on injection may occur.

QUICK FLICK M

4 Like thiopentone, it is contraindicated in some types of porphyria.
See Porphyria.

Dose
1–1.5 mg/kg IV, 6.6 mg/kg IM or 15–20 mg/kg PR.

◐ Methoxamine

Synthetic sympathomimetic amine drug, acts as a selective α_1 receptor agonist producing vasoconstriction. It is used for the treatment of hypotension.

Dose
Adult 1 mg IV boluses to a maximum of 5–10 mg. Acts within 1–2 min and effects last for 1 h IM dose 5–20 mg.

◐ Methylene Blue

See Methaemoglobin above.

◐ Metoclopramide

Metoclopramide (Maxolon) is a chlorinated procainamide derivative used for:
1 The prevention and treatment of nausea and vomiting.
2 To increase the rate of gastric emptying.
Acts mainly by antagonising central and peripheral dopaminergic receptors (DA2) and has a direct action on gastrointestinal smooth muscle.

Dose
Adult 10 mg IV, IM or PO as required up to 8 h.
Child 0.12 mg/kg/dose to a maximum of 15 mg IV, IM or PO.

Disadvantages
1 Extrapyramidal side effects may occur. **See** Dystonic Reaction, Acute.
2 Not suitable for patients with Parkinson's disease.
3 Low efficacy. There is little evidence that metoclopramide is an effective antiemetic at the usual adult dose of 10 mg.[26]

◐ Metoprolol

β_1 selective β adrenergic receptor blocking drug used for the treatment of:
1 Supraventricular tachycardia.
2 Hypertension.
3 Angina.
4 Premature ventricular ectopics.

Dose
Adult 1–2 mg IV boluses minutely to a maximum total dose of 15–20 mg.
Child 0.1 mg/kg (max 5 mg) over 5 min, repeat 5 minutely to a max of 3 doses. Consider infusion 1–5 µg/kg/min.

◗ Midazolam

A water soluble benzodiazepine with a fast onset and short duration of action. Useful for:

1 Premedication, due to its sedating, amnesic and anxiolytic effects.
2 Sedation for procedures, usually combined with other drugs e.g. fentanyl + propofol.
3 Seizure control.
4 Intrathecally to potentiate the analgesic effects of local anaesthetic agents.[27]

Dose Adult

Sedation for Procedures Inject 1–2 mg IV increments until patient is tolerant of procedure but still able to maintain verbal contact.

Premedication 0.07–0.08 mg/kg IM 30–60 min prior to the procedure.

Infusion for Prolonged Sedation Give LD of 2–5 mg/kg then 0.1–0.2 mg/kg/h titrated to clinical effect.

Dose Child

Premedication 0.1–0.2 mg/kg IV. A dose up to 0.5 mg/kg IV can be considered. Can give midazolam PO mixed with a sweet drink (midazolam is very bitter) 30–60 min before procedure.

Infusion 3 mg/kg in 50 mL of N/S run at 2 mL/h.

Intrathecal Midazolam

It is well established that intrathecal midazolam enhances the analgesic effects of intrathecal LA and opioids in humans and no human studies have indicated evidence of neurotoxicity.[28] However several rabbit studies have indicated neurotoxicity.[29,30,31] This controversy remains unresolved. The intrathecal dose is 1–2 mg of preservative free midazolam. Use the 1 mg mL solution. This prolongs analgesia from bupivacaine for about 4.5 h.[32] A continuous infusion of up to 6 mg/day has been given without apparent ill effects, for chronic pain.[33] The midazolam used should be the hydrochloride form and not contain preservatives such as benzoate and should be at a concentration not exceeding 1 mg/mL.

Note: Midazolam should be used with caution in patients on efavirenz, an antiviral drug, due to similar metabolic pathways. The anticholesterol drug atorvastatin results in a prolongation of midazolam's drug effects.[34]

◗ Milrinone

Second generation phosphodiesterase III inhibitor. Effects include positive inotropy and vasodilatation resulting in increased cardiac output without compromising myocardial O_2 supply-demand ratio. This is due to a reduction of preload and afterload and the lack of a significant tachycardia. Used for the treatment of cardiac failure e.g. post bypass or as a bridge to transplantation.

Dose

Give an IV loading dose of 37.5–50 µg/kg over 10 min then infusion 0.375–0.75 µg/kg/min.[35]

Advantages

1　Does not cause thrombocytopenia with chronic use, unlike amrinone.
2　The inotropic effect of milrinone is 20 × that of amrinone.[36]
3　Less prodysrhythmic than β stimulants.

Disadvantages

1　Vasodilation may cause significant hypotension.
2　Dysrhythmias may occur.
3　Dosage should be reduced in renal failure.[35]

◐ Minute Volume

Defined as the volume of gas leaving the lung per minute.
This volume = tidal volume × respiratory rate.
Adult 85–100 mL/kg
Child 100–200 mL/kg

◐ Mitral Incompetence (Regurgitation)

Mitral incompetence results in regurgitation of blood into the left atrium. The left ventricle (LV) is thus subjected to an increased workload leading to dilatation and hypertrophy. LV failure may occur. Left atrial dilatation develops and atrial fibrillation may occur in mixed lesions (mitral stenosis and mitral incompetence) or chronic mitral incompetence. Pulmonary hypertension and RV failure may also occur. There is a slow deterioration in exercise tolerance. If mitral incompetence occurs acutely, pulmonary oedema may occur and rapid decompensation and death may follow. Echocardiography will help define the cause and severity of mitral incompetence. A regurgitant fraction > 0.6 indicates severe disease.[37]

Management Aims During Anaesthesia

1　Consider antibiotic prophylaxis against bacterial endocarditis.
　　See *Bacterial Endocardarditis (BE) Prophylaxis*.
2　Consider invasive monitoring (arterial line, CVP, PA catheter, transoesophogeal echocardiography) depending on the severity of the condition and the extent of surgery.
3　Avoid increasing systemic vascular resistance (SVR), which will increase the regurgitant fraction and decrease the cardiac output (CO). Decreasing SVR in a controlled fashion can significantly increase CO.

4 A mild tachycardia can improve CO by preventing over distension of the LV and mitral valve distortion. Conversely avoid bradycardia.

5 Avoid hypovolaemia so that left atrial filling pressure is maintained. A well filled left atrium leads to less blood regurgitating back into this chamber and improved left ventricular filling.

6 Be aware of the risk of systemic emboli and/or complications of patient's anticoagulant drugs.

7 Avoid myocardial depressant drugs such as N_2O.

Mitral Regurgitation and Obstetrics

A carefully administered epidural anaesthetic should be well tolerated as long as:

1 Appropriate monitoring is used depending on the severity of the patient's condition.

2 Left atrial filling must be maintained with adequate fluid volume loading.

3 Ephedrine is preferable to aramine for treating hypotension.[38]

4 General anaesthesia is usually well tolerated as long as the above management aims are followed.

▶ Mitral Stenosis (MS)

MS is almost always caused by rheumatic fever. About 75% of patients will have other heart valve lesions. The normal mitral valve area is 4–6 cm². Symptoms occur when the valve area is reduced to 2.5 cm² and symptoms become severe at a valve area of < 1 cm². The normal atrial-ventricular diastolic pressure gradient across the mitral valve is < 5 mm Hg. Severe disease is present if this pressure is > 10 mm Hg. When the valve area is < 1 cm² the diastolic pressure across the valve may be > 25 mm Hg. Symptoms include exertional dyspnoea, orthopnoea and occasionally angina.

To compensate for the stenosed valve, the left atrium contracts more forcefully leading to left atrial dilatation and hypertrophy. Left atrial pressure is increased and if it exceeds colloid osmotic pressure (25–30 mm Hg) pulmonary oedema may occur. Some patients develop irreversible pulmonary hypertension with right ventricular hypertrophy which may lead to right ventricular failure. *See Pulmonary Hypertension*. Pulmonary and tricuspid valve incompetence may also occur secondary to pulmonary hypertension. Atrial fibrillation (AF) may develop which can produce sudden cardiac decompensation and emboli. For non-cardiac elective surgery, pre-operative mitral valve replacement is only indicated if this will prolong survival and decrease complications unrelated to the proposed non-cardiac surgery.[39] The patient may benefit from balloon valvuloplasty or valve replacement for high-risk surgery.

Aims of Anaesthetic Management

1 Consider invasive monitoring (CVP), intra-arterial BP monitoring, PA catheter, transoesophogeal echocardiography depending on the severity of the condition and the nature of the surgery.

2 Consider bacterial endocarditis prophylaxis. *See Bacterial Endocarditis (BE) Prophylaxis*.

3 Aim for normal to slow heart rate to allow time for LV filling through the stenosed valve. Avoid tachycardia, new AF or fast AF as this will decrease LV filling time and lead to a fall in CO. Therefore avoid atropine, glycopyrronium, ketamine and pancuronium. Cardiovert the patient if AF develops intraoperatively.

4 Prevent decreases in SVR as hypotension and decreased organ perfusion may result due to the relatively fixed CO.

5 Avoid or use cautiously drugs that are myocardial depressants e.g. volatile anaesthetic drugs.

6 Avoid factors which may increase pulmonary hypertension including N_2O, hypoxia and acidosis. *See Pulmonary Hypertension*. These may be unsafe if pulmonary vascular resistance is already elevated. If pulmonary hypertension is present, the pulmonary capillary wedge pressure may not correlate well with left atrial filling pressure.

7 Maintain preload to maintain LV filling but do not fluid overload the patient due to the risk of pulmonary oedema.

8 Hypovolaemia must be corrected promptly.

9 Avoid the Trendelenburg position which may lead to pulmonary oedema.

Mitral Stenosis and Obstetrics

1 Asymptomatic patients without pulmonary oedema are at minimally increased anaesthetic risk.[40] A mitral valve area > 1.5 cm^2 and a gradient < 5 mm Hg also suggests a low risk.

2 Patients with severe symptoms and a mitral valve area < 1 cm^2 should be considered for balloon mitral valvuloplasty during the second trimester.[41] This can be done under TOE guidance to avoid radiation to the fetus.

3 Mitral valve replacement may be necessary during pregnancy but is associated with a fetal loss rate of 10–30%.[41]

4 Epidural anaesthesia has been used successfully in patients with mitral stenosis. It is very important to avoid overfilling or underfilling the patient. Avoid adrenaline containing solutions. Neuroaxial block must be introduced cautiously.

5 Appropriate monitoring, depending on the severity of the lesion, must be instituted.

6 Cardioversion, if required, is safe for the fetus. For AF of sudden onset start with 25 J. *See Cardioversion*.

7 If hypotension occurs, metaraminol is preferred to ephedrine.

○ Mitral Valve Prolapse

Mitral valve prolapse is usually a benign condition and occurs in about 2.4–10% of the population depending on diagnostic criteria.[42] The condition is due to billowing of the posterior mitral valve leaflet into the left atrium during systole. In a minority of patients, usually with abnormal mitral valves, this lesion can result in strokes, endocarditis, significant or severe mitral valve regurgitation, dysrhythmias such as supraventricular tachycardia and sudden death. Mitral valve prolapse can be associated with other heart conditions such as hypertrophic cardiomyopathy and WPW.[43] Suspect this diagnosis in patients who develop unexpected atrial or ventricular dysrhythmias intra-operatively.

Aims of Anaesthetic Management

1 Increased ventricular emptying can increase the degree of prolapse and lead to acute regurgitation. Therefore avoid factors which increase contractility such as increased sympathetic nervous system activity. Also avoid decreasing systemic vascular resistance, and the head up or sitting position.
2 Consider antibiotic prophylaxis against bacterial endocarditis. **See** *Bacterial Endocarditis (BE) Prophylaxis*.
3 Avoid hypovolaemia which can lead to decreased preload and decreased ventricular filling.
4 Avoid tachycardia which may result in increased LV emptying which may increase the degree of prolapse.
5 Avoid high airway pressures which may accentuate prolapse.

○ Mivacurium

Benzylisoquinolinium diester non-depolarising neuromuscular blocking drug (NDNMBD), with a short duration of action. It is metabolised primarily by plasma cholinesterases. It is cleared from the plasma in about 3 minutes but its effects last much longer than this.[44]

Advantages

1 Shorter duration of action than other currently available NDNMB drugs (14–16 min)[44] making it useful for brief procedures. This situation will change when sugammadex becomes available for the rapid reversal of rocuronium.[45]
2 It does not require reversal drugs and routine reversal of mivacurium may not be necessary.[46] Can be given to patients with renal or liver failure.
3 Mivacurium can be given by infusion.

Disadvantages

1 Relatively slow onset of paralysis (3–4 min).[44]

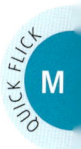

2 Recovery time may be delayed in some individuals possibly due to variations in plasma cholinesterase activity. In patients with atypical plasma cholinesterase recovery may be delayed > 6 h.[47]

3 Neostigmine may not effectively reverse blockade in these patients.[48] Neostigmine reversal of profound mivacurium neuromuscular blockage may cause prolongation of block due to impairment of plasma cholinesterase activity. Endophonium may be preferable to neostigmine for reversal due to this inhibition effect.[46]

4 Histamine release can occur causing flushing and hypotension, especially if the drug is given rapidly (<10–15 sec).[46]

Dose

Adult 0.2–0.25 mg/kg[48]

Top-Up-Dose 0.1 mg/kg required at ≈ 15 min intervals.

Infusion Dose 0.36–0.42 mg/kg/h.

Child 0.1–0.2 mg/kg

Top-Up-Dose 0.1 mg/kg

Infusion Dose 0.6–1 mg/kg/h.

◗ Monoamine Oxidase (MAO) Inhibitor Drugs

These drugs are used in the treatment of severe depression when other drugs are unsuccessful, and in the treatment of Parkinson's disease (selegiline).[49] These medications are of 2 types: non-selective MAO inhibitors and selective drugs for inhibition of MAO B or A.

Non-selective MAOI Drugs

These include phenelzine and tranylcypromine. These medications are associated with hypertensive crises if tyramine or phenylethylamine-containing foods are ingested. Drug interactions include:

1 Use of indirectly acting sympathomimetic drugs such as ephedrine, metaraminol and phenylephrine can precipitate a sympathetic discharge leading to life-threatening hypertension and/or hyperthermia. Direct acting sympathetic drugs such as adrenaline are not contraindicated.

2 Pethidine administration can lead to severe hypotension, profound respiratory depression, agitation, hypertension, seizures and coma.[50] Fentanyl and morphine can be used safely.

3 Reserpine, methyldopa and guanethidine may also precipitate hypertension.[51]

4 Levodopa and imipramine are also contraindicated.

5 Cocaine should also be avoided as it inhibits reuptake of noradrenaline leading to a build-up.

If elective surgery is planned consider stopping MAOI drugs 2 weeks prior to anaesthesia.[51]

However some authors suggest that the risk of suicide is greater than the risk of avoidable drug reactions and recommend continuance.[50]

Treatment of Hypertensive Crisis
Give phentolamine 2.5–5 mg IV boluses and titrate to blood pressure.

Selective MAOI Drugs
These drugs include selective MAO B inhibitors such as selegiline, and MAO A inhibitors such as moclobamide. Selegiline and moclobamide are associated with much less potential for hypertensive crisis after exposure to tyramine or phenylethylamine orally.

Moclobamide has a half life of only 4 h. *Use with pethidine is contraindicated.* Indirectly acting sympathomimetic drugs such as ephedrine should *NOT* be used with moclobamide.[52]

◐ Morphine

See also *Morphine, Extended Release Epidural* below. Morphine is an alkaloid of opium used for:

1 analgesia (agonist at mu 1, delta and kappa opioid receptors). **See** *Opioid Receptors*.
2 cough suppression and control of diarrhoea.
3 treatment of pulmonary oedema.

Dose Adult
IM/Subcut 0.1–0.2 mg/kg up to 4 h as required. Subcutaneous morphine is less painful for patients and is the preferred route.

IV 2–2.5 mg 5 min (up to 10–15 mg) until pain is controlled.

IV Infusion 1 mg/kg morphine in 500 mL N/S. Run the infusion at 10–40 mL/h (10–40 µg/kg/h).

Epidural Use preservative free morphine. In adults give 3 mg. This provides analgesia for about 12 h. However it takes about 1 h for the pain relief to be effective.[53]
Note: there is a risk of delayed respiratory depression with epidural morphine.

Intrathecal Use preservative free morphine. A suitable dose for e.g. hip replacement or CS is 100 µg.[54,55] Analgesia lasts 12 h or longer. Increasing the dose of intrathecal morphine increases the incidence and severity of pruritis but not nausea and vomiting.[55]
Note: there is a risk of delayed respiratory depression with intrathecal morphine.

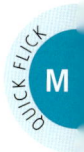

Oral For every 10 mg IM of morphine use 30 mg PO. Oral forms of morphine and average starting doses for adults and frequency include:

1   Kapanol capsules—sustained release 20 mg 12–24 h.
2   MS Contin-controlled release 30 mg 12 h.
3   Ordine (morphine oral liquid) immediate release 5–20 mg 4 h.

If converting morphine immediate release to sustained release preparation, divide the total daily dose of immediate release preparation by 2. For example if taking oridine 100 mg/day give MS contin 50 mg 12 h.

Dose Child

IM or Subcutaneously 0.1–0.15 mg/kg via a subcutaneous cannula (preferably placed intraoperatively).

IV Load 0.15 mg/kg morphine in 10 mL N/S in a syringe. Give incrementally 1 mL per 5 min to control pain.

IV Infusion Load 1 mg/kg morphine in 50 mL of 5% glucose. Run the infusion at 0.5–2.5 mL/h = 10–50 μg/kg/h.

Important Side Effects of Morphine

1   Drowsiness, sedation and euphoria (kappa receptor agonist effects). There is a risk of dependence due to these effects.
2   Respiratory depression (mu 2 agonist). This can be delayed in the case of intrathecal/epidural morphine.
3   Pruritus, nausea and vomiting.
4   Spasm of the sphincter of Oddi may occur increasing bile duct pressure.
5   Urinary retention.
6   Epidural morphine may reactivate herpes simplex labialis virus in obstetric patients.[56]
7   Morphine causes histamine release and is traditionally avoided in asthmatic patients. ***See*** *Asthma*.

Treatment of Side Effects

1   For life threatening respiratory depression in adults give naloxone 100 μg increments. For children give naloxone 2 μg/kg/dose repeated every 2 min. ***See*** *Naloxone*.
2   For pruritus consider the following strategies:
    a) Naloxone in small incremental doses e.g. 40 μg bolus IV repeated 5 min as needed × 5 doses.
    b) For patients with treatment-resistant pruritis on PCA morphine consider changing the patient to fentanyl PCA.
3   For nausea and vomiting from morphine PCA consider adding droperidol 2.5 mg per 100 mg PCA morphine.[57]

Morphine and Renal/Liver Failure

Use morphine cautiously in renal failure due to the accumulation of the metabolite morphine-6-glucuronide which can cause severe respiratory depression and decreased level of consciousness. Also use morphine cautiously in liver failure as hepatic encephalopathy may be precipitated.

◗ Morphine, Extended Release Epidural

This drug (DepoDur) is morphine bound to multivesicular lipid particles and is administered to adults epidurally in the lumbar or lower thoracic region. The morphine is released slowly from the lipid particles providing analgesia for 48 h.[58]

Indications

DepoDur is indicated for epidural injection in the lumbar and lower thoracic region only. This drug cannot be used with LA solutions in the epidural space because this causes premature release of the drug. A test dose of 2% lignocaine 3 mL can be used epidurally, but a period of at least 15 min must elapse and the catheter flushed with 1 mL of N/S before DepoDur is injected.

Dose

The maximum dose is 10 mg.[59] A dose of 7.5 mg or less should be considered in the elderly. Do not inject DepoDur through the epidural filter.

Side effects/Precautions

1 Do not use DepoDur with epidural LA solutions as this will cause premature release of the morphine. DepoDur cannot be used in association with CS if epidural LA has been used for labour pain. When DepoDur has been used for CS it has been injected after the cord was clamped. If performing CS under regional anaesthesia, use a CSE technique with LA injected intrathecally only.
2 As with standard morphine epidurally, respiratory depression can occur with DepoDur and patients require appropriate monitoring for 48 h.
3 Pruritis may occur.

◗ Muscarinic Receptors

See *Cholinergic Receptors*.

◗ Multifocal Atrial Tachycardia

See *Supraventricular Tachycardias (SVT)*.

◗ Myasthenia Gravis

Myasthenia gravis (MG) is a progressive autoimmune disease in which acetylcholine receptors at the neuromuscular junction are inactivated by anti-acetylcholine receptor antibodies and T-cells. This results in weakness and rapid fatigue of the affected skeletal muscle. The disease is associated

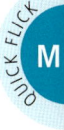

with thymus gland abnormalities, and thymectomy is frequently beneficial. The incidence of this condition is 1 per 30 000.[60] About two-thirds of sufferers are female.[60] Types of MG (as described by Osserman and Genkins)[61] are:

1. TYPE I—only involves extraocular muscles.
2. TYPE IIA—slowly progressive mild muscle weakness. Muscles of respiration spared.
3. TYPE IIB—severe and rapidly progressive muscle weakness. Muscles of respiration may be involved.
4. TYPE III—fulminant form of MG with rapid progression and high mortality.
5. TYPE IV—severe disease resulting from a progression of type I or II.

The disease may be exacerbated by conditions such as pregnancy, surgery and viral illness.[62]

Conditions Associated with Myasthenia Gravis

1. Cardiomyopathy and cardiac dysrhythmias.
2. Other autoimmune conditions such as rheumatoid arthritis and SLE.
3. Thymoma. This neoplasm can cause airway or vascular obstruction. **See** *Mediastinal Mass and Anaesthesia*.

Treatment of MG

1. Anticholinesterase inhibitor drugs such as pyridostigmine.
2. Corticosteroids.
3. Plasmapheresis.
4. IV immunoglobulin.
5. Immunosuppressive drugs such as azathioprine and cyclophosphamide.
6. Thymectomy.
7. Patients may take propantheline to block the muscarinic effects of anticholinesterase drugs.

Cholinergic Crisis and Myasthenic Crisis

An overdosage of anticholinesterase drugs can result in a cholinergic crisis. Effects include:

1. Muscle fasciculation and severe weakness.
2. Sweating and salivation.
3. Pallor.
4. Bradycardia.
5. Constricted pupils.

Myasthenic crisis is the development of severe weakness due to an exacerbation of MG. These conditions can be distinguished by injection of edrophonium 2 mg IV. In cholinergic crisis the muscle weakness will get worse and in a myasthenic crisis the weakness should improve. Treat cholinergic crisis with antimuscarinic drugs (atropine) and respiratory support.

Anaesthetic Considerations

1 Patients on immunosuppressive drugs and/or steroids should be considered for prophylactic antibiotic therapy.

2 Provide increased corticosteroid dosage to patients on long-term steroid therapy to cover the stress of surgery. **See** *Steroid Cover*.

3 In poorly controlled patients consider preoperative plasmapheresis.

4 Continue pyridostigmine up to the time of surgery.

5 Be prepared for the potential need to ventilate patients postoperatively. It is suggested that the need for postoperative ventilation is more likely in patients with:[63]

  a) duration of disease > 6 years.

  b) history of coexisting respiratory disease.

  c) daily dose of of pyridostigmine > 750 mg/day.

  d) vital capacity < 2.9 L.

6 Although initially stable postoperatively, patients may suffer respiratory impairment some hours after surgery. Therefore monitor these patients in a high dependency area.

7 Use opioids with caution due to inhibitory effects on ventilation.

8 The patient's anticholinesterase inhibitor medication may have to be given IV until oral intake is re-established. Equivalent doses are:[64]

  a) neostigmine   1 mg IV = 30 mg PO

  b) pyridostigmine 4 mg IV = 120 mg PO

  c) neostigmine   1 mg IV = pyridostigmine 30 mg PO.

Myasthenia Gravis and Neuromuscular Blocking Drugs

1 Patients with MG may require an increased dose of suxamethonium (1.5–2 mg/kg) but the effects of suxamethonium may last longer than in other people.

2 MG patients may be exquisitely sensitive to non-depolarising neuromuscular blocking drugs (NDNMBD). Consider titrating small doses of intermediate duration NMBD to assess their effects. Do not use long-acting NDNMBDs such as pancuronium.

3 A NDNMBD may not be necessary for intubation and ventilation in these patients when anaesthetised. Modern volatile agents such as sevoflurane and desflurane can depress neuromuscular transmission in myasthenics.[60]

4 Cisatracurium may produce more predictable results than vecuronium.[65]

5 Mivacurium may have a prolonged action in patients taking pyridostigmine.

6 NMBDs can be reversed by atropine and neostigmine but this can precipitate a cholinergic crisis. The best course of action is a controversial and unresolved issue. It may be preferable to await spontaneous recovery. Sugammadex may prove to be useful in this situation if rocuronium is used.

7 Only extubate the patient when there is evidence of adequate muscle strength for ventilation.

Myasthenia Gravis and Non-anaesthetic Drugs

1 Aminoglycoside antibiotics may exacerbate weakness in myasthenics.

2 β adrenergic blocking drugs can also cause increased weakness.

Myasthenia Gravis and Pregnancy

1 About 30% of women with MG experience a worsening of their condition during pregnancy.[66]

2 About 12% of infants born to mothers with MG will suffer weakness lasting about 18 days due to placental transfer of maternal antibodies.[66]

⟡ Myocardial Infarction (MI)

Topics Covered in this Section

▶ Effects of Recent MI on Peri-operative Risk

▶ Diagnosis of Peri-operative MI

▶ Management of Peri-operative MI

Effects of Recent MI on Peri-operative Risk

An acute MI is defined as an MI within the past 7 days. A recent MI is defined as an MI >7 days but <4 weeks ago. A recent MI is an 'active cardiac condition' and thus a major predictor of cardiac risk for non-cardiac surgery.[67] These patients should have referral to a cardiologist and coronary revascularisation prior to non-cardiac surgery. A history of MI (or abnormal Q waves on the ECG) is a 'clinical risk factor' for non-cardiac surgery, indicating intermediate risk. If a recent stress test does not indicate residual myocardium is at risk then the risk of reinfarction is low and non-cardiac surgery can be undertaken 4–6 weeks post infarct. *See Cardiovascular Peri-operative Risk Prediction for Non-cardiac Surgery* and *Coronary Artery Revascularisation Procedures and Subsequent Non-cardiac Surgery*.

Diagnosis of Peri-operative MI

1 Chest pain/diaphoresis in awake patients.

2 ECG changes. For 12-lead ECG changes *see Electrocardiography*. May see ST segment elevation > 1 mm measured 0.04 s after the J point, T wave inversion, new onset LBBB. With posterior MI may see ST depression in leads V1–V4. Priebe noted that most pre-operative myocardial infarcts occur early after surgery, and are associated with ST-segment depression rather than elevation.[68] Most are non-Q wave infarcts.

3 Biochemical evidence of peri-operative MI includes elevated troponin levels. A troponin level of 0.05–0.1 μg/L suggests minor cardiac damage, while a reading of >0.1 μg/L indicates significant cardiac damage/infarction.

Management of Peri-operative MI

Aims of Treatment

1 Optimise oxygen delivery to the myocardium.

2 Reduce myocardial oxygen demand.

3 Reperfusion of the ischaemic myocardium. Options include urgent angioplasty, stenting or coronary artery bypass grafts. Thrombolytic therapy should be considered but will usually be contraindicated after significant surgery.

4 Adequate analgesia in the awake patient. Obtain urgent cardiological opinion. Ideally stenting should be undertaken within 90 min of myocardial infarction.[69]

5 Continuous ECG monitoring to detect dysrhythmias particularly VF.

Optimising myocardial oxygenation and reducing myocardial oxygen demand are discussed below in the section on peri-operative myocardial ischaemia.

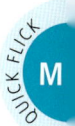

▷ Myocardial Ischaemia, Peri-operative

Topics Covered in this Section

▶ Factors Determining Myocardial O_2 Supply

▶ Factors Determining Myocardial O_2 Demand

▶ Prevention of Myocardial Ischaemia

▶ Detection of Myocardial Ischaemia

▶ Treatment of Myocardial Ischaemia

Factors Determining Myocardial O_2 Supply

Myocardial ischaemia occurs when O_2 supply to the myocardium fails to meet O_2 demand. The main determinants of O_2 supply are coronary blood flow and O_2 content of arterial blood. Coronary blood flow is determined by heart rate, diastolic blood pressure (80% of total flow occurs during diastole), coronary artery calibre, cardiac output and blood viscosity.

Factors Determining Myocardial O_2 Demand

Myocardial O_2 demand is determined by heart rate, myocardial wall tension and basal metabolic requirements. Oxygen demand is thus increased if afterload and/or preload increases or contractility increases or heart rate increases. Myocardial O_2 demand is nearly proportional to the tension time index (= tension in heart muscle during contraction × duration of contraction).

Prevention of Myocardial Ischaemia

The underlying principles in preventing myocardial ischaemia are to optimise factors which improve myocardial O_2 supply and reduce O_2 demand. Strategies include:

1 β blockers used to control heart rate (**see** *Beta-blocker Therapy and Reduction of Cardiac Risk*).

2   Alpha-2 adreno-receptor agonists such as clonidine and mivazerol have also been shown to reduce the incidence of peri-operative ischaemia.[70] These drugs should be considered for peri-operative control of hypertension in patients with known IHD or at least one risk factor undergoing surgery.[67]

3   Statin therapy. Peri-operative statin therapy (e.g. atorvastatin) reduced mortality by 44% in a meta-analysis by Hindler and colleagues.[71] *See Statin Therapy*.

4   Severe cardiac valve lesions should be considered for repair or replacement.

5   Peri-operative arrhythmias such as rapid AF should be corrected or controlled. Anti-dysrhythmia pacing/cardio version/defibrillation via an implanted pacemaker/defibrillator may also be beneficial.

6   Patients with major cardiac conduction defects e.g. complete heart block should be considered for pacemaker therapy prior to surgery. *See Pacing, Pacemakers and Anaesthesia*.

7   There is some evidence that calcium channel blocker drugs may be of benefit.[67]

8   Patients with unstable coronary syndromes or other evidence of severe IHD may benefit from coronary artery revascularisation procedures e.g. angioplasty, stenting, CABG. *See Cardiovascular Peri-operative Risk Prediction for Non-cardiac Surgery*.

9   Aspirin therapy preoperatively may be of benefit.[68]

10 Continue patient's antianginal drugs throughout the peri-operative period.

11 Volatile anaesthetic agents may precondition and post condition the heart against infarction.[67]

12 Prophylactic IV nitroglycerin is probably not effective for the prevention of myocardial ischaemia.[72]

13 Correct anaemia. Aim for a Hb of about 10 g/100 mL.

14 Prevent/correct hypothermia which is associated with postoperative myocardial ischaemia.[68]

15 Minimise peri-operative pain. Pain activates sympathetic tone which may lead to myocardial ischaemia.[68]

16 Continue supplementary O_2 therapy well into the postoperative period.

Detection of Myocardial Ischaemia

1   Chest pain/diaphoresis in awake patients.

2   ECG and ST segment analysis. *See ST Segment Analysis* for a description of the ECG changes associated with ischaemia. For lead positions to optimise detection of ischaemia *see Electrocardiography*.

Pulmonary Artery Catheter Findings

Pulmonary capillary wedge pressure typically rises significantly with myocardial ischaemia to > 15 mm Hg. In addition, V waves > 20 mm Hg may occur.

Transoesophageal Echocardiography
May show wall motion abnormalities and wall thickening.

Treatment of Myocardial Ischaemia

Myocardial ischaemia is treated by maximising oxygen supply to the myocardium and optimising preload, afterload, heart rate and myocardial contractility. Steps in management include:

1 Notify the surgeon and request that surgery be cancelled or expedited if possible.
2 Maximise O_2 delivery to the myocardium by ventilation with 100% O_2.
3 Correct anaemia. Transfuse to a haemoglobin of 10 g/100 mL.
4 Optimise heart rate to 60–80 bpm. Sinus tachycardia may be due to nocioceptive stimuli or light anaesthesia.
5 Ensure adequate anaesthesia and analgesia. Treat dysrhythmias as described in the relevant sections.
6 Use nitrates if pre-load is adequate or excessive to reduce pre-load and to dilate epicardial coronary vessels. Use GTN. *See Glyceryl Trinitrate*. Sublingual nitroglycerine 0.3 mg can be used while a GTN infusion is being organised.
7 If pre-load is inadequate e.g. due to haemorrhage, fluid load the patient.
8 Correct afterload issues. If inadequate afterload is causing hypotension treat with a vasoconstrictor e.g. metaraminol. If excessive afterload is causing or contributing to myocardial ischaemia ensure adequate anaesthesia and analgesia. Consider afterload reduction with an arterial vasodilator e.g. SNP. *See Sodium Nitroprusside (SNP)*.
9 Insertion of an intra-aortic balloon pump will improve myocardial perfusion during diastole.
10 Plan for urgent cardiologist review and possible ICU admission.
See Myocardial Infarction (MI) above.

REFERENCES

1 Gomez MN. Magnesium and cardiovascular disease. *Anesthesiology* 1988; 89: 222–40.
2 Donovan KD, Hockings BEF. Antiarrhythmic Drugs. In: Oh TE, ed. *Intensive Care Manual*, 4th edn. Butterworth–Heinemann, Oxford 1997: 102.
3 Fagan C, Phelan D. Severe convulsant hypomagnesaemia and short bowel syndrome. *Anaesth Intensive Care* 2001; 29: 281–3.
4 Bramwell S. Preterm Labour. In Datta S, ed. *Common Problems in Obstetric Anaesthesia*, 2nd edn. Mosby-Year Book Inc, St Louis Missouri 1995: 301–5.
5 Kowal A, Panaszek B, Barg W, Obojski A. The use of magnesium in bronchial asthma: a new approach to an old problem. *Achivum Immunologiae et Therapiae Experimentalis* 2007; 55: 35–9.

6   Patteson SK, Chesney JT. Anesthetic management for magnetic resonance imaging: problems and solutions. *Anesth Analg* 1992; 74: 121–8.

7   Gomillion M, Han JH. Magnetic Resonance Imaging. In Yao F-S, Fontes ML, Malhotra V, eds. *Yao and Artusio's Anesthesiology: Problem-Orientated Patient Management*, 6th edn. Lippincott Williams and Wilkins, Philadelphia, Pennsylvania 2008: 1231–48.

8   McBrien ME, Winder J, Smyth L. Anaesthesia for magnetic resonance imaging: a survey of current practice in the UK and Ireland. *Anaesthesia* 2000; 55: 737–43.

9   Rosewarne F. *Anaesthetic equipment*, 2nd edn. Self Published 1999; 259–65.

10 Langton JA, Wilson I, Fell D. Use of the laryngeal mask airway during magnetic resonance imaging. *Anaesthesia* 1992; 47: 532–3.

11 Gronert GA. Malignant hyperthermia. *Anesthesiology* 1980; 53: 396.

12 Brand JC. Preoperative diagnosis of malignant hyperthermia. *South African J Anaesth Analges* 2003 Feb: 10–13.

13 Ellis FR, Halsall PJ. Malignant hyperthermia. *Anaesthesia and Intensive Care Medicine* 2002; 3: 222–5.

14 Strazis KP, Fox AW. Malignant hyperthermia: A review of published cases. *Anesth Analg* 1993; 77: 297–304.

15 *Guidelines from the Malignant Hyperpyrexia Association of the United States*—MH protocol poster current May 2008, www.medical.mhaus.org (accessed July 2008).

16 Sims C. Masseter spasm after suxamethonium in children. *Br J Hosp Med* 1992; 47: 2: 139–43.

17 Slinger P, Karsli C. Management of the patient with a large anterior mediastinal mass: recurring myths. *Curr Opin Anaesthesiology* 2007; 20: 1–3.

18 Mackie AM et al. Anaesthesia and mediastinal masses. *Anaesthesia* 1984 39; 899–903.

19 Pullerits J, Holzman R. Anaesthesia for patients with mediastinal masses. *Can J Anaesth* 1989; 36: 681–8.

20 Neumann GG, Weingarten AE, Abramowitz RM et al. The anesthetic management of the patient with an anterior mediastinal mass. *Anesthesiology* 1984; 60: 144–7.

21 Lewer BMF, Torrance JM. Anaesthesia for a patient with a mediastinal mass presenting with acute stridor. *Anaesth Intensive Care* 1996; 24: 605–8.

22 Azizkhan RG, Dudgeon DL, Buck JR et al. Life threatening airway obstruction as a complication to the management of mediastinal masses in children. *J Pediatr Surg* 1985; 20: 816–22.

23 Peng PWH, Tumber PS, Gourlay D. Review Article: Perioperative pain management of patients on methadone therapy. *Can J Anesth* 2005; 52: 513–23.

24 Johnson D. Editorial: Methemoglobinaremia. *Can J Anesth* 2005; 52: 665–8.

25 Hirshman C. Perioperative management of the asthmatic patient. *Can J Anaesth* 1991; 38: 4: 26–32.

26 Henzi I, Walder B, Tramér MR. Metoclopramide in the prevention of postoperative nausea and vomiting—a quantitative systemic review of randomized placebo-controlled studies. *Br J Anaesth* 1999; 83: 761–71.

27 Kim MH, Lee YM. Intrathecal midazolam increases the analgesic effects of spinal blockade with bupivacaine in patients undergoing haemorrhoidectomy. *Br J Anaesth* 2001; 86: 77–9.

28 Tucker AP, Lai C, Nadeson R, Goodchild CS. Intrathecal midazolam I: a cohort study investigating safety. *Anesth Analg* 2004; 98: 1512–20.

29 Bozkurt P, Tunali Y, Kaya G, Okar I. Histological changes following epidural injection of midazolam in the neonatal rabbit. *Paediatr Anaesth* 1997; 7: 385–9.

30 Erdine S, Yucel A, Ozyalcin S et al. Neurotoxicity of midazolam in the rabbit. *Pain* 1999; 80: 419–23.

31 Demirel E, Ugur HC, Dolgun H et al. The neurotoxin effects of intrathecal midazolam and neostimine in rabbits. *Anaesth Intensive Care* 2006; 34: 218–23.

32 Kim MH, Lee YM. Intrathecal midazolam increases the analgesic effects of spinal blockade with bupivacaine in patients undergoing haemorrhoidectomy. *Br J Anaesth* 2001; 86: 77–9.

33 Borg PA, Krijinen HJ. Long term intrathecal administration of midazolam and clonidine. *Clin J Pain* 1996; 12: 63–8.

34 Donnell CG, Harte S, O'Driscoll J et al. The effects of concurrent atorvastatin therapy on the pharmacokinetics of intravenous midazolam. *Anaesthesia* 2003; 58: 874–910.

35 Skoyles JR, Sherry KM. Pharmacology, mechanisms of action and uses of selective phosphodiesterase inhibitors. *Br J Anaesth* 1992; 68: 293–302.

36 Jaski BE, Fifer MA, Wright RF et al. Positive inotropic and vasodilator actions of milrinone in patients with severe congestive heart failure. Dose-response relationships and comparison to nitroprusside. *J Clin Invest* 1985; 75: 643–9.

37 Stoelting RK, Dierdorf SF. *Anesthesia and Co-existing disease*, 4th edn. Churchill Livingstone, New York 2002: 32–5.

38 Mangano DT. Anesthesia for the Pregnant Cardiac Patient. In Hughes SC, Levinson G, Rosen MA, eds. *Shneider and Levison's Anaesthesia for Obstetrics*. Lippincott Williams & Wilkins, Philadelphia, 2002: 455–86.

39 Report of the American College Cardiology/American Heart Association Task Force on Practice Guidelines. ACC/AHA 2007 Guidelines on perioperative cardiovascular evaluation and care for non cardiac surgery. *Circulation* 2007; 116: e418–e499.

QUICK FLICK

M

40 Ngan Kee WD, Shen J, Chui ATO et al. Combined spinal epidural anaesthesia in the management of labouring patients with mitral stenosis. *Anaesth Intensive Care* 1999; 27: 523–6.

41 Reimold SC, Rutherford JD. Valvular heart disease in pregnancy. *N Eng J Med* 2003; 349: 52–9.

42 Stoelting RK, Dierdorf SF. *Anesthesia and Co-existing Disease*, 4th edn. Churchill Livingstone, New York, 2002: 32–5.

43 Reich DL, Mittnacht A, Kaplan JA. Uncommon Cardiac Diseases. In: Fleisher LA ed. *Anesthesia and Uncommon Diseases*, 5th edn. Saunders Elsevier, Philadelphia Pennsylvania 2006: 29–76.

44 Feldman S. Drug focus—mivacurium. *Br J Hosp Med* 1997; 57: 199–200.

45 Bettelli G. Which muscle relaxants should be used for day surgery and when. *Curr Opin Anaesthesiol* 2006; 19: 600–5.

46 Bevan DR. The new relaxants: are they worth it? (refresher course outline). *Can J Anesth* 1999; 46: R88–R94.

47 Goudsouzian NG, d'Hollander AA, Viby-Morgensen J. Prolonged neuromuscular block from mivacurium in two patients with cholinesterase deficiency. *Anesth Analg* 1993; 77: 183–5.

48 Cade L, Kakulas P. Mivacurium in daycase surgical patients. *Anesth Intensive Care* 1997; 25: 133–7.

49 Morris JGL. Selective monoamine oxidase inhibitors—clinical applications in neurology. *Australian Prescriber* 1993; 16(3): 57–8.

50 Malhotra V. Brachial plexus block. In Yao FSF, Artusio JF, eds. *Anesthesiology; Problem Orientated Patient Management,* 4th edn. JB Lippincott-Raven Philadelphia,1998: 535.

51 Lippman S, Nash K. Monoamine oxidase inhibitor uptake—potential adverse food and drug reactions. *Current Therapeutics* 1991 (February): 76–82.

52 Mcfarlane HJ. Anaesthesia and the new generation of monoamine oxidase inhibitors. *Anaesthesia* 1994; 49: 597–9.

53 Cousins MJ, Mather LE. Intrathecal and epidural opioids. *Anesthesiology* 1984; 61: 276–310.

54 Murphy PM, Stack D, Kinirons B, Laffey JG. Optimising the dose of intrathecal morphine in older patients undergoing hip arthroplasty. *Anesth Analg* 2003; 97: 1709–15.

55 Palmer CM, Emerson S, Volgoropolous D. Dose-relationship of intrathecal morphine for postcesarean analgesia. *Anesthesiology* 1999; 90: 437–44.

56 Chaney MA. Review Article: Side effects of intrathecal and epidural opioids. *Can J Anaesth* 1995; 42: 891–903.

57 Tramér MR. A rational approach to the control of postoperative nausea and vomiting: evidence from systemic reviews. Part II. Recommendations

for prevention and treatment, and research agenda. *Acta Anaesthesiol Scand* 2001; 45: 14–19.

58 Viscusi ER, Martin G, Hartrick CT et al. Forty-eight hours of postoperative pain relief after total hip arthroplasty with a novel, extended-release epidural morphine formulation. *Anesthesiology* 2005; 102: 1014–22.

59 DepoDur Product Information, Pacira Pharmaceuticals Inc, December 2007.

60 Lien CA, Poznak AV. Myasthenia Gravis. In Yao FSF, Artusio JF, eds. *Anesthesiology: Problem Orientated Patient Management*, 4th edn. JB Lippincott-Raven Philadelphia,1998: 867–77.

61 Osserman KE, Genkins G. Studies in myasthenia gravis: review of a twenty-year experience in over 1200 patients. *Mt Sinai J Med* 1971; 38: 497–538.

62 Kaldindi M, Ganport S, Tahmesebi F et al. Myasthenia gravis and pregnancy. *J Obstet Gynaecol* 2007; 27: 30–2.

63 Eisenkraft JB, Papatestas AD, Kahn CH et al. Predicting the need for postoperative mechanical ventilation in myasthenia gravis. *Anesthesiology* 1986; 65: 760–3.

64 Mason R. *Anaesthesia Databook: A Perioperative and Peripartum Manual* 3rd edn. Greenwich Medical Media Ltd, London 2001: 343.

65 Alley C, Dierdorf SF. Myasthenia gravis and muscular dystrophies. *Curr Opin Anaesthesiol* 1997;10: 248–53.

66 Urban MK, Lahlou S. Muscle Diseases. In: Fleisher LA ed. *Anesthesia and Uncommon Diseases* 5th edn. Saunders Elsevier, Philadelphia Pennsylvania 2006: 303–25.

67 Report of the American College Cardiology/American Heart Association Task Force on Practice Guidelines. ACC/AHA 2007 Guidelines on perioperative cardiovascular evaluation and care for non cardiac surgery. *Circulation* 2007; 116: e418–e499.

68 Priebe H-J. Review article: Perioperative myocardial infarction—aetiology and prevention. *Br J Anaesth* 2005; 95: 3–19.

69 DeGeare VS, Dangas G, Stone GW, Grines CL. Interventional procedures in acute myocardial infarction. *Am Heart J* 2001; 131: 15–24.

70 Wijeysundera DN, Naik JS, Beattie WS. Alpha-2 adrenergic agonists to prevent perioperative cardiovascular complications: a meta-analysis. *Am J Med* 2003; 114: 742–52.

71 Hindler K, Shaw A, Samuels J et al. Improved postoperative outcomes associated with preoperative statin therapy. *Anesthesiology* 2006; 105: 1260–72.

72 Dodds TM, Stone JG, Coromilas J et al. Prophylactic nitroglycerin infusion during noncardiac surgery does not reduce perioperative ischaemia. *Anesth Analg* 1993; 76: 705–13.

QUICK FLICK

M

N

○ N-acetyl Cysteine (NAC)

NAC is the treatment of choice for paracetamol poisoning. NAC therapy is also possibly useful for the prevention of peri-operative renal failure in at-risk patients having procedures associated with potential kidney insult. It may act by attenuating oxidative stress on the kidney by scavenging oxygen free radicals. It may also inhibit tumour necrosis factor by increasing glutathione concentrations. NAC has been shown to reduce contrast associated nephropathy in patients having radiological procedures by up to 90%.[1] However, some studies have shown no apparent benefit with NAC treatment.[2,3]

Dose
200 mg PO 12 h × 4 doses before the procedure. For patients at risk of renal failure having an emergency procedure, e.g. cardiac catheterisation, give NAC 150 mg in 500 mL N/S over 30 min immediately before IV contrast, then 50 mg/kg in 500 mL N/S over 4 h.[4]

Points to Note
N-acetyl cysteine appears to improve survival rates in early hepatorenal syndrome. **See** *Hepatorenal Syndrome (HRS)*.

○ Naloxone

Opioid receptor antagonist used to reverse the effects of opioid drugs, especially respiratory depression, nausea and vomiting as well as pruritus.

Dose for Respiratory Depression
Adult IV Bolus Dose 50–100 μg. Acts within 2 min and effects last for 20 min. Additional doses may therefore be required.
IV Infusion Dose 4 μg/kg/h.
Child 2 μg/kg/dose, repeat every 2 min.

Dose for Pruritis Due to Opioids in Adults
40 μg IV 5 min × 5 doses as needed.
Note: Naloxone should not be used as part of the initial resuscitation of newborns in the delivery suite until appropriate ventilation is given based on the infant's colour and heart rate.[5] Naloxone should not be given to newborns whose mothers are suspected or known to abuse opioids as this may precipitate abrupt withdrawal in the newborn.[5]

○ Nasal Anaesthesia

See *Awake Fibre-optic Intubation*.

○ Nasal Mucosa Vasoconstrictors

Include the following:
1 Cocaine. **See** *Awake Fibre-optic Intubation and Cocaine*.
2 Cophenylcaine forte spray.
3 Drixine drops (oxymetazoline HCl).

○ Nausea and Vomiting, Postoperative (PONV)

The overall incidence of postoperative nausea and vomiting (PONV) is about 20–30%.[6]

Patient Factors Associated with PONV
1 females, paediatric patients
2 history of PONV and/or motion sickness
3 non-smokers.

Surgical/Anaesthetic Factors Associated with PONV
1 use of volatile agents and/or N_2O
2 laparoscopic surgery, intra-abdominal surgery
3 opioids
4 doses of neostigmine > 2.5 mg
5 long surgical procedure.

Prevention Strategies for PONV
1 Routine prophylactic anti-emetic therapy is not cost effective. For more information on each drug see individual entries.
2 Consider prophylactic antiemetic therapy for at risk patients using a 5-hydroxytryptamine 3 (5-HT_3) receptor antagonist drug such as ondansetron combined with dexamethasone. These drugs are superior to the more traditional anti-nausea drugs such as metoclopramide.
3 Generous IV hydration.
4 Aggressive pain control with non-opioid analgesic drugs.
5 Avoidance of N_2O.[7]
6 Total IV anaesthesia with propofol with avoidance of volatile anaesthetic drugs.[8]
7 Postoperative O_2 therapy.[9]
8 New agents coming onto the market include aprepitant, a neurokinin-1 antagonist. The dose is 40 mg PO 1–3 h before surgery. Several trials have shown this drug to be superior to ondansetron. [10]

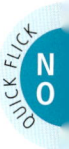

Treatment of PONV

1 ondansetron 4 mg
2 droperidol 0.625 mg

◖ Neck Haematoma

Seen most commonly after thyroid surgery and carotid endarterectomy. Neck haematoma can result in fatal airway compression and make direct laryngoscopy impossible.

Management

1 Notify the surgeon and arrange for an operating theatre urgently.
2 If the airway is threatened by significant haematoma, attempt to release the haematoma under LA infiltration (open up the incision). This can be life saving.[11]
3 If the above measure is not successful, spray tongue and pharynx with LA and attempt awake direct laryngoscopy. If able to see the vocal cords easily, administer GA and muscle relaxants and intubate.
4 If not able to see the vocal cords, decide whether the cause for this is likely to be reversible, i.e. the patient is uncooperative. If the cause is reversible, conduct a gaseous induction of general anaesthesia and perform laryngoscopy when the patient is 'deep'. The surgeon should be scrubbed and ready for urgent tracheostomy. If able to see the vocal cords, paralyse and intubate. If unable to see vocal cords but the patient is easy to ventilate proceed with surgery.
5 If airway difficulties occur during gaseous induction or the decision is made that direct laryngoscopy is likely to fail, perform an awake intubation using either:
   a) Fibre-optic technique. *See* Awake Fibre-optic Intubation.
   b) Retrograde technique. *See* Difficult Airway Management.
   c) Consider using an optical laryngoscope. *See* Airtraq.
6 Alternatively direct the surgeon to perform a tracheostomy under LA infiltration.

◖ Needle-stick Injury

General Measures after Needle-stick Injury

1 Promoting active bleeding from the wound.
2 Clean the wound thoroughly with soap and water.
3 Notifying appropriate 'staff health' personnel if available for documentation of injury, management of infection prevention and counselling.

Human Immunodeficiency Virus (HIV) Infection

Overall the risk of HIV infection from a single needle-stick injury is ≈ 3 per 1000.[12] Apart from blood, high-risk fluids include CSF, pleural, peritoneal, synovial fluid and breast milk. Low-risk fluids are vomit, urine, faeces and saliva.[13]

HIV Infection Prophylaxis

Post-exposure prophylactic therapy should ideally commence within 1 h of injury and be continued for 4 weeks. Five classes of drugs are available:

1   nucleoside reverse transcriptase inhibitors, e.g. zidovudine.
2   nucleotide analogue reverse transcriptase inhibitor, e.g. tenofovir.
3   non-nucleoside reverse transcriptase inhibitors, e.g. efavirenz.
4   protease inhibitors, e.g. indinavir.
5   fusion inhibitor, e.g. enfuvirtide.
6   integrase inhibitors.

Usually 3 or more antiviral drugs in various combinations are taken, e.g. triple therapy with zidovudine, lamivudine and indinavir.[13] Treatment should be under the guidance of an HIV physician. Resistance to certain antiviral drugs in the needle-stick source patient will influence drug choice for prophylaxis. Further information on this complex issue can be obtained from the website of the Centers for Disease Control and Prevention. Appropriate prophylaxis should reduce the incidence of HIV seroconversion after needle stick to 1 per 1 000 000.[14] A rapid test for HIV is available providing results in 20 min with a sensitivity and specificity of about 99.8%.[14]

Hepatitis B

The risk of seroconversion after a needle-stick injury in a non-immunised individual is ≈ 30%. The non-immunised individual can be given a rapid Hep B vaccination course plus Hep B immunoglobulin after needle-stick injury. A chronic carrier state occurs in 10% of patients infected with Hep B. Of this group about 20% will die from complications of Hep B such as cirrhosis and hepatocellular carcinoma.[15] Hep B immunisation has greatly reduced the risk of this illness for health care workers.

Hepatitis C

The risk of Hep C transmission from a needle-stick injury is probably about 1.8%.[16] There is no effective infection prophylaxis at the time of writing. About 50% of people infected with Hep C develop chronic hepatitis and an estimated 20% of these will progress to cirrhosis.[17] Some of these patients will progress to hepatocellular carcinoma. The current recommendations are to observe the needle-stick victim for seroconversion for Hep C. If Hep C is transmitted, early treatment with interferon is highly effective in preventing chronic Hep C from developing.[18]

◗ Negative Pressure Pulmonary Oedema

Negative pressure pulmonary oedema is defined as transudation of fluid into the alveoli due to intense negative pressure produced by vigorous inspiratory

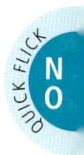

effort in the presence of upper airway obstruction, e.g. laryngospasm or biting the endotracheal tube. Maximum inspiratory effort against an upper airway obstruction can produce an intrathoracic pressure of 50–100 cm H_2O.[19] This condition can occur with a single breath and can cause significant hypoxia.

Treatment

1 Relieve the upper airway obstruction.
2 High concentration oxygen therapy.
3 CPAP in spontaneously breathing patients.
4 Diuretic therapy with lasix.

In severe cases mechanical ventilation with IPPV + PEEP may be required.

The pulmonary oedema normally resolves after 12–24 h with supportive therapy.[19]

▷ Neonatal Resuscitation

See *Newborn and Neonatal Resuscitation*.

▷ Neopuff

This device is essentially a T-piece circuit attached to an oxygen–air blender with a pressure gauge for measuring airway pressure. It is used for ventilation of the newborn. ***See*** *Newborn and Neonatal Resuscitation*. To set up the device:

1 Connect the gas supply to the inlet connection on the Neopuff casing. Ideally connect to medical air and oxygen. If only oxygen is available use this. Set the gas flow to 8 L/min. Start with air initially if available.
2 Adjust the inspiratory pressure control knob on the front panel to set the desired level of peak inflating pressure (≈ 30 cm H_2O). This is done by occluding the outlet aperture and turning the inspiratory pressure control knob clockwise until the desired pressure is achieved on the pressure gauge.
3 Next set the PEEP by twisting the knob on the distal end of the T-piece. Start with 5–8 cm H_2O.

Ventilate the newborn by occluding the outlet aperture (opposite the facemask) with a thumb or finger at a rate of 60 per minute with an inspiratory time of 0.5 sec. If after 90 s of effective ventilation HR < 90 change to 100% O_2.

▷ Neostigmine

This quaternary amine functions as a reversible, acid transferring cholinesterase inhibitor. Acts by binding to acetylcholinesterase, thus competing with acetylcholine binding. Used for the reversal of the effects of non-depolarising neuromuscular blocking drugs (NDNMBD) and in the treatment of myasthenia gravis. ***See*** *Myasthenia Gravis*.

IV Dose

For the reversal of NDNMBD: 50 µg/kg IV is given with an appropriate dose of anticholinergic drug. The maximum dose of neostigmine which can be used is 60–80 µg/kg.

Side Effects of IV Neostigmine

These can include bradycardia, excess salivation, abdominal cramps, bronchoconstriction and nausea/vomiting.

Intrathecal Use

Neostigmine has been used intrathecally in a dose of 25–100 µg. It is an effective analgesic agent but is associated with a high incidence of nausea and vomiting.[20] It can also cause bradycardia and agitation.

◗ Nerve Stimulator Positions

Common Peroneal Nerve

Attach the negative electrode (black) to the skin just behind the most lateral portion of the head of fibula and positive electrode (red) over the patella.

Facial Nerve Branches

Place the negative electrode just above and lateral to the orbit, and the positive electrode just lateral and below the orbit.

Ulnar Nerve

Place the negative electrode over the volar surface of the distal wrist on the ulnar side and the positive electrode just proximal to this. Stimulation results in adductor pollicis muscle activation.

Posterior Tibial Nerve

Place the negative electrode just posterior and distal to the medial malleolus and the positive electrode just posterior and proximal to medial malleolus. With stimulation plantar flexion of the toes is seen.

◗ Neuroanaesthesia

See also Cerebral Aneurysm Surgery.

Monitoring and Pre-operative Preparation

For major intracranial procedures such as removal of tumours:

1 Large bore IV access, e.g. 16 G cannula.
2 Peripherally placed central venous access.
3 Arterial line.
4 Precordial Doppler probe, if the risk of air embolus is high, such as when the sitting position is used. The Doppler probe should be placed over the right side of the heart (to the right of the sternum) between the third and sixth intercostal spaces.
5 Urinary catheter, temperature probe, nerve stimulator.

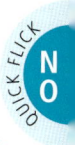

Induction and Maintenance

1 Alfentanyl 5–30 µg/kg is useful for attenuating the hypertensive response to intubation. Fentanyl ≈ 3 µg/kg can also be used but its onset time is slower. A remifentanil infusion can also be used with a bolus 0.5–1 µg/kg bolus prior to intubation.

2 Thiopentone—appropriate induction dose.

3 Give lignocaine 1–2 mg/kg at least 2 min before intubation.

4 Non-depolarising muscle relaxant of choice

5 Prior to intubation, spray the vocal cords and larynx with 3 mL of 4% topical lignocaine (adult). Do not intubate until the nerve stimulator indicates complete paralysis.

6 Secure the endotracheal tube carefully. An armoured tube is required if the patient is placed prone, in the sitting position or supine if the head is not in the neutral position. This is to prevent kinking of the endotracheal tube.

7 Maintain anaesthesia with isoflurane, sevoflurane and/or a propofol infusion. Desflurane, halothane and enflurane are not recommended for neuroanaesthesia (**see** *Desflurane and Halothane*). Nitrous oxide should not be used; it can cause an increase in ICP due to cerebral vasodilatation.[21] **See** *Nitrous Oxide*.

8 Maintain paralysis with a cisatracurium infusion 0.06–0.1 mg/kg/h.

9 Boluses of fentanyl as required. A remifentanil infusion can also be used.

10 The surgeon will frequently request the following:

   a) Mannitol 20% solution 0.25–1 g/kg IV.

   b) Phenytoin 15 mg/kg in N/S (not glucose). Max rate of administration 50 mg/min IV.

   c) Dexamethasone up to 20 mg IV.

11 Antibiotic cover such as cephazolin 1 g.

12 Ventilate, aiming for optimal oxygenation and moderate hypocapnia of ≈ 30 mm Hg CO_2. A lower $PaCO_2$ may cause cerebral ischaemia.[22] Check $PaCO_2$ formally on arterial blood gas sample.[22] It is preferable not to use positive end-expiratory pressure (PEEP) as it may cause increased intracranial pressure and a reduction in mean arterial pressure. PEEP does not protect against venous air embolism during neurosurgery in the sitting position.[23]

13 Do not infuse glucose containing solutions as elevated blood glucose levels can worsen cerebral ischaemic injury. Use N/S, which has a higher osmolarity than Hartmann's solution (300 mOsm/L vs 274 mOsm/L) and may therefore result in less brain swelling.[24]

14 If the patient is or becomes hypertensive, antihypertensive drugs to consider include the following:

   a) Thiopentone boluses are effective for treating sudden hypertension, e.g. at intubation.[25]

b) Clonidine 50 μg increments to a max of 300 μg.

c) β blocker, e.g. atenolol or esmolol.

d) Trimetaphan is a rapidly acting therapy with a similar onset time to sodium nitroprusside but causing less cerebral vasodilatation. However trimetaphan use is associated with a high incidence of bladder and bowel dysfunction and tachyphylaxis develops rapidly.

e) Sodium nitroprusside or glyceryl trinitrate may be used for hypertension unresponsive to the above drugs or when controlled hypotension is required. However both agents can cause increased intracranial pressure.[26]

15 Mild intra-operative hypothermia provides significant cerebral protection against ischaemia. The patient can be allowed to passively cool to ≈ 35°C until surgery is completed and closure begins. Active rewarming should then commence aiming for normothermia on emergence.[26]

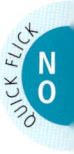

Emergence

Give 1–2 mg/kg lignocaine IV at least 2 min before extubation and consider extubating the patient 'deep' in order to minimise coughing.

○ Neuroleptic Malignant Syndrome (NMS)

This syndrome can be severe and potentially life threatening. It is triggered by drugs such as butyrophenones (haloperidol, droperidol), phenothiazines and thioxanthenes. NMS can also occur with the withdrawal of levodopa in Parkinson's disease.[27] The syndrome resembles, but is in no way related to, malignant hyperthermia. NMS is thought to be due to dopamine receptor blockade in the basal ganglia and the hypothalamus.[27] NMS has a high mortality ranging from 14% with oral drugs to 38% with parenteral drugs.[27]

Factors Predisposing to the Development of NMS

These include:

1 acute hyponatraemia[28]

2 pre-existing fever

3 stress/exhaustion

4 dehydration

5 pre-existing brain damage or dysfunction.

Clinical Presentation

NMS is characterised by:

1 Hyperpyrexia.

2 Muscle rigidity with excessive heat production. May see 'lead pipe' rigidity. The rigidity is a central effect, whereas in malignant hyperthermia the muscle rigidity is a direct peripheral effect.

3 Autonomic dysfunction.

4 Altered mental state.

5   Renal failure due to rhabdomyolysis.
6   Dyspnoea, respiratory failure.
7   Myocardial infarct and cardiac arrest.
8   Evidence of muscle damage (elevated creatine kinase levels and myoglobinuria).
9   Peripheral neuropathy.[29]
10 Disseminated intravascular coagulopathy.

Treatment

1   Ensure an adequate airway, that ventilation is occurring and the patient is well oxygenated. Intubate the patient if indicated.
2   Check pulse and blood pressure and ensure circulation is adequate. Support the patient's circulation if required.
3   Cease the causative drug.
4   Give IV fluids and ensure hydration is optimal.
5   Cool the patient (cooling blankets, cooled IV solutions).
6   Dantrolene. This drug relieves muscle spasms and helps reduce muscle related heat production.[29] *See* *Dantrolene*.
7   Bromocriptine mesylate is given orally to reduce creatinine kinase levels, reduce confusion and alleviate extra-pyramidal effects.[28] It acts via its dopamine receptor agonist effect. Amantadine is an alternative.
8   Circulatory and respiratory support.
9   Plasmapheresis has been used successfully in an intractable case of NMS.[27]
10 Other drugs to consider include levadopa-carbidopa, anticholinergics and calcium channel blocker drugs.[29]
11 Troller and Perminder reported that electroconvulsive therapy can be useful treatment of NMS, when the NMS is associated with catatonia and/or psychotic depression.[30]

◗ Newborn and Neonatal Resuscitation

A newborn refers to an infant in the first minutes to hours following birth. A neonate is a baby in the first 28 days of life.

Topics Covered in this Section

▶ The Apgar Score
▶ Normal Values
▶ Approach to Neonatal Resuscitation

The Apgar Score

The Apgar score was developed by Dr Virginia Apgar in 1952 for rapid assessment of newborns (A-appearance, P-pulse, G-grimace, A-activity, R-respiration).

Table N1 Apgar scoring

Characteristic	Description	Score
Colour	Cyanosed generally	0
	Body pink limbs blue	1
	Pink 'all over'	2
Pulse	Nil	0
	<100	1
	>100	2
Grimace due to catheter in nose	Nil	0
	Grimacing	1
	Cough	2
Muscle tone	Limp	0
	Some flexion	1
	Active motion	2
Respiratory effort	Nil	0
	Weak cry	1
	Strong cry	2

Apgar scores are measured at 1 and 5 min. The 5 min score correlates with the degree of neonatal depression and aids in predicting neonatal mortality.[31]

Normal Values

Normal heart rate for the newborn is 110–160 bpm. Normal tidal volume is 5–10 mL/kg. Pulse oximetry can be used to determine HR but is not a reliable indicator of ventilation. HR is a better indicator. Normal oxygen saturation in the newborn is initially 60% and this may take 10 or more minutes to rise to 90%. Cyanosis of the hands and feet with pink mucous membranes is a normal finding in the newborn.

Approach to Neonatal Resuscitation

This approach is based on the recommendations of the Australian Resuscitation Council and are current at the time of printing.

Basic Life Support Phase

The initial approach to newborn resuscitation involves simultaneous assessment and treatment. The steps in newborn BLS are:

1 Keep the baby warm preferably with an overhead radiant heater. Dry the baby off with a towel which will also provide stimulation. Infants with a gestational age < 28 weeks should not be dried and should be placed in a polyethylene bag (except the head) such as a Glad® Zip-Lock bag. The head should be dried as usual.

2 If the baby's HR > 100 bpm the baby's breathing efforts are likely to improve. Persistent apnoea and a HR < 100 bpm are indications for more aggressive resuscitation. Determine heart rate by listening to the heart

with a stethoscope or by feeling pulsations in the base of the umbilical cord. A pulse oximeter applied to the hand can also be used.

3 Position the newborn on their back with the head in a neutral position or slightly extended. Suction the pharynx with caution as this can cause laryngospasm and bradycardia. Use a 10–12 G suction catheter inserted no more than 5 cm from the lips and for no more than 5 s. The maximum suction pressure that should be used is 100 mm Hg.[32]

4 If meconium stained liquor is present and the baby is vigorous do not suck out the newborn's pharynx. If the meconium is thick and breathing effort is weak or absent, perform immediate laryngoscopy and suck away all visible meconium. Intubate the trachea, apply suction to the ET tube, then reintubate with a fresh tube. The appropriate ET tube sizes are:

   a) Pre-term Infant   2.5
   b) Term Infant   3.0
   c) Large Term Infant   3.5

5 If the baby does not establish effective breathing provide ventilation with either a Neopuff Infant Resuscitator or a similar device or a self inflating bag. *See Neopuff* for instructions. In short, set the peak inspiratory pressure to 30 cm H_2O and the PEEP to 5–8 cm H_2O. Ventilate at a rate of 40–60 per min with a 0.5 s inspiratory phase. It is unclear from the literature whether air or 100% O_2 should be used initially. The clinician performing the resuscitation should use his or her best judgement with regard to how the resuscitation is progressing. Consider using air initially but if after 90 s HR < 100 change to 100% O_2. Initial breaths may require a higher inflation pressure than subsequent breaths. The newborn that gasps will require lower inflation pressures than one who has made no respiratory effort.

6 If using a self-inflating bag, it should have a 240 mL capacity and a pressure release valve set to 40 cm H_2O by the manufacturer. This valve can be overridden by pressure on it with the thumb or finger. Use room air initially. If after 90 s HR < 100 use 100% O_2 (8 L/min) and an O_2 reservoir bag attachment.

7 Use an appropriate size facemask as follows: Preterm 0, Term 1, Large Newborn 2.

8 Effective ventilation is indicated by an increase in HR > 100, a rise in the chest with inflation and pinking up of the baby. Intubate the baby if effective ventilation cannot be achieved with a facemask. For the correct tube size see above. Listen to the chest to detect correct placement of the endotracheal tube and exclude endobronchial intubation. Measure/detect expired CO_2 if possible using for example the Pedi-Cap® CO_2 detector. The distance in cm from the tube tip to the patient's lips should be ≈ 6 cm + patient's weight in kg. If unable to intubate the neonate consider insertion of a size 1 LMA.

9 If HR < 60 after 30 s of effective ventilation with 100% O_2 commence chest compression with 3 compressions for each ventilation. Depress the chest one third of the anterior-posterior diameter. The compression point is 1 cm below a line drawn between the nipples. Use either two fingers with the other hand supporting the back or 2 thumbs with the fingers surrounding the chest and supporting the back. Use a ratio of 3 compressions:1 ventilation aiming for 90 compressions and 30 ventilations per minute. Do not pause compressions to ventilate. Instead coordinate the ventilation with the relaxation phase of the compression duty cycle. Continue chest compressions until the HR > 60 and rising.

Advanced Life Support Phase

IV drugs and fluids are rarely required for newborn resuscitation. The best access is via the umbilical vein using a 3.5–5.0 Fr umbilical vein catheter with a single end hole.

Technique for Umbilical Vein Catheterisation

1 The cord needs to be cut between the cord clamp and the umbilical skin, leaving about 2 cm of cord attached to the neonate. The two umbilical arteries will be seen to pout slightly. The single umbilical vein has a larger lumen than the arteries and will ooze a small amount of blood.

2 Fill the umbilical vein catheter with saline via a 3-way tap prior to insertion to reduce the possibility of air embolus.

3 Insert the catheter into the umbilical vein about 4–5 cm. Note that the umbilical vein turns sharply in a cephalad direction just below the skin. If the catheter is inserted too far it may enter a hepatic vein. The liver can be damaged by direct infusion of vasoactive drugs or bicarbonate. Attempt to enter the ductus venosus by having the tip of the catheter turned anteriorly (the ductus venosus branches from the anterior wall of the umbilical vein). Free flow of blood should be present. If an umbilical catheter is not available use a 8–10 FG neonatal feeding tube. Fix the catheter in place with tape.

4 When practical place a purse string silk suture around the base of the cord to prevent subsequent haemorrhage.

Note: A peripheral vein can also be used.

Drugs that should be used include:

1 *Adrenaline.* Give 10–30 μg/kg (0.1 mL/kg of adrenaline 1:10 000) if HR absent or < 60. Repeat this dose every 3 min unless HR >60. If unable to obtain IV access give 30–100 μg/kg adrenaline down the ET tube.

2 *IV fluids.* Give N/S 10 mL/kg if blood loss is suspected or the infant appears shocked (pale, poor perfusion). Repeat this dose as needed. If blood loss is strongly suspected give O –ve blood 10 mL/kg and assess the response.

QUICK FLICK

NO

3 *Naloxone*. This can be considered if the mother has received recent opoids and after initial resuscitation has been undertaken. Give 10 µg/kg IV or IM. Do not give naloxone to the baby if the mother is or suspected to be an abuser of opioids. This is because of the risk of a severe withdrawal response, such as neonatal seizures.[32]

4 *Sodium Bicarbonate*. Dilute the 8.4% solution to 4.2% with sterile water (1 mmol/mL to 0.5 mmol/mL). Give 1–2 mmol/kg (2–4 mL/kg of diluted solution). Inject sodium bicarbonate over at least 2 min to decrease the risk of intraventricular haemorrhage.[32]

5 If low cardiac output persists despite adrenaline, start a dopamine infusion at 5 µg/kg/min initially.

6 Treat hypoglycaemia (blood sugar level <2.2 mmol/L) with an IV bolus of 10% glucose 5 mL/kg, then an infusion of 60–100 mL/kg/day to prevent rebound.

Cessation of Resuscitation Attempts

If no response to resuscitation has occurred after 20 min and after consultation with the neonatal intensivist, consider the discontinuation of resuscitative efforts. If there has been no 'gasp' after 20 min (excluding drug effects) then the outlook is usually extremely poor i.e. death or severe morbidity.

Calling for Help

For a baby requiring ongoing resuscitation and transfer in New South Wales contact NETS on 1300 362 500 24 h per day. Other Australian states have similar systems in place.

◖ New York Heart Association (NYHA) Functional Classification of Patients with Heart Failure

The main symptoms referred to in this classification are dyspnoea and fatigue.

Table N2 NYHA classification of heart failure

Class	Description
1	Asymptomatic at rest, symptoms with heavy exercise
2	Symptoms with ordinary activity but comfortable at rest
3	Symptoms with minimal activity but comfortable at rest
4	Symptoms at rest

◖ Nicardipine

Dihydropyridine calcium channel antagonist drug used IV for the treatment of angina and hypertension and for inducing intra-operative hypotension. IV nicardipine has a rapid onset, is short acting and produces only slight myocardial depression.[33]

Dose
For the treatment of hypertension or induction of hypotension; IV bolus 0.017 mg/kg.[33]

Nifedipine

Dihydropyridine calcium channel antagonist used for the treatment of hypertension, angina and coronary artery spasm during coronary angiography or angioplasty. It is a potent arterial vasodilator with minimal venodilating effects.

Dose
Adult 10–40 mg PO 12 h for moderate to severe hypertension. If reduction in blood pressure is urgent a 10 mg tablet can be chewed then swallowed.[34]

Nifekalant

Class III antiarrhythmic drug useful for treating tachydysrhythmias. Pure potassium channel blocker with no significant negative inotropic effects.

Dose
0.3 mg/kg then infusion 0.4 mg/kg/h.

Nimodipine

Calcium channel antagonist drug which preferentially causes smooth muscle relaxation of cerebral arteries. It is used for the prevention and treatment of vascular spasm after subarachnoid haemorrhage (SAH). In SAH patients, nimodipine decreases the incidence of cerebral infarction by one third.[35]

Dose
Adult 60 mg 4 h PO starting within 4 days of SAH and continued for 3 weeks OR 1 mg/h IV via a central venous line for 2 h increased to 2 mg/h if the patient's blood pressure is not significantly compromised. Start as soon as possible and continue for 5–14 days (continue for at least for 5 days after surgery). ***See*** *Cerebral Aneurysm Surgery*.

Nitrous Oxide

The use of nitrous oxide in anaesthesia is in rapid decline. This is because of an increased risk of complications as described in the ENIGMA trial and listed in the disadvantages section below.[36] The ENIGMA II trial is currently in progress.

This gas is (or was) used for:

1 Supplementation of general anaesthesia usually at a concentration of 70%.
2 As an analgesic for labour and painful procedures.
3 For laparoscopic surgery to provide pneumoperitoneum.

Presented as a liquid in blue cylinders at a pressure of 44 bar at 15° C.

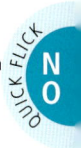

Physical Properties and MAC

Blood:gas solubility coefficient	0.47
Oil:Gas Solubility Coefficient	1.4
Boiling point	88°C
Critical Pressure	71.7 atmospheres
Critical temperature	36.5°C
MAC	105

Advantages

1 Potent analgesic properties equivalent to 10–15 mg of morphine in the adult.[37]
2 Effective sedative properties without respiratory depression.[37]
3 Decreases the MAC of volatile anaesthetic agents and accelerates the uptake of these agents.
4 It appears to be safe in patients with malignant hyperthermia susceptibility.
5 Inexpensive to produce.
6 Rapid onset and offset of action due to its relative insolubility.
7 When used with volatile agents it may decrease the risk of awareness.

Disadvantages

The ENIGMA trial found that for patients having major surgery there was an increased risk of wound infection, pneumonia and pulmonary atelectasis if N_2O was used.[36] However, the duration of hospital stay was not affected.

Specific Disadvantages of Nitrous Oxide Include:

1 Increased incidence of nausea and vomiting.[38,39]
2 N_2O use significantly reduces methionine synthetase activity after a few hours of exposure. This effect is due to N_2O oxidising cobalamin in vitamin B12. Chronic use can lead to megaloblastic anaemia and subacute combined degeneration of the spinal cord. N_2O anaesthesia has resulted in subacute combined degeneration of the spinal cord after a single exposure in patients with pernicious anaemia and/or vitamin B12 deficiency.[40]
3 N_2O decreases myocardial contractility, although this is offset by a stimulating effect on the sympathetic nervous system increasing peripheral vascular resistance. It also causes increased pulmonary vascular resistance in patients with pre-existing pulmonary hypertension.[38,39]
4 N_2O is 635 times more soluble than nitrogen in blood, thus causing a rapid increase in the size of air filled spaces e.g. pneumothorax, and in the size of gas emboli. This property also leads to diffusion hypoxia when N_2O administration is ceased. Supplementary O_2 is thus required at this time.
5 Supports combustion and thus can contribute to fires.
6 May increase intracranial pressure by increasing cerebral blood flow.[38,39]

Cerebral vascular reactivity to CO_2 is impaired with N_2O use. **See** *Neuroanaesthesia*.

7 Contributes to greenhouse gases and the destruction of ozone.[41]

8 Teratogenicity is suspected from animal studies[42,43] but N_2O has never been conclusively shown to be teratogenic in human pregnancy.[44] The Australian Drug Evaluation Committee currently rates N_2O as a Category A drug i.e. no proven long-term harmful effects on the human fetus despite extensive use.

9 N_2O lacks potency and there is a high risk of awareness if it is used as a sole anaesthetic agent.

10 N_2O anaesthesia causes elevated blood homocysteine levels which may increase the risk and incidence of myocardial ischaemia.[45]

WARNING: Nitrous Oxide and Ocular Surgery

Intraocular gas such as perfluoropropane (C_3F_8), or sulfurhexaflouride (SF_6) may be used therapeutically for the treatment of conditions such as retinal detachment and vitrectomy. Intraocular gas bubbles can exist for up to 10 weeks.[46] If N_2O is used for subsequent non-eye surgery during this time, sudden blindness may occur in the treated eye, due to expansion of the intraocular gas. N_2O is therefore contraindicated in this situation.

⊙ Non-steroidal Anti-inflammatory Drugs (NSAIDs)

General Comments

NSAIDs inhibit cyclo-oxygenase which catalyses the production of prostaglandin and thromboxane. They are anti-inflammatory and analgesic. Non-selective NSAIDs inhibit both COX-1 and COX-2 subtypes. COX-1 inhibition can result in side effects such as impaired renal function, platelet inhibition and gastric ulcers. Selective COX-2 inhibitor drugs, which have been available since 1999 produce the desired therapeutic effects without platelet inhibition. There is also a decreased risk of peptic ulcers. However selective COX-2 inhibitors have prothrombotic effects due to reduced prostacyclin generation. This has led to an increased incidence of coronary thrombosis and the worldwide withdrawal of rofecoxib due to increased myocardial infarction risk. Celecoxib, another selective COX-2 inhibitor, is thought to be less harmful in this regard than rofecoxib and is still available. Parecoxib and lumiracoxib (prexige) are more recent selective COX-2 inhibitors that are useful peri-operatively. Prexige was recalled in August 2007 due to liver side effects resulting in liver transplantation and death.

Precautions Applicable to both Selective and Non-selective NSAIDs

1 These drugs are contra-indicated in patients with:
   a) Peptic ulcer disease (past or present)
   b) Gastrointestinal bleeding or bleeding diathesis (past or present)

   c) Allergy to NSAIDs or aspirin.

   d) Pregnancy. These drugs may cross the placenta and cause premature closure of the fetal ductus arteriosus. NSAIDs increase the risk of miscarriage in early pregnancy.

2 These drugs are relatively contraindicated in patients with:

   a) Renal impairment. Acute renal failure can be precipitated by NSAIDs such as ketorolac. Patients on ACE inhibitor may be at increased risk of renal failure if given NSAIDs.[47]

   b) Patients with pre-eclampsia, hypovolaemia or uncontrolled hypertension.[48]

3 Use NSAIDs with caution in:

   a) The elderly.

   b) Patients with diabetes or vascular disease.

   c) Patients with heart failure on diuretics. NSAIDs cause sodium retention and may precipitate heart failure or hypertension in predisposed patients.[49]

   d) Patients on cyclosporin or triamterene.

   e) Patients who are taking renally cleared drugs with a low therapeutic index such as digoxin or aminoglycoside.

4 NSAIDs can cause severe hepatic toxicity leading to fulminant liver failure and death.[48]

Side Effects of Non-selective NSAIDs

1 These drugs increase bleeding time and blood loss in some studies due to platelet inhibition. For example, they should be avoided in tonsillectomy and plastic surgery patients. Platelet inhibition ceases 1–2 days after ceasing non-selective NSAIDs.

2 Non-selective NSAIDs vary in their risk profile in causing peptic ulcers. High-risk agents include piroxicam and ketoprofen, while lower risk agents include diclofenac and ibuprofen.[50]

3 Non-selective NSAIDs are contraindicated in patients with aspirin sensitive asthma. Other asthmatics are not at increased risk.

4 Non-selective NSAIDs are associated with a moderate increase in the risk of thrombo-embolic events such as MI.[51] **See** *Diclofenac* and *Ketorolac*.

COX-2 Selective Inhibitor Side Effects

1 Lower incidence of gastroduodenal ulcers than non-selective NSAIDs.[52] However these drugs should be not be used in patients with known PUD.

2 The undesirable effects of NSAIDs on the kidney may be similar for both selective and non-selective agents. There have been reports of renal failure occurring in association with the selective drugs.[53]

3 Chronic rofecoxib use is associated with increased risk of myocardial infarction and death. It was withdrawn globally in September 2004.

4 Lumiracoxib use has been associated with liver failure and death. It was withdrawn from the Australian market in August 2007.

5 Celecoxib and parecoxib are contraindicated in patients allergic to sulfonamides.

6 COX-2 selective NSAIDs do not appear to exacerbate aspirin sensitive asthma.[54]

7 COX-2 inhibitors may affect bone healing at high doses.

See Celecoxib and Parecoxib.

○ Noradrenaline

A catecholamine sympathomimetic agent acting mainly on α and β1 adrenoreceptors with almost no effect on β2 (vasodilating) adrenoreceptors. Used mainly as a vasoconstrictor to treat refractory hypotension, such as occurs in septic shock. Increases both systolic and diastolic blood pressure and diverts blood flow from the skin, liver, kidney and bowel to the brain and heart. There is thus a risk of ischaemia to the organs from which blood is diverted.

Dose

Give by central line only. Add 6 mg to 100 mL N/S or 5% glucose. Run at 0.05–0.30 µg/kg/min (titrate to desired effect). For a 70 kg patient this equals 3–20 mL/h. Start infusion at 5 mL/h.

Note:

1 If extravasation occurs, infiltrate the area of extravasation with 5–10 mg of phentolamine in 10–15 mL of N/S. This may reduce the risk of tissue necrosis.[55]

2 Do not administer noradrenaline in IV lines containing alkaline solutions as the noradrenaline may be inactivated.[55]

○ Normal Saline

Crystalloid intravenous solution containing the following properties:

Sodium	150 mmol/L
Chloride	150 mmol/L
Osmolarity	300 mOsm/L
pH	4.0–7.0.

Only 25% of infused saline remains in the intravascular space. Infusion of large volumes of normal saline can result in hyperchloraemic acidosis and pulmonary oedema due to decreased colloid osmotic pressure.

○ Normovolaemic Haemodilution

See Acute Normovolaemic Haemodilution (ANH).

�‍◗ NovoSeven

See *Recombinant Activated Factor VII (rFVIIa)*.

◗ Nupercaine

See *Spinal Anaesthesia*.

REFERENCES

1   Tepel M, van der Geit M, Schwarzfeld C et al. Prevention of radiographic-contrast-agent-induced reductions in renal function by acetylcysteine. *N Eng J Med* 2000; 34: 180–4.

2   Haase M, Hasse-Fielitz A, Bagshaw S, et al. Phase II, randomized, controlled trial of high-dose N-acetylcysteine in high risk cardiac surgery patients. *Crit Care Med* 2007; 35: 1324–31.

3   Hynninen MS, Niemi TT, Poyhia R, et al. N-acetyl cysteine for the prevention of kidney injury in abdominal aortic surgery: a randomized, double-blind, placebo-controlled trial. *Anesth Analg* 2006; 102: 1638–45.

4   Baker CS, Wragg A, Kumar S et al. A rapid protocol for the prevention of contrast-induced renal dysfunction: the RAPPID study. *J Am College Cardiol* 2003; 41: 2114–18.

5   *Australian Resuscitation Council Guidelines 13.1*. Feb 2006.

6   Tramér MR. A rational approach to the control of postoperative nausea and vomiting: evidence from systemic reviews. Part 1. Efficacy and harm of antiemetic interventions, and methodological issues. *Acta Anaesthesiol Scand* 2001; 45: 4–13.

7   Divatia J, Vaidya JS, Badwe RA, Hawaldar RW. Omission of nitrous oxide during anaesthesia reduces the incidence of postoperative nausea and vomiting. A meta-analysis. *Anesthesiology* 1996; 85: 1055–62.

8   Sneyd JR, Carr A, Byron WD, Bilski AJT. A meta-analysis of nausea and vomiting following maintenance of anaesthesia with propofol or inhalational agents. *Eur J Anaesthesiol* 1998; 15: 433–45.

9   Harmon D, Bajwa S. Supplemental oxygen for the prevention of nausea and vomiting. *Anesthesiology* 2000; 93: 584–5.

10 Diemunsch PA, Apfel CC, Philip B et al. NK1 antagonist apreptant vs. ondansetron for prevention of PONV: combining data from two large trials. *Anesthesiology* 2006; 105 : A125 (abstract).

11 Wilkes M, Hickey N. Anaesthesia for carotid surgery. *Br J Hosp Med* 1995; 53: 31–4.

12 Marcus R. Surveillance of health care workers exposed to blood from patients infected with human immunodeficiency virus. *N Eng J Med* 1988; 89: 1362–72.

13 Diprose P, Deakin CD, Smedley J. Ignorance of post-exposure prophylaxis

guidelines following HIV needlestick injury may increase the risk of seroconversion. *Br J Anaesth* 2000; 84(6): 767–70.

14 Levison J. The ostrich syndrome: obstetrician-gynecologists and human immunodeficiency virus exposure. *Obstets Gynecol* 2008; 111: 183–6.

15 Shoret LJ, Bell DM. Risk of occupational infection with blood-borne pathogens in operating and delivery room settings. *Am J Infect Control* 1993; 21: 343–50.

16 Updated US Public Health Services *Guidelines for the Management of Occupational Exposures to HBV, HCV, and HIV and Recommendations for Postexposure Prophylaxis* (2001). Centers for Disease Control and Prevention website: http://www.cdc.gov/ (accessed July 2008)

17 Liddle C. Hepatitis C. *Anesth Intensive Care* 1996; 24: 180–3.

18 Haber PS, Young MM, Dorrington L et al. Transmission of hepatitis C virus by needle-stick injury in community settings. *Gastroenterology and Hepatology* 2007; 22: 1882–5.

19 Duke J. Airway Management. In Duke J ed. *Anesthesia Secrets*, 2nd edn. Hanley and Belfus, Philadelphia 2000; 33–42.

20 Van de Velde M. What is the best way to provide analgesia after Caesarean section? *Curr Opin Anesthesiol* 2000; 13: 267–70.

21 Craen RA, Gelb AW. The anaesthetic management of neurosurgical emergencies. *Can J Anaesth* 1992 May; 39 (5 Part 2) : R29–R39.

22 Isert P. Control of carbon dioxide levels during neuroanaesthesia: current practice and an appraisal of our reliance on capnography. *Anaesth Intensive Care* 1994; 22: 435–41.

23 Giebler R, Kollenberg B, Pohlen G, Peters J. Effect of positive end-expiratory pressure on the incidence of venous air embolism and on the cardiovascular response to the sitting position during neurosurgery. *Br J Anaesth* 1998; 80: 30–5.

24 Young WL. Cerebral aneurysms: management and future horizons. *Can J Anaesth* 1998; 45: R17–R24.

25 Traill R. Neurosurgical anaesthesia. *Baillière's Clinical Anaesth* 1993; 7: 2: 399–422.

26 Abe K. Vasodilators during cerebral aneurysm surgery. *Can J Anaesth* 1993; 40: 775–90.

27 Gaitini L, Fradis M, Vaida S et al. Plasmapheresis in neuroleptic malignant syndrome (Case report). *Anaesthesia* 1997; 52: 165–8.

28 Tomson CRV. Neurolept malignant syndrome associated with inappropriate antidiuresis and psychogenic polydipsia. *Br Med J* 1986: 292: 171.

29 Shaw MB. Postoperative neuroleptic malignant syndrome. *Anaesthesia* 1995; 50: 246–7.

30 Troller JN, Perminder SS. Electroconvulsive treatment of neuroleptic

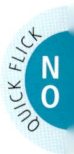

malignancy syndrome: a review and report of cases. *Aust NZ J Psychiatry* 1999; 33: 650–9.

31 Roy RN, Betheras R. The Melbourne chart—a logical guide to neonatal resuscitation. *Anaesth Intensive Care* 1990; 18: 348–57.

32 Elliott RD. Neonatal resuscitation: the NRP guidelines. *Can J Anaesth* 1994; 41: 742–53.

33 Nishiyama T, Matsukawa T, Hanaoka K, Conway CM. Interactions between nicardipine and enflurane, isoflurane, and sevoflurane. *Can J Anaesth* 1997; 44: 10: 1071–6.

34 *Cardiovascular Drug Guidelines*. 2nd edn. Published by the VMPF Therapeutics Committee on behalf of the Victorian Drug Usage Advisory Committee,1995: 68.

35 Sutcliffe AJ. Subarachnoid haemorrhage due to cerebral aneurysm. *Br J Anaesth CEPD Review* 2002; 2: 45–9.

36 Myles P, Leslie K, Chan M et al. Avoidance of nitrous oxide for patients undergoing advanced surgery: a randomized controlled trial. *Anesthesiol* 2007; 107: 221–31.

37 Stenqqvist O, Husum B, Dale O. Nitrous oxide: an ageing gentleman. *Acta Anaesthsiol Scand* 2001; 45: 135–7.

38 Dale O, Husum B. Nitrous oxide: from frolics to global concern in 150 years. *Acta Anaesthesiol Scand* 1994; 38: 749–50.

39 Brandt L. Nitrous oxide—no laughing matter? *Thoracic Cardiovasc Surg* 1990; 38: 79–80.

40 Hadzic A, Glab K, Sanborn KV, Thys DM. Severe neurological deficit after nitrous oxide anaesthesia. *Anesthesiol* 1995; 83: 863–6.

41 Logan M, Farmer JG. Anaesthesia and the ozone layer. *Br J Anaesth* 1989; 63:645–6.

42 Keeling PA, Rocke DA, Ninn JF et al. Folinic acid protection against nitrous oxide teratogenicity in the rat. *Br J Anaesth* 1986; 58: 1469–70.

43 Lane GA, Nahrwold ML, Tait AR et al. Anesthetics as teratogens: nitrous oxide is fetotoxic, xenon is not. *Science* 1980; 210: 899–901.

44 Hawkins JL. Anesthesia for the pregnant patient undergoing nonobstetric surgery. In: *Annual Refresher Course Lectures, American Society of Anesthesiologists*, 1997: 235.

45 Myles PS, Leslie K, Silbert B et al. A review of the risks and benefits of nitrous oxide in current anaesthesia practice. *Anesth Intensive Care* 2004; 32: 165–72.

46 Vote BJ, Hart RH, Worsely DR et al. Visual loss after nitrous oxide gas with general anaesthetic in patients with intraocular gas still persistent up to 30 days after vitrectomy. *Anesthesiology* 2002; 9: 1305–8.

47 Tarkkila P, Rosenberg PH. Perioperative analgesia with non-steroidal analgesics. *Curr Opin in Anaesthesiol* 1998; 11: 407–10.

48 Guidelines for the use of non-steroidal anti-inflammatory drugs in the perioperative period. Issued by The Royal College of Anaesthetists, January 1998.

49 Mashford ML, Andreoli T, Cosolo W et al. *Therapeutic Guidelines: Analgesic*, 3rd edn. Therapeutic Guidelines Limited 1997; 14.

50 McManus P, Henry DA, Birkett DJ. Recent changes in the profile of prescription NSAID use in Australia. *Med J Aust* 2000; 172: 188.

51 Kearney PM, Baignent C, Goodwin J et al. Do selective cyclo-oxygenase-2 inhibitors and traditional non-steroidal anti-inflammatory drugs increase the risk of atherothrombosis? Metaanalysis of randomized trials. *Br Med J* 2006; 332: 1302–5.

52 Cryer B. Nonsteroidal anti-inflammatory drug gastrointestinal toxicity. *Curr Opin Gastroenterology* 2001; 17: 503–12.

53 Ahmad SR, Kortepeter C, Brinker A et al. Renal failure associated with the use of celecoxib and rofecoxib. *Drug Safety* 2002; 25: 537–44.

54 Australian and New Zealand College of Anaesthetists and Faculty of Pain Medicine: Acute Pain Management: Scientific Evidence. 2nd edn, 2005: 47–9.

55 Guidelines 2000 for cardiopulmonary resuscitation and emergency cardiovascular care. *Circulation* 2000; 102 (suppl I): 1–131.

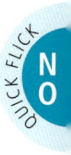

QUICK FLICK

N
O

O

Obesity

See *Body Mass Index (BMI) and Obesity*.

Obstructive Sleep Apnoea (OSA) Syndrome

This common disorder is characterised by recurrent and often prolonged episodes of apnoea/hypopnoea and hypoxaemia during sleep which can produce severe and potentially fatal physiological effects.

Clinical Manifestations

These may include:

1 pulmonary and systemic hypertension
2 right and left ventricular hypertrophy and failure
3 dysrhythmias
4 polycythaemia
5 excessive daytime sleepiness
6 respiratory failure

Note: There is often associated obesity.

Diagnosis

The 'gold standard' for diagnosis of OSA is full overnight polysomnography. A detailed description of sleep study diagnosis of OSA is beyond the scope of this manual. Most patients with OSA are undiagnosed at the time of anaesthesia.[1]

General Treatment Measures

1 Avoid sedating drugs such as alcohol and benzodiazepines.
2 Avoid supine sleep posture (e.g. sleep laterally).
3 Reduce weight if obese.
4 Drug therapy (progesterone, protriptyline) is helpful in some patients.[2]
5 Surgery to reduce airway obstruction e.g. uvulopalatopharyngoplasty.
6 Nasal continuous positive airway pressure (CPAP) machine.
7 Tracheostomy may be considered for life threatening OSA.[2]

Anaesthetic Implications

Pre-operative Aspects

1 Consider investigating patients for cardiorespiratory complications of OSA, e.g. CXR looking for cardiomegaly and evidence of pulmonary hypertension. Echocardiography may be appropriate.

2 Check FBC for polycythaemia. Phlebotomy should be considered if Hct > 0.65. **See** *Polycythaemia*.

3 Consider regional anaesthesia if appropriate for the procedure.

4 Avoid sedating premedication such as benzodiazepines and opioids.

5 OSA patients may also be difficult to intubate and may be at risk of aspiration due to associated obesity and gastro-oesophageal reflux.[3]

6 Consider the need for awake fibre-optic intubation, pre-operative drying agents and antacid therapy.

Intra-operative Management

See *Difficult Airway Management*.

1 Due to possibly associated aspiration risk, consider rapid sequence induction. Make adequate preparations for failed intubation should this occur. Make sure the patient is well preoxygenated prior to induction.

2 If the patient has pulmonary hypertension, **see** *Pulmonary Hypertension* for details of management.

3 Minimise intra-operative opioids if possible. Use short-acting opioids preferably. Use non-sedating analgesics such as paracetamol and NSAIDs.

4 Ensure NMBDs are fully reversed prior to emergence. Extubate the patient when he/she is fully awake/alert.

5 Consider extubation in the half-sitting position.[4]

Postoperative Management

1 This phase may be a particularly 'at risk' period for the OSA patient due to reduced supervision and monitoring. Unsupervised OSA patients on PCA or morphine infusions may be at increased risk of death and hypoxic brain damage.[1]

2 Nurse patients sitting up in bed, or laterally, rather than in a supine position.

3 Supplementary oxygen therapy is usually desirable but this is a debated issue.[5] Oxygen therapy may be detrimental in patients relying on hypoxic drive to maintain ventilation. Close postoperative observation will help reduce risk.

4 Consider regional anaesthesia for postoperative analgesia to avoid the sedating effect of systemic opioids.

5 Consider non-opioid analgesia such as NSAIDs.

6 Patients should use their nasal CPAP machines during sleep periods while in hospital.

7 Nursing in a high-dependency unit with pulse oximetry monitoring may be prudent. Continue to intensively monitor until opioid requirements are minimal.

◖ Occipital Nerve Block

See *Scalp Block*.

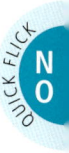

◯ Oculogyric Crisis

See *Dystonic Reaction, Acute*.

◯ Ondansetron

An antagonist at the 5-HT$_3$ (serotonin) receptor, both peripherally and centrally, ondansetron is used for the treatment/prevention of nausea and vomiting. It lacks the extrapyramidal side effects seen with dopamine receptor antagonist drugs such as metoclopramide.[6]

Dose
Adult 4–8 mg IV up to 8 h as required.
Child 0.1–0.2 mg/kg to a max of 8 mg.

Disadvantages
1 There is an increased risk of postoperative headache and constipation with ondansetron.[7]
2 Can cause decreased efficacy of tramadol.

◯ One Lung Ventilation

Topics Covered in this Section
▶ Indications for One Lung Ventilation
▶ Double Lumen Endotracheal Tubes (DLT)
▶ Bronchial Blockers
▶ Predictors of High Risk for One Lung Ventilation/Pneumonectomy
▶ Physiology of One Lung Ventilation
▶ Optimisation of Oxygenation During One Lung Ventilation

Indications for One Lung Ventilation
The indications for one lung ventilation include:
1 Prevention of spillage of blood or pus from one lung to the other.
2 Isolation of the lung which is causing leakage of ventilating gases. Causes of a leak from one lung include bronchopleural fistula and surgical or traumatic opening of a main conducting airway.
3 Unilateral bronchopulmonary lavage.
4 Improving exposure of the operative site for the surgeon.

Double Lumen Endotracheal Tubes (DLT)
One lung ventilation is usually achieved by insertion of a DLT. A left-sided tube is easier to place than a right-sided tube and is usually adequate for left or right lung ventilation unless there is pathology in the left main-stem bronchus.

DLT Sizes
Vary from 28 to 41 Fr. Adult male 39–41 Fr, Adult female 35–37 Fr.

Placement of a Left-sided Mallinckrodt BronchoCath™ DLT

This disposable plastic DLT has two curves: a distal curve for insertion into the left main bronchus and a proximal curve. Ensure the cuffs are well lubricated prior to insertion.

1　Induce anaesthesia, paralyse and ventilate.

2　Insert the DLT with the distal curve concave anteriorly. Once the distal part of the DLT has passed through the vocal cords, remove the stylet, and rotate the tube 90° so that the proximal curve is now concave anteriorly.

3　Advance the DLT until slight resistance felt, usually at ≈ 29 cm (27–31cm).[8]

4　Inflate the tracheal cuff with ≈ 5 mL of air and the bronchial (blue) cuff with ≈ 1.5 mL of air.

5　Ventilate the patient and ensure that both lungs are being inflated. If only one lung inflates, both tube lumens may be in one bronchus.

6　Clamp the bronchial lumen tube connection, open the bronchial lumen to air, and then assess ventilation. The right lung only should inflate. If both lungs inflate, deflate both cuffs and gently and incrementally insert the DLT further into the trachea. Repeat steps 4, 5 and 6.

7　Clamp tracheal lumen tube connection, open the tracheal lumen to air, and assess ventilation. Only the left lung should inflate. If only the right lung inflates, the right bronchus has been intubated. Deflate both cuffs, withdraw the DLT and reinsert the DLT with the head turned to the right and DLT rotated to the left.[8]

8　Ensure that the left lung apex is being ventilated i.e. bronchial lumen may obstruct the left upper lobe bronchus.

9　If there are persistent problems with placement, insert a fibre-optic bronchoscope down the tracheal lumen to check the position of the DLT. A 3.6–4.2 mm external diameter paediatric bronchoscope will fit through all sizes of DLT.[9] A 4.9 mm external diameter scope will pass through 41–39 DLTs.

10　Repeat steps 6 and 7 when the patient is repositioned.

A Second 'Blind' Technique of DLT Placement[10]

1　Select the DLT which will be long enough to extend from the lips to 1 cm below the carina. This is estimated by placing the DLT with the proximal curve facing posteriorly. The bifurcation point of the tube should lie just below the anterior border of the ear lobe and the bronchial cuff should be 1 cm below the manubrio-sternal junction.

2　Insert the tube as described in steps 1 and 2 above into the trachea just below the cords and inflate the bronchial cuff with 3–5 mL of air. Clamp the tracheal lumen tube connection, open the tracheal lumen to air, so that ventilation is through the bronchial lumen only. Ventilate the patient ensuring both lungs inflate evenly.

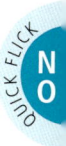

QUICK FLICK NO

3   Advance the DLT gradually until only one side of the chest is moving (the left side with correct placement). If only the right side inflates, withdraw the tube back into the trachea and rotate tube 180° anti-clockwise, then reinsert. If again unsuccessful repeat the manoeuvre but with the cuff deflated.
4   When the left bronchus is entered, indicated by left lung inflation only, deflate the cuff and insert the DLT 1 cm further plus the width of cuff. Reinflate the bronchial cuff with sufficient air to make a seal.
5   Test ventilate each lung separately as described above.

Troubleshooting

If unable to deflate the appropriate lung despite several attempts at repositioning the DLT, consider the following steps:

1   Pass the fibre-optic bronchoscope (FOB) down the bronchial lumen while continuing to ventilate the tracheal lumen.
2   Deflate both cuffs and pull the DLT into the trachea until the carina can be visualised.
3   Intubate the left main bronchus with the FOB.
4   Railroad the bronchial part of the DLT into the left main bronchus.

Bronchial Blockers

These devices enable the occlusion of the left or right bronchus to cause collapse of the appropriate lung.

Univent™ Tubes

An example of such a device is the Univent™ tube which consists of a single endotracheal tube with a separate channel for a manoeuvrable bronchial blocker that can be positioned in the left or right bronchus. The Univent™ has an oval lumen and adult sizes range from 6.0–9.0 mm internal diameter. Oxygen can be supplied to the deflated lung via the lumen of the bronchial blocker tube.

Technique for Placement of the Univent™[11]

1   Test the bronchial and tracheal cuffs and ensure that the tube is well lubricated. When fully inflated the bronchial cuff requires 6–8 mL of air.
2   Withdraw the blocker into its channel.
3   Intubate the patient in the conventional manner.
4   Use a fibre-optic bronchoscope to ensure accurate placement of the bronchal blocker into the right or left bronchus. In the left bronchus the optimal position is when the inflated cuff (6–8 mL of air) can just be visualised 5 mm distal to the carina. In the right bronchus correct placement is when the cuff is just proximal to the origin of the right upper lobe bronchus.

Advantages of the Univent™ Tube Compared with the DLT

1 The Univent™ tube is much more like a conventional endotracheal tube.
2 It is able to be used as an effective lobar blocker.
3 The Univent™ does not need to be replaced at the end of the case if ongoing ventilation is required.
4 The Univent™ tube is easier to insert in the patient who is a difficult intubation than a DLT. It can also be inserted using an awake fibre-optic intubation technique.
5 A bronchial blocker can be used in a patient who is too small for a DLT.

Disadvantages of the Univent™ Tube Compared with the DLT

1 Placement requires a fibre-optic bronchoscope due to the risk of trauma to the trachea or bronchus.
2 Inflation of the bronchial cuff can traumatise the trachea or bronchus.
3 During right upper lobe lobectomy the bronchial blocker may be caught in the suture line.
4 Inflation of the bronchial lumen may result in obstruction of the tracheal lumen.

Predictors of High Risk for One Lung Ventilation/Pneumonectomy

For predictors of poor tolerance of One Lung Ventilation and or pneumonectomy *see* *Respiratory Function Tests*.

Physiology of One Lung Ventilation

Blood flow to the dependent lung is ≈ 60% of the total pulmonary blood flow. If both lungs are ventilated, ventilation preferentially goes to the non-dependent lung. If the chest is opened this increases the mismatch of ventilation and perfusion. When the non-dependent lung is not ventilated, hypoxic vasoconstriction increases the blood flow to the dependent lung to 80% of the total. However volatile anaesthetic agents decrease hypoxic vasoconstriction. At 1 MAC isoflurane, the dependent lung blood flow is reduced to ≈ 75% of the total pulmonary blood flow.

Optimisation of Oxygenation During One Lung Ventilation

Optimisation of oxygenation can be achieved by applying the following measures:

1 Ensure position of DLT is optimal i.e. that left upper lobe is being ventilated. Suck out the lumens to remove secretions and identify and correct kinking of the tube. If any doubt exists at any stage check the position of the DLT with the fibre-optic bronchoscope.
2 It is difficult to predict the optimal tidal volume and ventilating pressure for the individual patient. Start with tidal volume of 10 mL/kg and limit the plateau airway pressure to 25 cm H_2O initially.[11] Increase the tidal volume to a maximum of 15 mL/kg if necessary. If the airway pressure

is excessive (>30 cm H_2O) decrease the tidal volume and increase the respiratory rate.

3   Set the respiratory rate so that $PaCO_2$ is maintained at 40 mm Hg.[8] It is usually necessary to increase respiratory rate by about 20%.[8] Consider permissive hypercapnia if barotrauma is a risk.

4   Apply continuous positive airways pressure (CPAP) of 5–10 cm H_2O to the non-dependent lung using a separate anaesthetic circuit.[12] Allow the non-dependent lung to inflate to a size that does not interfere with surgery. CPAP is most effective if commenced before the lung is deflated[12] or after a large tidal volume inflation to overcome critical opening pressures in the collapsed lung.[9] Alternatively O_2 can be insufflated into the non-dependent lung via tubing such as a suction catheter placed in the correct lumen.

5   Consider applying 5 cm positive end-expiratory pressure to the dependent lung if oxygenation is not satisfactory with CPAP. This will reduce atelectasis but may divert blood to the non-dependent lung and worsen oxygenation.

6   Increase FiO_2, up to 100%. The use of N_2O can result in increased dependent lung atelectasis. Therefore air/O_2 mixtures are preferable if less than 100% O_2 is used.

7   Intermittent reinflation of non-dependent lung or return to 2-lung ventilation may be required.

8   Clamping of pulmonary artery to the non-dependent lung will cease shunting of blood to that lung.

9   Ensure that cardiac output (CO) remains adequate as a decreased CO will contribute to hypoxaemia.

10 Treat any other reversible causes of hypoxaemia such as bronchospasm.

11 Intravenous anaesthesia with propofol has no effect on hypoxic vasoconstriction and may be of benefit.[13]

12 Adrenaline, noradrenaline, phenylephrine and dopamine all cause vasoconstriction in the dependent lung worsening ventilation/perfusion mismatch. However, if a vasopressor is required, dopamine may be the agent of choice as it has the least effect on hypoxic vasoconstriction.[13]

○ Opioid Receptors

These are classified as:

1   *Mu1* stimulation cause miosis, euphoria and supraspinal analgesia but has abuse potential.[14,15]

2   *Mu2* respiratory depression, inhibition of gut motility and bradycardia.[16]

3   *Kappa* ventilatory depression, sedation and spinal analgesia.

4   *Sigma* dysphoria, hallucinations, mydriasis, respiratory stimulation and tachycardia.

5   *Delta* ventilatory depression and modification of mu receptor activity.[14]

○ Opioids: Relative Potencies[14,17]

IV Opioids

Morphine 10 mg IV is equivalent to (all doses are IV):

Alfentanil	500 µg
Buprenorphine	300 µg
Carfentanil	40–50 µg
Codeine	120 mg
Fentanyl	80–100 µg
Heroin	5 mg
Hydromorphone	2 mg
Lofentanil	10–20 µg
Methadone	10 mg
Oxycodone	15 mg
Papaveretum	16 mg
Pethidine	75–100 mg
Remifentanil	80–100 µg
Sufentanil	20 µg

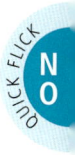

Oral Opioids

Morphine 10 mg IM is equivalent to 30 mg PO
Morphine 30 mg PO is equivalent to:

Codeine	240 mg PO
Dextromoramide	15 mg PO
Dextropropoxyphene	300 mg PO
Hydromorphone	7.5 mg PO
Methadone	20 mg PO
Oxycodone	30 mg PO
Pethidine	240 mg PO

○ Oxycodone

Synthetic opioid oral analgesic drug.

Dose

Adult For immediate release oxycodone (e.g. endone, oxynorm) start with 5 mg–10 mg PO 6 h, increase as required. If using sustained release (e.g. oxycontin) give 10 mg 12 h.
Child 0.1–0.2 mg/kg immediate release oxycodone e.g. endone PO 4–6 h max 10 mg.

○ Oxygen Content of Blood

Calculated from the equation: O_2 content/100 mL $= 1.34 \times O_2$ Saturation $\times$ Hb concentration/100 mL $+ 0.003 \times PaO_2$.

Oxymetazoline

Sympathomimetic used to constrict the arteriolar network of the nasal mucosa. Drixine contains a 0.05% solution of oxymetazoline.

Oxytocin

A naturally occurring polypeptide secreted by the hypothalamus and stored in the posterior pituitary gland. The synthesised form (syntocinon) is free of vasopressin, and is used for induction and augmentation of labour, and to cause and maintain uterine contraction post-partum. It is also used to cause uterine contraction in the setting of miscarriage.

Dose

1. For augmentation of labour 1.5–12 mUnits/min titrated to response. Do not infuse with glucose because of the risk of water intoxication due to the anti-diuretic effects of oxytocin. Infuse with Hartmann's solution or N/S.
2. For uterine contraction after delivery or evacuation of the uterus after miscarriage 10 units IV or IM. Effects last for ≈ 1 hr.

Note: Do not infuse oxytocin in the same line as blood or plasma because the drug will be inactivated by plasma oxytocinase. Oxytocin causes vasodilatation and if used in large amounts can cause hypotension and tachycardia.

REFERENCES

1. Benumof JL. Sleep apnoea and the obese patient. *Audio Digest: Anesthesiology* 2000: 42.
2. Boushra NN. Review article: Anaesthetic management of patients with sleep apnoea syndrome. *Can J Anaesth* 1996; 43: 599–616.
3. Kerr P, Shoenut JP, Millar T et al. Nasal CPAP reduces gastroesophageal reflux in obstructive sleep apnea syndrome. *Chest* 1992; 101: 1539–44.
4. den Herder C, Schmeck J, Appelboom DJ, de Vries N. Risks of general anaesthesia in patients with obstructive sleep apnoea. *Br Med J* 2004; 329: 955–9.
5. Loadsman JA, Hillman DR. Review article: Anaesthesia and sleep apnoea. *Br J Anaesth* 2001; 86: 254–66.
6. Watcha MF, White PF. Postoperative nausea and vomiting—its aetiology, treatment and prevention. *Anesthesiology* 1992; 77: 162–84.
7. Tramér MR, Reynolds DJM, Moore RA, McQuay HJ. Efficacy, dose response and safety of ondansetron in prevention of postoperative nausea and vomiting: A quantitative systematic review of randomized placebo-controlled trials. *Anesthesiology* 1997; 87: 1277–89.
8. Brodsky JB, Macario A, Cannon WB, Mark JBD. Blind placement of plastic left double-lumen tubes. *Anaesth Intensive Care* 1995; 23: 583–6.

9 Benumof JL, Alfery DD. Anesthesia for thoracic surgery. In: Miller RD, ed. *Anesthesia*, 3rd edn. Churchill Livingstone, New York 1990; 1517–603.

10 Russell W. A blind guided technique for placing double lumen endotracheal tubes. *Anaesth Intensive Care* 1992; 20: 71–4.

11 Campos JH. Current techniques for perioperative lung isolation in adults. *Anesthesiology* 2002; 97: 1295–301.

12 Slinger P, Triolet W, Wilson S. Improving arterial oxygenation during one lung ventilation. *Anesthesiology* 1988; 68: 291–5.

13 Eastwood J, Mahajan R. One-lung anaesthesia. *Br J Anaesth CEPD Reviews* 2002; 3: 83–7.

14 Philbin DM. Opioids. *Ballière's Clinical Anaesthesiology* 1989; 3 (1): 205–14.

15 Wilkinson DJ. Opioid agonist/antagonists in general anaesthesia. *Br J Hosp Med* 1987 Aug: 130–2.

16 Mather LE. Pharmacology of opioids—part 1. Basic aspects. *Med J Aust* 1986; 144: 424–7.

17 Mashford ML, Andreoli T, Cosolo W et al. *Therapeutic Guidelines: Analgesic* 3rd edn. Therapeutic Guidelines Limited 1997: 15.

QUICK FLICK

NO

P

◯ Pacing, Pacemakers and Anaesthesia

Topics Covered in this Section
- ▶ Classification of Permanent Pacemakers
- ▶ Anaesthetic Management of Patients with Permanent Pacemakers (Except AICDs)
- ▶ Anaesthesia and AICDs
- ▶ Pacemakers and Emergency Surgery (Pacemaker Technician Unavailable)
- ▶ External Defibrillation and Pacemakers
- ▶ Pacemakers and Specific Procedures
- ▶ Temporary Pacemaker Wire Insertion and Pacing
- ▶ Transcutaneous Pacing
- ▶ Transoesophageal Pacing
- ▶ Fist (Percussion) Pacing
- ▶ Biventricular Pacing

Classification of Permanent Pacemakers

More than 1500 types of pacemaker have been produced in the USA.
A code describing pacemaker function was devised in 1987 (and revised in 2002) by the North American Society of Pacing and Electrophysiology (NASPE) and the British Pacing Electrophysiological Group (BPEG). The code relies on 3–5 letters and their position in a sequence as follows:

1. Position 1—chamber paced i.e. **A**trium, **V**entricle, **D**ual or **O** (nil)
2. Position 2—chamber sensed **A, V, D** or **O** (pacemaker discharges without sensing)
3. Position 3—response to sensing, either **T**riggered, **I**nhibited, **D**ual response or **O** (nil)
4. Position 4—indicates rate modulation (programmability) either **O** (nil) or **R**ate modulation
5. Position 5—indicates multisite pacing capability either **O** (nil), **A**trial (one or both atrias), **V** (one or both ventricles), **D** (combinations of A and V)

In addition some pacemakers can provide anti-tachycardia pacing and defibrillation termed Automatic Implantable Cardioverter Defibrillators or AICDs. The code for these pacemakers is:

1. Position 1—chamber shocked either **A**trium, **V**entricle, **D**ual or **O**
2. Position 2—chamber to which anti-tachycardia pacing is administered, either **A, V, D** or **O**

3 Position 3—detection method of intrinsic cardiac rhythm either **E**lectrogram or **H**aemodynamic

4 Position 4—chamber to which anti-bradycardia pacing is administered either **A, V, D** or **O**

Common terms used to describe pacemakers include:

1 *Asynchronous* (VOO) Uses no sensing circuitry. It discharges continuously regardless of the patient's intrinsic rhythm. Almost all pacemakers will revert to asynchronous mode if a magnet is placed over the pacemaker.

2 *Demand* e.g. VVI paces when it does not sense R waves from the ventricular electrode. Thus this type of pacemaker does not interfere with intrinsic cardiac rhythm above a predetermined rate.

3 *Sequential/Dual Chamber* This type maintains the atrio-ventricular contraction sequence. DDD pacemakers sense the patient's P and R waves and pace the atria and ventricles sequentially.

4 *Programmable* This type can have their functions such as rate, output, sensing changed.

Most pacemakers are VVI, VVIR, DDD or DDDR.

Anaesthetic Management of Patients with Permanent Pacemakers (except AICDs)

The main issues with pacemakers and surgery are:

1 Electromagnetic interference e.g. diathermy can cause pacemaker malfunction e.g. failure to pace or inappropriate pacing.

2 The pacemaker may fail intra-operatively.

3 Programmable pacemakers may interact with cardiac monitors and interpret erroneously that the patient is exercising and inappropriately increase heart rate.

4 Electrocautery currents can be transmitted down pacing wires and cause myocardial injury and loss of capture or sensing.

5 External defibrillation of the patient can result in internal myocardial burns from the wires and damage or reprogramme the pacemaker.

Steps to be undertaken for anaesthetic management include:

1 The pacemaker should be checked preoperatively to see if it is functioning appropriately unless this has been done within the last 3 months.[1] The battery life should be checked by the technician and the battery replaced if required.

2 Discuss the peri-operative management of the patient's pacemaker with the cardiologist and pacemaker technician. The advice in this manual is not a substitute for their expertise. In many cases there will be no need to alter pacemaker function e.g. peripheral surgery, surgery without diathermy, patient not pacemaker dependent.

3 Determine whether the patient is pacemaker dependent. If yes then an alternative form of pacing needs to be available e.g. transcutaneous

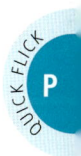

QUICK FLICK **P**

pacing.

4   Whether the programmable features are switched off depends on several factors including:

   a) If minute ventilation rate responsiveness is present program this off.

   b) Program all rate enhancements off (e.g. dynamic atrial overdrive, sleep rate etc.).

   c) Consider increasing the pacing rate to optimise O_2 delivery to the tissues e.g. 70 bpm.

   d) In patients that are pacemaker dependent consider programming the pacemaker to asynchronous (VOO or DOO) with the rate set greater than the patient's underlying rate. However VOO/DOO competition between paced and spontaneous beats could lead to sustained tachycardia or fibrillation particularly in the diseased heart.

   e) If the patient has a good intrinsic heart rate consider VVI mode and keep diathermy bursts short if they lead to bradycardia or asystole.

5   Although endocarditis has been reported with pacing wires[2] prophylactic antibiotics are not indicated unless additional risk factors are present.[3]

6   The risk of diathermy effects can be reduced by:

   a) Short irregular bursts of diathermy current at the lowest acceptable power output.

   b) Avoid the use diathermy within 15 cm of pacemaker or heart.

   c) Place the indifferent plate as far away from the heart and as close to the cutting blade as possible.

   d) The direction of the diathermy current (blade to plate) should be at right angles to the pacemaker system and not cross it.

   e) Use bipolar diathermy (the current flows through the 2 points of forceps) rather than unipolar (blade to plate). If unipolar diathermy is used, 'pure cut' is better than 'blend' or 'coag' settings.

7   'Pacemaker syndrome' may occur in patients with VVI pacemakers and consists of sudden hypotension with the onset of ventricular pacing.[3] It is due to the loss of atrioventricular synchrony and reflex vasodilatation due to atrial stretch-receptor stimulation. It is treated by a reduction in pacemaker rate so that sinus rhythm predominates, or increasing the sinus rate with atropine or isoprenaline.

8   The pacemaker should be rechecked postoperatively and reprogrammed by qualified staff if needed.

9   If pacemaker failure occurs during anaesthesia consider the following options to maintain heart rate:

   a) atropine.

   b) transcutaneous pacing.

   c) isoprenaline infusion.

10 Place nerve stimulators well away from the pacemaker.

Anaesthesia and AICDs

AICDs can provide anti-tachycardia pacing, synchronised shocks or unsynchronised shocks depending on the rate and rhythm detected. They can also provide anti-bradycardia pacing. AICDs can be affected by diathermy resulting in inappropriate anti-tachycardia pacing or shocks. AICDs can also be affected by insertion of a central line and should be disabled for this procedure. Some considerations include:

1 The defibrillating and anti-tachycardic functions should be deactivated prior to anaesthesia by appropriate technical staff.[4]

2 External defibrillation pads and connections should be applied before anaesthesia. If external defibrillation is required place the pads in an anterior/posterior position unless the pacemaker box is in the way. A higher than normal defibrillation energy may be required. DO NOT DEFIBRILLATE OVER THE AICD.

3 Medical staff are not at risk if in contact with a patient during AICD defibrillation.[4]

Emergency Surgery (Pacemaker Technician Unavailable)

The same considerations apply as outlined above. In addition:

1 A pacemaker magnet should be immediately available. If significant pacemaker malfunction occurs during surgery, application of a magnet to the pacemaker may convert it to a fixed rate mode. However, application of an external magnet to a pacemaker can also produce unwanted, unpredictable results.

2 Contact the cardiologist urgently if life-threatening pacemaker malfunction occurs that is not responsive to application of a magnet. Once a magnet is placed over the pacemaker, it should not be removed until a pacemaker technician is available. If the magnet is removed, a new program may become apparent. If the effects of the new program are deleterious then reapply the magnet and contact the cardiologist urgently.

3 Turn off the respiratory rate monitor in case the pacemaker responds to this with a tachycardia.

4 Suxamethonium is best avoided as muscle fasciculations may result in pacemaker malfunction.[3]

5 The pacemaker should be checked postoperatively by qualified staff as soon as practical.

6 If inappropriate defibrillation occurs with an AICD consider placement of an external magnet over the unit. This may deactivate the AICD and audible tones may be heard from the AICD. Removal of the magnet may reactivate the unit.

External Defibrillation and Pacemakers

External defibrillation can result in severe damage to the pacemaker and burns to the myocardial endothelium. If defibrillation is required place

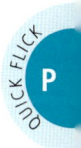

defibrillation pads as far away as possible from the pacemaker (>10 cm). The device must be checked for damage and accidental reprogramming as soon as it is practical to do so.

Pacemakers and Specific Procedures

1 Magnetic Resonance Imaging is, in general, contraindicated in patients with pacemakers. If MRI is considered essential, discuss the implications with the cardiologist.

2 Lithotripsy can be performed in patients with a pacemaker unless the pulse generator (or 'can') is abdominally placed. The above precautions should be used and a programmer should be available throughout the procedure. Contralateral lithotripsy can probably be safely perfomed in patients with AICDs.[4]

Temporary Pacemaker Wire (TPW) Insertion and Pacing

A typical unit used is a Medtronic 5375 Demand Pulse Generator. The steps are:

1 Insert a central venous sheath as described for *Internal Jugular Vein (IJV) Catheterisation*.

2 Insert a pacing wire towards the apex of the right ventricle either under X-ray guidance or use a flotation guided cardiac pacing wire.

3 Connect the pacing leads to the corresponding red and black leads and ask an assistant to connect these to the pacing box. The settings to be adjusted are:

   a) Stimulation Output—the pacing current strength.

   b) Sensitivity—the pacemaker's ability to sense the patient's QRS complexes.

   c) Rate—the pacing rate.

4 With the generator switched off, set the stimulation output to 5 mA and the 'rate' at (at least) 10 bpm > than the patient's intrinsic rate. Set the sensitivity control half way between 1.5 and 3 mV.

5 Turn the generator on. Advance the wire until ventricular 'capture' occurs (paced beats are seen on the ECG monitor). Deflate the balloon if using a flotation guided wire. Decrease the stimulation output until capture is lost, usually at about 1.5 mA. Then gradually increase the stimulation until the stimulation threshold is determined. Set the output current at 5 mA or at least 2 × the stimulation threshold.

6 Determine the sensitivity threshold by turning the rate control to 10 bpm < patient's intrinsic rate. Pacing should stop and the sense indicator light should flash with each R wave. Gradually turn the sensing control counterclockwise until the pacemaker starts to pace (pacing light flashes). Turn the sensitivity control clockwise until it is 2–3 × more sensitive than the sensing threshold.

Transcutaneous Cardiac Pacing (TCP)

1 The optimal transcutaneous pacing electrode pad placement is the anterior/posterior position. Apply the anterior electrode to the left of the sternum over the precordium. Apply the posterior electrode immediately behind the anterior electrode to the left of the spine. Alternatively the apex/right subclavian position can be used. *See Cardioversion*.

2 The pads are connected to the pacing unit and the desired rate set. The default rate is typically 80 per minute.

3 The strength of the pacing signal is gradually increased until 'capture' occurs e.g. 50–90 mA in patients with spontaneous circulation, up to 140 mA in cardiac arrest patients.[5] *See Cardiac Arrest*. Pace at a current that is 10% above the capture threshold.

4 With effective pacing you should see a wide QRS complex and a T wave after the pacing spike, and be able to feel a pulse.

5 If capture does not occur with maximum output (usually 140 mA) try repositioning the electrodes.

6 As well as treating bradycardia and asystole, transcutaneous pacing can be used to treat ventricular tachycardia and supraventricular tachycardia by either 'underdrive' pacing (pacing at a rate less than the tachycardia) or 'overdrive' pacing (pacing at a rate faster than the tachycardia). Although the latter is more successful, it is not possible to do if the tachycardia rate is >170 bpm (the maximum pacing rate).[6]

Transoesophageal Pacing

This is another non-invasive form of pacing but it is not as reliable as transcutaneous pacing.[6] Transoesophageal pacing can be used to provide atrial pacing (TAP) which preserves atrial priming pump function,[7] and to provide atrial overdrive pacing in the treatment of torsades de pointes, supraventricular tachycardia and atrial flutter.[6] This technique involves insertion of an oesophageal electrode which can be incorporated into an oesophageal stethoscope and placement of an external grounding electrode on the patient. Typical settings are square wave pulses of 10 ms at a current of 10 mA.

Fist Pacing

Mechanical stimulus to the heart can result in a myocardial electrical impulse leading to ventricular contraction. Fist pacing is indicated for haemodynamically unstable bradyarrhythmia as a stopgap measure until electrical pacing can be provided.[8]

This technique involves:

1 Serial rhythmic blows to the left lower edge of the sternum. These blows are of a lesser force than a precordial thump.

2 Apply 50–70 blows per minute.

Biventricular Pacing

Patients with advanced heart failure and evidence of intraventricular dyssynchrony may benefit from cardiac resynchronisation therapy in the form of biventricular pacing. Several studies have shown a decrease in mortality and decreased risk of sudden death with this technique.[9] Biventricular pacing results in improved ventricular contraction and relaxation dynamics, optimises co-ordination of the right and left ventricle and significantly improves the functional capacity of the patient. These devices are frequently combined with an AICD.

◐ Packed Cells

See Red Cells.

◐ Pancuronium

This drug is a long-acting non-depolarising, bis-quaternary aminosteroid neuromuscular blocking drug.

Dose

0.1 mg/kg IV. Effects last 45–60 min. Give top up doses of 0.03 mg/kg.

Advantages

Its long duration of action is useful for long operations and for patients who are being ventilated postoperatively.

Disadvantages

1   Pancuronium causes an increased heart rate, mean arterial pressure and cardiac output via a vagolytic action and enhanced sympathetic activity. This may be deleterious for patients in whom an increased heart rate is undesirable e.g. severe ischaemic heart disease.
2   It is metabolised in the liver (≈ 40%) and also excreted in the urine as the unchanged drug (≈ 50%). The dose should therefore be reduced in the presence of renal or liver impairment.

◐ Paracetamol

Acetanilide derivative analgesic antipyretic drug. Its actions are thought to be due to its selective inhibition of COX-3, a splice variant of COX-1, found in mature spinal cord and brain.[10] Paracetamol is also theorised to be a potent inhibitor of prostaglandin E synthesis in the central nervous system and peripherally reduces chemoreceptor function responsible for nociceptive impulse generation. It is not anti-inflammatory at normal dosages.

Dose

Adult 500–1000 mg 4–6 h PO or PR, max 4 g per day.
Child 20 mg/kg PO or PR initially then 15 mg/kg PO or PR. Subsequent doses 4–6 h, max 60 mg/kg per day.[11]

Precautions

1 Hepatotoxicity. This is the main risk factor with paracetamol use. This is due to the limited ability of hepatic glutathione to conjugate the toxic metabolite N-acetyl-p-benzo-quinone imine. Treatment of paracetamol overdose is with N-acetyl cysteine or methionine. Paracetamol should be used cautiously in patients with liver impairment due to such causes as chronic alcoholism, extensive liver resection and glucose-6-phosphate dehydrogenase deficiency.[12]

2 Muscular dystrophy and liver failure. There have been a few reports in the literature of fulminant hepatic failure in patients with muscular dystrophy receiving paracetamol perhaps related to decreased muscle mass.[13]

3 IV Paracetamol risks. There has been at least one death due to air embolus during the administration of IV paracetamol.[14] As the drug is contained in a glass bottle an airway needle is required to be inserted for the fluid to flow. Therefore the paracetamol infusion must be carefully observed to ensure air embolus does not occur.

◯ Paravertebral Block

Anatomy

This technique involves the blocking of nerve roots as they leave the spinal canal through the intervertebral foramina. These foramina are positioned midway between adjacent transverse processes and 2 cm anterior to the plane of the transverse processes. In the thoracic region the nerve root enters a triangular space (the paravertebral space) bounded by the vertebral body, the plane of the transverse process and the pleura.

Technique

Thoracic Paravertebral Blocks

These are useful for acute herpes zoster infection of the chest, rib fractures and unilateral operations such as breast surgery.[15] The technique is as follows:

1 Identify the spinous process one level above the chosen nerve root.
2 Sterilise the area around the entry point which is 3 cm lateral to the superior margin of this spinous process.
3 Anaesthetise the skin and deeper tissues at this point then insert a 10 cm 22 G spinal needle 90° to the skin.
4 Advance this needle onto the rib or transverse process (which will be at a depth of ≈ 3cm).
5 Walk the needle in a cephalad direction over the cephalad edge of the transverse process/rib.
6 Attach a 10 mL syringe (filled with saline or air) to the needle and test for loss of resistance as the needle point passes through the costo-transverse ligament into the triangular space described above.

7 Aspirate for blood, air or CSF. If negative inject 5–10 mL of LA e.g. bupivacaine 0.25%.

Lumbar Paravertebral Block

1 Identify the spinous process at the level of the nerve to be blocked.
2 The needle entry point is 3 cm lateral to the superior edge of the spinous process.
3 Prepare the skin as described above and insert a 10 cm spinal needle 10–30° cephalad. The transverse process should be contacted at a depth of 2.5–5 cm.
4 The needle is repositioned to walk off the lower medial edge of the transverse process (i.e. angled medially and more caudad). Advance the needle 2 cm.
5 After careful aspiration inject 5–10 mL of LA solution. A larger volume e.g. 20 mL can be injected at a single level which will block 3 or more levels.[16]

Risks of Paravertebral Block

The main risks are:
1 pneumothorax (at the thoracic levels)
2 Horner's syndrome (at thoracic levels)
3 subarachnoid or epidural block
4 intravascular injection.

◐ Parecoxib (Dynastat)

Parenteral COX-2 selective NSAID useful for treating acute pain. It is a prodrug for valdecoxib and can be given IV or IM.

Dose

40 mg IV or IM by slow deep injection. It is approved for single use only. Reduce dose to 20 mg for elderly patients less than 50 kg or patients with moderate-to-severe renal impairment. With IV injection effects start in 7–14 min and last up to 24 h.

Advantages

Like other COX-2 selective NSAIDs, parecoxib has little or no effect on platelet function or gut mucosa. ***See*** *Non-steroidal Anti-inflammatory Drugs (NSAIDs)*.

Disadvantages

1 Parecoxib is contraindicated in patients with sulfonamide allergy.
2 This drug is also contraindicated for use in cardiac surgery, in patients with severe or unstable IHD and major vascular surgery.
3 The drug should be avoided in patients with renal impairment.
4 Parecoxib is not approved for use in children.
5 Although a potent analgesic (superior to morphine 4 mg), it is inadequate as the sole analgesic for severe pain.

6 Catergory C drug in pregnancy—may cause harmful effects on the human fetus not including malformations.

○ Parkinson's Disease

Parkinson's disease is due to the loss of dopaminergic neurons in the substantia nigra of the brain. It is characterised by rigidity, tremor and bradykinesis. Patients may suffer from a variety of other complaints such as orthostatic hypotension and cardiac arrhythmias.

Treatment

Drugs used to treat Parkinson's disease include:

1 Dopamine precursors such as levodopa. Levodopa has a short half-life of 1–3 h.
2 Dopamine agonists e.g. ropinirole, apomorphine.
3 Monoamine oxidase B inhibitors e.g. selegeline.
4 Atypical agents e.g. amantadine (mechanism of action not understood).
5 Peripherally acting dopa decarboxylase inhibitors such as benserazide.
6 Catechol-o-methyl transferase inhibitors (inhibit dopamine breakdown) such as entacapone.
7 Anticholinergic drugs such as benzhexol.

Pre-anaesthetic Management

1 Place patient first on the operating list to ensure medication timing is optimal.
2 Continue drug therapy preoperatively up to the time of surgery. Give drugs through a nasogastric tube if necessary.
3 Patients that are having planned surgery who will be unable to take their medication for a prolonged period after surgery should be considered for apomorphine subcut therapy. As this drug is severely emetogenic consider domperidone 20 mg tds for 3 days PO prior to a subcutaneous infusion dose of apomorphine ≈ 30–40 mg over 16 h.[17] Apomorphine can also cause significant hypotension. Domperidone can be continued PR postoperatively.
4 Diphenhydramine can be useful for sedation in patients requiring premedication.[18]

Intra-operative Management

1 Levodopa can be given intraoperatively by naso/orogastric tube.
2 Use of succinylcholine may precipitate hyperkalaemia.[19] However this advice has been questioned by Muzzi et al. who found no potassium rise in 7 patients with Parkinson's disease given succinylcholine.[20]
3 Patients may be on selegeline which can interact with pethidine. *See* Monoamine Oxidase (MAO) Inhibitor Drugs.
4 Opioids may worsen rigidity.

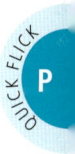

5 Propofol may have dopamine-like effects causing improved tremor control or dyskinesia. Do not use propofol if patients are having stereotactic surgery for Parkinson's disease.[21]

6 Atropine may cause central anticholinergic syndrome. Use glycopyrrolate instead.[17]

7 Keep patients well hydrated perioperatively.

Postoperative Management

1 NSAIDs and paracetamol can be used with the usual precautions.

2 Postoperative nausea and vomiting should not be treated with centrally acting antidopaminergic drugs such as metoclopramide and prochlorperazine.[17] Also avoid droperidol.

3 Continue oral therapy as soon as possible after surgery, by nasogastric tube if necessary.

4 Patients with Parkinson's disease are more prone to postoperative confusion and hallucinations.[22] Do not use haloperidol to treat postoperative confusion in Parkinson's patients.[17] Benzodiazepine sedation may be useful in this situation.[18]

◗ Partial Pressure of Gases

In Fully Humidified Inspired Air O_2—149 mm Hg (19.8 kPa), CO_2—0.3 mm Hg (0.04 kPa), H_2O—47 mm Hg (6.25 kPa) N_2—564 mm Hg (75 kPa)

Expired Gas O_2—116 mm Hg (15.4 kPa), CO_2—26.8 mm Hg (3.6 kPa), H_2O—47 mm Hg, N_2—569.9 mm Hg (75.7 kPa)

Alveolar Gas O_2—100 mm Hg (13.3 kPa), CO_2—40 mm Hg (5.3 kPa), H_2O—47 mm Hg, N_2—573 mm Hg (76.2 kPa)

Arterial Blood O_2—95 mm Hg (12.6 kPa), CO_2—40 mm Hg (5.3 kPa), N_2—570 mm Hg (75.8 kPa)

Venous Blood O_2—40 mm Hg (5.3 kPa), CO_2—46 mm Hg (6.1 kPa)

◗ Patient Controlled Analgesia (PCA) and Patient Controlled Epidural Anaesthesia (PCEA)

Adult Dosages

1 *Morphine* (120 mg in 60 mL N/S) Start with 1–2 mg boluses with a 5 min lockout. Use 1 mg for average patient, 2 mg for large fit male. Do not mix ketamine with morphine in the same PCA syringe as there is no added benefit.

2 *Fentanyl* (1200 µg in 60 mL N/S) Start with 10–20 µg bolus IV with 5 min lockout (10 µg for older frailer patient, 20 µg for fitter patient). PCA intranasal fentanyl has been used in adults with a dose of 25 µg and a 6 minute lockout.[23]

3 *Tramadol* (300 mg in 60 mL N/S) Start with 10–20 mg IV bolus with a 5 min lockout period.

4 *Remifentanil* There has been research into the use of IV PCA remifentanil for patients in labour. Various regimens have been used e.g. a background infusion of 0.025–0.1 μg/kg/min plus 0.25 μg/kg boluses with a 2 minute lockout. Patients must be observed very closely for excessive respiratory depression and sedation.[24]

5 *Pethidine—Used Epidurally* (300 mg in 60 mL N/S) 50 mg loading dose then 20 mg bolus with a 10 min lockout.

6 *Bupivacaine—Used Epidurally In Labouring Patients* Epidural bupivacaine can be administered with or without a basal infusion rate. For example use bupivacaine 0.125% 6 mL/h basal rate with a PCEA dose of 5 mL with a 15 min lockout period.

Child Dosages[25]

PCA techniques are not usually suitable for a child < 5 yrs.

1 *Morphine* 1 mg/kg loaded into 50 mL 5% glucose. Program 1 mL bolus (20 μg/kg) with a 5 min lockout + background infusion of 0.5 mL/h.

2 *Fentanyl* 50 μg/kg loaded into 50 mL 5% glucose. Program 0.5 mL bolus (0.5 μg/kg) with a 5 min lockout + background infusion of 1 mL/h.

⬥ Penetrating Eye Injury

See Eye Injury, Penetrating.

⬥ Penile Block

Useful for circumcision, hypospadias repair and penile trauma analgesia.

Anatomy

The penis is innervated by the dorsal nerves of the penis and the perineal nerves (both of which are branches of the pudendal nerves). The injection is made into a triangular space bounded by the symphysis pubis above, corpora cavernosa below and Bucks (Scarpa's) fascia anteriorly.

Technique (Do Not Use Adrenaline Containing LA)

1 Sterilise the skin at the dorsal base of the penis. Insert 23 G 32 mm needle at the 1030 and 0130 clock positions, just under the symphysis pubis. Direct the needle through the tough Bucks fascia at an angle of 10–15° to the midline. Alternatively, insert the needle in the midline, then redirect the needle to perform a paramedian injection on each side.

2 Aspirate prior to injection. If no blood is aspirated, inject LA on each side.
Child Inject 1 mL + 0.1 mL/kg each side. Use bupivacaine 0.25%.[26]
Adult Inject 20 mL of LA; use bupivacaine 0.5% 15 mL + lignocaine 2% 5 mL.

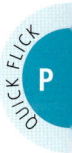

3 Also inject a bleb of LA at the penile scrotal junction extending to each side of the midline to block ventral branches of the perineal nerves. This greatly improves the reliability of the block.[27]

Alternative Technique

Simply inject LA subcutaneously around the base of the penile shaft (1–2 mL of bupivacaine 0.5% or 1.5–5 mL of 0.25%).[28] Do not use adrenaline containing solutions.

Note: The use of ropivacaine for penile block has been associated with ischaemia of the glans.[29]

Complications of Penile Block

1 Haematoma deep to Buck's fascia causing compression of dorsal veins and arteries with penile ischaemia.

2 Arterial vasospasm due to inadvertent injection of adrenaline containing solutions.

3 Intravascular injection of LA.

Treatment of Penile Ischaemia due to Penile Block

Penile ischaemia following penile block may be due to inadvertent use of adrenaline containing solutions or compression of penile blood vessels by haematoma formation. Treatments that have possibly been effective include:

1 Caudal anaesthesia to provide sympathetic blockade.[30]

2 Iloprost, a prostaglandin I_2 analogue, can be given by IV infusion.[29] A dose of 0.5–2 µg/h was used to treat penile ischaemia in an adult.[29]

⊙ Pentasaccharide

See Fondaparinux.

⊙ Pentax·AWS Video Laryngoscope

This device is very similar to Airtraq in terms of shape and design, and was developed in Japan in 2006. *See Airtraq.* It is used for laryngoscopy and intubation without the need to align the oral, pharyngeal and laryngeal axes, as is required for direct laryngoscopy. However the patient must be able to open his/her mouth $\simeq$ 3 cm. The handle contains disposable or rechargeable AA batteries, a light source and 5.3 cm high resolution LCD screen. It is connected to a 12 cm cable with a camera at the distal end. This cable is inserted into a disposable transparent lock-on blade which has a guide on the right hand side for the ET tube and there is a suction port through the blade.

Advantages

1 The device is intuitive and very easy to use.

2 The image quality on the screen is excellent and the screen can be rotated through 120° for comfort.

3 Intubation is very fast.
4 There is a sighting device on the screen which accurately predicts the initial trajectory of a PVC tube. Other types of ET tube e.g. reinforced tubes may pass posterior to the target marker.

Disadvantages
1 The batteries in theory could expire during the intubation although there is a warning signal.
2 There is no specific antifogging device.
3 The device is expensive at AUS$8500.
4 The device can be wiped clean but cannot be autoclaved.

○ Percutaneous Transluminal Coronary Angioplasty

See *Coronary Artery Revascularisation Procedures and Subsequent Non-cardiac Surgery*.

○ Perfluorocarbons

Artificial oxygen carrying solutions.
See *Blood Substitutes*.

○ Pericardial Effusion

See *Cardiac Tamponade*.

○ Pericardial Tamponade/Pericardiocentesis

See *Cardiac Tamponade*.

○ Peripartum Cardiomyopathy

Diagnosis
Peripartum cardiomyopathy is diagnosed if cardiac failure occurs in the last trimester of pregnancy or within 5 months of delivery and no other cause can be identified.[31] It is a rare condition, with an incidence of 1 per 3000–4000 pregnancies.[31] Interestingly in Haiti the incidence may be 1 per 299 live births.[32] The aetiology is unknown by definition but thought to be possibly related to viral and/or an abnormal immune response to pregnancy. There is no specific test for peripartum cardiomyopathy.

Pre-anaesthetic Management for Caesarean Section
Management of these patients involves optimisation of preload, afterload and contractility as with all other forms of heart failure. *See* *Congestive Cardiac Failure (CCF)*.
Important strategies include:
1 Assessment by obstetric, cardiac and anaesthetic specialists.

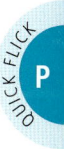

2 Appropriate investigations including ECG and cardiac echocardiography.

3 Supportive measures including bed rest and oxygen supplementation.

4 Preload optimisation. This may include fluid restriction, diuretics and venodilation agents such as GTN for reducing preload or fluid therapy to increase preload.

5 Afterload reduction with arterial vasodilators such as hydralazine or sodium nitroprusside. ACE inhibitors can be used postpartum but are contraindicated during pregnancy due to teratogenicity.

6 Enhancement of cardiac contractility with inotropic agents such as digoxin and/or dobutamine, milrinone. Intra-aortic balloon pump support may be required. An AICD may be required for malignant arrhythmias.

7 β-blockers can be helpful but are potentially harmful to the fetus. β-blockers may adversely affect uteroplacental and fetal haemodynamics causing such effects as decreased placental blood flow.[33] β-blockers should be ceased before labour.

8 Appropriate monitoring including arterial line, central line + PA catheter, TOE and fetal cardiotocograph.

9 Thromboembolic prophylaxis.

Anaesthetic Management

The aims of anaesthetic management are to provide cardiovascularly stable anaesthesia in addition to the requirements outlined in the section on *Caesarean Section (CS)*. The type of anaesthesia chosen will depend on the severity of the cardiomyopathy, and the skill and experience of the anaesthetist involved.

General Anaesthesia

GA for CS may be preferred in cases of severe peripartum cardiomyopathy, due to the risk of potential cardiovascular instability with regional blockade.[34,35] In addition to the points made in the section on *Caesarean Section (CS)* the following should be noted:

1 The IV induction drug used for rapid sequence e.g. thiopentone or propofol should be used in an appropriately reduced dose to decrease the risk of excessive myocardial depression.

2 One case report recommended maintenance of anaesthesia with a propofol/remifentanil infusion.[31]

Regional Anaesthesia

Epidural anaesthesia may be of benefit in some patients due to the reduction in afterload without reduced contractility. However, epidural anaesthesia must be induced slowly and carefully with appropriate invasive monitoring, depending on the severity of the condition. For example one patient requiring CS had an epidural block established to a T4 level over 6 hours with an infusion of bupivacaine and fentanyl.[31] Subarachnoid block anaesthesia is generally not recommended in these patients although 'low dose' combined spinal epidural anaesthesia has been used successfully.[36]

Postanaesthetic Care

Mortality is difficult to estimate but is probably around 15% due to cardiac failure, dysrhythmias and thromboembolic complications.[37] About 30% of women recover fully and up to 10% require a heart transplant.[38]

◗ Pethidine

Synthetic phenylpiperidine opioid receptor agonist used for analgesia and the treatment of postoperative shivering. ***See*** *Shivering Postoperatively*.

Dose

Adult IV/IM 25–100 mg IM as required up to 3 h. For IV analgesia, give 20–25 mg increments 5 min up to 150 mg.

Adult Epidural Dose 25–50 mg. ***See*** *Patient-controlled Analgesia (PCA) and Patient-controlled Epidural Anaesthesia*.

Child 1 mg/kg IM or same dose in 10 mL N/S, give in 1 mL increments IV 5 min prn.

Advantages

1 Pethidine may cause less nausea than morphine.[39]
2 Pethidine has little effect on coughing.[39]
3 Although once thought to cause less spasm of the sphincter of Oddi than morphine, this effect is unlikely to be clinically significant.[40]
4 Pethidine has local anaesthetic effects and has been used as a sole anaesthetic agent epidurally for surgery in critically ill patients.[41]

Disadvantages

1 Pethidine is inferior to morphine for analgesia at equivalent dosages. It is also shorter acting.
2 Pethidine can produce severe reactions in patients taking monoamine oxidase inhibitor drugs. ***See*** *Monoamine Oxidase (MAO) Inhibitor Drugs*.
3 It is not suitable for subcutaneous injection due to stinging.
4 Use pethidine with caution in renal failure as accumulation of the metabolite norpethidine may occur. Accumulation of norpethidine may also occur when pethidine is used in high dose over days. Norpethidine is a potent convulsant and may also cause tremors, twitches and myoclonus. Symptoms of norpethidine toxicity can occur below the 600 mg/day recommended safety level.[40]

5   Pethidine causes more euphoria and is much more likely to be abused than morphine.[40]
6   Pethidine is inferior to hydromorphone for the treatment of ureteric colic.[42]

◔ Phaeochromocytoma

Phaeochromocytomas are rare catecholamine secreting tumours and 90% arise from the adrenal medulla. About 10% are bilateral and about 10% are malignant.[43] They may also secrete other substances such as enkephalins, somatostatin and calcitonin.

Pre-operative Assessment
The main clinical features are due to secretion of noradrenaline, adrenaline and dopamine. They include:
1   Paroxysmal hypertension often associated with dysrhythmias, headaches, sweating and tremor.
2   Postural hypotension due to volume depletion.
3   Hyperglycaemia due to α_2 adreno-receptor stimulation decreasing insulin release and promoting glycogenolosis.
4   Catecholamine induced cardiomyopathy/cardiac failure.
5   Anxiety, psychosis and visual disturbances may occur.

Pre-operative Investigation and Preparation
In addition to routine investigations patients must be evaluated for cardiac dysfunction including ECG and echocardiography. Preparation for surgery takes about 2 weeks. The aims of pre-operative preparation are to:
1   Control blood pressure, dysrhythmias and heart failure.
2   Normalise intravascular volume.
3   Normalise blood glucose levels.
Recommended treatment and preparation strategies are:
1   α adreno-receptor blockade should be initiated with a drug such as phenoxybenzamine (*see* *Phenoxybenzamine*). Commence with 20 mg PO bd increasing by 10–20 mg/day. The aims of treatment are to prevent blood pressure rises above 165/90 and to have a mild postural hypotension. Doxazocine is an alternative to phenoxybenzamine. Prazosin can be added if α blockade is inadequate with phenoxybenzamine.[43]
2   Beta adreno receptor blockade is indicated for tachydysrhythmias and tachycardia.
Note: β adreno-receptor blockade therapy must NEVER be commenced in the absence of α receptor blockade. This is because of the risk of blocking β adreno-receptor mediated vasodilatation resulting in exacerbation of hypertension. Also β blockade without α blockade may result in myocardial

depression sufficient to result in cardiac failure in the presence of elevated SVR. **See** *Adrenergic Receptors*.

3 Alpha methylparatyrosine inhibits catecholamine synthesis by up to 80% and can be useful pre-operatively and intra-operatively to help control blood pressure.[43]

4 Beta blockade results in vasodilatation of the chronically vasoconstricted intravascular space. Ensure normovolaemia is re-established. A fall in haematocrit of 5% is suggestive of intravascular repletion.

5 Control blood glucose levels. Insulin is rarely required.

Pre-anaesthetic Phase

1 Consider a benzodiazepine premedication.

2 Establish large bore IV access and intra-arterial blood pressure measurement. Use LA liberally for line insertion to reduce nociceptive stimulation which can precipitate hypertension.

3 Insert a CVP line or PA catheter. This can be inserted after induction of GA. Transoesophageal echocardiography should be considered in patients with significant cardiomyopathy.

4 Thoracic epidural anaesthesia to supplement GA is useful to attenuate the adrenergic response to surgery and for postoperative pain control post-operative. However epidural anaesthesia does not block the hypertensive effects of catecholamine release due to tumour handling. Epidural blockade may also complicate interpretation of extremes of hypertension and hypotension during and after surgery.[44]

5 Avoid morphine and hydromorphone, which cause histamine release and may therefore induce catecholamine release.[43] Opioids with minimal histamine releasing properties include fentanyl, alfentanil and buprenorphine.

6 Do not use droperidol pre-operatively or intra-operatively.[43] This drug can block α_2 receptors and inhibit catecholamine reuptake. Droperidol can also interact with dopamine receptors resulting in increased catecholamine release.

7 Sodium nitroprusside is often required for severe refractory hypertension and should be pre-prepared and ready for immediate infusion. Brief episodes of hypertension can be treated with IV phentolamine.

Induction and Maintenance Phase

1 Aim for cardiovascular stability and deal with hypertension and hypotension promptly.

2 Induce anaesthesia with appropriate dosages of midazolam, fentanyl, and propofol or thiopentone. Consider measures to reduce the hypertensive response to intubation. **See** *Hypertensive Response to Intubation (Attenuation of)*. Do not use ketamine because it stimulates the sympathetic nervous system.

3 Use a muscle relaxant devoid of histamine release such as rocuronium or vecuronium. Avoid pancuronium due to its tendency to cause tachycardia, and suxamethonium which may release histamine. Also fasciculations due to suxamethonium may cause abdominal compression and release of tumour catecholamines.[43]

4 Maintain anaesthesia with isoflurane or sevoflurane. Do not use halothane which sensitises the myocardium to catecholamines. Desflurane may cause sympathetic nervous system stimulation at higher doses so it is not an ideal choice in this situation.

5 Consider using a magnesium sulphate infusion. A loading dose of 40–60 mg/kg can be used then an infusion of about 2 g/h.[45] Magnesium reduces catecholamine release, and is an antagonist at alpha-adrenergic receptors. It is also an arteriolar dilator and anti-arrythmic.[46] Magnesium prolongs the effects of NDNMBDs and the dose of these drugs should therefore be modified appropriately.

6 Phentolamine boluses (1–2 mg) or an infusion can be useful for controlling hypertension. For severe hypertension use a sodium nitroprusside infusion.

7 The use of a remifentanil infusion has been associated with significant hypotension and bradycardia in patients who are undergoing phaeochromocytoma surgery and who are α and β adrenoreceptor blocked.[47]

8 Consider β blocker drugs such as metoprolol or an esmolol infusion for intra-operative tachydysrhythmias. In one study 2 patients with persistent tachycardias resistant to β blockers (and adenosine in one case) responded well to a carefully titrated dose of neostigmine.[48] Nicardipine has also been used.[49]

9 Hypertension is particularly likely to occur on intubation, at the time of pneumoperitoneum (in laparoscopic surgery) and when the tumour is manipulated.

10 Hypotension can occur with removal of the tumour. Treat this with liberal IV fluids. Use a noradrenaline infusion for persistant hypotension unresponsive to adequate fluid loading.

11 Blood loss tends to be poorly tolerated by these patients and blood transfusion should be considered early.

12 Monitor blood glucose levels. Commence glucose containing IV fluids once the tumour is removed.[43]

13 Reverse neuromuscular blockade with neostigmine and glycopyrrolate. Avoid atropine which may cause an excessive increase in heart rate.[43]

Advantages of Laparoscopic Surgery[48]
Some phaeochromocytomas are resectable laparoscopically. Advantages include:

1 Possibly less blood loss.

2 Shorter hospital stay.

3 Less postoperative pain and better cosmetic result.

Disadvantages of Laparoscopic Surgery[49]

1 The creation of pneumoperitoneum can be particularly hazardous and precipitate an adrenergic crisis. Sood et al. reported much less haemodynamic disturbance when low intra-abdominal pressures (8–10 mm Hg) were used.[50]

2 Longer operation time.

3 Tendency to greater cardiovascular instability with an increased requirement for sodium nitroprusside.

Post-anaesthetic Phase

The patient should be monitored in a high dependency or intensive care unit. Problems to anticipate and treat include:

1 Hypoglycaemia. Give glucose containing solutions postoperatively.

2 Hypotension. This may require vasopressor/inotropic therapy (but exclude hypovolaemia/haemorrhage).

3 Hypertension persists postoperatively in up to 50% of patients. Consider residual tumour or renal ischaemia as possible aetiological factors.

Mortality

The peri-operative mortality for well prepared patients is 0–3%.[51] For undiagnosed or ill prepared patients with phaeochromocytoma the mortality approaches 50%.[52] Five-year survival for malignant tumours is about 46%.[53]

○ Phenoxybenzamine

Tertiary amine (a halo-alkylamine) used for the treatment of hypertension including the management of phaeochromocytoma. Acts by producing irreversible (non competitive) α receptor blockade. Its actions therefore last 3–4 days after a single dose.

Dose

Adult 10–60 mg PO in divided doses or 10–40 mg IV over 1 h. Effects take ≈ 1 h to manifest.

Child 0.2–1 mg/kg 12–24 h oral or 1 mg/kg over 1 h IV then 0.5 mg/kg/dose 6–12 h.

○ Phentolamine

Antihypertensive imidazoline agent. Acts by competitive α_1 adreno-receptor blockade and to a lesser extent α_2 adreno-receptor blockade resulting in arterial vasodilatation with little venodilatation. Used for the treatment of hypertension, including the peri-operative management of patients with phaeochromocytoma.

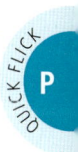

Dose
Adult 5–10 mg IM or 1 mg boluses IV. Effects last 10–30 min. Can also be given by IV infusion at a rate of 1–20 µg/kg/min.
Child 0.1 mg/kg IV then infusion 5–50 µg/kg/min IV.

◐ Phenylephrine

Powerful synthetic direct acting α_1 adreno-receptor agonist with weak β adreno-receptor activity. It is similar in action to noradrenaline but is less potent and has a longer duration of action. As stated by Levy it is now widely regarded as the vasopressor of choice in obstetric anaesthesia.[54]

Indications
Useful for the treatment of:
1   Hypotension due to its vasoconstrictor action.
2   As a nasal decongestant used topically.
3   For producing mydriasis without cycloplegia.
4   To overcome paroxysmal supraventricular tachycardia.

Dose for Hypotension
Give by IV infusion. Dilute 10 mg in 500 mL 5% glucose (20 µg/mL). Run at 0.15–0.7 µg/kg/min. For a 70 kg patient give 30–150 mL/h. If giving IV boluses use extremely cautiously e.g. increments of 50–100 µg.

Precautions/Contraindications
Phenylephrine is contraindicated in patients with:
1   severe hypertension
2   ventricular tachycardia.
The drug should be used with caution in patients with:
1   hyperthyroidism
2   bradycardia/partial heart block
3   ischaemic heart disease/severe atherosclerosis.

◐ Phenytoin

Hydantoin derivative used for:
1   Prophylaxis and treatment of seizures.
2   Class 1 anti-arrhythmic drug useful for the treatment of dysrhythmias associated with digoxin toxicity.

Dose for Seizure Control and Prevention
Loading Dose 10–15 mg/kg IV loaded into N/S (not glucose). Give no faster than 50 mg/min with ECG monitoring. Give 3–4 mg/kg/day for maintenance.
Therapeutic Level 40–80 µmol/L.
Note: Patients treated with phenytoin have increased dose requirements of vecuronium and pancuronium but not cisatracurium or atracurium.

⟡ **Physostigmine**

Alkaloid anticholinesterase drug from the West African calabar bean. It crosses the blood–brain barrier and is useful for the treatment of:
1 Glaucoma.
2 Atropine intoxication.
3 Trycyclic antidepressant poisoning.
4 Central anticholinergic syndrome (**see** *Central Anticholinergic Syndrome*).

⟡ **PICC Line**

PICC stands for Peripherally Inserted Central Catheter. This is a useful device for long-term venous access.

Technique for Insertion
1 Using aseptic technique, insert a 20 G cannula into a suitable large vein in the antecubital fossa.
2 Insert the guide wire through the cannula then remove the cannula.
3 Insert the introducer over the guide wire, then remove the introducer.
4 Insert the banana catheter over the guide wire then remove the guide wire.
5 Insert the catheter through the banana catheter, then remove the banana catheter by splitting it while it is gradually withdrawn.
6 Suture the PICC line into place.

⟡ **Placental Abruption**

See *Abruptio Placentae*.

⟡ **Placenta Accreta/Increta/Percreta**

The following terms refer to invasion by placental tissue into the myometrium of the uterus:
1 Accreta is invasion through the decidua, to the inner surface of the myometrium.
2 Increta is invasion into the myometrium.
3 Percreta is invasion into the full thickness of the myometrium. Other organs such as the bladder may be involved.

The term placenta accreta is used in this section to cover all the histiological types described above.

Placenta accreta has an incidence of about 1 per 2500 deliveries.[55] This condition is associated with placenta praevia (see below), previous CS or repeated uterine curettage. Due to increasing CS rates the incidence of placenta accreta is increasing. A patient with placenta praevia and a history of 2 or more CS has a 48% risk of placenta accreta.[56]

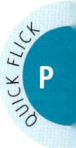

Diagnosis

This condition is usually diagnosed at the time of delivery or at CS when there is failure of the placenta to separate from the uterine wall, associated with severe haemorrhage. Uterine inversion may occur. The condition may be diagnosed prior to delivery by transvaginal ultrasound.[57] MRI imaging can be used to identify the extent of trophoblastic invasion.

Management of Placenta Accreta

1 If the condition is diagnosed pre-operatively, elective CS hysterectomy is required and preparation must be made for massive blood loss. Consider pre-operative autologous blood donation. Anaesthetic options are general anaesthesia, epidural anaesthesia or CSE. Spinal anaesthesia as a single-shot technique may not last long enough for this procedure.

2 In one reported case of known placenta percreta an aortic balloon was placed pre-CS and used to control severe intra-operative haemorrhage.[58] Interventional radiology with balloon occlusion of the Iliac or uterine arteries has an increasingly important role in diminishing blood loss. Sheaths and access catheters may be placed pre-operatively or intra-operatively.

3 Management of undiagnosed placenta accret at the time of delivery or CS follows the same principles as other conditions associated with massive blood loss. **See** *Blood Loss Assessment and Initial Management* and *Blood Transfusion*.

◖ Placenta Praevia

This condition is defined as implantation of the placenta in the lower uterine segment over or near the internal os of the uterus. Placenta praevia occurs in about 0.5% of deliveries with a recurrence risk of about 5%. Diagnosis is usually by antenatal ultrasound. Painless PV bleeding may occur. Caesarean section (CS) is required for patients with placenta praevia.

Placenta praevia is associated with an increased risk of placenta accreta, being ≈ 5% if no previous CSs have occurred. This risk increases in association with the number of previous CSs rising to 67% with 4 or more previous CS operations.[59] **See** *Placenta Accreta/Increta/Percreta* above.

Anaesthetic Management for Elective Caesarean Section

Traditionally general anaesthesia was advocated for elective Caesarean section because of concern over the hypotensive effects of regional anaesthesia combined with potentially massive blood loss. However regional anaesthesia has been used in many centres without any increase in adverse outcome rates.[60] Preparations must be made for massive blood loss including large bore IV access and the immediate availability of cross-matched blood. As noted above the risk of haemorrhage is increased by a past history of CS due to the increased risk of placenta accreta. The use of radiologically placed balloon catheters inserted prophylactically into the uterine arteries should be considered if facilities are available.

Anaesthetic Management of the Haemodynamically Unstable Patient

1 Ensure adequate airway and breathing.
2 Replace the patient's intravascular volume with appropriate fluid (crystalloid, colloid, blood).
3 *See* Blood Loss Assessment and Initial Management.
4 *See* Caesarean Section. General anaesthesia will be required in almost all cases.

◗ Plasmalyte A

A type of isotonic crystalloid fluid formulated without calcium to prevent clotting in transfused blood. It contains per 100 mL NaCl 526 mg, Sodium Gluconate 502 mg, Sodium Acetate Trihydrate 368 mg, KCl 37 mg, MgCl 37 mg. It should not be given to patients at risk of or who are suffering from hyperkalaemia e.g. renal failure patients.

◗ Platelet Adenosine Diphosphate (ADP) Receptor Antagonists

These thienopyridine drugs are potent inhibitors of platelet aggregation. Examples of these drugs include clopidogrel (Plavix) and ticlopidine (Ticlid).

Description and Mechanism of Action
These drugs act on platelet surface glycoproteins to irreversibly inhibit platelet adhesion and aggregation. The action of these drugs is delayed for 24–48 h and becomes maximal in 3–5 days.[61] The antiplatelet effect of these drugs is synergistic with aspirin.

Indications
These drugs are used to treat patients with ischaemic heart disease to reduce the incidence of ischaemia and infarction, to prevent coronary artery stent occlusion, and other thrombo-embolic disorders. They are often used with aspirin or as an alternative to aspirin in patients who cannot tolerate aspirin. Platelet glycoprotein antagonists are used acutely in patients undergoing percutaneous coronary interventions or in patients with unstable coronary syndromes unresponsive to conventional therapy.

Anaesthesia and Surgery
These drugs increase the risk of haemorrhage during surgery. However ceasing these drugs may result in such effects as coronary artery stent occlusion or myocardial infarction. *See* Coronary Artery Revascularisation Procedures and Subsequent Non-cardiac Surgery.

QUICK FLICK

P

If in consultation with the patient's surgeon and cardiologist/neurologist the decision is made to cease clopidogrel it should be stopped 7 days before surgery. Ticlopidine needs to be stopped 14 days before surgery. Neuraxial anaesthesia can be used after the same cessation times. Ticlopidine can cause neutropenia and thrombocytopenia.

Elective Surgery and Ongoing Clopidogrel Therapy *see Coronary Artery Revascularisation Procedures and Subsequent Non-cardiac Surgery.*

Emergency Surgery
In emergency surgery, platelet transfusion is the only effective treatment for haemorrhage due to clopidogrel/ticlodipine.[61] With clopidogrel, transfused platelets will be effective a few hours after the last dose.

◑ Platelet Glycoprotein IIb/IIIa Receptor Antagonists

Drug Description and Indications
These drugs act by inhibiting glycoprotein IIb and IIIa receptors on platelets thus reducing their ability to aggregate. They are always used in combination with other anti-clotting drugs such as heparin and aspirin. Examples include abciximab (RePro), eptifibatide and tirofiban. These drugs are administered intravenously for such indications as:

1 Patients undergoing percutaneous coronary artery interventions.

2 Patients with angina unresponsive to conventional therapy.

The effects of these drugs can be monitored by activated clotting time or more accurately by turbidometric aggregometry or the platelet function analyser.

Adverse Effects
These include bleeding, allergic reactions and thrombocytopenia.

Platelet GP IIb/IIIa Antagonists and Emergency Surgery
1 Cease all anti-platelet therapy as soon as possible before surgery.

2 Consider prophylactic platelet transfusion in patients on abciximab if the drug is ceased less than 12–24 h before surgery.[62]

3 Check platelet count and activated coagulation time.

4 Delay surgery in patients on eptifibatide and tirofiban for 4–6 h if possible.[63] Platelet transfusions are not effective in patients who have received eptifibatide or tirofiban.[64]

5 Consider using an anti-fibrinolytic drug such as aminocaproic acid.

◑ Platelet Therapy

The normal platelet count is $150–400 \times 10^9$/L (150 000–4 000 000/mm³). An increased risk of surgical bleeding occurs if the platelet count is

<50–80 × 10⁹/L, and spontaneous bleeding can occur below a platelet count of about 20 × 10⁹/L. Patients produce about 10% of their platelet count per day.

Storage of Platelets for Transfusion

Platelet concentrates are stored at 20–24°C and last about 5 days. The bags must be agitated gently and continuously during storage. Compatibility testing is not necessary routinely for transfusion.

Platelet Bag

A platelet bag contains >55 × 10⁹ platelets in 40–70 mL of plasma and is collected from a single unit of whole blood.[65] The pH at expiry is 6.8–7.4.

Pooled Platelets

Pooled platelets are obtained from a pool of ABO-identical donors and are contained in a volume of 160 mL. This equates to about 240 × 10⁹ platelets. Pooled platelets reduce the risk of recurrent febrile non-haemolytic transfusion reactions in multitransfused patients. These pooled platelets can also be leukocyte depleted to reduce the risk of HLA alloimmunisation and transmission of lymphocyte-born viral infections such as CMV.

Apheresis Platelets

Platelets obtained by an apheresis machine. These platelets may then undergo leukocyte depletion for the same reasons as pooled platelets.

Indications

The indications for platelet therapy are:

1 Decreased platelet numbers (thrombocytopenia) due to causes such as haemorrhage and diseases such as leukaemia, bone marrow failure. Platelets may be given to treat haemorrhage (platelet count < 50 000/mm³) or prevent spontaneous haemorrhage as follows:
   a) platelet count < 10 000/mm³ if no other risk factors
   b) < 20 000/mm³ if other risk factors present e.g. fever.
   Platelets may also be indicated if platelet count <100 000/mm³ and there is microvascular bleeding, or high risk from bleeding e.g. neurosurgery.
2 Impaired platelet function and bleeding e.g. clopidogrel therapy.

A unit of platelets increases platelet count in the adult by about 5–10 000/mm³. In children 10 mL/kg of platelets increases platelet count by about 30–40 000/mm³. Do not use a filter with a pore size <170 µm. A standard blood giving set filter is acceptable. Transfused platelets have a reduced lifespan of 1–3 days. Transfusion can proceed as fast as tolerated and should not exceed 4 h.

ABO Compatability and Platelets

Use ABO-Rh type compatible platelets to increase their lifespan. ABO incompatible platelets may be used in an emergency but reactions may

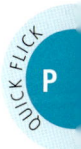

occur such as low-grade haemolysis. If Rh +ve platelets are given to a Rh –ve female with child bearing potential, Rh(D) immunoglobulin should be considered (250 IU per platelet treatment dose).

When Not to Give Platelets

1 Immune-mediated platelet destruction.
2 Thrombotic thrombocytopenic purpura.
3 Haemolytic uraemic syndrome.

◐ Pleural Catheter

***See** Chest Drain*.

◐ Pneumothorax

***See** Chest Drain*.

◐ Polycythaemia

Definition

Hb level >17 g d/L (Hct >0.51) in men and > 16 g/dL (Hct >0.47) in females. This condition can be divided into:

1 *Relative Polycythaemia* Red cell mass is normal but plasma volume is reduced.
2 *Apparent or Stress Polycythaemia* Can be due to smoking, alcohol, obesity and other causes. Hb is increased but red cell mass is normal.
3 *Absolute Polycythaemia* Can be primary (Polycythaemia Vera) or secondary due to causes such as congenital heart disease and inappropriate production of erythropoietin. Polycythaemia vera (PV) is a myeloproliferative disorder characterised by increased Hb levels, leukocytosis and increased platelet count. These patients are prone to impaired haemostasis and thrombo-embolic complications.

Anaesthetic Considerations in the Patient with Polycythaemia Vera

Patients with PV that is newly diagnosed or untreated should have elective surgery delayed until the condition is controlled medically for 4 months or longer due to the high incidence of thrombo-embolic and haemorrhagic complications. Haemorrhagic complications can be due to thrombocytopenia, platelet dysfunction and/or impaired fibrinolysis. Venesection should be considered if the Hct > 0.65 and there are symptoms of hyperviscosity. These include headache, faintness, vision disturbances, muscle pain and weakness, peripheral paraesthesia and depressed mentation. ***See** Hyperviscosity Syndrome*. To treat, remove one unit of blood replacing it with 500 mL of normal saline. Aim for a pre-operative Hct of <0.45 in males and <0.42 in females.

Emergency Surgery

Venesection should be performed pre-operatively if the Hct > 0.65.

◐ Popliteal Fossa Block

The popliteal block is used to block the common peroneal and tibial nerves via a single injection in the popliteal fossa. This is effectively equivalent to a sciatic nerve block.

Anatomy

The popliteal fossa is diamond shaped. The upper medial side is formed by semitendinosus; the lateral side by biceps femoris. The lower medial and lateral sides are formed by the medial and lateral heads of gastrocnemius. The sciatic nerve lies at the apex of the diamond and at this point it bifurcates into the common peroneal nerve which runs down on the lateral side of the fossa and the tibial nerve which runs through the popliteal fossa just medial to the midline.

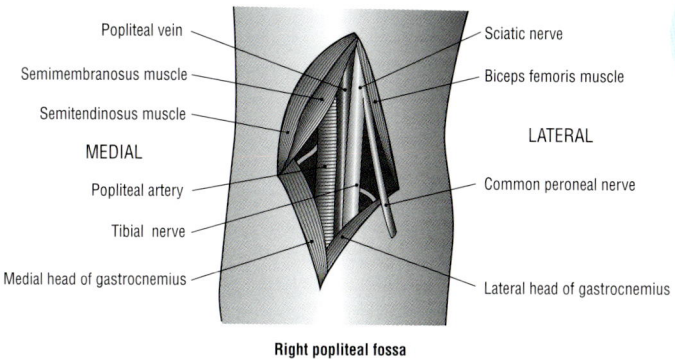

Right popliteal fossa

Figure P1 Anatomy of the popliteal fossa

Common Peroneal (Lateral Popliteal) Nerve (L4, L5 & S1) Supplies:

1 Forms the sural nerve with a branch of the tibial nerve supplying the posterolateral calf and lateral side of foot to the fifth toe.
2 Skin over the anterolateral and posterolateral calf.
3 Forms the superficial and deep peroneal nerves. *See Ankle Blocks and Innervation of the Foot.*

Tibial (Medial Popliteal) Nerve (L4, L5,S1, S2 & S3) Supplies:

1 Forms part of sural nerve (see above).
2 Branches into medial calcaneal and medial and lateral plantar nerves.
Note: The medial side of the leg and foot are supplied by branches of the femoral nerve.

Technique in the Adult[66]

1   Position the patient prone. Draw a triangle formed by the semitendinosus, biceps femoris and the skin crease of the popliteal fossa.

2   Bisect the triangle with a perpendicular line from base to apex.

3   Identify the point 5–6 cm cephalad from the skin crease (popliteal fold) along this bisecting line and 1 cm lateral to it. Mark this point with an X. This is the insertion point.

4   Using aseptic technique, insert 7.5 cm 22 G spinal needle through anaesthetised skin at point X at a 45–60° cephalad angle and seek paraesthesia. If a nerve stimulator is available use an insulated stimulation needle and seek a motor response. Start with a stimulating current of 2 mA with an end-point for injection of muscle reaction just being lost at 0.3 mA. A search pattern perpendicular to the nerve may be required to find it.

5   Inject 30–40 mL of LA (lignocaine 1% or bupivacaine 0.25%).

6   To anaesthetise the medial side of the calf and foot the femoral branches can be blocked by injecting 10 mL of LA over the medial tibial head just below the knee. **See also** *Saphenous Nerve Block*.

Note: The onset of the block takes 20 min or more.

Technique in the Child[67]

1   In children, the insertion point can be calculated as follows. Again the triangle formed by the popliteal fold and the apex of the popliteal fossa is bisected with a perpendicular line. The distance from the popliteal fold to the point of insertion is 1 cm cephalad per 10 kg of body mass (e.g. in a 25 kg child the distance is 2.5 cm).

2   Insert the insulated stimulation needle at a 45° angle to the skin lateral to the midline.

3   Inject bupivacaine 0.25% using a dose of 1 mL/kg.

Ultrasound Guided Technique[68]

1   Position the patient supine with the leg to be blocked flexed at the knee

2   The linear array ultrasound probe is placed in the popliteal fossa at right angles to the long axis of the leg (short axis view of the nerves).

3   Identify the politeal artery (pulsatile, difficult to compress) and the popliteal vein (compressible and non-pulsatile). The vein is closer to the skin surface and lateral to the artery.

4   Identify the sciatic nerve by following the tibial and common perineal nerves up the leg until the point of division is reached.

5   Move the probe to the lateral edge of the popliteal fossa. Insert a 10 cm short bevel block needle using a lateral in plane approach above the biceps femoris tendon and advance the tip to the sciatic nerve. Inject 20 mL of LA e.g. 1% ropivacaine.

◗ POR 8

POR 8 is 8-ornithine vasopressin. Used for skin and tissue vasoconstriction to decrease surgical bleeding. Dilute to 0.1–0.2 units/mL. Do not administer >0.5 units/kg.

Side Effects

These include hypertension and dysrhythmias. The drug is teratogenic and is therefore contraindicated in pregnancy (POR 8 product information).

◗ Porphyria

Topics Covered in this Section

▶ Acute Intermittent Porphyria
▶ Variegate Porphyria
▶ Hereditary Coproporphyria
▶ Types of Porphyria Not Requiring Avoidance of Triggering Drugs

The porphyrias are a group of inherited or acquired enzymatic defects involving haem synthesis characterised by an overproduction of porphyrins and their precursors. These diseases can be classified into hepatic and erythropoietin types.

Acute Intermittent Porphyria

Pathophysiology

Acute intermittent porphyria is a form of hepatic porphyria more common in females.[69] This illness is associated with attacks of severe abdominal pain and neurotoxity manifesting as psychoses, cranial and peripheral nerve dysfunction and autonomic dysfunction. Hypertensive complications and renal failure are the most frequent causes of death in this group. A significant proportion of pregnant women with porphyria will experience an attack during pregnancy.[69]

Symptoms and Signs of Acute Attacks

About 1% of acute attacks are fatal. Clinical manifestations include:

1 severe abdominal pain
2 autonomic instability (tachycardia, hypertension or hypotension)
3 dehydration and electrolyte disturbances
4 neuropsychiatric manifestations, seizures
5 muscle weakness.

Pharmacological Triggering Agents

The following drugs can, or are suspected of being able to, precipitate an acute attack as described above:

1 Thiopentone and other barbiturates and etomidate.
2 Endogenous steroids and drugs with a steroid structure. Pancuronium and vecuronium are unsafe.

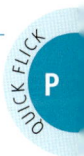

QUICK FLICK

P

3 Enflurane is possibly unsafe. It is contentious but likely that isoflurane and halothane are safe.[70]

4 Imipramine and tolbutamide are unsafe.

5 Alpha methyl dopa, hydralazine and phenoxybenzamine are also contraindicated.

6 Pentazocine. Other opioids are safe.

7 Oral contraceptive pill and griseofulvin are unsafe.

8 Of the benzodiazepines, nitrazepam and flunitrazepam are considered unsafe and diazepam is unsafe (but see below). Midazolam is considered safe.[69]

9 Phenytoin is unsafe.[71]

10 Avoid diclofenac, ibuprofen and fenoprofen.

11 Amiodarone is contraindicated.

Pre-anaesthetic Considerations

1 Avoid prolonged fasting and consider a glucose-saline drip to minimise starvation stress.

2 Acute intermittent porphyria is not a contraindication to regional anaesthesia. Bupivacaine is considered safe and lignocaine is probably safe.

Drugs Considered Safe

1 Propofol (probably safe),[69] ketamine (probably safe),[70] droperidol (safe). Avoid propofol infusions which may not be safe.[72]

2 Opioids (except pentazocine) are safe.

3 N_2O is safe. Isoflurane and halothane are probably safe but controversy exists.[69,70]

4 All muscle relaxants are safe **except** steroid based ones e.g. vecuronium and pancuronium.

5 Anticholinergic and anticholinesterase drugs.

6 Antiemetics such as droperidol and prochlorperazine are safe but metoclopramide should probably be avoided.

7 Aspirin, naproxen and Indomethacin are all safe.

8 Heparin is safe.

Treatment of an Acute Exacerbation of Porphyria

1 *Hypertension and Tachycardia* commonly occur during an acute attack and β blockers are the treatment of choice especially propranolol.

2 *Seizures* All commonly used anticonvulsants are porphyrogenic. However some of the new antiepileptic drugs such as gabapentin and vigapentin appear to be effective and safe. Diazepam has been used.[73] Check for hyponatraemia as a cause of the seizures. Magnesium sulphate is effective in porphyric patients who are hypomagnesaemic.[69]

3 Keep the patient well hydrated. If an acute attack occurs, give glucose 20 g/h. Haem arginate (haematin) can produce dramatic clinical improvement during an acute attack by reducing the synthesis of aminolaevulinic acid.[69] The dose of haem arginate is 3 mg/kg/day over 15 min by IV infusion through a central venous line. Give haematin for 4 days. Tin protoporphyrin, an inhibitor of haem oxygenase, may also be useful.

4 Treat severe pain with opioids such as morphine or pethidine.

Variegate Porphyria

Affects both sexes. Avoid triggering drugs as described above. Patients exhibit severe photosensitivity and thin fragile skin.

Hereditary Coproporphyria

Avoid the above triggering agents. This type also exhibits skin manifestations. Acute attacks tend to be less severe than in acute intermittent porphyria.

Types of Porphyria not Requiring Avoidance of Triggering Drugs

1. Porphyria cutanea tarda.
2. Erythropoietic uroporphyria.
3. Erythropoietic protoporphyria.

QUICK FLICK P

Postanaesthetic Confusion

See *Confusion, Agitation, Decreased Level of Consciousness, Postanaesthetic*.

Postdural Puncture Headache

See *Epidural Anaesthesia*.

Posterior Cutaneous Nerve of Thigh Block (Posterior Femoral Cutaneous Nerve Block)

Anatomy

(S1, S2 & S3) The posterior cutaneous nerve of the thigh is a branch of the sacral plexus. It supplies skin over the lower lateral part of gluteus maximus, back and medial side of thigh, popliteal fossa and upper part of the back of leg.

Technique

1. With the patient in the lateral position (with the side to be blocked uppermost) identify the greater trochanter and the ischial tuberosity and draw a line between them.
2. Identify the point one quarter of the distance along this line from the medial end and mark it with an X.
3. Flex the hip to 90°. The site of entry is just above point X on the gluteal fold.
4. Using aseptic technique insert a short bevelled needle and feel for loss of resistance with penetration of the superficial fascia. Attach a saline-filled

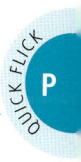

syringe and feel for a second loss of resistance as the needle penetrates the fibrous fatty tissue and gluteus maximus.

5 Inject 4 mL bupivacaine 0.5% for child of 1 year, add 0.5 mL for each subsequent year up to a total of 12 mL.

◗ Postpartum Haemorrhage

Mean blood loss with vaginal delivery is about 500 mL and with CS is about 1000 mL.[74] Postpartum haemorrhage (PPH) is defined as post-partum loss of greater than 600 mL of blood. Generally speaking PPH of up to 1000 mL is usually well tolerated. Major PPH can be defined as greater than 40% of blood volume or >2 L.[75] The incidence of PPH is 3–7% of vaginal deliveries.[76] Causes of PPH include:

1 Uterine atony.
2 Retained placenta or products.
3 Trauma to the uterus or birth canal.
4 Uterine inversion. This may be associated with placenta accreta.
    See *Uterine Inversion* and *Placenta Accreta/Increta/Percreta*.
5 Coagulation abnormalities.

Treatment of PPH

1 Ensure adequate airway and ventilation of the patient.
2 Obtain large bore IV access.
3 Give appropriate resuscitation fluids (crystalloid/colloid/blood).
    See *Blood Loss Assessment and Initial Management* and *Blood Transfusion*. Transfuse red cells, platelets and clotting factors as needed.
4 Uterine massage and/or bimanual compression of the atonic uterus may reduce blood loss.
5 Appropriate surgical intervention ie. ensuring uterus is empty, repair of birth canal trauma.
6 Pharmacotherapy to contract the uterus if uterine atonia is the cause. Appropriate drugs include (see individual entries):
    a) Oxytocin 10 IU IV stat + infusion of 40 IU in 1000 mL N/S, with the infusion rate titrated to effect. Alternatively use carbetocin 100 µg IV over 1 min.
    b) Ergometrine 100–500 µg IV or 200–500 µg IM. An alternative ergot type drug is methergine in a dose of 200 µg IM or 20 µg IV.
    Note: Severe hypertension can occur if the patient has received ephedrine or other vasoactive drug in addition to an ergot alkaloid.
7 Prostaglandin F_2 alpha 250 µg IM or intramyometrially. This drug can cause bronchospasm, acute pulmonary oedema and myocardial infarction from coronary artery spasm.[77]
8 Consider external abdominal aortic compression to temporarily reduce blood loss while more definitive treatment is organised.[76] Compression of

the aorta can be achieved because postpartum the abdominal wall is lax and the rectus abdominis muscles are diastatic. This technique involves pressing a fist into the abdomen in the midline just above the umbilicus. This results in the abdominal aorta being compressed between the fist and the vertebral column.

9 Consider vaginal/uterine packing.

10 Uterine balloon tamponade with e.g. Rusch catheter balloon, or a Sengstaken-Blakemore oesophageal catheter.[78]

11 Arterial occlusion/embolisation (iliac, uterine, aortic) by an interventional radiologist should also be considered and may be lifesaving. Embolic agents include gel foam pledgelets, polyvinyl acetate particles and platinum coils. These techniques appear to be safe with a low incidence of short-term or long-term complications.[79]

12 If the above treatment is unsuccessful, laparotomy is required. Surgical options include the B-Lynch uterine compression suture, progressive ligation of the uterine arteries, tubal branches of the ovarian arteries and finally internal iliac arteries. Hysterectomy is usually required if arterial ligation fails. Consider recombinant activated factor VII therapy prior to committing to hysterectomy.[80] ***See*** *Recombinant Activated Factor VII (rFVIIa)*. Give 90 µg/kg initially then repeat this dose at 20 min if needed. Perform hysterectomy if this treatment fails.[80]

13 DIC may occur. **See** *Disseminated Intravascular Coagulation (DIC)*.

◁ **Potassium**

Potassium is the major intracellular cation and is very important in the function of excitable tissue. NR in serum 3.2–5.5 mmol/L.

Hypokalaemia

This is severe if K^+ level is <2.5 mmol/ L and is associated with:

1 Characteristic ECG changes include prolongation of the PR interval, T wave inversion and prominent U waves.

2 Dysrhythmias including atrial and ventricular tachycardias such as torsades de pointes.

3 Weakness, hypotonicity, ventilatory failure and prolongation of NDNMBD effects.

4 Rhabdomyolysis (if prolonged, severe hypokalaemia).

Treatment of Hypokalaemia

1 IV potassium chloride. Do not exceed 40 mmol/h.[81] For rapid correction give 10 mmol in 100 mL 5% glucose over 30 min. Measure K^+ each hour and repeat this dose until serum K^+ reaches 4.0 mmol/L. Rapid correction of hypokalaemia is not without risk ($\approx$ 0.5% morbidity).[82] It should only be done in urgent situations.

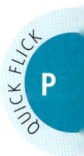

QUICK FLICK **P**

2 Treat the cause of the hypokalaemia.

Hyperkalaemia

This is severe if serum K^+ is >6.5 mmol/L and very severe at 7 mmol/L or greater. Hyperkalaemia may cause:

1 Characteristic ECG changes such as flattening of the P wave, tall peaked T waves and widening of the QRS complex and the PR interval. Development of deep S waves, sinus arrest with nodal rhythm, sine wave ECG pattern and asystole may also be seen.

2 Cardiac dysrhythmias may occur including ventricular ectopic beats, atrial arrest, atrioventricular block, ventricular tachycardia and ventricular fibrillation.

3 The effects of NDNMBDs drugs are antagonised.

4 Tingling, weakness and flaccid paralysis may occur.

5 Hypotension.

Treatment of Hyperkalaemia

Emergency management includes:

1 Calcium chloride 5–10 mL of 10% solution IV (or calcium gluconate 10 mL IV). This is to stabilise the myocardium against the effects of hyperkalaemia and does not reduce serum K^+ levels.

2 Glucose 50 mL of a 50% solution + 10 u actrapid. Anticipate and treat hypoglycaemia. In children give 0.1 u/kg actrapid with 1 mL/kg 50% glucose.

3 Salbutamol 10–20 mg nebulised over 10 min or subcut terbutaline 7 µg/kg.[83]

4 Frusemide 20–40 mg IV.

5 Haemodialysis.

6 Sodium bicarbonate is no longer recommended for the treatment of hyperkalaemia, but is indicated if there is a co-existing metabolic acidosis.[84]

7 Subsequent management (and for less severe hyperkalaemia):
   a) Resonium A or calcium resonium 15 g PO 6 h or 30 g PR 8 h.
   b) Treat the cause if possible.
   Note: SUXAMETHONIUM IS CONTRAINDICATED IF HYPERKALAEMIA IS PRESENT.

◖ Prazosin

Quinazoline derivative used for the treatment of hypertension, phaeochromocytoma and prostatism. Acts by competitively inhibiting α_1 adreno-receptors resulting in arterial and venous vasodilatation.

Dose

Adult 1 mg 8-12 h, gradually increased to up to 20 mg/day.
Note: Prazosin can cause postural hypotension.

○ **Pre-eclampsia/Eclampsia**

Topics Covered in this Section
▶ Pre-eclampsia and Eclampsia Defined
▶ Aetiology of Pre-eclampsia/Eclampsia
▶ Clinical Features
▶ Treatment Aims
▶ Management of Hypertension
▶ Prophylaxis/Treatment of Seizures
▶ Optimising Intravascular Volume and Renal Function
▶ Management of Coagulopathy
▶ Anaesthetic Management
▶ Post-partum Management

Pre-eclampsia and Eclampsia Defined

Pre-eclampsia can be defined as the onset of hypertension after the 20th week of pregnancy in association with proteinuria (> 300 mg/24 h). The disease may occur rarely prior to the 20th week of pregnancy associated with such conditions as a hydatidiform mole.[85] Pre-eclampsia can be sub-classified into:

1 Mild—systolic blood pressure (SBP) >140 mm Hg, diastolic blood pressure (DBP) >90 mm Hg.
2 Severe—SBP >160 mm Hg, DBP >110 mm Hg.

If seizures occur during pre-eclampsia (and up to 10 days following birth) eclampsia is diagnosed. The mortality of pre-eclamsia/eclampsia is 2–4%. Up to 7% of pregnant women develop pre-eclampsia[85] and eclampsia occurs in up to 0.12% of pregnancies.[86]

Aetiology of Pre-eclampsia/Eclampsia

During normal pregnancy at about weeks 14–16, secondary trophoblastic invasion from the placenta into the inner third of the myometrium results in uterine spiral arteries undergoing autonomic denervation. There is a diminishment of the musculo-elastic portions of these arteries and they become large-calibre low-resistance vessels. In pre-eclampsia, this secondary invasion does not occur leading to high resistance in the myometrial spiral arteries which remain responsive to vasomotor stimuli. In turn this leads to placental ischaemia and infarcts and increased release of uterine renin, stimulation of aldosterone secretion and breakdown of placental architecture.

These abnormalities lead to:

1 Widespread maternal endothelial injury.
2 Decreased production of vasodilating substances such as prostacyclin and an overproduction of vasoconstrictors such as thromboxane A_2.

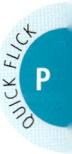

QUICK FLICK **P**

3   Arterial vasospasm, increased platelet aggregation and increased capillary permeability.
4   Intrauterine growth retardation of the fetus.

Clinical Features

Cardiovascular and Respiratory Effects

An increased systemic vascular resistance, circulatory volume contraction and increased left ventricular work occurs. Cardiac dysfunction may supervene resulting in cardiogenic pulmonary oedema. Non-cardiogenic pulmonary oedema may also develop due to leaky pulmonary capillaries and decreased plasma oncotic pressure. There can be marked pharyngeal and laryngeal oedema making intubation difficult.

Central Nervous System Effects

Headache, visual disturbances, irritability, hyper-reflexia, clonus and seizures may occur. If seizures do occur eclampsia is diagnosed. About 40% of seizures occur post-partum.

Intracranial haemorrhage may also occur accounting for 30–40% of deaths from pre-eclampsia.

Renal Effects

Proteinuria (>300 mg/day) may occur. Oliguria/renal failure may also develop but usually recovers if the patient survives. Hyperuricaemia >0.35 mmol/L may be a marker of potential fetal risk.[87]

Hepatic Effects

Hepatocellular damage, liver swelling and liver rupture can occur. Patients may complain of epigastric pain.

Haematological Effects

Haemolysis, coagulopathy and increased blood viscosity may occur. The patient may develop disseminated intravascular coagulation.

Utero/Placental/Fetal Effects

Uteroplacental blood flow may be greatly decreased leading to intra-uterine growth retardation and increased risk of placental abruption. Reverse diastolic flow on umbilical artery flow studies is an indication for urgent CS.

HELLP Syndrome

This syndrome is characterised by the presence of haemolysis, elevated liver enzymes and low platelet count in the pre-eclamptic or eclamptic patient. HELLP syndrome occurs in 4–2% of pre-eclampsia cases.[88] It is not a separate disease entity but rather a type of presentation of severe pre-eclampsia/eclampsia.

Treatment Aims

1 Control hypertension.
2 Prevent/treat seizures.
3 Treatment of other complications such as renal impairment and pulmonary oedema.
4 Optimise delivery time to avoid fetal compromise without unduly endangering the mother.

Management of Hypertension

Aim for a blood pressure of 120–140 SBP and 80–90 mm Hg DBP.

Mild Pre-eclampsia

For less severe hypertension (SBP 140–159 mm Hg, DBP 90–109 mm Hg) use oral therapy:

1 Methyldopa is considered first line treatment.[89] Use 250 mg 12 h up to 750 mg 6 h.
2 Labetalol should be added if methyldopa is inadequate. Use 100 mg 12 h up to 300 mg 6 h.
3 The next drug to add is nifedipine 10–20 mg orally 12 h, maximum dose 40 mg 12 h. If nifedipine or other Ca channel blocker drug is used with magnesium therapy there is an increased risk of hypotension and neuromuscular blockade. Therefore blood pressure and neuromuscular function need to be carefully monitored.

Do not use ACE inhibitors or angiotensin 2 receptor antagonists. These drugs may increase the risk of fetal death. Atenolol, esmolol, acebutalol and metoprolol should be avoided as they may cause fetal bradycardia and hypotension.

Severe Pre-eclampsia

A blood pressure >159 mm Hg systolic or 109 mm Hg diastolic should be treated as an emergency. The main risk of severe hypertension is intracerebral haemorrhage.[85] Drugs to consider are:

1 Hydralazine 5–10 mg IV bolus. Repeat at 15 min intervals up to a maximum dose of 40 mg.
2 Labetalol in doses of 5–10 mg IV. IV labetalol is not available in Australia at the time of writing. This can be repeated at 5 min intervals up to 1 mg/kg. The total dose required may vary from 20–300 mg.[90] Labetalol is not thought to adversely affect the fetal heart rate or uteroplacental blood flow.[90,91]
3 Diazoxide 30 mg IV minutely to a maximum of 300 mg.
4 Sodium nitroprusside (SNP) infusion. Pre-eclamptic patients may be extremely sensitive to SNP.[90] SNP may cause fetal cyanide or thiocyanate toxicity and fetal bradycardia.[90] Use invasive blood pressure monitoring.

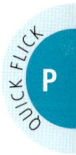

QUICK FLICK P

For patients in labour with severe hypertension, in addition to the above treatments:

1 Monitor CTG continuously for fetal distress.
2 Consider epidural analgesia which in addition to treating labour pain may assist in blood pressure reduction.

Prophylaxis/Treatment of Seizures

Treatment of Seizures

1 Diazepam IV 5–10 mg increments up to 20 mg or midazolam 2.5–5 mg.
2 Magnesium 2 g IV bolus (see below).
3 Intubate the patient if the seizure is prolonged or there is a significant period of loss of consciousness. This will require precautions as outlined in the section on general anaesthesia below. Organise urgent cerebral CT scan and/or urgent CS.
4 Ensure left lateral tilt or full lateral positioning is used at all times.
5 Add phenytoin if seizures continue despite magnesium.[85]

Prevention of Seizures

Magnesium therapy indicated for:

1 Persistent severe hypertension.
2 Pre-eclampsia with signs of impending eclampsia e.g. hyper-reflexia, clonus, headaches, visual disturbances.

Magnesium is a potent anticonvulsant which also reduces systemic vascular resistance improving uterine blood flow and lowering blood pressure.[90]

Magnesium Dose

1 Loading dose of 4 g (8 mL of a 50% solution of magnesium sulfate in 250 mL N/S) over 20 min via a central line. Magnesium sulfate can be given via a peripheral cannula initially in an emergency until central venous access is obtained.
2 Maintenance infusion of 1 g/h. Continue the magnesium infusion for 24 h after delivery or after the last seizure. Up to 3 g/h can be used.
3 If the initial dose of 4 g does not prevent convulsions give a second loading dose of 2–4 g over 20 min.
4 Monitor magnesium blood levels every 6 h. The therapeutic level is 2–3.5 mmol/L.[92] Cease the infusion if the blood level of Mg^{2+} >3.5 mmol/L. Monitor knee jerk reflexes. Stop the infusion and check the Mg^{2+} level if these disappear. Decrease or stop the magnesium infusion if urine output <30 mL/h (Mg^{2+} is renally excreted).

Table P1 Effects of magnesium therapy

| Clinical effects | Mg^{2+} (units in common use) | | |
	mmol/L	mEq/L	mg/dL
Normal serum level	0.75–1.0	1.5–2.0	1.8–2.4
Therapeutic anti-convulsant level	2–3.5	4–7	4.8–8.4
Loss of patellar reflexes	3.5–5	7–11	8.4–12
Skeletal muscle relaxation	6	12	14.4
SA and AV block/respiratory paralysis	6–7.5	12–15	14.4–18
Cardiac arrest	>12	>25	>30

Magnesium Toxicity

In addition to supportive measures for airway breathing and circulation, treat gross magnesium toxicity with:

1 Calcium chloride 1 g slow IV injection.
2 Fluid loading and diuretic therapy to increase renal excretion.
3 Glucose and insulin to increase Mg^{2+} entry into cells.
4 Dialysis.
5 Pacing should be considered if asystole occurs and does not respond to the above treatment in addition to the management outlined in *Cardiac Arrest*.[93]

Magnesium Therapy and Anaesthesia

1 Magnesium therapy potentiates the effects of NDNMBDs. Dosages of NDNMBDs should be reduced as guided by neuromuscular monitoring. Fasciculations may not be seen with suxamethonium.
2 Magnesium 40 mg/kg given immediately after induction of anaesthesia appears to be effective in reducing the hypertensive response to intubation in pre-eclamptic patients.[94]

Optimising Intravascular Volume and Renal Function

Although these patients tend to be intravascularly depleted, the main causes of death in pre-eclampsia/eclampsia are pulmonary oedema and cerebral haemorrhage. Persistent renal failure rarely occurs. Optimum fluid management in these patients is difficult to predict and excess IV fluid can precipitate pulmonary oedema in severe pre-eclampsia cases. A suggested approach is:

1 If there is no evidence of pulmonary oedema and urine output >0.5 mL/kg/h give total daily IV fluids (oral and IV) 1–1.5 mL/kg/h.
2 If urine output <0.5 mL/kg/h consider a cautious fluid challenge of Hartmann's solution 250–500 mL. If urine output does not improve consider CVP monitoring aiming for a CVP of 6–8 mm Hg.[95] This is controversial because the gradient between CVP and PCWP can be as high as 10 mm Hg. Therefore a CVP of 4 mm Hg or less may be safer.[95,96] If urine output does not improve consider a PA catheter.

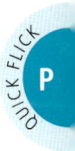

QUICK FLICK

P

3   If pulmonary oedema is present on chest auscultation and clinical grounds, consider a PA catheter and ICU admission. Carefully titrate IV fluids to a PCWP of 5–8 mm Hg. Consider starting with IV fluids at a rate 0–0.5 mL/kg/h.

Management of Coagulopathy

Give a platelet transfusion if the platelet count $< 20 \times 10^9$/L (20 000/mm³) Also give platelets if the count is $20–40 \times 10^9$/L and there is active bleeding and/or severe hypertension.[87] Give FFP if coagulopathic.

Anaesthetic Management

Epidural Anaesthesia for Labour and CS

Pre-eclamptic patients are often hypovolaemic and careful fluid loading with 500 mL of crystalloid followed by 100 mL/h is reasonable if there is no evidence of fluid overload. Epidural blockade should be achieved gradually and significant hypotension treated with small doses of ephedrine (3–6 mg) and IV fluid boluses if appropriate. It is also essential to exclude significant thrombocytopenia and coagulopathy prior to epidural insertion. If the platelet count is $> 100 \times 10^9$/L (100 000/mm³) significant coagulopathy is unlikely.[97] If the platelet count is > 75 000/mm³, the platelet count is not falling precipitously, coagulation studies are normal and the patient does not have clinical evidence of a bleeding tendency e.g. bruises, it is probably reasonable to proceed with epidural block. Epidural anaesthesia should not be done if the platelet count is > 50 000/mm.[3] In between these numbers is a grey area. It may be safer not to use adrenaline containing LA solutions for epidural blockade but this is debateable.[90]

Spinal Anaesthesia for CS

SAB used cautiously has become an acceptable approach for patients without epidural catheters with the same precautions and preparations as above. CSE can also be used. There may be slightly more hypotension than with epidural block but this is easily dealt with.[98]

General Anaesthesia

In addition to the recommendations in the section *Caesarean Section (CS)* also consider:

1   Invasive monitoring. In patients with moderate or severe pre-eclampsia an arterial line should be sited if not already present. A central venous line should be considered but can be sited after the baby is delivered.
2   Airway oedema may make intubation difficult and preparations for failed intubation must be made. Have smaller ET tubes readily available.
3   It is imperative to prevent/control the hypertensive response to intubation pharmacologically. However no drug protocol available at present is totally reliable. Although opioids may result in fetal respiratory depression,

this is much easier to treat than intracranial haemorrhage in the mother. Suggested drug strategies include:

a) Alfentanil bolus 2–3 mg (40 μg/kg) IV just prior to induction.
b) Fentanyl 8 μg/kg IV just prior to induction, noting that some respiratory depression of the newborn may occur.[99]
c) Remifentanil infusion of 1–1.5 μg/kg/min IV run for 60–90 s prior to induction. Consider a bolus of 1–2 μg/kg IV in addition to the infusion.
d) Lignocaine 1 mg/kg IV just prior to induction.
e) Hydralazine 5–10 mg IV at least 10 min before induction.
f) Magnesium bolus 30–60 mg/kg IV. Note that magnesium therapy may result in NDNMBDs having an exaggerated response.

All Types of Anaesthetic

Do not give ergometrine in the presence of eclampsia/pre-eclampsia, due to the risk of precipitating a hypertensive crisis.[85] Oxytocin is acceptable but administer the drug very slowly to avoid CVS collapse. Also consider prophylaxis for thromboembolic disease. *See Deep Venous Thrombosis (DVT) Prophylaxis.*

Postpartum Management

1 If epidural anaesthesia has been used pre-delivery, consider continuing the epidural post delivery with an infusion of bupivacaine or ropivacaine (plus fentanyl) to maintain peripheral vasodilation.
2 Patients should be monitored in a high dependency area or the intensive care unit.
3 Pre-eclampsia may become more severe in the post-partum period and ongoing vigilance is required. Of the patients who suffer convulsions about 40% of these begin in the post-partum period.
4 Although controversial, NSAIDs can be considered after 24 h postpartum if renal function is normal and urine output is good.

▷ Pregabapentin

See Gabapentin and Pregabalin.

▷ Pregnancy and Non-obstetric Surgery—Anaesthetic Considerations

It is estimated that during 1–2% of pregnancies non-obstetric surgery and anaesthesia is perfomed.[100] The most likely procedures to be performed are laparoscopy and appendicectomy.[100] There is a slightly increased risk of spontaneous abortion associated with anaesthesia and surgery in the first and second trimester of pregnancy.[101] Preterm labour in the postoperative period is also more likely. It is not possible to separate anaesthesia, the disease requiring surgery, or the surgery itself, as the main causative factor. Some older studies have suggested an increased risk of CNS defects in the fetus if the mother has anaesthesia in the first trimester.[102] Elective surgery should be avoided if possible during pregnancy due to the increased risks of miscarriage, fetal abnormalities and premature labour. All female patients of childbearing age should be asked about the possibility of pregnancy prior to anaesthesia and surgery. However this is a very controversial medico-legal issue. At one extreme in some hospitals there is routine mandatory pregnancy testing in all females of childbearing age having anaesthesia.[103] Another approach is to ask the patient if she is or might be pregnant. If the patient thinks they may be pregnant offer a urine pregnancy test. This approach raises many issues including the cost of pregnancy testing, the problems of false positive and false negative results and theatre delays.

Non-teratogenic Effects of Anaesthetic Drugs

1 Ketamine in doses > 1.1 mg/kg can significantly increase uterine tone.
2 Avoid giving inhalational agents above 2 MAC as this can decrease cardiac output and adversely affect fetal perfusion.

Cardiovascular Issues

1 *Supine Hypotensive Syndrome*—Aorto-caval compression, resulting in hypotension when supine, can occur after the first trimester. At term, when supine, 10% of patients have symptoms but 90% have complete aorto-caval compression by the gravid uterus.[104] The compression is relieved by left lateral displacement of the uterus i.e. place a wedge under the right hip producing left lateral tilt.
2 *Increased Thrombo-embolism Risk*—Mobilise the pregnant patient early after surgery and use other precautions against deep venous thrombosis. ***See*** *Deep Venous Thrombosis (DVT) Prophylaxis*.
3 *Maintain adequate blood pressure*, as maternal hypotension may lead to fetal asphyxia due to decreased uterine blood flow.
4 *Vasoactive drugs* such as phenylephrine and dopamine may significantly reduce uterine blood flow.

Respiratory Issues

1 *Aspiration Risk*—Patients are at increased risk for aspiration from as early as ≈ 12th week and especially from the 20th week,[101] up until 2–3 days postpartum. ***See*** *Aspiration, Prevention and Treatment*. Patients at risk of aspiration should receive antacid medication and a rapid sequence induction if a general anaesthetic is used. ***See*** *Rapid Sequence Induction (RSI)*.
2 *Lung Function Changes*—Functional residual capacity is decreased from about the second trimester while closing capacity and oxygen consumption are increased. Thus pregnant patients undergo rapid O_2 desaturation if apnoea or airway obstruction occurs.
3 *Increased vascularity and oedema of airway mucosa* may result in the need

for a smaller than expected endotracheal tube size, and bleeding with instrumentation of the airway e.g. nasal intubation.

4   *Hyperventilation* should be avoided in the pregnant patient as this can result in fetal hypoxia and acidosis.

Regional Anaesthesia

Pregnant patients tend to be more sensitive to local anaesthetic agents than non-pregnant patients. It is recommended to reduce the dose of LA used by 25–30%. Ensure there is adequate IV fluid loading and treat hypotension promptly.

Teratogenicity of Anaesthetic Drugs

Major birth defects occur in about 3% of the population. The fetus is most vulnerable to teratogenic drugs during the period of organogenesis (second to the 12th week). Agents of concern include:

1   Nitrous oxide has been shown to decrease uterine blood flow in animal studies but has never been conclusively shown to cause adverse effects in human pregnancy. *See Nitrous Oxide*. Nitrous oxide should be avoided in prolonged surgery during early pregnancy due to its inhibitory effect on methionine synthetase. This enzyme is required for DNA synthesis in humans.

2   Benzodiazepine drugs should be avoided in early pregnancy. They have been anecdotally associated with cleft lip anomalies.[105] Congenital inguinal hernia has also been associated with benzodiazepine use in early pregnancy.[106]

3   Cocaine use has been associated with microcephaly and other congenital abnormalities.

4   Propofol has, in animal studies, resulted in delayed ossification and abnormal cranial ossification in the fetus and an increased incidence of subdural haematomas (Propofol Product Information). Although the manufacturer advises against the use of propofol in pregnancy, there is no evidence of teratogenicity in humans.

5   Non-steroidal anti-inflammatory drugs should be avoided due to concerns regarding premature constriction of the ductus arteriosus and the development of oligohydramnios.[107]

Fetal Monitoring and Welfare

The most important factors in maintaining fetal wellbeing during anaesthesia are avoiding maternal hypotension, hypovolaemia, hypocarbia and hypoxia. Consider intermittent or continuous fetal monitoring after ≈ 20th week intraoperatively. If monitoring indicates a non-reassuring fetal heart trace consider measures such as:

1   Increasing maternal oxygenation.

2   Increasing maternal blood pressure.

QUICK FLICK

P

3 Changing the site of surgical traction.

4 Increasing uterine displacement.

Radiological Issues in Pregnancy

The effects of X-rays on the fetus depend upon the dose of radiation measured in rad or rem (1 rem = 1 rad) and the gestational age of the fetus. The most dangerous period for malformations is between 4 and 17 weeks.[108]

Prior to 4 weeks the fetus is either destroyed by X-rays or no malformation occurs (all or nothing).[108] The threshold dose for producing fetal malformation is thought to be 12–20 rad. To minimise the risk of X-ray injury:

1 Use fetal lead shielding.

2 Avoid single or cumulative X-ray dosage > 5 rad.

Table P2 Amount of rad dosage to fetus from various X-ray procedures

Estimated fetal rad dosage[109]	X-ray procedure
0.0001	C spine 3 views
0.00007	CXR
0.05	CT head
2.6–9	CT abdomen

Table reproduced with permission from the authors of: Weinberg et al. The pregnant trauma patient. *Anaesth Intensive Care* 2005; 33: 167–80.

◐ Pressure Units

1 mm Hg = 0.133 kPa = 1.36 cm H_2O = 100 Pa.

1 bar = 100 kPa, 1 kPa = 1% of an Atmosphere.

1 kPa = 7.50 mm Hg, 1 torr = 133 Pa.

1 lb/sq. inch (PSI) = 6.89 kPa.

1 Atmosphere = 760 mm Hg = 14.7 PSI = 1.013 bar.

1 Atmosphere = 760 torr = 101.3 kPa.

◐ Procainamide

Class Ia anti-arrythmic drug useful for the treatment of:

1 atrial flutter, atrial fibrillation, supraventricular tachycardia

2 unsustained ventricular tachycardia

3 Wolff-Parkinson-White associated atrial fibrillation.

Dose

IV 50 mg/min until the dysrhythmia is controlled or the QRS widens or SBP falls below 85 mm Hg up to a maximum dose of 1000–1500 mg. Then provide an infusion of 2–4 mg/min.

Precautions

1 Procainamide is contraindicated in prolonged QT syndrome.

2 Procainamide can worsen muscle weakness in myasthenia gravis.

3 Non-depolarising muscle relaxant drugs have a prolonged effect in the presence of procainamide.

Prochlorperazine

A phenothiazine of the piperazine subclass, this drug is useful for the treatment of:

1 nausea and vomiting
2 vertigo

Prochlorperazine acts by a central antidopaminergic receptor effect.

Dose

Adult PO 5–20 mg 8–12 h.

Adult IM 12.5 mg IM up to 6 h. Although not recommended by the manufacturer, prochlorperazine can be given IV safely at a rate not exceeding 5 mg/min.[109]

Disadvantages

1 This drug is unsuitable for patients with Parkinson's disease.
2 Prochlorperazine can cause dystonic reactions (**see** *Dystonic Reaction, Acute*).
3 This drug can precipitate the neuroleptic malignant syndrome. **See** *Neuroleptic Malignant Syndrome (NMS)*.

Promethazine

Promethazine is a phenothiazine anti-histamine drug with sedative and anti-emetic properties. Acts mainly by blocking H_1 histaminergic receptors and also has some anti-cholinergic, anti-dopaminergic and anti-serotoninergic properties. Promethazine is used for the treatment of:

1 allergic reactions
2 pruritus
3 emesis.

Dose

Adult 25–50 mg IV or 25–75 mg PO daily in divided doses.
Child 0.2–0.5 mg/kg/dose 6–8 h IV, IM or PO.

Sedation Dose 0.5–1.5 mg/kg, maximum 100 mg.

Propacetamol

Intravenous form of paracetamol. 1 g of propacetamol IV is equivalent to 500 mg of paracetamol PO.

Propofol

Propofol is a 2,6-diisopropyl phenol (a hindered phenol) used as an intravenous anaesthetic agent for induction + maintenance of anaesthesia and also for sedation. Presented as a white emulsion of soya bean oil and egg phosphatide containing 1% propofol.

Dose for Induction of Anaesthesia
Adult 2–2.5 mg/kg.
Child 3–3.5 mg/kg.

Dose for Total Intravenous Anaesthesia
1 For unpremedicated patient—12 mg/kg/h for 10 min, then 10 mg/kg/h for 10 min, then 8 mg/kg/h for 10 min, then 6 mg/kg/h.
2 For premedicated patient as above but start at 10 mg/kg/h. Titrate the infusion rate to the patient's physiological response. The usual maintenance dose for anaesthesia is 6–12 mg/kg/h.

Total Intravenous Anaesthesia Using the Diprifusor® Technique (Target-controlled Infusion)[110]
This technique involves the use of computer-controlled propofol infusion pump called a Diprifusor™. The computer program includes the Marsh pharmokinetic model to estimate actual patient blood concentrations of propofol. The patient's weight and age are entered into the pump's computer and the desired blood concentrations are 'dialled up' on the Diprifusor™ which is able to adjust infusion rates appropriately to achieve this level. A misleading feature of the Diprifusor is that the age value entered has no effect on the amount and rate of propofol delivery.[111] The Diprifusor™ has not as yet been recommended for use in children. The age range available on the Diprifusor™ is 16–100 yrs and the weight range 30–150 kg.

Table P3 Suggested blood propofol concentrations for various stages of anaesthesia (ZENECA 'Guide for Anaesthetists' Product Information 1999)

Stage of anaesthesia	Blood concentration in μg/ml
Induction with	(Initial Target Concentration)
Midazolam 2 mg and Fentanyl 100 μg	*Young healthy adult patient:* Unpremedicated 6 μg/mL Premedicated 4 μg/mL (Range 4–8 μg/mL) *For older, sicker patient* use a target concentration of 3–4 μg/ml
Maintenance of anaesthesia (with O$_2$ and N$_2$O)	*Young, healthy patient:* 3.5–5.3 μg/mL *Older, sicker patient:* 2.8–3.5 μg/mL

Notes

1 Induction times for the initial target blood concentrations outlined above are ≈ 60–120 s.
2 For a gradual induction of anaesthesia in patients who are elderly or unwell begin with 3 μg/mL, then increase concentration gradually in steps of 0.5–1 μg/mL 1 minutely.
3 The target concentration to maintain anaesthesia is 3.0–6.0 μg/mL, depending on factors such as the amount of surgical stimulation and what other drugs are used.
4 Patients will wake up at a propofol concentration of ≈ 1–2 μg/mL.
5 Use entropy or a BIS monitor to measure levels of anaesthesia.

Dose for Sedation

Adult give boluses of 20–50 mg or an infusion at a rate of 1–4 mg/kg/h titrated to clinical effect. Alternatively aim for a blood concentration of 0.5–2 μg/mL via the Diprifusor™.

The Orchestra System

This is a new device that enables highly sophisticated computerised IV delivery of up to 8 infusions including propofol and remifentanil. Weight and age both influence the amount and rate of propofol delivery. Another advantage of this system is that the expensive glass propofol Diprifusor syringes are not required.

Advantages

1 Propofol is the only satisfactory practical drug for total intravenous anaesthesia. Rapid redistribution and elimination results in a short duration of action even after prolonged periods.
2 It has less hangover effect and less nausea and vomiting compared with thiopentone.[112]
3 Propofol does have some anxiolytic effects.[110]
4 Propofol has anticonvulsant properties and has been used to successfully treat status epilepticus in humans[110] (but see below).
5 Safe to use in patients with malignant hyperpyrexia susceptibility.
6 Propofol is probably safe as a single dose for patients with porphyria but may not be safe if given as an infusion. **See** *Porphyria*.

Disadvantages

1 Pain on injection.
2 Seizure-like movements and seizures have occurred with propofol administration. Seizure incidence has been estimated to be 1 in 47 000 administrations.[113] Propofol should probably be avoided in epileptics although this is more for medico-legal than scientific reasons.[114]
3 Causes a 20% drop in mean arterial pressure and a 20% decrease in systemic vascular resistance.[110] This effect is more pronounced in the

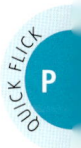

QUICK FLICK P

elderly[115] and hypovolaemic. Propofol must be used with extreme caution in the elderly.

4 Abuse potential.

5 Allergic reactions are rare. However patients with a history of significant egg allergy or allergy to soya bean oil should not be given propofol.[116]

6 Propofol infusions in ICU for prolonged sedation have been associated with rhabdomyolysis, metabolic acidosis, cardiac arrythmias and death in children and adults (termed Propofol Infusion Syndrome).[117] The mechanism of this syndrome is unknown but thought to be related to propofol-induced disruption of fatty acid metabolism leading to cardiac and skeletal muscle cell death.[117] Propofol is contraindicated for paediatric sedation in ICU and its use in adults limited. Rosen et al. suggest that infusion rates be <5 mg/kg/h and no longer than 48 h.

�‣ Propranolol

Propranolol is an aromatic amine non-selective β receptor blocker without intrinsic sympathomimetic activity. Used for the treatment of:

1 Angina, hypertension and tachydysrhythmias.

2 Hypertrophic cardiomyopathy.

3 Phaeochromocytoma, thyrotoxicosis, migraine and acute exacerbations of porphyria.

Dose
Adult 1–10 mg IV titrated to desired clinical response.

◊ ProSeal™ Laryngeal Mask Airway

See *Laryngeal Mask Airway (including ProSeal™, Fastrach™ and C-Trach™).*

◊ Prostate Surgery

See *Transurethral Resection of Prostate (TURP).*

◊ Prostin F$_2$ alpha

Prostin F$_2$ alpha is the methylated analogue of prostaglandin F$_2$ alpha. It is used to cause uterine contraction for therapeutic abortion and the treatment of postpartum haemorrhage (PPH) due to uterine atony. **See** *Postpartum Haemorrhage.*

Dose for Uterine Atony with PPH
Give 250 μg IM or intramyometrially for refractory uterine atony. Repeat dose every 15–30 min up to a total dose not exceeding 2 mg.

Note: Prostaglandin F$_2$ alpha increases airway resistance and is relatively contraindicated in asthma.[118] Overdose of this drug may cause cardiovascular collapse.[119]

�‌ Protamine

Obtained from fish sperm, protamine is a mixture of cationic proteins used to neutralise the anticoagulant effect of heparin. It is also ≈ 60% effective in reversing the effects of low molecular weight heparin.

Dose for Reversing Heparin

1 mg of protamine neutralises 100 units of heparin. Give slowly (over minutes), as it can cause acute hypotension, bradycardia and anaphylactoid/ anaphylactic reactions. Can also cause pulmonary vasoconstriction/ hypertension acutely.

Dose for Reversing Low Molecular Weight Heparin

Only about 60% of the activity of LMWH can be reversed by protamine.
1 Dalteparin (Fragmin) give protamine 1 mg/100 u of dalteparin.
2 Enoxaparin (Clexane) give protamine 1 mg/1 mg of enoxaparin.

Adverse Effects of Protamine

1 Protamine can cause anaphylactic or anaphylactoid reaction with hypotension, bronchospasm and pulmonary oedema. Patients who have fish allergy, vasectomy, insulin exposure or previous protamine exposure may have an allergic reaction to protamine.[120]
2 Protamine can also cause pulmonary hypertension, possibly through the release of complement.
3 In patients in whom protamine is contraindicated alternative drugs to reverse heparin include fresh frozen plasma, recombinant platelet factor 4, heparinase–I and other experimental drugs.[120]

◌ Prothrombin Time

See *International Normalised Ratio (INR)*.

◌ Prothrombinex-HT

Prothrombinex-HT is a concentrate of the human coagulation factors II, IX and X. It is used for the urgent reversal of warfarin. It is recommended to consult with a haematologist in this situation. **See** *Warfarin*.

Prothrombinex-HT is contraindicated in patients with thrombosis or DIC.

◌ Pruritus, Due to Opioids

See *Morphine*.

◌ Pseudocholinesterase Deficiency

See *Sux Apnoea*.

In patients with pseudocholinesterase deficiency the effects of the following drugs may be prolonged:

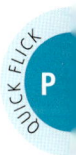

1 suxamethonium
2 mivacurium.

◑ Pulmonary Artery (PA) Catheter

Topics Covered in this Section
▶ PA Catheter Measurements and Normal Values
▶ Technique of PA Catheter Placement
▶ Diagnostic Patterns
▶ Cardiac Output Studies
▶ Factors Affecting the Accuracy of PCWP and Cardiac Output Studies

PA Catheter Measurements and Normal Values

Central Venous Pressure (CVP)	0–6 mm Hg
Mean Pulmonary Artery Pressure (MPAP)	9–16 mm Hg
Pulmonary Capillary Wedge Pressure (PCWP)	8–12 mm Hg
Cardiac Output (CO)	4–8 L/min
Cardiac Index (CI)	$2.5–4$ $L.min^{-1}.m^{-2}$
Stroke Volume (SV)	60–130 mL
Right Ventricular Stroke Work (RVSW)	$4–8$ $g.m.m^{-2}.beat^{-1}$
Left Ventricular Stroke Work (LVSW)	$44–68$ $g.m.m^{-2}.beat^{-1}$
Stroke Volume Index (SVI)	$35–70$ $mL.beat^{-1}.m^{-2}$
Systemic Vascular Resistance (SVR)	1000 $dyne.s.cm^{-5}$
Systemic Vascular Resistance Index (SVRI)	$1760–2600$ $dyne.s.cm^{-5}.m^{-2}$
Pulmonary Vascular Resistance (PVR)	100 $dyne.s.cm^{-5}.m^{-2}$
Pulmonary Vascular Resistance Index(PVRI)	$44–225$ $dyne.s.cm^{-5}.m^{-2}$

Technique for PA Catheter Placement

Insertion measurements quoted are for the right internal jugular approach. For a much more detailed description of insertion technique refer to Kong and Singer's article listed in the references.[121] The technique is as follows:

1 Insert the pulmonary artery (PA) catheter sheath (8.5 F) as for an internal jugular or subclavian central line insertion (**see** *Internal Jugular Vein (IJV) Catheterisation* and *Subclavian Vein Central Line*).

2 After flushing all the lumens and testing the flotation balloon, attach the proximal end of the distal (balloon) lumen to the pressure transducer and calibrate ('zero'). Ensure none of the lumens is open to air at their proximal ends. Insert the PA catheter through the sheath haemostasis valve and transduce the pressure measured at tip of balloon lumen. Once the tip of the PA catheter is in the vein (at ≈ 20 cm insertion distance) inflate the balloon with 1.5 mL of air and measure the pressure as the catheter is advanced. With correct placement 4 types of pressure wave are seen:

   a) SVC and right atrial (0–4 mm Hg).

b) Right ventricle, at ≈ 30 cm (25/30 mm Hg)

c) Pulmonary artery (PA), entered at about 40–50 cm (25/9 mm Hg). A dicrotic notch appears on the waveform. The PA diastolic pressure can be falsely elevated if the heart rate exceeds 120 bpm due to insufficient time for the pressure to return to baseline.[122] A mean PA pressure >20 mm Hg is diagnostic of pulmonary hypertension.

d) Pulmonary artery wedge pressure (8–12 mm Hg). Also called pulmonary capillary wedge pressure (PCWP). This pressure is used to approximate left ventricular end diastolic pressure (LVEDP). The PCWP should be equal to, or less than, the PA diastolic pressure.

3 When the balloon is deflated the PA pressure trace should reappear. If it does not, withdraw catheter a few cm.

Diagnostic Patterns

Table P4 Some common diagnostic patterns

Condition	PCWP	CO	SVR
Hypovolaemic shock	Low	Low	High
Cardiogenic shock	High	Low	High
Vasogenic shock	Low	High	Low

PA Catheter Findings with Some Specific Conditions

1 *Cardiac Tamponade* There tends to be equalisation of all cardiac diastolic pressures i.e. RA = RVD = PAD = PCWP.

2 *Myocardial Ischaemia* See elevation in PCWP typically to >15 mm Hg and V waves >20 mm Hg.

3 *Right Ventricular Infarction* Typically see high RA pressure, poor RVSW and normal or low PCWP.

4 *Mitral Incompetence* V waves on recording of the pulmonary artery occlusion pressure. The size of the V wave correlates with the degree of regurgitant flow.

Conditions Causing Elevation of the PCWP

1 Left ventricular failure.

2 Mitral stenosis and mitral incompetence.

3 Cardiac tamponade and constrictive pericarditis.

4 Volume overload.

Cardiac Output Studies

1 Enter patient's weight and height into the cardiac output studies program. Enter the patient's CVP and PCWP.

2 Inject cold saline into the right atrial port of the PA catheter at the end-expiration point of the patient's ventilatory cycle.

3 Repeat 4–6 times aiming for a consistent cardiac output result.

4   Enter the averaged cardiac output value and initiate the calculations function.

Factors Affecting the Accuracy of PCWP and Cardiac Output Studies

1   Thermodilution CO may be inaccurate in patients with tricuspid incompetence, intracardiac shunts and atrial fibrillation.

2   PCWP will be greater than LVEDP in patients with conditions such as mitral stenosis and prolapsing left atrial tumours.[123] PCWP will be less than LVEDP in conditions such as decreased left ventricular compliance and LVEDP >25 mm Hg.[123]

3   In the presence of pathologically large 'a' waves (as occurs with mitral stenosis, complete heart block, atrial myxoma and early acute heart failure) use the end-exhalation diastolic PCWP measurement.

4   If there are pathological large 'v' waves (as can occur with mitral regurgitation, left atrial enlargement and VSD) again use the diastolic end-expiration PCWP measurement.

5   The tip of the PA catheter should lie in West Zone 3 of the lung (where venous and arterial pressure exceed alveolar pressure 95% of the time).[124]

6   Peak end-expiratory pressure (PEEP) by increasing pleural pressure will artificially elevate the measured PCWP value. To correct for PEEP >10 cm H_2O subtract half the PEEP pressure from the measured PCWP or use the following formula:[123]

$$\text{Actual PCWP (mm Hg)} = \text{Measured PCWP (mmHg)} - \frac{\text{PEEP} \times 0.75}{3}$$

◗ Pulmonary Embolism (PE)

Pulmonary embolism is the commonest cause of preventable death in hospitals. One per cent of hospital admissions will die from PE.[125] In pregnant patients who develop DVT and are not treated, 24% will suffer a PE and 15% die. In treated patients 4.5% develop a PE and <1% die.[126]

Diagnostic Features

1   Dyspnoea, pleuritic chest pain, cyanosis.

2   Tachycardia.

3   Confusion.

4   Friction rub, wheezing, pleural effusion.

5   Evidence of elevated pulmonary artery pressure i.e. accentuation of pulmonary valve closure sound, widened splitting of the second heart sound, palpable right ventricular heave, raised CVP.

6   Hypotension and cardiovascular collapse and death may occur. Overall mortality is about 10%.[127]

Investigations

1 ECG changes may occur such as ST depression and T wave inversion in anterior leads, deep S wave in lead I and a Q wave and inverted T wave in lead III.
2 CXR may show an enhanced pulmonary artery shadow, lung oligaemia in the area affected by the embolus and a wedge-shaped area on the pleural surface suggesting infarction.
3 Echocardiography may indicate RV dilatation and hypokinesis with apical sparing suggesting PE. Thrombus may be seen in the cardiac chambers and an estimate of pulmonary artery pressure can be made. A negative echocardiogram does not exclude PE.
4 Arterial blood gases may show hypoxaemia and hypocarbia.
5 Serum D-dimer may be elevated.
6 Ventilation/perfusion scan.
7 Pulmonary angiography may provide a definitive diagnosis.
8 Spiral CT scan (contrast-enhanced spiral volumetric CT scan) can provide rapid, accurate diagnosis of PE.

Treatment

Management of PE is determined by the patient's clinical conditions and available resources.

Cardiovascularly Unstable Patient

1 Resuscitate the patient i.e. ensure adequate airway and ventilation, provide 100% O_2. Ensure adequate cardiac rhythm and blood pressure and support the circulation as required. *See Cardiac Arrest*. Intravascular volume expansion and inotropic support may be required.
2 Consider thrombolytic therapy with e.g. Streptokinase 250 000 units IV over 30 min then 10 000 units/h for 24–72 h or Tissue Plasminogen Activator 15 mg IV bolus then 45 mg/h for 2 h.

Or Alternatively:

3 Consider surgical embolectomy + immediate femoral–femoral bypass and pump oxygenation until conventional cardiopulmonary bypass can be established. Percutaneous embolectomy is performed in some specialist centres.
4 Use noradrenaline if a vasopressor is required. Intra-aortic balloon counterpulsation may be helpful.
5 Inhaled selective pulmonary vasodilators such as nitric oxide or prostacyclin may be of benefit in addition to the other measures discussed.[128,129]

Cardiovascularly Stable Patient

For less critical situations heparinise the patient using either unfractionated or low molecular weight heparin as follows:

1 *Heparin* Give a loading dose 5000 IU then infuse heparin at 18 units/kg/h. Maintain the activated partial thromboplastin time (APTT) at 1.5–2.5 × control i.e. at 50–90 s. The NR for APTT is 25–30 s.

2 *Low Molecular Weight (LMW) Heparin*
  a) Dalteparin 100 u/kg/12 h subcutaneously or 200 u/kg/day.
  b) Enoxaparin 1 mg/kg/12 h subcutaneously or 1.5 mg/kg/day.

Therapy with unfractionated heparin or LMW heparin should be continued for at least 5 days overlapping with oral warfarin therapy from day 1. The International Normalised Ratio (INR) must be in the therapeutic range (2.0–3.0) for at least 2 days before ceasing heparin therapy. If patients cannot be heparinised e.g. ongoing bleeding consider insertion of an inferior vena caval filter.

⊙ Pulmonary Hypertension

Pulmonary hypertension is diagnosed when mean pulmonary artery pressure > 25 mm Hg at rest with a PCWP <12 mm Hg.[130] Pulmonary hypertension is considered moderately severe when mean pulmonary artery pressure (PAP) > 35 mm Hg, and right ventricular (RV) failure is unusual unless mean PAP >50 mm Hg.[131] It may be primary or secondary to such causes as pulmonary emboli, congenital cardiac disease with left-to-right shunts, mitral stenosis, morbid obesity and sickle cell anaemia.

Pathophysiology

Pulmonary hypertension results in:

1 Right ventricular (RV) hypertrophy and dilatation with eventual RV failure. There is increased RV end-diastolic pressure with subsequent elevated central venous pressure (CVP).

2 Pulmonary valve regurgitation.

3 Right atrial enlargement and tricuspid regurgitation.

4 Dyspnoea, haemoptysis and chest pain.

5 Further increases in pulmonary vascular resistance (PVR) result in increased RV failure and/or decreased venous return to the left ventricle with systemic hypotension. Cardiac output is low and fixed.

6 Acute rises in PAP can cause RV failure, bulging of the intraventricular septum with reduced LV filling and decreased LV output. This can lead to a vicious cycle of reduced coronary blood flow, further reduction in right and left ventricular function, bradycardia due to myocardial hypoxia and cardiac arrest.[132]

Treatment

The main treatment options are:

1 Vasodilators such as high dose calcium channel blockers.

2 Anti-proliferative prostanoids such as prostacyclin IV infusions.

General Considerations

Factors which (in the presence of pulmonary hypertension) increase PVR must be avoided. These include:

1 N_2O.
2 Adrenaline, dopamine and other α adreno-receptor agonists.
3 Protamine, serotonin, thromboxane A_2 and prostaglandins such as PGF_2 alpha and PGE_2.
4 Hypoxia, hypercarbia, acidosis.
5 Positive end-expiratory pressure and lung hyperinflation.
6 Cold, anxiety and stress.

PVR, when elevated, can be decreased by:

1 Hyperventilation to produce hypocarbia.
2 Correction of hypoxia.
3 Drugs such as nitric oxide, morphine, glyceryl trinitrate, sodium nitroprusside, tolazoline and inhaled or IV prostacycline (PGE_2). Also isoprenaline and other β adreno-receptor agonists, aminophylline and ganglion blocking drugs. Epoprosterol may also be useful.

To maintain cardiovascular stability:

1 Avoid marked decreases in venous return. This will cause decreased RV filling leading to decreased RV output. Correct fluid and blood loss rapidly.
2 Avoid marked decreases in SVR. Cardiac output is restricted by a fixed RV output. If SVR falls the patient may not be able to maintain blood pressure by increasing cardiac output.
3 Avoid drugs which cause myocardial depression.
4 Maintain heart rate. Bradycardia may result in reduced cardiac output with hypotension and right ventricular failure.

These patients are at high risk of thromboembolic phenomenon and require pre- and postoperative anticoagulant therapy.

Specific Anaesthetic Management
Monitoring

Invasive arterial blood pressure and CVP monitoring will usually be required for anaesthetised patients with pulmonary hypertension. The use of pulmonary artery catheter monitoring is controversial due to the risk of pulmonary artery rupture, dysrhythmias and difficulty interpreting the data obtained especially in the presence of anatomical shunts.[133] If a PA catheter is used it may provide a useful warning of a sudden rise in PAP. If this occurs attempt to reduce PAP, and aim to decrease PVR more than SVR. This should lead to an increase in cardiac output.[132] Consider evaluating the effects of planned drug strategies prior to anaesthesia.

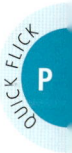

Intra-operative exacerbation of pulmonary hypertension

This may result in acute RV failure with progressive elevation in CVP, falling LV output and hypotension. In addition to strategies described above different drugs have been used in various case reports which successfully reduced pulmonary artery pressure. These include:

1 Sodium nitroprusside.[134]
2 Isoprenaline.[135]
3 Isoflurane.[136] This may be the preferred inhalational anaesthetic drug in this condition.
4 Inhaled prostacycline 20 μg 4 h.
5 Inhaled iloprost.[130]
6 IV prostacycline 4 ng/kg/min.[132]
7 Inhaled nitric oxide.[130]
8 Noradrenaline may be the most appropriate inotrope in this condition due to its ability to increase SVR without causing a tachycardia. PVR has been shown to decrease in animals given noradrenaline.[116]
9 Antibiotic prophylaxis for bacterial endocarditis is required for patients with associated heart valve or other structural abnormalities. *See Bacterial Endocarditis (BE) Prophylaxis*.

Obstetric Implications

Pregnancy complicated by pulmonary hypertension is associated with a high incidence of death (30–50%) and pregnancy is not recommended in these patients.[130] Neonatal survival is much higher at about 85%.[130] Ideally these patients require a multi-disciplinary approach with early involvement of the cardiologist, haematologist, neonatologist, obstetrician and anaesthetist.

Vaginal Delivery

1 Epidural blockade for labour can be used but must be carefully titrated with small increments of LA and opioids. Patients must be closely monitored, including invasive arterial and central venous blood pressure measurement.[137] Patients should receive continuous oxygen therapy. Use ephedrine for hypotension. Consider intrathecal morphine as an alternative to epidural anaesthesia for labour.
2 It is important to prevent pushing/ Valsalva manoeuvre at the time of delivery. Forceps or vacuum extraction should be used.
3 Oxytocin used for induction and/or augmentation of labour was considered safe in the Smedstad et al. patient series.[133] However oxytocin may cause an acute rise in PVR leading to reduced cardiac output and some clinicians advise avoiding the drug or giving it very cautiously.[138,139]

Caesarean Section (CS)

Epidural anaesthesia can be used for CS and may be preferable to GA but there is insufficient experience to recommend one technique over another.[133]

Single shot spinal anaesthesia is contraindicated but CSE techniques with a low dose spinal component have been used successfully.[130] If GA is selected or is mandatory an opioid based anaesthetic may be appropriate by providing cardiovascular stability.

◐ **Pulmonary Oedema**

Simultaneously with resuscitation, identify the cause of pulmonary oedema and treat if possible. Causes of pulmonary oedema include:

1 Fluid overload (e.g. IV fluids, glycine).
2 Acute myocardial dysfunction.
3 Neurogenic pulmonary oedema.
4 Post-obstruction pulmonary oedema (forced inspiration against a closed upper airway). *See Negative Pressure Pulmonary Oedema.*
5 Increased pulmonary capillary permeability as occurs with Adult Respiratory Distress Syndrome.

Treatment Strategies

1 Ensure adequate airway. Intubate the patient if necessary.
2 Ensure adequate ventilation. Administer 100% O_2. Continuous Positive Airways Pressure (CPAP), Bi-level Positive Airway Pressure (BiPAP), intermittent positive pressure ventilation (IPPV) + positive end-expiratory pressure (PEEP) may be required depending on the severity of respiratory distress. These treatment modalities are of benefit by reducing the work of breathing and by decreasing left ventricular afterload due to decreased transmural pressure as a consequence of increased positive intra-thoracic pressure.[140] Extravascular lung water is not decreased by these treatments.[141]
3 Ensure circulation is adequate *see Cardiac Arrest*. Reduce cardiac preload by sitting patient upright or reverse Trendelenburg position.
4 Drug therapy includes:
    a) Frusemide 40–120 mg.
    b) Morphine 2 mg increments at 2 min intervals to a total of 10 mg (relieves agitation and probably causes venodilation decreasing preload).
    c) If the cause of pulmonary oedema is LV failure, commence glyceryl trinitrate (GTN) infusion (*see Glyceryl Trinitrate*).
    Consider sublingual nitroglycerine 600 µg while preparing the GTN infusion. GTN will reduce LV filling pressure decreasing LV wall tension and O_2 consumption.
5 Consider inotropic support e.g. dobutamine may be appropriate due to its effects on β adreno-receptors causing reduced afterload and a greater effect on inotropy than chronotropy. *See Dobutamine.*
6 Consider using a phosphodiesterase III inhibitor. *See Amrinone* and *Milrinone.*

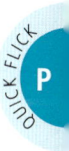

7 Consider the use of a mechanical circulatory assist device such as an intra-aortic balloon pump. **See** *Congestive Cardiac Failure (CCF)*.

8 Establish invasive monitoring i.e. arterial line, central venous line and consider insertion of a PA catheter.

9 Initial investigations include ECG, CXR, arterial blood gases. A transoesophageal TOE may be readily available in some institutions and helpful in diagnosis. Obtain urgent cardiology consultation.

◯ Pulmonary Valve and Subvalvular Stenosis

Pulmonary valve stenosis is considered severe if the pressure gradient across the pulmonary valve is > 50 mm Hg with a normal cardiac output.[142]
The stenosed valve eventually causes right atrial and right ventricular (RV) hypertrophy. RV output is maintained until the pressure gradient across the valve exceeds about 80 mm Hg. The RV will begin to fail and RV output decreases. This decreases LV preload and thus cardiac output, leading to fatigue, syncope and angina. SVR increases in an attempt to compensate for low cardiac output. LV stroke volume is low and fixed and dependent on HR.

Secondary infundibular hypertrophy can occur with dynamic right ventricular outflow obstruction as occurs in hypertrophic cardiomyopathy.[143]
See *Hypertrophic Cardiomyopathy (HCM)*.

Management Aims

1 Avoid factors which increase right ventricular O_2 requirements such as tachycardia and increased myocardial contractility.

2 Avoid factors decreasing right ventricular O_2 supply such as hypotension. Treat hypotension promptly with a vasoconstrictor.

3 Venous return must be maintained. Replace fluid and blood loss promptly.

4 Avoid marked decreases in systemic vascular resistance.

5 Marked increases in RV filling pressure are not well tolerated. Do not overfill the patient's intravascular space

6 Avoid bradycardia and drugs which decrease myocardial contractility.

7 Consider balloon valvuloplasty of the stenosed pulmonic valve preoperatively.

8 Provide antibiotic prophylaxis for bacterial endocarditis. **See** *Bacterial Endocarditis (BE) Prophylaxis*.

Anaesthesia and Pulmonary Valve Stenosis

Asymptomatic patients without decompensation tolerate anaesthesia well. In decompensated patients the following is required:

1 Invasive monitoring (arterial blood pressure and CVP). CVP prior to anaesthesia will indicate the patient's usual RV filling pressure. Maintain this filling pressure throughout the peri-operative period.

2 Maintain systemic vascular resistance, preload, contractility and a reasonable heart rate (90–110 bpm).[137]

Obstetrics and Pulmonary Valve Stenosis

Mild-to-moderate pulmonary valve stenosis is in general associated with a low fetal and maternal risk.[144]

Vaginal Delivery

In decompensated patients epidural anaesthesia must be provided with extreme caution. Invasive monitoring is required to maintain a 'normal' CVP for the particular patient. Consider intrathecal morphine or other opioid as a possible alternative to epidural blockade. Ransom and Leicht reported on the management of a pregnant patient with severe pulmonary stenosis for labour and delivery. They used an intrathecal sufentanil infusion with LD 10 µg then an infusion of 5 µg/h, supplemented by 1.5 mL of 1% lignocaine at the time of delivery.[143]

Caesarean Section

There is little information from the literature to guide management. Mangano recommends GA following the principles outlined above.[137]

REFERENCES

1 Allen M. Pacemakers and implantable cardioverter defibrillators. *Anaesthesia* 2006; 61: 883–90.

2 Bryan CS, et al. Endocarditis related to transvenous pacemakers: syndromes and surgical implications. *J Thorac Cardiovasc Surg* 1978; 75: 758.

3 Bloomfield P, Bowler MR. Anaesthetic management of the patient with a permanent pacemaker. *Anaesthesia* 1989; 44: 42–6.

4 Kam PCA. Anaesthetic management of a patient with an automatic implantable cardioverter defibrillator in situ. *Br J Anaesth* 1997; 78: 102–6.

5 Otto CW. Clinical utilisation of pacemakers and defibrillators for the anesthesiologist. 48th Annual Refresher Course Lectures, American Society of Anesthesiologists. 1997; 216: 1–6.

6 Cooper J. What's new in temporary pacing? *Br J Hosp Med* 1994; 52: 9: 437–8.

7 Szafranski JS, Obberoi MP, Chetty PK, Dabiri MD. Use of transesophageal atrial pacing during electroconvulsive therapy. *Anesthesiology* 1996; 84: 211–14.

8 *Australian Resuscitation Council Policy Statement 11.3*, February 2006.

9 Rivera Dee Ann, Bristow M. Cardiac resynchronisation—a heart failure perspective. *Annals of Noninvasive Cardiol* 2005; 10: 16–23.

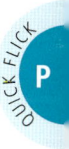

10 Pleuvry BJ. Non-opioid analgesics. *Anaesthesia and Intensive Care Medicine* 2005; 6: 25–9.

11 Peutrell JM, Wolf AR. Pain in children. *Br J Hosp Med* 1992; 47 (4): 289–93.

12 Australian and New Zealand College of Anaesthetists and Faculty of Pain Medicine: *Acute Pain Management: Scientific Evidence*. 2nd edn, 2005: 45.

13 Pearce B, Grant IS. Case Report: Acute liver failure following therapeutic paracetamol administration in patients with muscular dystrophies. *Anaesthesia* 2008; 63: 89–91.

14 Pierson R, Coupe M. (Letter) Reducing the risk of air embolism following administration of intravenous paracetamol. *Anaesthesia* 2008; 63: 96–107.

15 Pusch F, Freitag H, Weinstabl C, Obwegeser R, Huber E, Wilding E. Single-injection paravertebral block compared to general anaesthesia in breast surgery. *Acta Anaesthesiol Scand* 1999; 43: 770–4.

16 Richardson J, Sabanathan S. Thoracic paravertebral anaesthesia. *Acta Anaesthesiol Scand* 1995; 39: 1005–15.

17 Errington DR, Severn A M, Meara J. Parkinson's disease. *Br J Anaesth CEPD Reviews* 2002; 2: 69–73.

18 Nicholson G, Pereira AC, Hall GM. Parkinson's disease and anaesthesia (Review Article). *Br J Anaesth* 2002; 89: 904–16.

19 Gravlee GP. Succinylcholine-induced hyperkalaemia in a patient with Parkinson's disease. *Anesth Analg* 1980; 59: 444–6.

20 Muzzi DA, Black S, Cucchiara RF. The lack of effect of succinylcholine on serum potassium in patients with Parkinson's disease. *Anesthesiology* 1989; 71: 322.

21 Anderson BJ, Marks PV, Futter ME. Propofol—contrasting effects in movement disorders. *Br J Neurosurg* 1994; 8: 387–8.

22 Golden WE, Lavender RC, Metzer WS. Acute postoperative confusion and hallucinations in Parkinson's disease. *Ann Intern Med* 1989; 111: 218–22.

23 Toussaint S, Maidl J, Schwagmeier R, Striebel HW. Patient-controlled intranasal analgesia: effective alternative to intravenous PCA for postoperative pain relief. *Can J Anesth* 2000; 47: 299–302.

24 Balki M, Kasodekar S, Dhumne S, Bernstein P, Carvalho JC. Remifentanil patient-controlled analgesia for labour: optimizing drug delivery regimens. *Can J Anesth* 2007; 54: 626–33.

25 Cooper MG. *The New Children's Hospital Acute Pain Treatment Manual*, 2nd edn, revised June 1996.

26 Serour F. Mori J. Optimal regional anaesthesia for circumcision. *Anesth Analg* 1994; 79: 129–31.

27 Brown TCK, Weidner NJ, Bouwmeester. Dorsal nerve of the penis block—anatomical and radiological studies. *Anaesth Intensive Care* 1989; 17: 34–8.

28 Irwin M, Cheng W. Comparison of subcutaneous ring block of the penis with caudal epidural block for post-circumcision analgesia in children. *Anaesth Intensive Care* 1996; 24: 365–7.

29 Burke D, Joypaul V, Thomson MF. Circumcision supplemented by dorsal penile nerve block with 0.75% ropivacaine: a complication. *Regional Anaesthesia and Pain Medicine* 2000; 25: 424–7.

30 Berens R, Pontus SP. A complication of circumcision and dorsal nerve block of the penis. *Reg Anesth* 1990; 15: 309–10.

31 George LM, Gatt SP, Lowe S. Peripartum cardiomyopathy: four case histories and a commentary on anaesthetic management. *Anaesth Intensive Care* 1997; 25: 292–6.

32 Fett JD, Christie LG, Carraway RD, Murphy JG. Five-year prospective study of the incidence and prognosis of peripartum cardiomyopathy at a single institution. *Mayo Proceed* 2005; 80: 1602–6.

33 Bricelj V. The use of adrenergic beta-blockers in pregnancy. *Heart Views* 1999; 1: 130–2.

34 Browa G, O'Leary M, Douglas J, Herkes R. Perioperative management of a case of severe peripartum cardiomyopathy. *Anaesth Intensive Care* 1992; 20: 80–3.

35 McCarroll CP, Paxton LD, Elliott P, Wilson DB. Use of remifentanil in a patient with peripartum cardiomyopathy requiring Caesarean section. *Br J Anaesth* 2001; 86: 135–8.

36 Pirlet M, Baird S, Pryn S et al. Low dose combined spinal-epidural anaesthesia for caesarean section in a patient with peripartum cardiomyopathy. *Internat J Obstetric Anesth* 2000; 9: 189–92.

37 Sliwa K, Fett J, Elkayam U. Peripartum cardiomyopathy. *Lancet* 2006; 368: 687–93.

38 Amos MA, Wissam AJ, Stuart DR. Improved outcomes in peripartum cardiomyopathy with contemporary treatment. *Am Heart J* 2006; 152: 509–13.

39 Sasada MP, Smith SP. Drugs in Anaesthesia and Intensive Care, 2nd edn. Oxford University Press, Oxford 1997: 288.

40 Latta KS, Ginsberg B, Barkin RL. Meperidine: a clinical review. *American J Therapeutics* 2002; 9: 53–68.

41 Ngan Kee WD. Epidural Pethidine:pharmacology and clinical experience. *Anaesth Intensive Care* 1998; 26: 247–55.

42 Jasani NB, O'Connor RE, Bouzoukis JK. Comparison of hydromorphone and meperidine for ureteric colic. *Acad Emerg Med* 1994; 1: 539–43.

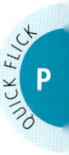

QUICK FLICK

P

43 Singh G, Kam P. An overview of anaesthetic issues in phaeochromocytomas. *Annals Academy of Medicine* 1998; 27: 843–8.

44 Roizen MF, Harrigan RW, Koike M. A prospective randomized trial of four anaesthetic techniques for resection of phaeochromocytoma. *Anaesthesiology* 1982; 57: A43.

45 Watson VF, Vaughan RS. Magnesium and the anaesthetist. *Br J Anaesth CEPD Reviews* 2001; 1: 16–20.

46 Morton A. Magnesium sulphate for phaeochromocytoma crisis (Letter). *Emergency Med Australia* 2007; 19: 482.

47 Breslin DS, Farling PA, Mirakhur RK. Case report: The use of remifentanil in the anaesthetic management of patients undergoing adrenalectomy: a report of three cases. *Anaesthesia* 2003; 58: 358–62.

48 Davies MJ, McGlade DP, Banting SW. A comparison of open and laparoscopic approaches to adrenalectomy in patients with phaeochromocytoma. *Anaesth Intensive Care* 2004; 32: 224–9.

49 Tauzin-Fin P, Hilbert G, Krol-Houdek M, Gosse P, Maurette P. Mydriasis and acute pulmonary oedema complicating laparoscopic removal of phaeochromocytoma. *Anaesth Intensive Care* 1999; 27: 646–9.

50 Sood J, Jayaraman L, Kumra V, Chowbey P. Laparoscopic approach to pheochromocytoma: is a lower intraabdominal pressure helpful? *Anesth Analg* 2006; 102: 637–41.

51 Roizen MF. Endocrine abnormalities and anaesthesia. ASA Refresher Course Lectures. San Francisco: American Society of Anesthesiologists. 1985; 253–65.

52 Apgar V, Papper EM. Phaeochromocytoma—anaesthetic management during surgical treatment. *Arch Surg* 1951; 62: 634–48.

53 Foo M, Burton BJL, Ahmed R. Phaeochromocytoma. *Br J Hosp Med* 1995; 54: 318–21.

54 Levy DM. Emergency Caesarean section: best practice (Review article). *Anaesth* 2006; 61: 786–91.

55 Read JA, Cotton DB, Miller FC. Placenta accreta: changing clinical aspects and outcome. *Obstet Gynecol* 1980; 56: 31–4.

56 Litwin MS, Loughlin KR, Benson CB et al. Placenta percreta invading the bladder. *Br J Urol* 1989; 64: 283–6.

57 Lerner JP, Deane S, Timor-Tritsch IE. Characterization of placenta accreta using transvaginal sonography and color Doppler imaging. *Ultrasound Obstet Gynecol* 1995; 5: 198–201.

58 Paull JD, Smith J, Williams L, Davison G, Devine T, Holt M. Balloon occlusion of the abdominal aorta during Caesarean hysterectomy for placenta percreta. *Anaesth Intensive Care* 1995; 23: 731–4.

59 Clark SL, Koonings P, Phelan JP, et al. Placenta praevia/accreta and prior Caesarean section. *Obstet Gynecol* 1985; 66: 89–92.

60 Parekh N, Husaini SWU, Russell IF. Caesarean section for placenta praevia: a retrospective study of anaesthetic management. *Br J Anaesth* 2000; 84: 725–30.

61 Kam PCA, Nethery CM. Review article: The thienpyridine derivatives (platelet adenosine diphosphate receptor antagonists), pharmacology and clinical developments. *Anaesthesia* 2003; 58: 28–35.

62 Kam PCA, Egan MK. Platelet glycoprotein IIb, IIIa antagonists. *Anesthesiology* 2002; 96: 1237–49.

63 Sreeram GM, Sharma AD, Slaughter TF. Platelet glycoprotein IIb/IIIa antagonists: perioperative implications. *J Cardiothoracic Vascular Surg* 2001; 15: 237–40.

64 Tcheng JE. Clinical challenges of platelet glycoprotein IIb/IIIa receptor inhibitor therapy: Bleeding, reversal, thrombocytopaenia and retreatment. *Am Heart J* 2000; 139: S38–S45.

65 Australian Red Cross Circular of Information, May 1994.

66 Mulroy MF. Regional Anesthesia: An Illustrated Procedural Guide. 2nd edn. Little, Brown and Company, Boston 1989: 209–10.

67 Konrad C, Jöhr M. Blockade of the sciatic nerve in the popliteal fossa: a system for standardization in children. *Anesth Analg* 1998; 87: 1256–8.

68 Scott DM, Chuan A. *Regional Anaesthesia, Pocket Guide*. Adrenaline Strategics Pty Ltd, Melbourne, Victoria 2007: 94.

69 Jensen NF. Fiddler DS, Striepe V. Anesthetic considerations in porphyrias. *Anesth Analg* 1995; 80: 591–9.

70 Ashley EMC. Anaesthesia for porphyria. *Br J Hosp Med* 1996; 56:1: 37–42.

71 Stoelting RK, Dierdorf SF. *Anesthesia and Co-existing Disease*, 3rd edn. Churchill Livingstone, New York, 1993: 375–8.

72 Elcock D, Norris A. Elevated porphyrins following propofol anaesthesia in acute intermittent porphyria. *Anaesthesia* 1994; 49: 957–8

73 Moore MR. International review of drugs in acute porphyrias—1980. *Int J Biochem* 1980; 12: 1089–97.

74 Sundaram R, Brown AG, Koteeswaran SK, Urquhart G. Anaesthetic implications of uterine artery embolisation in management of massive obstetric haemorrhage. *Anaesthesia* 2006; 61: 248–52.

75 Thomas C, Madej T. Obstetric emergencies and the anaesthetist. *Br J Anaesth CEPD Reviews* 2002; 2: 174–7.

76 Riley DP, Burgess RW. External aortic compression: a study of a resuscitation maneuver for postpartum haemorrhage. *Anaesth Intensive Care* 1994; 22: 571–5.

77 Krumnikl JJ, Toller WG, Prenner G, Metzler H. Beneficial outcome after prostaglandin-induced post-partum cardiac arrest using levosimendan and extracorporeal membrane oxygenation. *Acta Anaesthesiol Scandi* 2006; 50 (6): 768–70.

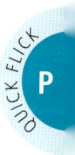

QUICK FLICK P

78 Doumouchtsis SK, Papergeorghiou AT, Arulkumaran S. Systematic review of conservative management of postpartum hemorrhage: what to do when medical treatment fails. *Obstet Gynecol Surv* 2007; 62: 540–7.

79 Eriksson LG, Mulic-Lutvica A, Jangland L, Nyman R. Massive postpartum haemorrhage treated with transcatheter arterial embolization: technical aspects and long-term effects on fertility and menstrual cycle. *Acta Radiologica* 2007; 48: 635–42.

80 Welsh A, McLintock C, Gatt S, Somerset D, Popham P, Ogle R. Guidelines for the use of recombinant activated factor VII in massive obstetric haemorrhage. *Austral and NZ J Obstets Gynaecol* 2008; 48: 12–16.

81 Worthley LIG. Fluid and Electrolyte Therapy. In: Oh TE, Bersten A, Soni N eds. *Oh's Intensive Care Manual.* Butterworth–Heinemann, UK 2003: 891–2.

82 Tetzlaff JE, Walsh MT. (Review article) Potassium and anaesthesia. *Can J Anaesth* 1993; 40 (3): 227–46.

83 Putcha N, Allon M. Management of hyperkalaemia in dialysis patients. *Sem Dial* 2007; 20: 431–9.

84 Hollander-Rodriguez JC, Calvert JF. Hyperkalemia. *Am Fam Physic* 2006; 73: 283–90.

85 Brown MA, Hague WM, Higgins J, Lowe S, McCowan L, Oats J, Peek MJ, Rowan JA, Walters BNJ. Consensus Statement: the detection, investigation and management of hypertension in pregnancy: executive study. *Aust NZ J Obstet Gynaecol* 2000; 40: 139–55.

86 Cheng AY, Kwan A. Perioperative management of intra-partum seizure. *Anaesth Intensive Care* 1997; 25: 535–8.

87 Consensus statement of the Australasian Society for the Study of Hypertension in Pregnancy. Management of hypertension in pregnancy: executive summary. *Med J Aust* 1993; 158: 700–2.

88 Crosby ET. Obstetrical anaesthesia for patients with the syndrome of haemolysis, elevated liver enzymes and low platelets. *Can J Anaesth* 1991; 38 (2): 227–33.

89 Rey É, LeLorier J, Burgess E et al. Report of the Canadian Hypertension Society Consensus Conference: 3. Pharmacological treatment of hypertensive disorders in pregnancy. *Can Med J* 1997; 157: 1245–54.

90 Boxer LM, Malinow AM. Pre-eclampsia and eclampsia. *Curr Opin Anaesthesiol* 1997; 10 (3): 188–97.

91 Malinow AM. Obstetric anaesthesia revisited: Anesthetic considerations for the pre-eclamptic patient. *Audio-Digest Anesthesiology* 1995: 37.

92 James MFM. Magnesium in obstetric anesthesia. *International J Obstetric Anesth* 1998; 7: 115–23.

93 Miller MA, Crystal CS, Helphenstine J, Young SE. Successful resuscitation of hypomagnesaemia asystolic cardiac arrest with the use of early transvenous cardiac pacemaker: a case report. *Emerg Med J* 2006; 23: e22.

94 Allen RW, James MFM, Uys PC. Attenuation of the pressor response to tracheal intubation in hypertensive proteinuric pregnant patients by lignocaine, alfentanil and magnesium sulphate. *Br J Anaesth* 1991; 66: 216–23.

95 Ramanathan J, Bennett K. Pre-eclampsia: fluids, drugs and anaesthetic management. *Anesthesiol Clin North Am* 2003; 21: 145–63.

96 Young P, Johansen R. Haemodynamic, invasive, and echocardiographic monitoring in the hypertensive patient. *Best Practice and Research Clinical Obstet Gynecol* 2001; 15: 605–22.

97 Schindler M, Gatt S, Isert P et al. Thrombocytopenia and platelet functional defects in pre-eclampsia: implications for regional anaesthesia. *Anaesth Intensive Care* 1990; 18: 169–74.

98 Visalyaputra S, Rodanant O, Somboonviboon W et al. Spinal versus epidural anesthesia for Cesarean delivery in severe preeclampsia: a prospective randomized, multicenter study. *Anesth Analg* 2005; 101: 862–8.

99 Morrison DH. Anaesthesia and preeclampsia. *Can J Anaesth* 1987; 34 (4): 415–22.

100 Kuczkowski KM. Nonobstetric surgery in the parturient: anesthetic considerations (Editorial). *J Clin Anesth* 2006;18: 5–7.

101 Blass N. Non-obstetric surgery during pregnancy. In: Datta S, ed. Obstetric Anesthesia, 2nd edn. Mosby, St Louis 1995: 427–38.

102 Sylvester GC, Khoury MJ, Lu X, Erickson JD. First trimester anaesthesia exposure and the risk of central nervous system defects: a population-based care control study. *Am J Public Health* 1994; 84: 1757–60.

103 Kotob F, Twersky RS. Is Routine Preoperative Pregnancy Testing Necessary? In: Fleisher LA, ed. *Evidence-Based Practice of Anesthesiology*. Saunders Philadelphia, Pennsylvania, 2004: 18–22.

104 Griffiths C, Agarwal R. Hypotension. In: Duke J, Rosenberg SG. *Anesthesia Secrets*. Hanley & Belfus, Inc Philadelphia, Mosby St Louis, 1996; 196–7.

105 Hawkins JL. Anesthesia for the pregnant patient undergoing nonobstetric surgery. In: *48th Annual Refresher Course Lectures*, American Society of Anesthesiologists, 1997: 235.

106 Rathmell JP, Viscomi CM, Asburn MA. Management of nonobstetric pain during pregnancy and lactation. *Anesth Analg* 1997; 85:1074–87.

107 Littleford J. Effects on the fetus and newborn of maternal analgesia and anesthesia: a review. *Can J Anesth* 2004; 51: 586–609.

108 Weinberg L, Steele RG, Pugh R, Higgins S, Herbert M, Story D. The pregnant trauma patient. *Anaesth Intensive Care* 2005; 33: 167–80.

109 Trissel LA. *Injectable Drugs Handbook*, 12th edn. American Society of Health System Pharmacists, 2003: 273.

110 Leslie K. Diprivan-based anaesthesia using Diprifusor™ TCI. Zeneca product literature, October 1998.

111 Ouattara A, Boccara G, Lemaire S et al. Target-controlled infusion of propofol and remifentanil in cardiac anesthesia: influence of age on predicted effect-site concentration, *Br J Anaesth* 2003; 90: 617–22.

112 Myles PS, Hendrata M, Bennett AM, Langley M, Buckland MR. Postoperative nausea and vomiting. Propofol and thiopentone: Does choice of induction agent affect outcome? *Anaesth Intensive Care* 1996; 24: 355–9.

113 Sutherland MJ, Burt P. Propofol and seizures. *Anaesth Intensive Care* 1994; 22: 733–7.

114 Sneyd JR. Propofol and epilepsy (Editorial). *Br J Anaesth* 1999; 82: 168–9.

115 Harwood TN. Optimizing outcome in the very elderly surgical patient. *Curr Opin Anaesthesiol* 2000; 13: 327–32.

116 Hofer KN. Possible anaphylaxis after propofol in a child with food allergy. *The Annals of Pharmacotherapy* 2003; 37: 398–401.

117 Rosen D, Nicoara A, Koshy N et al. Too much of a good thing? Tracing the history of the propofol infusion syndrome. *J of Trauma* 2007; 63: 443–7.

118 Douglas MJ. New drugs, old drugs and the obstetric anaesthetist (Refresher Course Outline). *Can J Anaesth* 1995; 42 (5): R3–R8.

119 Douglas MJ, Farquharson DR, Ross PL et al. Cardiovascular collapse following an overdose of prostaglandin $F_2 \alpha$: A case report. *Can J Anaesth* 1989; 36: 466.

120 Mukadam ME, Pritchard P, Riddington D, et al. Case conference: Case 7 2001 Management during cardiopulmonary bypass of patients with presumed fish allergy. *J Cardiothoracic Vascular Anesthesia* 2001; 4: 512–19.

121 Kong R, Singer M. Insertion of a pulmonary artery flotation catheter: how to do it. *Br J Hosp Med* 1997; 57: 9: 432–5.

122 Bouchard RJ, Gault JH, Ross J Jr. Evaluation of pulmonary arterial end-diastolic pressure as a measurement of left ventricular end-diastolic pressure in patients with normal and abnormal left ventricular performance. *Circulation* 1971; 44: 1072–9.

123 Lehr S. Pulmonary artery catheterization. In: Parsons P, Wiener-Kronish JP, eds. *Critical Care Secrets*. Mosby, St Louis 1992: 53–8.

124 Bowyer MW. Invasive cardiac monitoring. In: Parsons P, Wiener-Kronish JP, eds. *Critical Care Secrets*. Mosby, St Louis 1992: 15–20.

125 The Australian and New Zealand Working Party on the Management and Prevention of Venous Thromboembolism (Booklet) *Prevention of Venous Thromboembolism*. Health Education and Management Innovations 2005.

126 Peters CW, Abraham JL, Edwards RK. Cardiac arrest during pregnancy. *J Clin Anesthes* 2005; 17: 229–34.

127 McGrath B, Fletcher SJ. Intensive care management of pulmonary embolism. *Anaesth Intensive Care* 2001; 2: 347–52.

128 Capellier G, Jacques T, Balvay P et al. Inhaled nitric oxide in patients with pulmonary embolism. *Intensive Care Med* 1997; 23: 1089–92.

129 Webb SA, Stott S, van Heerden PV. The use of inhaled aerosolized prostacyclin (IAP) in the treatment of pulmonary hypertension secondary to pulmonary embolism. *Intensive Care Med* 1996; 22: 353–5.

130 Bonnin M, Mercier FJ, Sitbon O et al. Severe pulmonary hypertension during pregnancy. *Anesthesiol* 2005; 102: 1133–7.

131 Stoelting RK, Dierdorf SF. *Anesthesia and Co-existing disease*, 3rd edn. Churchill Livingstone, New York 1993: 103.

132 Myles PS. Anaesthetic management for laparoscopic sterilization and termination of pregnancy in a patient with severe primary pulmonary hypertension. *Anaesth Intensive Care* 1994; 22: 465–9.

133 Smedstad KG, Morison DH. Pulmonary hypertension and pregnancy: a series of eight cases. *Can J Anaesth* 1994; 41(6): 502–12.

134 Roessler P, Lambert TF. Anaesthesia for Caesarean section in the presence of primary pulmonary hypertension. *Anaesth Intensive Care* 1986; 14: 317–20.

135 Slomka F, Salmeron S, Zetlaoui P, et al. Primary pulmonary hypertension and pregnancy: anaesthetic management for delivery. *Anesthesiol* 1988; 68: 959–61.

136 Cheng DCH, Edelist G. Isoflurane and primary pulmonary hypertension. *Anaesthesia* 1988; 43: 22–4.

137 Mangano DT. Anesthesia for the pregnant cardiac patient. In: Schnider SM, Levinbson G eds, *Anesthesia for Obstetrics*, 2nd edn. Williams and Wilkins, Baltimore 1987: 123–41.

138 Roberts NV, Keast PJ. Pulmonary hypertension and pregnancy—a lethal combination. *Anaesth Intensive Care* 1990; 18: 366–74.

139 Takeuchi T, Nishii O, Okamura T, Yaginuma T. Primary pulmonary hypertension in pregnancy. *Int J Gynecol Obstet* 1998; 26: 145–50.

140 Lapinsky SE, Mount DB, Mackey D, Grossman R. Management of acute respiratory failure due to pulmonary edema with nasal positive pressure support. *Chest* 1994; 105: 229–31.

141 Rizk NW, Murray JF. PEEP and pulmonary oedema. *Am J Med* 1982; 72: 381–3.

142 Boon NA, Fox AA. Diseases of the cardiovascular system. In: Edwards CRW, Bouchier IAD, Haslett C, Chilvers ER, eds, *Davidson's Principles and Practice of Medicine*, 17th edn. Churchill Livingstone, Edinburgh 1995: 29–5.

QUICK FLICK

P

143 Ransom D, Leicht C. Continuous spinal analgesia with sufentanil for labour and delivery in a patient with severe pulmonary stenosis. *Anesth Analg* 1995; 80: 418–21.

144 Reimold SC, Rutherford JD. Valvular heart disease in pregnancy. *N Eng J Med* 2003; 349: 52–9.

Quadraplegia/Paraplegia (Chronic) and Anaesthesia

See *Spinal Cord Injury (Pre-existing) and Anaesthesia.*

R

▶ Raised Intracranial Pressure

See *Intracranial Pressure (ICP) and Treatment of Raised ICP*.

▶ Rapid Infusion Catheter Exchanger Set

Used to obtain large bore peripheral IV access. The set contains either a
7 Fr 5 cm catheter or an 8.5 Fr 6.4 cm catheter with a dilator, a 0.64 mm
diameter spring-wire guide and a scalpel.

Technique

1 Aseptically insert a cannula (at least a 20 G) into a suitable large peripheral
   vein. Anaesthetise the insertion site if the patient is awake.
2 Release the tourniquet and insert the guide wire through the cannula,
   then remove the cannula.
3 At the site of wire entry use the scalpel to incise the skin sufficiently to
   enable the dilator and catheter to pass easily into the vein.
4 Insert the catheter with dilator using a twisting motion. When the catheter
   is in place remove the dilator and the guide wire. *Never lose visual contact
   with wire.*
5 Suture the catheter to the skin.

▶ Rapid Sequence Induction (RSI)

This is a technique for the induction of anaesthesia designed to reduce the
possibility of aspiration prior to intubation. A skilled assistant is mandatory for
this technique.

The steps are:

1 Check the anaesthetic machine and breathing circuit and ensure suction is
   available and within easy reach. Ensure aids to intubation are within easy
   reach, such as a Teflon introducer.
2 Always have a prepared plan if intubation fails. **See** *Difficult Airway
   Management*.
3 Have all the required anaesthetic and emergency drugs drawn up. Decide
   on drug dosages before the anaesthetic begins.
4 Attach all appropriate monitoring to the patient and position the patient
   for intubation (head extended on a firm pillow, neck flexed).
5 Preoxygenate (denitrogenate) the patient for 3–5 min. If time is critical
   rapid preoxygenation can be achieved by 4 vital capacity breaths.
6 Induce anaesthesia with thiopentone 3–5 mg/kg or propofol 2–2.5 mg/kg IV

followed immediately by suxamethonium 1.5 mg/kg. Ask the patient to keep his/her eyes open. Cricoid pressure is applied by the assistant as the patient begins to lose consciousness (eyes begin to close). Cricoid pressure involves the assistant pressing on the cricoid cartilage with the thumb and index finger. To identify the cricoid cartilage *see* *Cricothyroid Puncture and Cricothyrotomy*. The force of cricoid pressure should be about 30 N.[1]

7 If a nasogastric (NG) tube is in situ it should be left in place. This is because the NG tube increases the efficiency of cricoid pressure and allows 'venting' of gastric gases and fluids.[1] Remember to apply suction to the NG tube prior to performing RSI to empty the stomach.

8 The patient will be paralysed after fasciculations occur or in 50–60 s if no fasciculations are seen.

9 If suxamethonium is contraindicated, use rocuronium 0.6–0.9 mg/kg. Good intubating conditions will be provided by rocuronium in 60 s but this drug is not the equal of suxamethonium for reliability of intubating conditions.

Intubate the trachea. Cricoid pressure is removed when the intubation is confirmed by end tidal CO_2 monitoring. The tracheal tube cuff is inflated when the assistant is instructed to do so by the anaesthetist.

◗ Recombinant Activated Factor VII (rFVIIa)

This is also referred to as activated factor VII, NovoSeven, eptagog alfa-activated and rFVIIa.

Description and Indications

Recombinant activated factor VII (rFVIIa) is manufactured from baby hamster kidney cells which express cloned human factor VII. First used in patients in 1988, this drug is useful for the prevention or control of bleeding during surgery or trauma in haemophiliac patients with inhibitors to factors VIII or IX. It has since been used 'off licence' to successfully treat non haemophiliacs with massive haemorrhage from various causes (trauma, surgical, DIC, sepsis), unresponsive to all other available coagulation factors. rFVIIa has also been used prophylactically to reduce bleeding in operations such as open prostatectomy.[2] rFVIIa can also be used to normalise INR in patients over-anticoagulated with warfarin.[3] This drug represents a major breakthrough in the management of blood loss as a universal haemostatic agent. Its half-life is about 2.7 h.

Mechanism of Action

rFVIIa enhances the process of haemostasis at the site of bleeding without systemic activation of coagulation.[4] This is because rFVIIa requires tissue factor (TF) to become active. TF is exposed at the site of injury and the TF-rFVIIa combination activates the coagulation cascade on activated platelet membranes adhering to the site of injury. Because of this localised action, systemic haemostasis does not occur.

Efficacy of rFVIIa

rFVIIa has been typically used in situations where there is:

1 Severe blood loss.
2 Transfusion of blood, platelets, FFP, cryoprecipitate and other clotting factors.
3 Coagulopathy (often dilutional) that may or may not correct with the above treatment.
4 Ongoing life-threatening haemorrhage.

Stage of Resuscitation when rFVIIa Should be Considered

Consider this therapy when:

1 Bleeding continues to be life threatening after maximal conventional therapy including at least 10 units of blood, 8–10 units of FFP, 8–10 units of platelets and 10 units of cryoprecipitate[5] (the 10/8/8/10 rule).
2 All surgical and/or embolisation options have been exhausted. Major vessel bleeding should be controlled.
3 Haematologist confirms optimal conventional therapy.
4 Hypothermia and acidosis have been reversed or minimised as much as possible. Aim for a pH > 7.1.
5 Platelet count must be adequate (>50 000/mm^3) for rFVIIa to work.

Dose

Dose for Acute Bleeding

1 90 μg/kg by IV bolus over 3–5 min. Round the dose up or down to the nearest vial size. Repeat this dose after 20 min if needed. Give 35–120 μg/kg IV every 3–12 h if continued treatment is required.
2 rFVIIa is presented in vials of 1.2–4.8 mg and a diluent (sterile water) is provided.

Dose for Prevention of Ongoing Blood Loss 35–120 μg/kg IV every 2–3 h for 1–2 days then every 2–6 h if ongoing treatment is required.

Dose for Prevention of Severe Blood Loss in Patients Without Coagulopathy 40–80 μg/kg IV.[3]

Dose to Reverse Warfarin Effects 80 μg/kg IV

Advantages

1 rFVIIa appears to have an excellent safety profile in both therapeutic dosages and overdose. The rate of fatal thrombo-embolic complications is low (0.07% in one report of 5522 patients).[4]
2 There is no infection risk.
3 Drug volume is not an issue compared with potentially large fluid loads with platelets, FFP and other clotting factors.
4 The drug can be given rapidly.

5 rFVIIa may improve platelet function.[6]
6 May be acceptable to Jehovah's Witness patients.

Disadvantages
1 rVIIa is extremely expensive.
2 There are rare reports of anaphylactoid reactions. rFVIIa is contraindicated in patients with hypersensitivity to mouse, hamster or bovine proteins.

○ Red Cells

Based on the *Australian Red Cross Circular of Information 2003*, with permission.

'Red cells' (or 'packed cells') means the red cell component of a unit of whole blood when most of the plasma has been removed. Packed cells for transfusion have the following characteristics.

Storage
Packed cells are stored at 2–6°C for up to 42 days. If removed from refrigeration, the blood should be returned to refrigeration or transfusion begun within 30 min. Once the packed cell container has been opened the contents are considered expired in 4 h.

Contents
Depending on the manufacturer packed cells contain varying amounts of glucose, mannitol, adenine, sodium chloride, sodium citrate and phosphate. The volume of a unit of red cells is about 240 mL and the haematocrit is 0.5–0.75. Haemolysis at expiry is less than 0.8% of cells. As stored blood ages the electrolyte and pH values change.

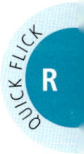

Table R1 Physiochemical properties of stored blood[7]

Physiochemical property	2 weeks storage	5 weeks storage
pH	7.2	6.6
Sodium (mmol/L)	168	156
Potassium (mmol/L)	30	48

2,3-diphosphoglycerate which is one of the regulators of oxygen unloading from haemoglobin is almost completely dissipated after 3 weeks of storage.[7] However, levels regenerate quickly after transfusion.

CMV Negative Cellular Products
These are blood products including red cells, from individuals free of CMV virus. If these are not available, leukocyte filtered blood is the best alternative. Patients that should receive CMV negative red cell units include:
1 All women transfused during pregnancy regardless of their CMV status.
2 All neonates.
3 CMV –ve patients with haematological malignancy.

4 HIV patients.

5 Solid organ transplant recipients.

Red Cells with Buffy Coat Removed

These are suspended red cells after centrifuging whole blood and removing plasma and the 'buffy coat layer' which contains platelets and white cells. Indications for this type of blood are the same as for leukocyte depleted whole blood. *See* *Whole Blood*. This technique is less effective than leukodepletion filters.

Leukocyte Depleted Red Cells

Blood is centrifuged, plasma is removed, and white cells are removed by a filter. The residual WBC count should be $<0.2 \times 10^9/L$. Indications are the same as for leukocyte depleted whole blood. *See* *Whole Blood*.

Red Cells Washed (Triple Washed Cells)

Red cells are washed with N/S to remove plasma proteins, antibodies and electrolytes. Red cells washed are indicated for patients with IgA deficiency with anti-IgA antibodies. Such patients may suffer allergic transfusion reactions including anaphylaxis after multiple transfusions of non-washed red cells. Washed cells are also used to prevent destruction of recipient cells by antibodies in the donor unit e.g. HEMPAS, and to prevent hyperkalaemia in neonates from transfused blood.

Irradiated Products

Blood irradiation prevents T cells from replicating and reduces the risk of graft-versus-host disease. Indications include:

1 Neonates in NICU.

2 Patients receiving directed donations from first degree relatives.

3 Patients with haematological malignancy.

4 Any other patient that is immunocompromised.

Risks of Red Cell Transfusion *see* *Blood Transfusion*.

◗ Reflexes

Table R2 Limb reflex nerve roots

Reflex	Nerve roots involved
Plantar	S1
Ankle	S1, S2
Knee	L3, L4
Biceps	C5, C6
Triceps	C7, C8

Remifentanil

This 4 anilidopiperidine opioid drug is a selective mu receptor agonist with extremely fast onset and offset times and a similar potency to fentanyl. Remifentanil is a derivative of fentanyl with an ester linkage that is rapidly metabolised by non-specific plasma esterases, resulting in a context sensitive half-life of ≈ 3 min.[8]

Uses

1. To provide intra-operative CVS stability and offset the effects of nocioceptive stimulation. The recommended dose range is 0.1–0.5 µg/kg/min. This rate can be increased for periods of extreme stimulation such as rigid bronchoscopy to a maximum of 2 µg/kg/min.
2. Can be used for intubation instead of a muscle relaxant (but with a suitable anaesthetic induction agent). The recommended dose in fit patients is 3–4 µg/kg.
3. To prevent the hypertensive response to intubation. For example for pre-eclamptic patients a dose of 1–1.5 µg/kg/min run for 60–90 s prior to induction. ***See*** *Pre-eclampsia/Eclampsia*.
4. Patient controlled analgesia. ***See*** *Patient Controlled Analgesia (PCA) and Patient Controlled Epidural Anaesthesia*.

QUICK FLICK R

Advantages

1. MAC of volatile agents and the effective anaesthetic infusion dose of propofol are reduced by 50–75% in the presence of a remifentanil infusion.
2. Clearance of remifentanil is independent of renal/hepatic function.
3. Rapidly titratable to desired clinical effect providing excellent cardiovascular stability.

Disadvantages

1. Formulated in glycine, an inhibitory neurotransmitter. *Remifentanil is not recommended for spinal or epidural administration*.[8]
2. The offset of remifentanil is so rapid that patients will be without analgesia within about 10 min of infusion cessation (unless regional anaesthesia or longer acting opioids are utilised). Also if the infusion of remifentanil stops unintentionally intraoperatively all opioid effects will rapidly disappear. Postoperative analgesia should be commenced well before the remifentanil infusion is stopped.
3. Blood pressure is reduced by 15–20% and a mild bradycardia is usual. Severe cardiovascular depression may occur in some patients.
4. When remifentanil is used for sedation there is a higher incidence of nausea and respiratory depression than with propofol.[9]

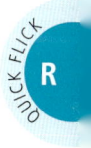

5 Remifentanil infusion particularly at high doses has resulted in opioid induced hyperalgesia in some studies,[10] but not in others.[11] The clinical significance of this effect is unclear.

○ Renal Protection

See *Abdominal Aortic Aneurysm Repair (AAA) Surgery, Fenoldopam* and *N-acetyl Cysteine (NAC)*.

○ Renal Transplant Surgery

Pre-operative Phase

1 Ensure the patient has received pre-operative immunosuppressive therapy including prednisone 20 mg PO, cyclosporin and azothioprine.

2 Pre-operative dialysis to within 0.5 kg of ideal body weight is desirable.[12] Aim for K^+ <6 mmol/L and pH >7.25. Treat pH <7.25 preferably with dialysis, otherwise give 50 mmol of sodium bicarbonate. For treatment of hyperkalaemia *see* *Potassium*.

3 Ensure arterio-venous fistulas are identified and protected with soft padding and kept warm. Place IV cannulas and blood pressure cuff on the other arm. Palpate the fistula at intervals to check patency.

4 Obtain large bore peripheral IV access. Do not use the cephalic vein if possible which should be preserved for future AV fistulas (*see* *Veins of the Upper Limb*). Central venous access is essential, but this can be obtained after induction. Invasive arterial blood pressure monitoring is not required unless indicated by the patient's co-morbid conditions.

5 Give antibiotic cover prior to surgery using a broad spectrum antibiotic e.g. cephazolin 1 g.

Intra-operative Phase

1 Consider a rapid sequence induction if delayed gastric emptying is suspected. Do not use suxamethonium in the presence of hyperkalaemia. Propofol or thiopentone can be used. The most appropriate muscle relaxant is cisatracurium although a single dose of rocuronium can be given. Maintain anaesthesia with O_2, air and isoflurane or desflurane. Sevoflurane can also be used as there is no evidence of nephrotoxicity despite theoretical concerns.[13] *See* *Sevoflurane*.

2 Monitor temperature and keep the patient normothermic.

3 Fentanyl at normal doses is the opioid of choice. Pethidine and morphine are unsuitable due to the accumulation of active metabolites (norpethidine and morphine-6-glucuronide).

4 Keep patients reasonably well filled intravascularly. This may require large volumes of fluid (60–100 mL/kg). The target CVP is around 10–12 mm Hg.[12] N/S is the IV fluid of choice. If colloid is required albumin solution may be preferable to gelatin and dextran solutions.[13]

5 If hypotension occurs during surgery discuss the management with the surgeon, but in general treat with intravascular volume expansion. If volume expansion is ineffective give a vasopressor. Consider inotropic support with dobutamine or dopexamine if hypotension persists.[12]

6 The surgeon may request drugs to optimise renal graft perfusion such as mannitol 0.5 g/kg + frusemide 80 mg IV. Dopamine may also be considered (200 mg in 100 mL 5% glucose) although there is little evidence of efficacy.[12] Start the dopamine infusion at 5 mL/h.

7 Prior to arterial unclamping of the graft kidney aim for a central venous pressure of ≈ 10–12 mm Hg.[12] Optimal intravascular fluid volume is essential for graft survival. N/S is the crystalloid of choice (no potassium or lactate).[14]

8 If a blood transfusion is required use a leucocyte reduction filter e.g. Sepacell.

9 Postoperative analgesia can be enhanced by performance of a TAP block. **See** *Transversus Abdominis Plane Block*.

Postoperative Phase

Use fentanyl IV via a PCA infusion pump for postoperative analgesia. Do not use morphine or pethidine due to the possible accumulation of harmful metabolites.[14] NSAIDs and paracetamol should not be used.[13]

○ Respiratory Function Tests

The most useful tests of respiratory function are:

1 *Exercise tolerance*

2 *Spirometry*. The most useful measurements are:

   a) *FEV_1*, forced expiratory volume in the first second. An FEV_1 of <1 L or <30% predicted is indicative of severe disease. A >10–15% increase in FEV_1 after a bronchodilator such as ventolin is administered indicates a significant response to that drug.[15]

   b) *FVC*, forced vital capacity.

   c) *Ratio of FEV_1 to FVC*. This ratio should normally be greater than 80% of predicted. A ratio <70% is indicative of obstructive lung disease e.g. asthma, chronic bronchitis and emphysema. A 60–70% ratio indicates mild disease, while a ratio of <50% indicates severe disease. An FEV_1:FVC ratio of >70%, with a FVC <80% of the predicted, is indicative of restrictive lung disease, as occurs with fibrosing alveolitis and chest wall abnormalities.

   d) *Vital capacity*. A vital capacity <50% predicted, or < 2 L indicates increased risk of pulmonary complications.

   e) *Arterial blood gases*. A PaO_2 < 60 mm Hg and/or a $PaCO_2$ > 50 mm Hg indicates respiratory failure.

   f) *Carbon monoxide (CO) diffusion capacity*. This test measures transfer of CO into the blood from the lungs (DLCO). The result is given as a percentage of predicted normal. Carbon monoxide transfer is reduced in patients with alveolar disease and pulmonary vascular obstruction such as pulmonary emboli. CO transfer is increased in such conditions as pulmonary haemorrhage and congestive cardiac failure. A DLCO <50% predicted is indicative of increased anaesthetic risk.

g) *Measurement of TLC, RV and VC.* Total lung capacity (TLC), residual volume and vital capacity (VC) can also be useful.

h) *Maximum breathing capacity (MBC).* MBC normally > 100 L/min. If MBC <50% predicted or less than 50 L/min, there is an increased anaesthetic risk for major surgery.

i) *Flow volume dynamics.* A discussion of this area is beyond the scope of this manual.

Respiratory Factors Predicting Increased Risk for Abdominal Surgery[16]

1 FEV_1 & FVC <70% predicted.
2 FEV_1/FVC <65% predicted.
3 MBC & DLCO <50% predicted.

Respiratory Factors Predicting Increased Risk for Pulmonary Lobectomy[17]

1 FEV1 <1 L or <40–50% of predicted.
2 MBC <40–70 L/min or <40% of predicted.

Lung Function Tests Indicating Increased Operative Risk for Pneumonectomy[17]

1 Postoperative predicted FEV_1 <0.85 L or pre-operative FEV_1 < 2 L + FEV_1 < 50% of FVC.
2 MBC < 70 L/min or < 55% of predicted.
3 Hypercapnia on room air ($PaCO_2$ > 45 mm Hg).
4 Temporary pulmonary occlusion of pulmonary artery on the planned operative side (with PA catheter) can be considered. Increased risk exists if $PaCO_2$ >60 mm Hg, PaO_2 <40 mm Hg or pulmonary artery pressure rises to greater than 40 mm Hg.

◯ Resuscitation of the Newborn

See Neonatal Resuscitation.

◯ Retained Placenta

See Uterine Relaxation for Retained Placenta.

◯ Retinal Detachment Surgery

During retinal repair surgery the surgeon may inject sulfur hexafluoride (SF_6) intravitreally. If N_2O is being used as part of the anaesthetic, it should be discontinued 15–20 min before injection of gas. This is because the N_2O can diffuse into the gas bubble and greatly increase intraocular pressure. N_2O should not be used in subsequent anaesthetics while the intravitreal gas is present.

◗ Retrograde Intubation

A basic technique for retrograde intubation is described below:

1 Attach a 5 mL syringe to an 18 G cannula, insert the cannula through the cricothyroid membrane in a cephalad direction. Once air is aspirated slide the cannula further into the trachea over the stylet.
2 Pass a guidewire through the cannula and retrieve this from the mouth.
3 Remove the cannula.
4 Use the guidewire to guide an ET tube into the trachea until resistance is felt.
5 Pass a Teflon bougie into the trachea through the ET tube.
6 Remove the wire and insert the ET tube further into the trachea over the Teflon bougie.

Use of the Cook Retrograde Intubation Set

1 Insert the 18 G introducer needle as described above with syringe attached.
2 Pass the guide wire through the needle and then remove the needle.
3 Retrieve the guidewire from the mouth and attach a needle holder to the guidewire at the skin incision.
4 Insert the guiding catheter into the mouth over the guidewire until resistance is felt (the guiding catheter is just in the trachea).
5 Pass the ET tube through the mouth over the guiding catheter until resistance is felt.
6 Remove the guiding catheter and wire and insert the ET tube further into the trachea.

◗ Rocuronium

Quaternary aminosteroid non-depolarising neuromuscular blocking drug. Rocuronium is an analogue of vecuronium.

Dose

0.6 mg/kg IV. Rocuronium has a duration of action of 30–40 min. Maintenance bolus doses of 0.15 mg/kg can be given.

Infusion Dose 3–5 μg/kg/min can be given, titrated to the measured twitch response.

Advantages

1 Rapid onset of action with adequate intubating conditions achieved in 60 s.

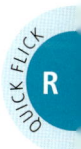

2 Minimal cardiovascular side effects. Rocuronium can cause some increase in heart rate.[18] It does not cause histamine release.

3 Suitable for use by continuous infusion.

4 Presented as a ready-to-use solution unlike vecuronium which is presented as a powder.

5 Can be rapidly reversed at any time after dosing by sugammadex (**see** *Sugammadex*).

Disadvantages

1 Rocuronium is cleared principally by uptake in the liver and secretion in the bile.[19] A small proportion is excreted in the urine. Effects of rocuronium may be prolonged in the presence of hepatic disease and, to a lesser extent, renal disease.[19]

2 Intubating conditions are often not ideal after 60 s; this drug is therefore less reliable than suxamethonium for this purpose.[20]

3 Rocuronium precipitates with thiopentone. This can result in the blockage of IV catheters and bronchospasm.[21] Flush thiopentone from the IV line before giving rocuronium.

4 Requires refrigeration (storage at 2–8°C). If removed from refrigerator the rocuronium ampoule should be discarded within 12 weeks.

5 Allergic reactions to rocuronium may be more common than with some other currently used NDNMBDs such as vecuronium.[21,22]

◖ Ropivacaine

Aminoamide local anaesthetic drug, presented as the pure s-enantiomer. Useful for all types of local and regional anaesthetic techniques except for Bier block.

Dose

Adult and Child Older Than 12 Years Maximum permissible dose depends on site: epidural 200 mg, intrathecal 20 mg, field block 187.5 mg, major nerve block 300 mg. The lowest effective dose should be used. A mg/kg dose advisory is not available.

Children Under 12 Years See below.

Lumbar Epidural Use (Adult) 15–25 mL of 0.75% solution for surgical anaesthesia. For labour analgesia use 10–20 mL of 0.2% solution. For postoperative analgesia an infusion of 0.2% can be run at 6–14 mL/h.

Thoracic Epidural Use (Adult) 5–15 mL of 0.75% mg/mL solution to establish the block then an infusion of 6–14 mL/h of 0.2% solution for postoperative analgesia. **See** *Epidural Anaesthesia*.

Subarachnoid Block Use (Adult) A 0.5% solution. For example 3.5 mL of 0.5% ropivacaine is effective for hip arthroplasty.[23]

Infusion for Continuous Peripheral Nerve Blockade (Adult) 5–10 mL/h 0.2% solution. Use for up to 48 h.

Caudal Epidural Dose (Child) 0.2% 2 mg/kg. Doses up to 3 mg/kg have been used safely.

Peripheral Nerve Block (Child) Use 0.5% up to 2 mg/kg.

Ropivacaine and Adrenaline

Adrenaline will not prolong the action of ropivacaine used for nerve blocks. However adrenaline can be added to ropivacaine used for local anaesthetic infiltration to reduce bleeding. Add 0.1 mL adrenaline 1:1000 solution (0.1 mg) to 20 mL of ropivacaine to produce a final concentration of 1:200 000.

Advantages

1 Less cardiotoxic than bupivacaine.
2 Some vasoconstrictor properties. The addition of adrenaline does prolong the duration of cutaneous analgesia but not the duration of peripheral nerve block.[23]
3 Ropivacaine produces a longer duration of cutaneous block than bupivacaine.[23]
4 For epidural blockade the duration of sensory block is similar for the two drugs. The duration of peripheral nerve block is shorter with ropivacaine than bupivacaine at equal concentrations.[23]

Disadvantages

1 Ropivacaine is more cardiotoxic than lignocaine. Cardiac arrest due to IV ropivacaine with successful resuscitation has been described in several reports.[24,25]
2 Ropivacaine has similar central nervous system toxicity to bupivacaine (see below for information on ropivacaine toxicity).
3 Ropivacaine is about 25% less potent than bupivacaine. A dose of 7.5 mg/mL ropivacaine is comparable to 6 mg/mL bupivacaine.
4 The vasoconstrictive properties of ropivacaine may potentially result in end organ ischaemia. For example the use of ropivacaine for penile block has resulted in a report of transitory ischaemia of the penile tip. ***See** Penile Block*.
5 Ropivacaine is contraindicated for IV regional anaesthetic technique (Bier Block).

Ropivacaine Toxicity

Ropivicaine cardiotoxicity is more amenable to treatment than bupivacaine cardiotoxicity. Ropivacaine toxicity typically manifests with:

1 dizziness, drowsiness

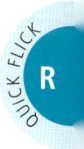

R

QUICK FLICK

2   loss of consciousness, seizure
3   progressive bradycardia, hypotension and asystole.
Note: Ventriclar fibrillation may occur.

Treatment of Ropivicaine Induced Cardiac Arrest

1   Supportive management of airway, breathing and circulation. If cardiac arrest occurs treat as per *Cardiac Arrest*.
2   Treat seizures with small doses of diazepam, midazolam, thiopentone or propofol.[26]
3   Calcium channel blockers and phenytoin are contraindicated.[26]
4   If the above measures are unsuccessful, use intralipid 20% as described in *Intralipid for the Treatment of Bupivacaine/Ropivacaine Toxicity.*
5   Evidence for the effectiveness of intralipid therapy was published by Litz et al. for a patient with asystole due to ropivacaine toxicity.[27]

REFERENCES

1   Gabbott DA. Recent advances in airway technology. *Br J Anaesthesiol CEPD Reviews* 2001; 1: 76–80.

2   Friedrich PW, Henny CP, Messelink EJ, et al. Effect of recombinant activated factor VII on perioperative blood loss in patients undergoing retro pubic prostatectomy: a double-blind placebo-controlled randomized trial. *Lancet* 2003; 18: 201–5.

3   Roberts HR, Monroe DM, Escobar MA. Current concepts in haemostasis. *Anesthesiology* 2004; 100: 722–30.

4   Martinowitz U, Kenet G, Segal E et al. Recombinant activated factor VII for adjunctive haemorrhage control in trauma. *J Trauma Injury Infection Crit Care* 2001; 51: 431–9.

5   Gowers CJD, Parr MJA. Recombinant activated factor VIIa use in massive transfusion and coagulopathy unresponsive to conventional therapy. *Anesth Intensive Care* 2005; 33: 196–200.

6   Tobias JD. Synthetic factor VIIa to treat dilutional coagulopathy during posterior spinal fusion in two children. *Anesthesiology* 2002; 96: 1522–5.

7   Lovric VA. Alterations in blood components during storage and their clinical significance. *Anesth Intensive Care* 1984; 12: 246–51.

8   Thompson JP, Rowbotham DJ. Editorial: Remifentanil—an opioid for the 21st century. *Br J Anaesth* 1996; 76 (3): 341–2.

9   Servin FS, Raeder JC, Merle JC et al. Remifentanil sedation compared with propofol during regional anaesthesia. *Acta Anaesthesiol Scand* 2002; 46: 309–15.

10 Guignard B, Bossard AE, Coste C et al. Acute opioid tolerance: intraoperative remifentanil increases postoperative pain and morphine requirement. *Anesthesiology* 2000; 93: 409–17.

11 Gustorf B, Nahlik G, Hoerauf KH, Kress HG. The absence of acute tolerance during remifentanil infusion in volunteers. *Anesth Analg* 2002; 94: 1223–8.

12 Rabey P. Anaesthesia for renal transplantation. *Br J Anaesth/CPED Reviews* 2001; 1: 24–7.

13 SarinKapoor H, Kaur R, Kaur H. Anaesthesia for renal transplant surgery. *Acta Anaesthesiol Scand* 2007; 51: 1354–67.

14 Moote CA. Anesthesia for renal transplantation. *Anesth Clin Nth America* 1994; 12(4): 691–711.

15 Apps MCP. A guide to lung function tests. *Br J Hosp Med* 1992; 48(7): 396–401.

16 Glass GD, Olsen GN. Preoperative pulmonary function testing to predict postoperative morbidity and mortality. *Chest* 1986; 89: 127–35.

17 Benumof JL, Alfery DD. Anesthesia for thoracic surgery. In: Miller RD, ed. *Anesthesia*, 3rd edn. Churchill Livingstone, New York 1990: 1520–1.

18 Epemolu O, Bom A, Hope F, Mason R. Reversal of neuromuscular blockade and simultaneous increase in plasma rocuronium concentration after intravenous infusion of the novel reversal agent Org 25969. *Anesthesiology* 2003; 3: 632–7.

19 Pollard BJ. Drug Focus: Rocuronium and cisatracurium. *Br J Hosp Med* 1997; 57: 346–8.

20 Patel N, Smith CE, Pinchak AC. Emergency surgery and rapid sequence intubation: rocuronium vs succinylcholine. *Anesthesiology* 1995; 83: A914.

21 Heier T, Guttormsen AB. Anaphylactic reactions during induction of anaesthesia using rocuronium for muscle relaxation: a report of 3 cases. *Acta Anaesthesiol Scand* 2000; 44: 775–81.

22 Laake JH, Røttingen JA. Rocuronium and anaphylaxis—a statistical challenge. *Acta Anaesthesiol Scand* 2001; 45: 1196–203.

23 McClure JH. Ropivacaine. *Br J Anaesth* 1996; 76: 300–7.

24 Chazalon P, Tourtier JP, Villevieille T. Ropivacaine-induced cardiac arrest after peripheral nerve block: Successful resuscitation. *Anesthesiology* 2003; 99: 1449–51.

25 Huet O, Eyrolle IJ, Mazoit JX, Ozier YM. Cardiac arrest and plasma concentration after injection of ropivacaine for posterior lumbar plexus blockade. *Anesthesiology* 2003; 99: 1451–3.

26 Finucane BT. Ropivacaine cardiac toxicity—not as troublesome as bupivacaine (Editorial). *Can J Anesth* 2005; 52: 449–53.

27 Litz RJ, Popp M, Stehr N, Koch T. Successful resuscitation of a patient with ropivacaine-induced asystole after axillary brachial plexus block using lipid infusion. *Anaesthesia* 2006; 61: 800–1.

QUICK FLICK

R

S

◊ 'Saddle' Block

See *Subarachnoid Block (SAB)*.

◊ Salbutamol

Synthetic sympathomimetic drug used for the treatment of
bronchoconstriction and premature labour. Salbutamol also has a role in the
treatment of hyperkalaemia. ***See*** *Potassium*. Acts by stimulating β_2 and, to a
lesser extent, β_1 adreno-receptors.

Dose for Bronchospasm
Adult
Puffer 200–400 µg inhaled 6–8 h.
Nebuliser 2.5–5 mg 4 h or more frequently up to every 20 min depending on
the severity of the bronchospasm.
IV 5 µg/kg bolus over 10 min then infusion 10–20 µg/min. Mix 15 mg
salbutamol with 250 mL N/S. 10 mL/h of this solution = 10 µg/min.

Child
Puffer 100–200 µg 4–6 h.
Nebuliser 0.03 mL/kg of 0.5% solution of salbutamol 4 h or more frequently
depending on the severity of the bronchospasm.

    Alternatively (using 0.5% solution):

Child <3y	0.3 mL
Child 3–6 y	0.4 mL
Child 6–12 y	0.5 mL

Make the volume up to 4 mL with N/S prior to nebulisation.
IV 5 µg/kg over 10 min then infusion 1–5 µg/kg/min which is equivalent to
$0.06 \times$ Wt mL/h of 1 mg/mL solution.

Dose for Uterine Relaxation to Halt Premature Labour
Load 25 mg of salbutamol in 1 L Hartmann's solution and infuse 60–100 mL
over 10–20 min.[2] Run the infusion at up to 50 µg/min, although tachycardia
usually prevents the infusion rate being safely increased above 20 µg/min.
As a general guideline, slow the infusion rate when the maternal pulse rate
reaches 120/min, and cease if the pulse rate reaches 140/min.[2]

Potential Side Effects
IV salbutamol therapy can cause:
1   Anxiety and tremor.

2 Widening of pulse pressure, tachycardia and hypotension.

3 Hyperglycaemia and hypokalaemia.

4 Prolonged use of salbutamol over days can cause pulmonary oedema.

5 Hyperinsulinaemia and hypoglycaemia can occur in the fetus.

�‣ Sander's Injector

See *Transtracheal Jet Ventilation*

�‣ Saphenous Nerve Block

Anatomy

The saphenous nerve is the cutaneous branch of the posterior division of the femoral nerve and supplies sensation to the medial side of the leg and foot.

Nerve Stimulator Technique[3]

1 Palpate the point 3.5 cm posterior to the centre of the bony prominence of the medial femoral condyle.

2 Sterilise and anaesthetise the skin at this point. Insert a 5 cm 22 G insulated block needle. Attach a nerve stimulator and set the stimulating current at 2 mA. Attempt to elicit paraesthesia over the medial malleolus.

3 Reduce the stimulation current and adjust the needle position to maintain paraesthesia, the end-point of nerve localisation being paraesthesia persisting at 0.4 mA. The depth of needle insertion on average is 2.8 cm.

4 Inject 10 mL of LA agent e.g. lignocaine 2% with adrenaline.

Loss of Resistance (LOR) Technique[3]

1 Identify the sartorius muscle on the medial side of the femur.

2 After sterilising and anaesthetising the skin just above the knee joint insert a 20 G Tuohy needle attached to a 10 mL syringe suitable for a LOR technique. Insert the needle until LOR occurs (identifying the subsartorial fat pad).

3 Inject LA e.g. 10 mL of lignocaine 2% with adrenaline. There is a 20% failure rate with this technique.

�‣ Scalp Block

The posterior scalp is innervated by the:

1 *Greater occipital nerve* (C2, C3): supplies the skin over the occiput to the vertex.

2 *Lesser occipital nerve* (C2): supplies the occipital area immediately above and behind the mastoid, and the skin over the mastoid process. It is derived from the cervical plexus.

3 *Third occipital nerve* (C3): supplies the skin of the lower occiput.

The anterior scalp is innervated by the supra-orbital and supra-trochlear nerves. These are branches of the frontal nerve (in turn a branch of the ophthalmic division of the V cranial nerve). There are also contributions from:

1 *Zygomaticotemporal nerves* (V2).
2 *Auriculotemporal nerves* (V3).
3 *Greater auricular nerves* (C2, C3).

Technique for Scalp Block[4]
1 Position the patient sitting with the head flexed. Identify the nuchal ridge on the posterior scalp.
2 Identify the point (X) over the occipital protuberance 2.5 cm lateral from the midline.
3 Sterilise the skin and insert a 23 G needle at point X to contact bone. Inject a ridge of 3 mL of LA to anaesthetise the *greater occipital nerve*.
4 To anaesthetise the *lesser occipital nerve*, angle the needle anteriorly and laterally along the back of skull. Inject subcutaneous anaesthesia from this point to the mastoid process. Use about 8 mL of LA.
5 To anaesthetise the entire scalp, perform the block bilaterally and extend a subcutaneous wheal around the entire scalp circumference. Inject subcutaneously above the ears and continue anteriorly at the same level.

See *Supraorbital and Supratrochlear Nerve Blocks*.

◖ Scalp Capillary pH Measurement

Fetal scalp capillary blood pH can help in the diagnosis of fetal hypoxia and acidosis. A pH of <7.2 may indicate the need for urgent delivery.[5]

Table S1 Fetal scalp pH and significance

pH value	Interpretation
≥ 7.25	Normal
7.20–7.24	Preacidotic
<7.20	Acidotic

◖ Sciatic Nerve Block

This block is useful for surgery on the foot and lower leg but note that the medial side of the leg, ankle and foot will not be anaesthetised. These areas are supplied by the saphenous branch of the femoral nerve.

Anatomy
The *sciatic nerve* is formed from the following sacral plexus nerve roots: L4, L5, S1–3. The nerve leaves the pelvis via the greater sciatic foramen and descends beneath gluteus maximus between the greater trochanter and the ischial tuberosity to enter the thigh behind adductor magnus. The nerve travels along the postero-medial aspect of the femur and divides at the apex of the popliteal fossa into the tibial nerve and common peroneal nerve. **See** *Popliteal Fossa Block*.

Supplies
Motor to the hamstring muscles and all the muscles of the leg and foot.

Sensory for all the leg and foot below the knee except for the medial side of the leg, over the medial malleolus and posterior thigh.

Techniques of Sciatic Nerve Block

There are many approaches to the sciatic nerve. 5 techniques will be described.

Anterior Approach

1 Position the patient supine and identify the anterior superior iliac spine (ASIS) and the pubic tubercle. Draw a line between these 2 landmarks.
2 Draw a second line parallel to the first extending from the greater trochanter in a medial caudad direction.
3 At the junction of the medial third and lateral two-thirds of the first line draw a perpendicular which intersects the second line. This is the entry point.
4 Sterilise (and if the patient is awake, anaesthetise) the skin and insert a 125 mm 23 G insulated needle attached to a nerve stimulator.
5 When the lesser trochanter of the femur is contacted walk off the medial border. The nerve will be located ≈ 2.5 cm deeper than this point. Start with a stimulating current of 3 mA at 2 Hz. Reduce the current to 0.2–0.6 mA when the nerve is located (preferably ankle movement is seen).
6 Inject 20 mL of 0.5% bupivacaine (or 30 mL of bupivacaine 0.25% or 30 mL of ropivacaine 5 mg/mL).

Posterior Approach[6]

1 Position patient in the lateral position with leg to be blocked uppermost and flexed at the hip and knee (Sim's position).
2 Identify the greater trochanter and the posterior superior iliac spine (PSIS) and draw a line between these two landmarks.
3 Draw a second line from the sacral hiatus to the greater trochanter. Drop a perpendicular from the midpoint of the first line and draw an X where it crosses the second line. This is the entry point. Prepare skin as above.
4 The X should overlie the U-shaped sciatic notch at its superior and lateral border. Insert 10 cm 23 G insulated needle until paraesthesia, a motor response or bone is encountered (usually the lateral border of the notch).
5 Withdraw and advance more medially. The nerve will lie just a little deeper than the bone.
6 Note that the nerve emerges from the upper medial border of the notch then curves down to lie equidistant from the ischial tuberosity and the greater trochanter. This may help identify the position of the nerve.
7 Inject LA in dosages described above.

QUICK FLICK S

Lithotomy Approach

This is a very simple and reliable approach.

1 Position the patient supine, with the leg to be blocked flexed at the hip.
2 Identify the greater trochanter and ischial tuberosity, and the midpoint between these two landmarks. This is the entry point.
3 Insert 10 cm insulated 23 G needle attached to nerve stimulator. Start with 4 mA at 2 Hz. Elicit movement in the foot which should persist when current is reduced to 0.3 mA.
4 Inject LA in dosages described above.

Lateral Approach

1 Identify the point 2 cm below and 2 cm posterior to the greater trochanter. Prepare the skin as above.
2 Insert a 10 cm 23 G insulated needle attached to a nerve stimulator, contact the femur, then reinsert so that needle passes just behind femur.
3 When the sciatic nerve is contacted, inject LA as described above.

Ultrasound-Guided Approach[7]

The authors used lignocaine 1% and ropivacaine 0.25% 50:50 mix with 1:400 000 adrenaline (total volume 30 mL).

1 Position the patient laterally with the side to be anaesthetised uppermost and the knee flexed.
2 Draw a line between the lateral margin of the greater trochanter and the ischial tuberosity.
3 Use the ultrasound probe parallel to this line to identify the sciatic nerve in the subgluteal space (which lies between gluteus maximus and quadratus femoris). The nerve is oval shape at this level and up to 2 cm in depth.
4 Using aseptic technique and LA to the skin, insert a 10 cm insulated nerve block needle (e.g. a Stimuplex) connected to a nerve stimulator set at 1 Hz and 1 mA.
5 Place the needle tip next to the nerve. Movement of the foot should be seen.
6 After an aspiration test, inject 2–5 mL of LA as a test dose. This should distend the subgluteal space.
7 Inject the rest of the LA incrementally over 2–3 min. Circumferential spread of the LA around the sciatic nerve should be observed.

▷ Sciatic Nerve Sheath Catheter

This is a technique for postoperative analgesia in which the surgeon inserts a catheter into the sciatic nerve sheath during surgery for an above knee amputation. The nerve block is established with 20 mL of bupivacaine 0.25% or ropivacaine 10 mg/mL. This is followed by an infusion of bupivacaine 0.25% run at 10 mL/h.

○ Seizures

See *Epilepsy, Status*.

○ Serotonin Syndrome

This syndrome is due to excessive serotonin in the central nervous system. It is usually due to overdose of a single drug or interaction between two different types of drug e.g. tramadol and sertraline. Examples of drugs that may cause this syndrome include:

1   Selective serotonin reuptake inhibitors such as sertraline, fluoxetine, paroxetine, venlafaxine
2   Monoamine oxidase inhibitors e.g. moclobamide.
3   Tramadol.
4   Prochlorperazine.
5   St John's wort.
6   Sibutramine: a centrally acting appetite suppressor that blocks the reuptake of noradrenaline, serotonin and dopamine. Serotonin syndrome can occur if fentanyl, pethidine, dextrorphan or pentazocine are given.

Symptoms and Signs
1   Mental state changes such as confusion, hypomania, agitation.
2   Motor disturbance such as incoordination, tremor, clonus, pyramidal rigidity.
3   Hyperreflexia.
4   Autonomic disturbances with diaphoresis, diarrhoea and fever.

Treatment
1   This condition is usually self limiting (under 24 h) once the causative drugs are ceased, but fatalities have occurred.
2   5-HT antagonists such as methysergide have been used to treat refractory or severe cases.

○ Sevoflurane

Volatile inhalational halogenated ether type anaesthetic agent.

Physical properties and MAC:

Blood:Gas Solubility Coefficient	0.69
Oil:Gas Solubility Coefficient	48
Saturated Vapour Pressure (20°C)	160 mm Hg (21.3 kPa)
Boiling Point	58.6°C
MAC	2.05%

Advantages
1   The absence of pungency coupled with low blood solubility makes sevoflurane the agent of choice for inhalational induction.

QUICK FLICK **S**

2 Low blood:gas solubility results in sevoflurane providing rapid induction of anaesthesia, and rapid emergence.

3 Cerebral autoregulation is preserved up to an inspired concentration of 1.5 MAC.[8]

4 Sevoflurane causes bronchodilation.

5 Ozone-friendly agent.

Disadvantages

1 Although concerns have been raised regarding potential renal toxicity with sevoflurane no evidence of renal damage has been detected clinically. Sevoflurane does not produce intrarenal fluoride ions as does methoxyflurane.[9]

2 Sevoflurane is degraded by CO_2 absorbers to produce several compounds including compound A which is toxic to rat kidney tissue. Compound A production is increased by high sevoflurane concentrations, low gas flow rates, high soda-lime temperature and the use of barium lime (baralyme).[10] Although no evidence of renal damage in humans has been attributed to compound A it is recommended that:

  a) Do not use sevoflurane in the presence of baralyme.

  b) Fresh gas flows should be > 2 L/min.[8]

3 Do not leave gases flowing through CO_2 absorbant between anaesthetic cases as this can lead to the absorbant becoming desiccated. Dessication of the absorbant in the presence of sevoflurane may result in smoke/fire, and significant carbon monoxide production. In patients this may cause airway irritation, difficult ventilation, severe airway oedema and erythema and elevated carboxyhaemoglobin levels (Abbott Australasia Communication 25 November 2003). An unusally delayed rise or unexpected decline of inspired sevoflurane concentration compared to the vaporiser setting may indicate significant heating of the CO_2 absorbant.

4 Sevoflurane causes prolongation of the Q-T interval (as does isoflurane and enflurane).[11] Sevoflurane has been implicated in causing torsades de pointes (polymorphic VT).[12] Q-T prolongation due to sevoflurane can be reversed by ceasing sevoflurane and maintaining anaesthesia with a propofol infusion.[13] *See Long QT Syndrome (LQTS)*.

5 Postoperative agitation may be more common in children after a sevoflurane anaesthetic compared with halothane.[14]

6 Can rarely cause convulsions at high inhalational dosages.[15]

7 Rarely sevoflurane can degrade in the storage bottle resulting in a 'hiss' when opening and an acrid odour.[15] Do not use the contents if this occurs.

8 Sevoflurane can induce malignant hyperthermia. Do not use in MH susceptible patients. *See Malignant Hyperthermia*.

⊙ **Shivering Postoperatively**

Shivering after a general anaesthetic is common (up to 60% of patients)[16] and usually benign but can lead to undesirable effects such as:[17]

1 increased O_2 consumption
2 raised intraocular pressure
3 disruption of delicate surgical repair
4 hypoglycaemia.

Prevention

1 Use of warming devices such as warm air filled blankets (e.g. Bair Hugger™) and a heating mattress.
2 Minimising the surface area of the patient that is exposed.

Treatment

1 Exclude causes of shivering other than anaesthesia such as hypoglycaemia, fever and hypothermia.
2 Exogenous heat.
3 Pethidine 0.5 mg/kg IV.[18]
4 Clonidine 1.5 µg/kg IV.[18]
5 Tramadol 1 mg/kg/IV.[19] Tramadol may be more effective than pethidine.[20]

⊙ **Sickle Cell Disease**

Topics Covered in this Section

▶ Spectrum of Sickle Cell Disease
▶ Diagnosis of Sickle Cell Disease
▶ Sickle Cell Anaemia (SCA)
▶ Anaesthetic Considerations for SCA
▶ Obstetric Anaesthesia and SCA
▶ Anaesthetic Considerations for Sickle Cell Trait
▶ Treatment of Sickle Cell Crisis

Spectrum of Sickle Cell Disease

Sickle cell disease is an inherited haemoglobinopathy due to a mutation on chromosome 11 that results in the production of an abnormal haemoglobin, HbS. This mutation is due to valine being substituted for glutamic acid at the sixth amino acid position of the β chain of the globin molecule. Deoxygenation of HbS results in the formation of insoluble globin polymers (long crystals). This gives the red blood cell (RBC) a sickled shape which results in increased RBC destruction and episodes of obstruction of blood vessels. Repeated cycles of sickling and unsickling eventually result in irreversible sickling. Patients suffer from a chronic haemolytic anaemia and episodes of *sickle cell crisis* in which vaso-occlusion results in tissue ischaemia and infarction with severe pain (see below). Other effects include pulmonary

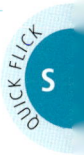

hypertension, cardiomegaly, CCF and renal failure. This disease affects mainly Africans and some Mediterranean races.

Types of sickle cell disease include:

1 *HbSS*, the homozygous form of the disease, associated with severe haemolytic anaemia. This variant is sickle cell anaemia (SCA). RBC contain 85–95% HbS.[21] Variable increases in HbF occur in patients with sickle cell anaemia which offers some protection from sickling, reducing complication rates and increasing survival. Levels of HbF above 20% are particularly effective.[21]

2 *HbSC*, sickle cell HbC disease. In this condition, in addition to the HbS gene, a mutant β chain gene causes cellular dehydration and increased intracellular HbS concentration. Most patients will eventually develop symptoms but median survival is longer than for HbSS.

3 *HbAS* (Sickle Cell Trait), heterozygous form. Patients are usually not anaemic. The red cell contains 20–45% HbS. Sickling starts at an O_2 saturation of 40% and the critical PaO_2 for irreversible sickling is 20 mm Hg. This disease does carry some risk e.g. splenic infarcts at altitude.[21] HbAS is thought to provide some survival advantage over normals in cases of malarial illness.

4 *Alpha thalassaemia and HbSS* sometimes coexist resulting in a less severe anaemia than in HbSS alone.[22]

Diagnosis of Sickle Cell Disease

A Sickledex test will detect HbS but does not identify the type of sickle cell disease. The genotype can be detected by haemoglobin electrophoresis.

Sickle Cell Anaemia (SCA)

Sickling occurs in response to reduced O_2 tension, acidosis, cold, dehydration and can occur with drug therapy in association with a glucose-6-phosphate dehydrogenase deficiency. **See** *Glucose-6-Phosphate Dehydrogenase (G6PD) Deficiency*. At 65% O_2 saturation, 75% of RBC are sickled. The critical PaO_2 for irreversible sickling is 42 mm Hg.[21] Patients have a chronic severe haemolytic anaemia, impaired renal concentrating ability and susceptibility to severe bacterial infections. Sickle cell crisis results in hypoxia/infarction of affected tissues. This leads to pain, renal impairment, haemolytic anaemia, fever, tachycardia and a self perpetuating cycle of acidosis and hypoxia. Patterns of attacks include the following:

1 *Chest syndrome* describes recurrent episodes of chest pain, fever and pulmonary infiltrates.

2 *Sickle cell lung disease* with progressive deterioration in lung function and cor pulmonale.

3 *Sequestration crisis* occurs particularly in young children, due to pooling of RBCs in the spleen and liver. This causes massive sudden enlargement of these organs.

4 *Aplastic crisis*, due to sudden severe bone marrow depression, is another potentially fatal complication. This can be precipitated by infection, typically viral.[22]

Anaesthetic Considerations for SCA

Pre-operative Measures

1 Pre-operative transfusion therapy to correct anaemia to 10 g/dL is recommended prior to intermediate- or high-risk surgery. It is no longer recommended to reduce HbS levels to < 30%.[23]

2 For minimally symptomatic patients having minor surgery, pre-operative transfusion is probably unnecessary.[23]

3 Keep the patient well hydrated peri-operatively. These patients tend to have renal impairment with reduced renal concentrating ability.

4 Do not perform elective surgery in the presence of infection as a crisis may be precipitated.[21]

Intra-operative and Postoperative Measures

1 It is imperative to prevent hypoxia, acidosis, dehydration and hypothermia. Maintain a mild respiratory alkalosis with intermittent positive pressure ventilation. Use higher than usual inhaled FiO_2 concentrations.

2 Use prophylactic antibiotic therapy. These patients are prone to overwhelming infections, particularly streptococcal infection, due to functional hyposplenism.

3 Prevent local circulatory stasis. Vasopressors should not be used if possible.[21]

4 SCA is a relative contraindication to tourniquet use. Tourniquets have been used safely in these patients but this technique should be undertaken very cautiously.[24] For example, Al-Ghamdi reported using exchange transfusion to reduce HbS from 82.6% to 47% prior to the sequential application of tourniquets for bilateral knee replacement.[25]

5 A cell-saver should probably not be used due to the high incidence of sickling in the washed cells.[26]

6 Ensure the above management continues postoperatively.

7 Regional anaesthesia is associated with higher incidence of painful crises compared with GA.[27]

Obstetric Anaesthesia and SCA

In addition to the general measures described above:

1 It is especially important to prevent aorto-caval compression in this group.

2 The incidence of CS is higher in this group than the normal population.[28]

3 The safety of epidural blood patch for post-dural puncture headache (PDPH) is unknown in this group. Chiron et al. used 30 mL of Plasmion® (a modified fluid gelatin) heated to 37.5°C injected into the epidural space, in a sickle cell disease patient with PDPH, with good results.[29]

Anaesthetic Considerations for Sickle Cell Trait

1   Extra special precautions should be taken to prevent hypoxia in the peri-operative period in these patients due to an increased risk of complications such as cerebral infarction and superior sagittal sinus thrombosis.[21]
2   A cell-saver should probably not be used due to the high incidence of sickling in the washed cells.[26]

Treatment of Sickle Cell Crisis

1   Provide adequate analgesia but observe closely for respiratory depression. Opioids will usually be required, at least initially.
2   Correct/prevent dehydration.
3   Treat infective complications with antibiotics.
4   Keep patient well oxygenated.
5   Blood transfusion should only be undertaken if pain is refractory to maximal opioid therapy, or the patient suffers a stroke or acute chest syndrome (see below).[23]
6   Hydroxyurea therapy. Hydroxyurea can increase HbF concentration and have other beneficial effects in this condition.[30]

Treatment of Acute Chest Syndrome

IV dexamethasone 0.3 mg/kg 12 h × 4 doses may be of benefit.[31]

◯ Single Ventricle Repair

See *Fontan Procedure*.

◯ Sleep Apnoea Syndrome

See *Obstructive Sleep Apnoea (OSA) Syndrome*.

◯ SLIPA

SLIPA stands for streamlined liner of the pharynx airway. This is a single use supralaryngeal airway used in a similar way to the LMA. It consists of a plastic preformed shape that lines the pharynx without requiring an inflatable cuff to provide a seal. The device resembles a shoe with the toe protruding into the oesophageal opening, the lumen behind the toe opening into the larynx, and the heel in the nasopharynx. It can be used to provide positive pressure ventilation. The correct size of SLIPA is deduced by matching the width across the thyroid cartilage with that of the bridge of the SLIPA. The hollow structure of the SLIPA is felt by the inventor to reduce aspiration risk by providing a 50 mL storage reservoir for regurgitated fluid.[32]

◯ Sodium Bicarbonate

Inorganic salt is used:
1   In the treatment of severe life-threatening metabolic acidosis.

2   In the treatment of cardiac arrest associated with pre-existing metabolic
    acidosis or after return of spontaneous circulation when there has been a
    prolonged period of cardiac arrest.
3   To reduce the availability of free drug in the serum in situations such
    as tricyclic antidepressant overdose. Sodium bicarbonate is also used
    to alkalinise the urine to increase drug excretion after, for example,
    barbiturate overdose.
4   In the treatment of severe life-threatening hyponatraemia if hypertonic
    saline is not available. Sodium bicarbonate is no longer used for the
    treatment of hyperkalaemia. **See** *Potasium*.

It is presented as an 8.4% solution (1 mmol/mL) with an osmolarity of
2000 mOsm/L.

Dose for Profound Metabolic Acidosis

To restore pH to normal:[33]

$$\text{Dose (mmol)} = \text{Base deficit (mEq/L)} \times \frac{\text{Body Wt (kg)}}{3}$$

Give half this dose then recheck acid–base status.

◖ Sodium Nitroprusside (SNP)

Direct-acting vasodilator of resistance and capacitance vessels (arterio-
and venodilator). SNP is 44% cyanide by weight. It acts by spontaneously
dissociating to form nitric oxide, which causes vasodilatation. SNP is used
for the treatment of severe hypertension (in conjunction with invasive blood
pressure monitoring) and for the control of blood pressure during surgery
such as cerebral aneurysm repair.

Dose

1   Mix 50 mg SNP powder with 100 mL of 5% glucose. The recommended
    dose range is 0.3–6 µg/kg/min. In order to minimise the risk of cyanide
    toxicity the lower dose range of 0.3 µg/kg/min–2 µg/kg/min is suggested.[34]
    The maximum permissible rate of SNP is 10 µg/kg/min and this should not
    be used for longer than 10 min.

Table S2 Infusion rate for sodium nitroprusside (500 µg/mL) for a 70 kg patient

Dose	Rate of infusion
0.3 µg/kg/min	2.5 mL/h
2 µg/kg/min	17 mL/h
6 µg/kg/min	50 mL/h
10 µg/kg/min	84 mL/h

2   If necessary add other hypotensive drugs to reduce SNP dose such as
    trimetaphan. SNP can also be given as a bolus of 1–2 µg/kg (in a 70 kg
    patient this = 0.14–0.28 mL of the above solution).

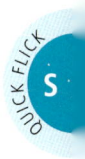

3 Protect the solution from light by measures such as foil wrapping. In room light 45% will decay in 6 h. If marked degradation does occur the solution changes to a blue colour.

Symptoms/Signs of Cyanide (CN⁻) Toxicity

1 Resistance to SNP therapy.
2 Metabolic acidosis/increased serum lactate.
3 Tachycardia, dysrhythmias, sweating and hyperventilation.
4 Cyanide poisoning occurs with CN⁻ serum levels of > 8 μg/mL.

Treatment of CN⁻ Toxicity

1 Cease SNP infusion. Ensure adequate airway, breathing and circulation and administer 100% O_2. Give sodium bicarbonate to correct acidosis (*see Sodium Bicarbonate*).
2 Give sodium thiosulphate 150 mg/kg IV over 15 min then an infusion of 30–60 mg/kg/h (converts CN⁻ to thiocyanate).[34]
3 Sodium nitrite 4–6 mg/kg very slowly IV.[34] This drug results in increased quantities of methaemoglobin to combine with the CN⁻.
4 Other alternative treatments include:
  a) Hydroxycobalamin IV. The dose is not firmly established although 100 μg/kg is suggested.[35]
  b) Cobalt ethylenediaminetetraacetic acid 600 mg IV over 1 min + 300 mg if no response to the initial dose. Give 25 mL of 50% glucose concurrently.

▷ Sotalol

Non-selective β adrenergic receptor blocker with marked Class 3 anti-arrhythmic properties, useful for:[36]
1 Second-line treatment of antrioventricular (AV) nodal and AV re-entrant tachycardias. Also used for the prevention of these dysrhythmias.
2 Termination of sustained ventricular tachycardia (VT)[37] and for the prevention of recurrent VT and ventricular fibrillation (VF).
3 The prevention of atrial fibrillation (AF) after cardioversion.

Adult PO Dose 160–640 mg daily in 2–3 divided doses.

Adult IV Dose 0.5–1.5 mg/kg over 5–20 min. In VT/VF associated cardiac arrest give 1 mg/kg over 1 min then 0.5 mg/kg over 1 min for breakthrough VT.

Problems

1 Sotalol can cause hypotension, bradycardia and AV block.
2 On rare occasions sotalol administration can cause the development of polymorphic VT or torsades de pointes.

3 Sotalol is contraindicated in asthma and long QT syndrome. **See** *Long QT Syndrome (LQTS)*.
4 Renally excreted. Reduce dosage in patients with renal impairment.
5 Sotalol has a long half life of 8–15 h.

Spinal Anaesthesia

See *Subarachnoid Block (SAB)*.

Spinal Anatomy

There are 33 vertebrae in total: 7 cervical, 12 thoracic, 5 lumbar, 5 sacral (fused) and 4 coccygeal (fused). There are occasionally 3 or 5 coccygeal vertebrae.

Landmarks
A line joining the illiac crests (Tuffier's line) passes through the lower part of L4 vertebra or the L4–5 disc space with some interpatient variation. C7 spinous process (*vertebra prominens*) is the first prominent spinous process when running the fingers down the nuchal furrow.

The angle of the scapulae are at the same level as the T7 spinous process.

Spinal Cord
Extends from the medulla to L1–2 disc space in the adult (range T12 vertebra to L2–3 disc).

Spinal Nerves
There are 31 pairs of nerves: 8 cervical, 12 thoracic, 5 lumbar, 5 sacral and 1 coccygeal.

Subarachnoid Space
Extends from the foramen magnum to S2 vertebra. At this level the dura continues (without a space) as part of the filum terminale which attaches to the coccyx.

Epidural Space
Extends from the foramen magnum to the sacral hiatus. **See** *Epidural Anaesthesia*.

Spinal Cord Injury (Pre-existing) and Anaesthesia

The main concerns with anaesthesia in patients with chronic spinal cord injury are:

1 autonomic dysreflexia
2 respiratory inadequacy
3 muscle spasms.

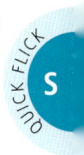

Autonomic Dysreflexia (AD)

Deregulation of the autonomic nervous system by spinal cord injury can result in episodes of autonomic dysreflexia (occasionally referred to as 'autonomic hyperreflexia' or 'mass reflex'). This condition is typically associated with lesions above the T6 vertebrae. These episodes are characterised by sudden severe hypertension, bradycardia, headache and sweating. The attacks are due to unopposed sympathetic activity causing severe vasoconstriction below the level of injury. AD can be fatal, due to intracerebral haemorrhage, and retinal haemorrhage can also occur. These episodes can be triggered by surgery, bladder distension, bowel distension, uterine contractions and other noxious stimuli. Attacks tend to start from 3 months to 12 years after the injury.[38]

Treatment of AD

AD must be treated cautiously as severe hypotension can occur.
1   Remove the noxious stimulus e.g. empty the bladder, deepen GA.
2   Drug therapy e.g. phenoxybenzamine, nifedipine, hydralazine and clonidine have all been used.[39]

Anaesthesia and AD

Important points are:
1   Patients with low complete spinal lesions with no history of autonomic dysreflexia, or symptomatic muscle spasms, having surgery below the level of spinal cord lesion do not require anaesthesia.[39]
2   GA does not always control AD unless deep GA is used. Spinal anaesthesia does reliably prevent AD, although epidural anaesthesia may not.[1,2] Spinal anaesthesia tends to be well tolerated.

Other Important Anaesthetic Considerations

1   Valsalva manoeuvre tends to cause a precipitous fall in BP in quadriplegics.
2   Patients with high lesions are prone to postural hypotension, so caution must be used with head up positioning.
3   These patients must not receive suxamethonium or hyperkalaemic cardiac arrest may be precipitated. Suxamethonium can be used within 72 h of the injury or after 9 months.[39]
4   Patients may require anaesthesia because reflex muscle spasms may prevent surgery occurring.
5   Patients with high spinal lesions may have significant respiratory impairment.
6   LA with adrenaline should be avoided due to the increased sensitivity of cord injured patients to adrenaline.

Obstetrics and Chronic Spinal Cord Injury
Labour
Patients with lesions below T10 are likely to feel pain with contractions. Uterine contractions can precipitate AD and AD can occur up to 48 h post delivery. Epidural anaesthesia is recommended for the control of AD in this situation.[39] If epidural and drug therapy are unable to control AD consider a magnesium sulfate infusion.[40] Proceed to GA and CS if all else fails.

CS
SAB or GA are both satisfactory forms of anaesthesia for CS.

▷ Spirometry

See *Respiratory Function Tests*.

▷ Statin Therapy

Cholesterol lowering drugs have anti-inflammatory and antithrombotic actions and have a stabilising effect on coronary artery plaques. They are recommended for patients with elevated cholesterol levels, unstable angina or MI. Peri-operative statin therapy reduced mortality by 44% in a meta-analysis by Hindler and colleagues.[41] For patients who are having non-cardiac surgery and are on statin therapy, this should be continued peri-operatively.[42] Statin therapy should be considered for all patients having vascular surgery with or without cardiac risk factors. Statin therapy should also be considered for patients with at least one cardiac risk factor undergoing intermediate risk surgery.

▷ Status Epilepticus

See *Epilepsy, Status*.

▷ Steroid 'Cover' for Surgery/Anaesthesia

Need for Supplementary Glucocorticoids for Patients on Long-term Glucocorticoid Therapy
Patients taking more than 10 mg/day of prednisone on a long term basis are at risk of peri-operative CVS collapse due to inadequate endogenous glucocorticoid production in response to the surgical 'stress'. This type of complication is probably extremely rare but must be prevented with peri-operative steroid supplementation. The dose of 'steroid' to be given is unresolved and steroid supplementation is not indicated if oral steroids have been ceased for more than 3 months.[43] Nicholson et al. make the following recommendations:[43]

1 *Minor Surgery*—Usual oral steroid dose preoperatively or 25 mg hydrocortisone on induction. Then resume normal oral steroid therapy.

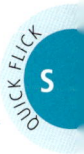

2 *Moderate Surgery*—Usual oral steroid dose preoperatively and 25 mg hydrocortisone on induction. Give an infusion of hydrocortisone 100 mg over 24 h. Restart oral therapy on day 2.

3 *Major Surgery*—Usual oral steroid dose preoperatively and 25 mg hydrocortisone on induction. Give an infusion of hydrocortisone 100 mg over 24 h for 2–3 days. Restart oral therapy when gastrointestinal function returns.

❍ Steroid Equivalents

Table S3: Relative potencies of glucocorticoids

Drug	Equivalent dose in mg
Hydrocortisone	80 mg
Dexamethasone	3 mg
Methylprednisolone	16 mg
Prednisone	20 mg

❍ ST Segment Analysis

Computerised automated monitoring of ST segments in leads II and V5 will detect about 80% of myocardial ischaemic episodes. Use the diagnostic ECG filtering mode. Ischaemia is associated with:

1 Transient tall T waves/T wave inversion.

2 A non-specific increase in R wave amplitude.

3 ST depression denoting endocardial ischaemia which is significant when > 1 mm from the baseline 60 ms after the J point and which lasts > 60 s. The J point is the end of the QRS complex, where the S wave becomes the ST segment. Down sloping and horizontal ST segment depression is considered more significant than upsloping ST segment depression.

4 ST segment elevation denoting transmural ischaemia is significant if ≥ 2 mm.

5 ST segment monitoring may not be helpful if there is intraventricular conduction delays, left bundle branch block, ventricular pacing, no P waves or the patient is taking digoxin.

❍ Subarachnoid Block (SAB)

Topics Covered in this Section

▶ Anatomy Relevant to Subarachnoid Anaesthesia
▶ Contraindications to the Use of SAB
▶ Technique for SAB
▶ Taylor's Approach to SAB
▶ Local Anaesthetic Solutions for SAB
▶ Subarachnoid Opioids
▶ SAB Needles

▶ 'Saddle' Block
▶ Combined Spinal Epidural Anaesthesia
▶ Anticoagulant Therapy and SAB
▶ Continuous Spinal Anaesthesia/Analgesia
▶ Complications of SAB

Anatomy Relevant to Subarachnoid Anaesthesia

In adults the spinal cord extends from the medulla to the L1, L2 interspace although in some individuals the cord can extend as far as the L2, L3 disc level. A line through the iliac crests passes through the lower part of L4 or the L4, L5 interspace.

Contraindications to the Use of SAB

The absolute contraindications to SAB anaesthesia are:
1 Patient refusal.
2 Significant coagulopathy.
3 Infection at the site of insertion.

Technique for SAB

1 Obtain large bore adequate IV access and load the patient with 500 mL–1 L of crystalloid IV.
2 Position the patient either sitting or laterally with maximum lumbar flexion.
3 Sterilise the skin over the lumbar spine and anaesthetise the site of insertion. Use the L3, L4 or the L4, L5 interspace. A midline or paramedian approach can also be used. See below for Taylor's Approach to SAB.
4 Insert the spinal needle into the subarachnoid space, as evidenced by the return of cerbrospinal fluid (CSF).
5 Inject the LA solution (see below for drug types and dosages), then place the patient in the supine position, unless intending to produce 'saddle' analgesia, which is described below under the heading 'Saddle Block'. Anticipate and treat hypotension with vasopressors such as ephedrine or metaraminol +/– further IV fluid loading.

Taylor's Approach to SAB[44]

1 After obtaining adequate IV access, place the patient in the lateral or sitting position.
2 The point of entry is 1 cm medial and 1 cm caudal to the lowermost prominence of the posterior superior iliac spine. The aim is to pass the spinal needle through the L5–S1 interspace via a lateral oblique approach. Sterilise and drape the skin around the entry site.
3 Anaesthetise the skin at the entry point

4 Direct the spinal needle medially in a cephalad direction aiming to enter the subarachnoid space laterally between L5 and S1. If bone is encountered walk the needle off the sacrum into the subarachnoid space.

Local Anaesthetic Solutions for SAB

1 *Bupivacaine*: Either bupivacaine plain 0.5% solution, or bupivacaine 0.5% heavy solution (containing glucose 80 mg/mL), can be used. Heavy bupivacaine, which is hyperbaric in CSF, demonstrates less cephalad spread than plain. These solutions provide subarachnoid blockade for 2–2.5 h. The dose for transurethral resection of prostate (TURP) surgery of either solution is ≈ 3 mL. The dose of heavy or plain bupivacaine 0.5% for LSCS is ≈ 2.4 mL with intrathecal opioid supplementation.

2 *Ropivacaine* is about 25% less potent than bupivacaine. For hip arthroplasty 3.5 mL of the 0.5% solution is effective.

3 *Cinchocaine* (Nupercaine, Dibucaine) heavy 0.5% solution contains 60 mg/mL glucose. Effects last ≈ 2 h. A suitable dose for TURP surgery is 1.8–2 mL. About 1.5 mL would be suitable for LSCS.

4 *Tetracaine* (Pontocaine): Duration of action longer than bupivacaine. A suitable dose for CS is 7–10 mg of hyperbaric solution.

Subarachnoid Opioids

Although prolonged effective analgesia is provided, there are significant side effects with intrathecal opioids. The most important of these is delayed respiratory depression.

1 *Morphine*: Give 0.1–0.3 mg depending on patient's size and physical condition. Onset of analgesia takes ≈ 15–45 min and the effects last about 12–24 h. Pruritus is common, especially in patients undergoing CS (70–85%).[45] 150 μg is effective for CS, hip and knee joint replacement.

2 *Diamorphine* (heroin): Give 0.3–0.8 mg depending on patient's size and physical condition. Effects last up to 22 h.[46]

3 *Fentanyl*: Small doses are useful for enhancing the intra-operative effect of LA solutions e.g. fentanyl 25 μg + 2.5 mL bupivacaine 0.5% heavy solution is a suitable dose for CS. Analgesic effects of intrathecal fentanyl have a rapid onset but there is little evidence for significant postoperative analgesia at a dose of 20–25 μg.[47]

4 *Pethidine*: This is the only opioid with significant LA properties in doses suitable for analgesia. Pethidine can be used as a sole agent for spinal anaesthesia. 1 mg/kg pethidine has been used for CS.[48] Subarachnoid pethidine is associated with a high incidence of nausea and vomiting in labouring women.

5 *Sufentanil*: 2.5–5 μg in adults.

Adverse Effects of Subarachnoid Opioids

These include:

1 pruritus
2 nausea and vomiting
3 delayed respiratory depression

SAB Needles

1 *Quincke*: Conventional sharp cutting edge needle. 25 and 26 G needles are available, but even with the 26 G needle the incidence of post-dural puncture headache (PDPH) is about 20–25% in the obstetric population.[49] It is recommended to orientate the needle bevel parallel to the longitudinal direction of the dural fibres.
2 *Whitacre*: Pencil point needle without a cutting edge, intended to reduce the incidence of PDPH. The rounded opening is on the side 2 mm from the tip. The incidence of PDPH with a 22 G Whitacre is ≈ 3.5%[50] and ≈ 1.2% with a 25 G needle.[51]
3 *Sprotte*: A pencil point variant with (compared to the Whitacre) a gentler conical point angle and a larger hole at the distal end of the shaft. The incidence of PDPH ≈ 3–10% with 24 G Sprotte in the obstetric population.[49]

'Saddle' Block

This is a type of SAB aimed at anaesthetising the sacral nerves only. SAB is performed in the sitting position with 1.5 mL of heavy bupivacaine 0.5% and the patient remains sitting for at least 5 min.

Combined Spinal Epidural Anaesthesia

These techniques can be undertaken in several different ways:
1 Siting an epidural catheter then performing a subarachnoid block at a more caudad vertebral interspace.
2 Using a 'kit' (e.g. Portex, Mallinckrodt™) containing a Tuohy needle with a Huber tip +/– a spinal needle 'back-eye' aperture for a 26 or 27 G pencil point spinal needle and a blind ended catheter with 3 lateral eyes. In another variation the epidural needle may have a separate barrel fused to it for the spinal needle.
3 Siting a spinal needle, then, while leaving the obturator in place, siting an epidural catheter at the same interspace.[52]

Use of a Combined Spinal Epidural Kit 'Needle-Through-Needle' Technique

1 It is recommended that the patient be positioned in the lateral decubitus position. This is to avoid/diminish the hypotensive effects of spinal anaesthesia while positioning and securing the epidural catheter.
2 Use the Tuohy needle to identify the epidural space in the usual way.
3 The spinal needle is then passed through the Tuohy needle into the subarachnoid space. A popping sensation may be felt and CSF should be seen returning through the spinal needle to confirm correct placement.

QUICK FLICK

S

4 Inject appropriate LA dose into subarachnoid space (depending on procedure). See above for dosages.

5 Remove the spinal needle and insert the epidural catheter through Tuohy needle then remove the Tuohy needle. Tape the epidural catheter securely.

6 Use epidurally administered LA to supplement subarachnoid block or for postoperative analgesia.

CSE and Labour

A suggested dose is bupivacaine 2.5 mg plus fentanyl 25 μg via the spinal needle. This is effective for about 90 min. This can be followed by an epidural infusion or top-ups as required. *See Epidural Anaesthesia*.

Advantages

1 Rapid onset of analgesia.

2 Little or no motor block.[53]

3 Epidural catheter placement may be more reliable when a CSE technique was used compared with the traditional epidural only technique.[54]

Disadvantages

1 An 18% incidence of fetal bradycardia has been noted when this technique is used. No increase in the emergency CS rate was seen.[54]

2 The risk of meningitis may be increased due to the proximity of the catheter to the breech in the dura.[55]

3 The risk of damage to the spinal cord and in particular the conus may be increased compared with traditional epidural anaesthesia.[56]

4 The incidence of urinary retention may be increased compared with epidural alone.

CSE and CS

CSE enables prolongation of anaesthesia due to unforeseen circumstances such as the need for post CS hysterectomy.[55]

However, there is no evidence that CSE is superior to a 'single shot' spinal for CS.[55] Recently DepoDur, an extended release formulation of morphine, has become available. It is given epidurally for CS at a dose of 10 mg and cannot be used with epidural LA but can be used with SAB LA. *See Morphine, Extended Release Epidural*.

Anticoagulant Therapy and SAB

See Epidural Anaesthesia (Anticoagulant Therapy and Epidurals) and use the same precautions as outlined in this section.

Continuous Spinal Anaesthesia/Analgesia

Continuous spinal anaesthesia/analgesia is very effective for anaesthesia and managing postoperative pain and cancer pain. This technique is not popular due to the high incidence of post-dural puncture headache (PDPH) and technical difficulties. For example, fine needles and catheters designed to reduce the incidence of PDPH have a tendency to kink and break. This treatment modality has also been associated with significant neurological injury such as cauda equina syndrome. To minimise the risks of neurological injury it is recommended to:[57]

1 Insert catheters no more than 3 cm into the subarachnoid space.
2 Avoid caudal placement.
3 Use small doses of plain isobaric LA solutions. Abandon the technique if up to 3 mL of LA is ineffective.[57]

Advantages

1 Excellent analgesia.
2 Good cardiovascular stability when small doses of plain solution are used. Hence this technique has been used in patients with severe aortic stenosis.
3 Continuous infusions of opioids can be very effective in treating labour pain in obstetric patients with severe cardiac lesions e.g. intrathecal sufentanil 10 μg followed by an infusion of 5 μg/h. **See** *Sufentanil*.

Disadvantages

1 Risk of cauda equina syndrome.
2 Risk of PDPH.
3 Increased risk of infection/meningitis.
4 Risk of catheter breakage.
5 Query increased risk of intrathecal bleeding.

Complications of SAB

1 Hypotension is the most common side effect. Ensure the patient is adequately hydrated, and treat hypotension promptly. Hypotension, severe bradycardia and/or asystole may occur even in young, healthy patients. Prompt treatment with atropine, ephedrine and/or adrenaline is usually effective.[58]
2 Headache.
3 Nerve injury. Transient radicular radiation may occur with mild-to-severe back pain radiating to the buttock usually lasting < 2 days. The incidence of this complication with bupivacaine is 0–3%.
4 Spinal cord injury and especially injury to the conus medullaris may also occur.[59] Do not inject solution through a spinal needle that has caused pain on entering the subarachnoid space.[59] If pain occurs when injecting anaesthetic solution cease injecting and resite the spinal needle. A space no higher than L3/4 should be selected.[56]
5 Spinal cord compression due to haemorrhage or infection. The risk of a spinal or epidural haematoma in association with a SAB is about 1:250 000.[60]

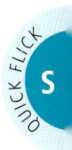

6 Transitory deafness can occur in up to 16% of patients having SAB.[61] This may be due to middle ear changes as a result of CSF loss and this complication may be more common in younger patients.[61]

Subarachnoid Haemorrhage

See *Cerebral Aneurysm Surgery*.

Subclavian Vein Central Line

Technique for Insertion:

1 Position patient supine with a rolled towel or bag of fluid between the shoulder blades. Tilt the trolley ≈ 10–15° head down.

2 Sterilise the skin above and below the clavicle, then palpate the inferior edge of the clavicle and identify the border of subclavius muscle (which runs from the first rib to the inferior surface of the clavicle). This border lies just lateral to the curvature at the midpoint of the clavicle.

3 Anaesthetise the skin and deeper tissues with a 23 G 32 mm needle, aiming towards the sternal notch and keeping the shaft of needle parallel to the floor.

4 Insert the Seldinger needle with the shaft parallel to the floor, aiming to pass the needle just under the clavicle and aiming towards the sternal notch.

5 If the subclavian artery is entered the needle needs to pass more anteriorly (the artery lies posterior to the vein). **See** *Brachial Plexus Block*—Figure B3: Anatomical relations of the superior surface of the first rib.

6 Aspirate while advancing the needle. If air is obtained, the needle has passed through the pleura.

7 Once the subclavian vein is punctured, remove the syringe and pass the guide wire into the vein and remove the Seldinger needle.

8 Incise the skin with a scalpel to enable the dilator to be passed over the wire, then insert the dilator into the vein thus allowing easy passage of the catheter. Remove the dilator then pass the catheter over the wire and into the vein. Remove the wire. Insert the catheter 12 cm for the average adult. Suture the catheter to the skin and cover with a sterile dressing.

9 Organise and review chest X-ray. The tip should lie in the SVC above the cephalic limit of the pericardial reflection.

Note: Never lose visual contact with the wire. Never leave a catheter lumen open to air.

Sub-Tenon's Block

See *Eye Blocks*.

Succinylcholine

See *Suxamethonium*.

○ Sufentanil

A synthetic opioid drug which is a derivative of fentanyl. Used for the induction and maintenance of anaesthesia and for postoperative analgesia. Sufentanil is about 5–10 × more potent than fentanyl and has a slightly shorter elimination half-life.

Dose

IV The appropriate dose required depends on the complexity of surgery e.g. appendicectomy 1–2 µg/kg, bowel resection 2–8 µg/kg.[62] For cardiac surgery 8–50 µg/kg (with postoperative ventilation).

Epidural Dose 20 µg for adults.

Intrathecal Dose In adults 2.5–5 µg. An intrathecal infusion of sufentanil can be considered for labour in obstetric patients with severe cardiovascular disease. A patient with severe pulmonary valve disease received intrathecal sufentanil 10 µg LD then an infusion of 5 µg/h with good effect.[62]

○ Sugammadex

Sugammadex is a cyclodextrin that fully reverses the effects of rocuronium within 2–3 minutes.[63] It acts by irreversibly encapsulating rocuronium and thus preventing its action on nicotinic acetylcholine receptors at the neuromuscular junction. It has no known significant side effects and a dose of up to 40 mg/kg was well tolerated.[64] This drug is also partially effective for reversing the effects of vecuronium and pancuronium but has no effect on atracurium or mivacurium.

Sugammadex is currently undergoing phase III clinical trials and is not yet (at the time of printing) approved for clinical use in the European Union.

Dose

The precise dose of sugammadex required depends on the degree of rocuronium induced neuromuscular blockade. Profound neuromuscular block due to rocuronium can be rapidly reversed by a dose of 8–16 mg/kg IV.

Incomplete rocuronium neuromuscular blockade can be reversed by 0.2 mg/kg IV.

Points to Note

1 Sugammadex and sugammadex/rocuronium complexes are excreted unchanged renally.[65]
2 If neuromuscular blockade needs to be re-established after sugammadex has been administered use suxamethonium or cisatracurium.

○ Superior Laryngeal Nerve (SLN) Block

Anatomy

A branch of the vagus nerve the *superior laryngeal nerve* divides into *external* and *internal* branches. The *external* branch supplies the cricothyroid muscle and the *internal* branch supplies sensation to the interior of the larynx as far down as the vocal cords. The *internal* branch passes around the inferior border of the greater cornu of the hyoid bone and through the *thyrohyoid membrane*.

Technique
1 Palpate the hyoid bone. Sterilise the skin and then use a 23 G 32 mm needle to 'walk' caudad off the hyoid bone's greater cornu near its posterior tip and just through the thyrohyoid membrane.
2 Inject 2–3 mL of LA e.g. lignocaine 2%.

◌ Superior Vena Cava Syndrome

In this condition the superior vena cava (SVC) is obstructed usually by malignant masses on the right side such as bronchogenic carcinoma or lymphoma. The effects of obstruction include:
1 Oedema of the head, neck and upper extremities.
2 Cerebral venous congestion with headaches, visual disturbances, raised ICP and altered mentation.
3 Proptosis may be present.
4 Dyspnoea, orthopnoea and cough, laryngeal oedema.
The condition is exacerbated if obstruction is below the azygous vein preventing collaterals forming.

Anaesthetic Implications
1 Management in a head up position may be helpful.
2 Keep patients well volume loaded to maintain preload but avoid overhydration.
3 Avoid venodilating drugs.
4 Give drugs and fluids into veins draining into the inferior vena cava. If central venous access is required use the femoral vein.
5 Laryngeal oedema due to venous engorgement may make intubation difficult.
6 The effects of the mediastinal mass causing the obstruction may also be deleterious. ***See*** *Mediastinal Mass and Anaesthesia*.

◌ Supine Hypotensive Syndrome
See *Pregnancy and Non-obstetric Surgery—Anaesthetic Implications*.

◌ Supraorbital and Supratrochlear Nerve Blocks
See *Forehead Block*.

Supraventricular Tachycardias (SVT)

These tachycardias are usually narrow complex and originate either in the atrium (atrial tachycardias) or the bundle of His (junctional tachycardias). However, some SVTs may demonstrate broad QRS complexes (**see** *Broad Complex Tachycardia*).

Atrial Tachycardias

Vagal manoeuvres and adenosine are usually ineffective. Atrial tachycardias include:

1. *Atrial Fibrillation*—Irregular tachycardia with no P waves.
2. *Atrial Flutter*—Flutter waves on ECG. The atrial rate is usually 300 and the ventricular rate is usually 150.
3. *Unifocal Atrial Tachycardia*—Regular tachycardia with identical abnormal P waves.
4. *Multifocal Atrial Tachycardia* (MAT)—Is an irregular tachycardia with P waves of different morphologies. It tends to be associated with significant cardio/respiratory illness.
5. *Junctional Tachycardias*—These dysrhythmias tend to be of abrupt onset (termed paroxysmal SVT) with palpitations, dizziness, chest pain and dyspnoea. They tend to respond to vagal manoeuvres and adenosine with sudden cessation of the SVT. Types of junctional tachycardias include:
   a) *AV Node Re-entry Tachycardia*. There are two conducting pathways in the AV node and perinodal tissue allowing re-entry. There are no P waves and the tachycardia is regular and typically there is an abrupt onset and offset.
   b) *AV Re-entry Tachycardia*. There is an accessory pathway allowing a re-entry tachycardia to occur separate to the AV node e.g. WPW. This may be termed an AV reciprocating tachycardia. **See** *Wolff-Parkinson-White (WPN) Syndrome*.

QUICK FLICK S

Treatment of Atrial Tachycardias

See *Atrial Fibrillation (AF), Acute* and *Atrial Flutter, Acute*.

For patients with unifocal or multifocal atrial tachycardia there is usually an underlying cause such as chronic airways limitation or electrolyte abnormality. Treatment of the cause may reverse the SVT.

Cardiovascularly Stable Patients

1. Magnesium is the drug of choice for acute control of MAT.[66]
2. Consider verapamil or β blockers to improve rate control by slowing AV conduction. These drugs may also revert the SVT. Do not use verapamil and a β blocker in the same patient.
3. Consider amiodarone or use amiodarone first if the patient has known underlying cardiac dysfunction (i.e. ejection fraction less than 40%).[67]

Cardiovascularly Unstable Patients

1   If significant cardiovascular compromise, use DC cardioversion.
2   Cardioversion may be ineffective in MAT.[68]

Treatment of Junctional Tachycardias
Cardiovascularly Stable Patients

1   Obtain a detailed clinical history, examine the patient and perform a 12-lead ECG. This will indicate the type of SVT (see above).
2   Ask the patient or patient's cardiologist what works best for that individual patient e.g. verapamil.
3   If this is a new junctional SVT try vagal manoeuvres. These include carotid sinus massage, Valsalva's manoeuvres, ice water on the face. These will terminate about 20% of paroxysmal SVTs.[69] Carotid sinus massage should not be performed if there is a carotid bruit or a CVA in the past 3 months.[69]
4   Use adenosine (*see Adenosine*). In patients with WPW; adenosine may cause a dangerously rapid ventricular response.[70] **See** *Wolff-Parkinson-White (WPW) Syndrome*.
5   If adenosine is ineffective consider an anti-arrythmic drug such as verapamil or a β blocker such as esmolol. Do not use verapamil and a β blocker in the same patient.
6   If the above treatment is ineffective consider amiodarone, rapid atrial pacing[68] and cardioversion (see below).

Cardiovascularly Unstable Patients

This can be defined as SBP< 90 mm Hg, chest pain, heart failure or heart rate > 200 bpm.[66] Use DC synchronised cardioversion under sedation. For monophasic defibrillators use energy settings of 50–100 J, 200 J, then 360 J.[67] For biphasic defibrillators about half this energy can be used. Use adenosine if cardioversion fails.

Cardiovascularly Unstable Child

1   Vagal manoeuvres can be used if they do not delay cardioversion.
2   Synchronised DC cardioversion. Use 0.5–1 J/kg initially then 2 J/kg (monophonic or biphasic energies).
3   If unsuccessful consider adenosine or amiodarone, repeat cardioversion and seek urgent expert paediatric cardiologist advice.

Treatment of Pulseless SVT

See *Cardiac Arrest*.

Give synchronised DC cardioversion shocks. For monophasic defibrillators in adults use energy settings of 100 J, 200 J then 360 J. For biphasic defibrillators about half this energy can be used. If unsuccessful give amiodarone then repeat cardioversion shocks. In the child use 0.5–1 J/kg monophasic or biphasic energy.

○ **Suxamethonium**

Depolarising neuromuscular blocking drug. It is a dicholine ester of succinic acid.

Dose

Adult 1.5 mg/kg IV, 2.5 mg/kg IM. For electroconvulsive therapy give ≈ 50–75 mg.
Child 2 mg/kg IV, 4 mg/kg IM.

Advantages

1 Produces rapid, profound, reliable paralysis in 30–60 s.
2 Short acting with a duration of action of 3–5 min. Metabolised by pseudocholinesterase.

Disadvantages

1 Suxamethonium causes a rise in the serum potassium. This rise is exaggerated in certain conditions associated with muscle denervation, which include serious burns and denervation illnesses such as Guillain-Barré, hemiplegia and paraplegia, tetanus and Duchenne's muscular dystrophy.
   Suxamethonium is contraindicated in these conditions as subsequent hyperkalaemia can precipitate cardiac arrest.
2 Suxamethonium is contraindicated in the presence of hyperkalaemia from any cause e.g. renal failure.
3 This drug can accentuate myotonia in myotonic dystrophy.
4 It is a potent trigger of malignant hyperthermia. ***See*** *Malignant Hyperthermia (MH)*.
5 Suxamethonium can cause prolonged paralysis in patients with deficient/abnormal pseudocholinesterase (plasma cholinesterase). ***See*** *Sux Apnoea*.
6 Muscle pains may occur especially in young women.
7 Suxamethonium can cause severe bradycardia, especially in children. This is most likely to occur when a second dose of suxamethonium is given.
8 Suxamethonium causes a small rise in intra-ocular pressure (IOP) which could, theoretically, place the eye with a penetrating injury at risk. Loss of intra-ocular contents due to suxamethonium has not been reported but loss of contents due to coughing is well recognised. ***See*** *Eye Injury, Penetrating*. Narrow angle glaucoma is another condition in which elevation of IOP is undesirable.
9 This drug also causes a rise in intracranial pressure but this is opposed by thiopentone.
10 If suxamethonium is given after the administration of neostigmine, muscle paralysis may last up to 50–90 min due to inhibition of plasma cholinesterase.[72]
11 Suxamethonium effects can be prolonged in the presence of some drugs such as ecothiopate iodide.

S
QUICK FLICK

12 Suxamethonium use has resulted in cardiac arrest and death in a number of children with occult myopathy.[73]

◗ Sux Apnoea

In this condition, paralysis due to suxamethonium is prolonged up to several hours. It is due to abnormal or deficient pseudocholinesterase (plasma cholinesterase). *See Suxamethonium*.

Incidence of Abnormal Pseudocholinesterase
In about 0.7% of the population suxamethonium induced paralysis will be slightly prolonged.[71] In about 1 in 2000 patients the effects of suxamethonium may last several hours.[71]

Investigation of Sux Apnoea: Dibucaine Numbers
The dibucaine number is a measure of the percentage inhibition by dibucaine (cinchocaine) of the activity of normal cholinesterase. The test is done by adding benzoylcholine to plasma which pseudocholinesterase breaks down. The addition of dibucaine inhibits the breakdown of benzolcholine to varying degrees depending on the type of pseudocholinesterase present. Normal pseudocholinesterase is inhibited the most. Fluoride or chloride can be used instead of dibucaine.

Table S4 Clinical significance of dibucaine number

Dibucaine Number	Patient Phenotype	Clinical Significance
80	Normal	Nil
40	Heterozygous	Paralysis Prolonged (minutes)
20	Homozygous	Paralysis Prolonged (hours)

Management
1 Maintain light anaesthesia and mechanical ventilation until paralysis spontaneously reverses as evidenced by a nerve stimulator.
2 Investigate the patient and near relatives for an inherited pseudocholinesterase abnormality.

Causes of Pseudocholinesterase Deficiency
1 Plasmapheresis, dialysis, cardiac bypass.
2 Drugs such as ecothiopate drops, cytotoxic drugs, chlorpromazine.
3 Exposure to organophosphate compounds.

◗ Syntocinon

See Oxytocin.

○ Syntometrine

See *Ergometrine Maleate*.

REFERENCES

1 Shann F. *Drug Doses*, 9th edn. Collective Pty Ltd, Melbourne 1996: 50–1.

2 Brinsmead M. Fetal and neonatal effects of drugs administered in labour. *Med J Aust* 1987;146: 481–5.

3 Comfort K, Lang SA, Ray W. Saphenous nerve anaesthesia—a nerve stimulator technique. *Can J Anaesth* 1996; 43: 8: 852–7.

4 Mulroy M. *Regional Anaesthesia: An Illustrated Procedural Guide*, 2nd edn. Little, Brown and Company, Boston 1996: 223–7.

5 Arkoosh VA. Neonatal resuscitation in the obstetric suite: what you need to know. In 48th Annual Refresher Course Lectures. *American Society of Anaesthetists* 1997; 236: 1–7.

6 Mulroy MF. *Regional Anesthesia: An Illustrated Procedural Guide*. 2nd edn. Little, Brown and Company, Boston 1996: 201–27.

7 Karmakar MK, Kwok WH, Ho AM. Ultrasound-guided sciatic nerve block: description of a new approach at the subgluteal space. *Br J Anaesth* 2007; 98: 390–5.

8 Smith I, Nathanson M, White PF. Sevoflurane—a long awaited volatile anaesthetic. *Br J Anaesth* 1996; 76: 435–45.

9 Patel S, Goa KL. Sevoflurane: A review of its pharmacodynamic and pharmacokinetic properties and its clinical use in general anaesthesia. *Drugs* 1996; 51: 658–00.

10 Frink EJ. Toxicologic potential of desflurane and sevoflurane. *Acta Anaesthesiol Scand* 1995; 39 (105): 120–1.

11 Kleinsasser A, Kuenszberg E, Loekinger A et al. Sevoflurane, but not propofol, significantly prolongs the Q-T interval. *Anesth Analg* 2000; 90: 25–7.

12 Abe K, Takada K, Yoshiya I. Intraoperative torsade de pointes ventricular tachycardia and ventricular fibrillation during sevoflurane anesthesia. *Anesth Analg* 1998; 86: 701–2.

13 Kleinsasser A, Loeckinger A, Lindner KH et al. Reversing sevoflurane-associated Q-Tc prolongation by changing to propofol. *Anaesthesia* 2001; 56: 248–71.

14 Beskow A, Westrin P. Sevoflurane causes more postoperative agitation in children than does halothane. *Acta Anaesthesiol* Scand 1999; 43: 536–41.

15 Eger E. Volatile Anaesthetics for the new millennium. *Audio-Digest Ancsthesiology*. 2000; 42: 15.

16 Horn E-P. Postoperative shivering: aetiology and treatment. *Curr Opin in Anaesthesiol* 1999; 12: 449–53.

17 Mahajan RP, Grover VK, Sharma SL, Singh H. Intraocular pressure changes during muscular activity after general anesthesia. *Anesthesiology* 1988; 66: 419–21.

18 Horn E-P, Standl T, Sessler DI, von Knobelsdorf G, Buchs C, am Esch JS. Physostigmine prevents postanesthetic shivering as does meperidine or clonidine. *Anesthesiolology* 1998; 88: 108–13.

19 Bamigbade TA, Langford RM. The clinical use of tramadol hydrochloride. *Pain Reviews* 1998; 5: 155–82.

20 Bhatnagar S, Saxena A, Kannan TR et al. Tramadol for postoperative shivering: a double-blind comparison with pethidine. *Anaesth Intensive Care* 2001; 29: 149–54.

21 Mason R. *Anaesthesia Databook: A Perioperative and Peripartum Manual*, 3rd edn. Greenwich Medical Media Limited 2001: 218–24.

22 Embury SH. The clinical pathophysiology of sickle cell disease. *Ann Rev Med* 1986; 36: 361–76.

23 Vijay V, Cavenagh JD, Yate P. The anaesthetist's role in acute sickle cell crisis. *Br J Anaesth* 1998; 80: 820–8.

24 Stein RE, Urbaniak J. Use of the tourniquet during surgery in patients with sickle cell haemoglobinopathies. *Clin Orthopaed Related Research* 1980; 151: 231–3.

25 Al-Ghamdi AA. Bilateral total knee replacement with tourniquets in a homozygous sickle cell patient. *Anesth Analg* 2004; 98: 543–4.

26 Brajtbord D, Johnson D, Ramsay M et al. Use of the cell saver in patients with sickle cell trait. *Anesthesiology* 1989; 70: 878.

27 Koshy M, Weiner SJ, Miller ST et al. Surgery and anaesthesia in sickle cell disease. *Blood* 1995; 86: 3676–84.

28 Denzer BI, Birnbach DJ, Thys DM. Anesthesia for the patient with sickle cell disease. *J Clin Anesth* 1996; 8: 598–602.

29 Chiron B, Laffon M, Ferrandiére M, Pittet J-F. Postdural puncture headache in a patient with sickle cell disease: use of an epidural colloid patch. *Can J Anaesth* 2003; 50: 812–14.

30 Steinberg MS. Management of sickle cell disease. *Drug Therapy* 1999; 340: 1021–30.

31 Bernini JC, Rogers ZR, Sandler ES et al. Beneficial effects of intravenous dexamethasone in children with mild to moderate severe acute chest syndrome complicating sickle cell disease. *Blood* 1998; 92: 3082–9.

32 Miller DM. Advantages of ProSeal and SLIPA airways over tracheal tubes for gynaecological laparoscopies. *Can J Anesth* 2006; 53: 188–93.

33 Sasada MP, Smith SP. *Drugs in Anaesthesia and Intensive Care*, 2nd edn. Oxford University Press, Oxford 1997: 334–5.

34 Friedrich JA, Butterworth JF. Sodium nitroprusside: twenty years and counting. *Anesth Analg* 1995; 81: 152–62.

35 Weekes JWN. Poisoning and drug intoxication. In: Oh TE, ed. *Intensive Care Manual* 4th edn. Butterworth–Heinemann, Oxford 1997: 667.

36 Donovan KD, Hockings BEF. Antiarrhythmic drugs. In: Oh TE, ed. *Intensive Care Manual* 4th edn. Butterworth–Heinemann Oxford 1997: 101.

37 Ho DSW, Zecchin RP, Richards DAB et al. Double-blind trial of lignocaine versus sotalol for acute termination of spontaneous sustained ventricular tachycardia. *Lancet* 1994; 344: 18–23.

38 Eldridge AJ, Kipling M, Smith J. Anaesthetic management of a woman who became paraplegic at 22 weeks gestation after a spontaneous spinal cord haemorrhage secondary to a presumed arteriovenous malformation. *Br J Anaesth* 1998; 81: 976–78.

39 Hambly PR, Martin B. Anaesthesia for chronic spinal cord lesions. *Anaesthesia* 1998; 53: 273–89.

40 Maehama T, Izena H, Kanazawa K. Management of autonomic hyperreflexia with magnesium sulfate during labour in a woman with spinal cord injury. *Am J Obstets Gynecol* 2000; 183: 492–3.

41 Hindler K, Shaw A, Samuels J et al. Improved postoperative outcomes associated with preoperative statin therapy. *Anesthesiology* 2006; 105: 1260–72.

42 Report of the American College of Cardiology/American Heart Association Task Force on Practice Guidelines. ACC/AHA 2007 Guidelines on perioperative cardiovascular evaluation and care for non cardiac surgery. *Circulation* 2007; 116: e418–e499.

43 Nicholson G, Burrin JM, Hall GM. Peri-operative steroid supplementation. *Anaesthesia* 1998; 53: 1091–104.

44 Pippa P, Barbagli R, Rabassini M et al. Postspinal headache in Taylor's approach: A comparison between 21 and 25-gauge needles in orthopaedic patients. *Anesth Intensive Care* 1995; 23: 560–3.

45 Yeh H–M, Chen L–K, Lin C–J et al. Prophylactic intravenous ondansetron reduces the incidence of intrathecal morphine-induced pruritus in patients undergoing cesarean delivery. *Anesth Analg* 2000; 91: 172–5.

46 Glynn CJ. Intrathecal and epidural administration of opiates. *Baillière's Clinical Anaesth* 1987; 1: 4: 915–32.

47 Dahl JB, Jeppesen SI, Jørgensen H et al. (Review article) Intraoperative and postoperative analgesic efficacy and adverse effects of intrathecal opioids in patients undergoing Caesarean section with spinal anaesthesia. *Anesthesiol* 1999; 91: 1919–27.

48 Nguyen Thi TV, Orliaguet G, Ngu TH, Bonnet F. Spinal anesthesia with meperidine as the sole agent for Caesarean delivery. *Reg Anesth* 1994; 19: 386–9.

49 Ross AW, Greenhalgh C, McGlade DP et al. The Sprotte needle and post

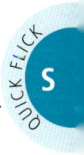

QUICK FLICK

S

dural puncture headache following Caesarean section. *Anaesth Intensive Care* 1993; 21: 280–3.

50 Gielen MJM. Postdural puncture headache (PDPH): a review. *Regional Anesthesia* 1989; 14: 101–6.

51 Spencer HC. Postdural puncture headache: what matters is technique. *Regional Anaesthesia and Pain Medicine* 1998; 23: 374–9.

52 Cook TM. Combined spinal epidural anaesthesia: a new technique. *International J Obstet Anesth* 1989; 8: 3–6.

53 Collis RE, Baxandall ML, Srikantharajah ID, et al. Combined spinal epidural (CSE) analgesia: technique, management, and outcome of 300 mothers. *International J Obstetric Anesthesia* 1994; 3: 75.

54 Maccarthur A. Management of controversies in obstetric anesthesia. *Can J Anesth* 1999; 46: R111–R116.

55 Levy DM. Anaesthesia for Caesarean section. *Br J Anaesth* 2001; 6: 162–7.

56 Holloway J, Seed PT, O'Sullivan GO, Reynolds F. Paraesthesia and nerve damage following combined spinal epidural anaesthesia: a pilot survey. *Internat J Obstet Anesth* 2000; 9: 151–5.

57 Burnell S, Byrne AJ. Continuous spinal anaesthesia. *Br J Anaesth CEPD Review* 2001; 1: 134–7.

58 Løvstad RZ, Granhus G, Hetland S. Bradycardia and asystolic cardiac arrest during spinal anaesthesia: a report of five cases. *Acta Anaesthesiol Scand* 2000; 44: 48–52.

59 Greaves JD. Serious spinal cord injury due to haematomyelia caused by spinal anaesthesia in a patient treated with low-dose heparin. *Anaesthesia* 1997; 52: 150–68.

60 Tryba M. Epidural regional anaesthesia and low molecular weight heparin: pro (German). *Anaesthesia Intensivmed Notfallmed Schmerzther* 1993; 28: 179–81.

61 Jenkins K. Baker AB. Review Article: Consent and anaesthetic risk. *Anaesthesia* 2003; 58: 962–84.

62 Ransom D, Leicht C. Continuous spinal analgesia with sufentanil for labour and delivery in a patient with severe pulmonary stenosis. *Anesth Analg* 1995; 80: 418–21.

63 Hunter JM, Flocton EA. Editorial: The doughnut and the hole: a new pharmacological concept for anaesthetists. *Br J Anaesth* 2006; 97: 123–6.

64 Molina AL, de Boer HD, Klimek M et al. Reversal of rocuronium-induced (1.2mg kg^{-1}) profound neuromuscular block by accidental high dose of sugammadex (40 mg kg^{-1}). *Br J Anaesth* 2007; 98: 624–7.

65 de Boer HD, Driessen J, Marcus M et al. Reversal of rocuronium-induced (1.2 mg/kg) profound neuromuscular block by sugammadex: a multicenter, dose-finding and safety study. *Anesthesiol* 2007; 107: 239–44.

66 Chauhan VS, Krahn AD, Klein GJ et al. Supraventricular tachycardia. *Med Clin North Am* 2001; 85:193–223.

67 Guidelines 2000 for Cardiopulmonary Resuscitation and Emergency Cardiovascular Care. *Circulation* 2000; 102 (suppl I): 112–28.

68 Donovan KD, Hockings BEF. Cardiac Arrhythmias. In Oh TE. *Intensive Care Manual*. 4th edn. Butterworth–Heinemann 1997; 73–81.

69 Xanthos T, Ekmektzoglou K, Vlachos I et al. A prognostic index for the successful use of adenosine in patients with paroxysmal supraventricular tachycardia in emergency settings: a retrospective study. *Am J Emerg Med* 2008; 26: 304–9.

70 Sanghavi S, Rayner-Klein J. Management of pre-arrest arrhythmia. *Br J Anaesth CEPD Reviews* 2002; 4: 104–12.

71 Whittaker M. Plasma cholinesterase variants and the anaesthetist. *Anaesthesia* 1980; 35: 174–97.

72 Stern R. *Drugs, Diseases and Anaesthesia*. Lippincott-Raven, Philadelphia 1997: 457.

73 Sullivan M, Thompson WK. Succinylcholine-induced cardiac arrest in children with undiagnosed myopathy. *Can J Anaesth* 1994; 41: 497–501.

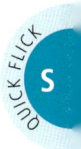

QUICK FLICK S

T

❍ Tachycardias

Attempt to make a specific diagnosis. If the QRS complexes are narrow *see* *Supraventricular Tachycardias (SVT)*. If the QRS complexes are broad *see* *Broad Complex Tachycardia* and *Ventricular Tachycardia (VT)*.

❍ Tap Block

See *Transversus Abdominis Plane Block*.

❍ Tension Pneumothorax

See *Chest Drain*.

❍ Tetralogy of Fallot

More than a brief overview of this complex topic is beyond the scope of this manual and larger texts should be consulted. This condition is the most common cyanotic heart disease encountered in adults and consists of:

1 large VSD
2 right ventricular outflow tract obstruction (valvular or infundibular)
3 right ventricular hypertrophy
4 a dilated aorta overriding the VSD.

These defects lead to right-to-left shunting and cyanosis. The usual initial treatment was a Blalock-Taussig shunt joining the systemic circulation to the pulmonary artery e.g. from the innominate artery to the pulmonary artery. A more definitive repair was then carried out at a later time with closure of the VSD and relief of the right ventricular outflow obstruction. Currently definitive repair is favoured in the neonatal period if the patient's anatomy is favourable.

Corrected Tetralogy of Fallot

In patients with repaired tetralogy of Fallot the main anaesthetic concerns are:

1 Dysrhythmias, especially VEBs, bigeminy and VT.
2 Conduction abnormalities especially RBBB, left anterior hemiblock, complete heart block hypoxia and polycythaemia if a Blalock-Taussig shunt was performed without subsequent definitive repair. These patients are also at risk of paradoxical embolism.
3 Right ventricular failure.
4 Pulmonary valve regurgitation.
5 Pulmonary artery stenosis.
6 Endocarditis risk.

Pregnancy and Corrected Tetralogy of Fallot

Patients with corrected tetralogy of Fallot without residual pulmonary stenosis or arrhythmia tend to cope with pregnancy and labour without major difficulty.[1]

Uncorrected Tetralogy of Fallot

This condition is associated with a high mortality with only 3% of patients surviving to age 40 yrs. Anaesthetic concerns are many and include:

1   Increased right-to-left shunting if systemic vascular resistance decreases.
2   Decreased cerebral perfusion if systemic vascular resistance increases.
3   Endocarditis prophylaxis.

The overall aim is to maintain CVS stability with normovolaemia, maintenance of SVR and avoidance of drugs which increase myocardial contractility.

❍ Thienopyridine Drugs

Examples include clopidogrel and ticlopidine. **See** *Platelet Adenosine Diphosphate (ADP) Receptor Antagonists.*

❍ Thiopentone

Thiobarbiturate intravenous general anaesthetic agent and anticonvulsant.

Dose for IV Anaesthesia

Adult 3–5 mg/kg IV. The drug acts within 1 arm–brain circulation time and its effects last 5–15 min.
Child 5 mg/kg.

Advantages

1   No pain on injection.
2   Inexpensive.
3   Potent anticonvulsant.
4   Cerebrovascular resistance increases with reduced cerebral blood flow, reduced intracranial pressure and reduced cerebral metabolic O_2 demand.

Disadvantages

1   Repeated doses or infusion of thiopentone result in prolongation of recovery time. Recovery becomes dependent on drug metabolism (rather than redistribution as with lower doses) which is slow (elimination half-life 3.4–22 h).
2   Thiopentone has negative inotropic effects; it decreases cardiac output by 20% and mean arterial pressure decreases.[2]
3   Thiopentone may have some bronchoconstrictive effects.[2] Use thiopentone with caution or avoid in asthmatics. **See** *Asthma.*

QUICK FLICK

T

4 Thiopentone can precipitate neurotoxicity in some types of porphyria. *See Porphyria*.

5 Extravasation of thiopentone may cause tissue necrosis.

6 Intra-arterial thiopentone can cause severe arterial constriction and distal limb gangrene. *See Intra-arterial Injection*.

7 Thiopentone is associated with a higher incidence of postoperative nausea and vomiting than propofol.[3]

8 Severe anaphylactoid reactions can occur with an incidence of about 1 per 20 000.[2]

◗ Thoracic Epidural

See Epidural Anaesthesia.

◗ Thoracoabdominal and Thoracic Aortic Aneurysm and Dissection Repair

More than a brief overview of this highly complex subject is beyond the scope of this manual. The incidence of thoracic aortic aneurysm is about 6 per 100 000.[4] Open surgical repair of thoracic aortic aneurysms is associated with significant mortality risk of 10–15%. In poor surgical candidates with multiple co-morbidities mortality can be as high as 50%.[5] During thoracic aorta cross-clamping the kidneys and spinal cord are subject to severe ischaemia. The incidence of paraplegia is about 3–15% and the incidence of renal failure is 18–27%.[6] Interruption of blood flow to the spinal cord due to obstruction of the artery of Adamkiewicz, which originates at about T9–T12 (range T5–L2) level, is of particular concern. Paraplegia has been reported to occur up to 8 days post repair.[5] As stenting technology improves an ever increasing percentage of descending thoracic aortic aneurysms are being repaired by the endovascular route with a reduced mortality rate compared with that of open repair.

The Crawford Classification of Thoracoabdominal Aneurysms[7]

1 *Type 1* extends from the proximal descending thoracic aorta (DTA) to the upper abdominal aorta but terminates proximally to the renal arteries.

2 *Type 2*—as above but the aneurysm extends beyond the renal arteries.

3 *Type 3*—begins in the distal half of the DTA and extends for a variable length into the abdomen.

4 *Type 4*—begins at the diaphragm and involves the entire abdominal aorta.

The DeBakey Classification of Aortic Dissections[8]

1 *Type I*—dissection begins near the aortic valve and extends down to the common iliac arteries.

2 *Type II*—dissection is limited to the ascending aorta.

3 *Type IIIa*—dissection begins distal to the left subclavian artery and ends in the descending thoracic aorta.

4 *Type IIIb*—begins as above and ends in the abdominal aorta.

Pre-operative Assessment and Preparation for Open Repair

The pre-operative assessment and preparation is similar to abdominal aortic aneurysm repair. ***See*** *Abdominal Aortic Aneurysm (AAA) Surgery* with the following qualifications:

1 Place arterial line and rapid infusion cannula in the right arm. This is because the left arm will be bent up and placed over the shoulders allowing a left chest approach to the aneurysm.

2 A double lumen tube will be required.

3 Heart bypass may be required.

4 TOE can be useful to help monitor heart function.

5 Consider using somatosensory evoked potentials to monitor spinal cord function.[9]

Physiological Effects of Thoracic Aorta Cross-clamping[6]

1 Thoracic aorta cross-clamping produces severe cardiovascular changes with:

  a) 50% increase in proximal aortic arterial pressure

  b) 40% reduction in ejection fraction and produces left ventricular wall motion abnormalities in 92% of patients.

  Central venous pressure, pulmonary artery pressure and pulmonary wedge pressure are all elevated. Myocardial ischaemia may be precipitated.

2 Preload consistently increases with clamping above the coeliac artery.

3 Renal blood flow is severely ($\approx$ 90%) decreased.

4 Blood flow to the spinal cord is greatly diminished. CSF pressure increases.

Physiological Effects of Thoracic Aorta Unclamping[6]

1 Systemic vascular resistance and arterial pressure decrease by 70–80%.

2 Cardiac output may increase, decrease or be unchanged.

Strategies to Protect Spinal Cord and Renal Function

The aims of these strategies is to maintain spinal cord blood flow and/or reduce spinal cord metabolic demands.

  Techniques include:

1 CSF drainage.

2 Distal aortic perfusion e.g. left atrial to left femoral vein bypass.

3 Hypothermia to 32–33°C. Do not cool below 32°C because of the risk of myocardial irritability and dysrhythmias.

4 Intercostal artery re-implantation.

5 Profound hypothermia with cardiopulmonary bypass and circulatory arrest.

QUICK FLICK **T**

6 Minimising cross-clamp time. Spinal cord injury increases dramatically after 30 min of cross-clamp time.

7 Prevent/treat hyperglycaemia.

CSF Drainage

CSF is drained via an intrathecal lumbar drain to lower CSF pressure. This reduces intraspinal pressure and therefore increases spinal cord perfusion pressure. Aim to keep CSF pressure at or below 10 mm Hg.[10] Continue CSF pressure control for 3 days postoperatively. If delayed paraplegia occurs CSF drainage may produce improvement. Risks of CSF drainage include:

1 Cerebral herniation.

2 Epidural haematoma.

3 Subdural haematoma.

4 Meningitis.

Thoracic Aortic Stent Grafts

Stent repair is an evolving technique and is usually confined to aneurysms distal to the origin of the left subclavian artery to prevent compromise of the cerebral circulation (descending thoracic aorta). This technique has also been used to treat dissections and rupture of the descending thoracic aorta. Stent repair is associated with a reduced mortality and a greatly decreased incidence of spinal cord injury.[11] Patients must be monitored post repair for endoleaks which necessitate further surgery.

Anaesthesia for Stent Repair

General anaesthesia, neuraxial block and local anaesthesia have all been used for stent repair. Usually a femoral artery approach is used. The important considerations for this type of surgery are:

1 The patient must be completely still for the precise positioning of the stent.

2 Preparation must be made to manage massive blood loss which can occur at any time.

3 The patient must be fully heparinised during the procedure.

○ Thromboelastography (TEG)

This technique is a test of coagulation, documenting the interaction of platelets, clotting factors and clot quality throughout the process of clot formation, strengthening, contraction and lysis. It has been used mainly in liver transplant and cardiac surgery but may find wider applications. The device and the technique involve the following steps:

1 Place 0.35 mL of freshly drawn blood in a cup which is heated to 37°C.

2 A pin suspended on a torsion wire has its tip in the blood sample.

3 The cup oscillates and while the blood is liquid the pin is not affected.

4 As clot starts to form the pin is twisted and this signal is amplified and recorded on heat sensitive paper.

TEG Measurements[12]

The following variables can be identified:

1 *Reaction time (r)*—time from sample placement to TEG amplitude reaching 2 mm (NR 6–8 min). This correlates to the time of initial fibrin formation.

2 *Clot formation time (K)*—time from r to TEG amplitude reaching 20 mm (NR 3–6 min). This is the time for a fixed degree of clot viscoelasticity to be reached.

3 *Alpha angle (α°)*—is the angle formed by the slope of the TEG tracing between r and K (NR 50–60°). This is an indication of the speed at which solid clot forms.

4 *Maximum amplitude (MA)*—is the widest point of the TEG (NR 50–60 mm). This reflects the absolute strength of the fibrin clot.

5 A_{60} is the amplitude of the tracing 60 min after MA is achieved (NR MA—5 mm). This is a measure of clot lysis or retraction.

6 *Clot lysis index (CLI)*—the A_{60} divided by (MA × 100) and expressed as a percentage. This value measures amplitude as a function of time and reflects lysis destruction of clot integrity.

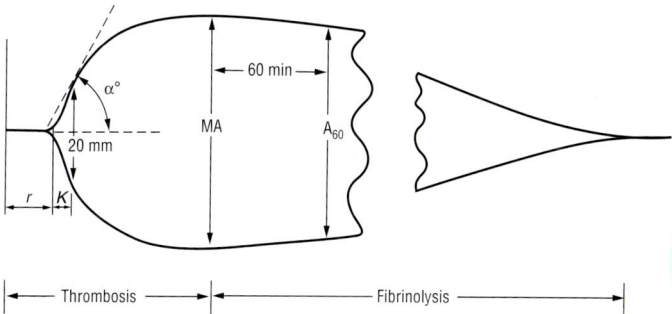

r = reaction time—time for tracing amplitude to reach 2 mm
K = clot formation time—time for tracing amplitude to reach 20 mm
alpha angle (α°) = angle formed by the shape of the TEG tracing from the r to the K value
MA = maximum amplitude of the TEG trace
A_{60} = amplitude of tracing 60 mm after MA is achieved

Figure T1 Thromboelastography (TEG) measurements

Interpretation of Results

1 Reaction time (r) prolongation may be due to coagulation factor deficiencies, anticoagulants or hypofibrinoginaemia. A short reaction time suggests a hypercoagulable state.

2 Coagulation time (K) reflects intrinsic clotting factors, fibrinogen and platelet function.

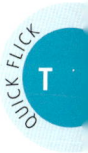

3 Alpha angle (α°)—a decreased value suggests hypofibrinoginaemia or thrombocytopenia.

4 Maximum amplitude (MA) is significantly reduced by platelet abnormalities or deficiency.

○ **Thrombolytic Therapy**

See *Pulmonary Embolus (PE)*.

○ **Thrombophilia**

See *Deep Venous Thrombosis (DVT) Prophylaxis*.

○ **Thyroid Storm/Thyrotoxic Crisis**

Thyroid storm is a hypermetabolic clinical syndrome resulting from excessive thyroid hormone causing life-threatening multi-organ dysfunction. These effects typically include:

1 Tachycardia and other tachydysrhythmias, hypertension, pulmonary oedema and congestive cardiac failure.

2 Tachypnoea and hypercarbia.

3 Delirium, stupor and comas—seizures may occur.

4 Respiratory and metabolic acidosis.

5 Electrolyte derangements such as hypokalaemia, hypercalcaemia, hypomagnesaemia and hyponatraemia.

6 Hyperthermia.

7 Nausea, vomiting, diarrhoea and abdominal pain.

Thyroid storm can be triggered by thyroid surgery, withdrawal of anti-thyroid drugs and intercurrent illness such as infection. It is more likely to occur postoperatively than intra-operatively.

Prevention of Thyroid Storm in Hyperthyroid Patients for Elective Thyroidectomy

1 Patients should be rendered euthyroid with a 6–8 week course of anti-thyroid drug, e.g. propylthiouracil.

2 Give potassium iodide for 1–2 weeks before surgery.

3 Add a β blocker drug for tachycardia if present.

Prevention of Thyroid Storm During Emergency Surgery[13]

In patients undergoing emergency surgery, the risk of thyroid storm can be reduced by:

1 β adrenergic blocker drugs such as propranolol or esmolol.

2 Anti-thyroid drugs such as propylthiouracil (PTU) 200–400 mg PO 6 h.

3 Hydrocortisone 40 mg IV 6 h. Glucocorticoids decrease peripheral conversion of T_4 to T_3.

4 Potassium iodide 5 drops PO 6 h or Lugol's solution 30 drops 6 h. These inhibit release of T_4 and T_3.

5 Do not give aspirin which displaces thyroid hormones from binding proteins.

Treatment of Thyroid Storm

Treatment can be divided into supportive measures and drug therapy.

1 Ensure adequate airway, breathing and circulation. Intubation and ventilation may be required.

2 IV fluid therapy, including glucose solution. Significant dehydration may occur.

3 Normalise glucose and electrolytes.

4 Treat hyperthermia with cooling blankets, ice-packs and cold lavage of body cavities. Paracetamol can be given but not aspirin.

5 Give an anti-thyroid drug such as propylthiouracil (PTU). Give 1 g PO then 200 mg PO 6 h. Alternatively use carbimazole 60–120 mg PO. These drugs can be given by a nasogastric tube. Effects usually begin in 1 h.

6 Potassium iodide or Lugol's solution. This can be given 1 h after the anti-thyroid drug. Give potassium iodide 500 mg PO 8 h or 200 mg in 500 mL N/S over 2 h every 12 h. Iodine can increase thyroid hormone release if it is not given *after* PTU. If a patient is allergic to iodine use lithium carbonate 300 mg PO 6 h.

7 Propranolol or other β adrenergic blocker drug. Give propranol 40 mg PO 8 h or 1 mg IV as required. Aim for a heart rate of 90 bpm.

8 Glucocorticoid drug such as hydrocortisone 100 mg IV 6 h. This will treat adrenal insufficiency and decrease T_4 release and conversion to T_3.

9 Guanethidine or reserpine therapy should be considered in propranolol-resistant thyroid storm or in patients unable to tolerate β blockers. The doses are reserpine 2.5–5 mg/kg 4–6 h or guanethidine 1–2 mg/kg/day in divided doses.

10 Consider plasmapheresis, plasma exchange, dialysis or charcoal haemoperfusion in refractory cases to remove thyroid hormone.

11 Consider dantrolene if the above measures are unsuccessful.

◯ Thyromental Distance

See *Difficult Airway Management*.

◯ Tibial Nerve Sheath Catheter

A technique for postoperative analgesia in which the surgeon inserts a catheter into the tibial nerve sheath during surgery for a below knee amputation. The nerve block is established with 20 mL of bupivacaine 0.25% or ropivacaine 10 mg/mL. This is followed by an infusion of bupivacaine 0.25% run at 10 mL/h.

⊘ Ticlopidine

Potent antiplatelet drug with significant anaesthetic and surgical implications. **See** *Platelet Adenosine Diphosphate (ADP) Receptor Antagonists*.

⊘ Tirofiban

Antiplatelet drug. **See** *Platelet Glycoprotein IIb/IIIa Receptor Antagonists*.

⊘ Tonsillectomy, Bleeding after Surgery

The main anaesthetic issues are:
1 Hypovolaemia and anaemia due to haemorrhage requiring resuscitation + blood transfusion.
2 'Full stomach' due to swallowing of blood.
3 Potential difficulty intubating the patient due to blood, oedema and distortion of airway anatomy.
4 Potential underlying bleeding disorder.

Pre-anaesthetic Phase
1 Adequately replace the patient's intravascular volume. Transfuse blood if required.
2 Obtain skilled assistance and notify the surgeon who must be present in the operating theatre.
3 Ensure at least 2 separate suction units are working and accessible.

Anaesthetic Phase
The main anaesthetic options are:
1 Gaseous induction with the patient in the left lateral position with intubation when the patient is 'deep' and still lateral.
2 Rapid sequence induction with thiopentone, suxamethonium and cricoid pressure. **See** *Rapid Sequence Induction (RSI)*.
3 Perform nasogastric drainage of blood from the stomach before extubation.

⊘ Torsades de Pointes

This is a polymorphic ventricular tachycardia. The QRS complexes appear to twist around the baseline on the ECG. When the patient is in sinus rhythm this condition is associated with a long Q-T interval and U waves. **See** *Long QT Syndrome (LQTS)* for causes. A ventricular beat during the Q-T interval initiates the ventricular tachycardia. Torsades de pointes frequently resolves spontaneously but ventricular fibrillation can occur.

Treatment
1 If the torsades de pointes is sustained and associated with haemodynamic instability or VF develops provide immediate non-

synchronised defibrillation. Use sedation prior to defibrillation if the patient is conscious. The patient will be unconscious if VF develops.

2 In less urgent circumstances e.g. recurrent short bursts of torsades de pointes give magnesium 2 g IV (4 mL of a 50% solution over 10–15 min) followed by an infusion of 2–4 mg/min.

3 Maintain serum K^+ in the high normal range.

4 Cease causative factors if possible e.g. sevoflurane. Propofol can be substituted to maintain anaesthesia.

5 If magnesium is ineffective and the patient is not cardiovascularly compromised use transvenous overdrive pacing. Pace at a rate of 90–110 bpm. An isoprenaline infusion can be used to chemically pace the patient while transvenous pacing is being organised. However isoprenaline is contraindicated in IHD and patients with congenital long QT syndrome.[14] *See* *Isoprenaline*.

6 *See* *Long QT Syndrome (LQTS)* for ongoing management.

◗ Total Intravenous Anaesthesia (TIVA)

See *Propofol*.

◗ Total 'Spinal'

See *Epidural Anaesthesia*.

◗ Tracheal Rupture

This condition can present as an airway emergency and can be intrathoracic or extrathoracic. Tracheal rupture can be due to:

1 Trauma (usually blunt). Oesophageal rupture can be confused with tracheal rupture.

2 Intubation e.g. due to stylet injury or over inflation of the tracheal cuff.[15]

3 Neck/tracheal surgery.

4 Malignancy.

5 Coughing.

Presentation

1 Subcutaneous emphysema (this can be massive).

2 Pneumothorax.

3 Respiratory compromise.

4 Stridor.

5 Haemoptysis.

6 CVS collapse/death.

Diagnosis

This can be made by clinical findings + investigations such as:

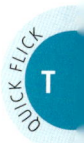

1 *Neck/chest X-rays*. Look for prevertebral air, subcutaneous and mediastinal emphysema. Pneumoperitoneum and pneumopericardium can develop.
2 *Neck/chest CT scan*. 3-D CT scans can be diagnostic.[15]
3 *Bronchoscopy*. This can indicate the site and extent of the lesion and whether surgery or conservative management is indicated.

Management

Management of this condition depends on the severity of the rupture, the site of rupture and the patient's level of compromise. In virtually all cases the site of rupture needs to be inspected by FOB.

Small extra thoracic tracheal tears in the absence of a gross air-leak may be treated conservatively with:
1 airway humidification
2 chest physiotherapy
3 antibiotics.

Intrathoracic tracheal ruptures will usually require surgical repair and may cause mediastinitis. If the patient's condition is deteriorating or there is impending asphyxia, the airway below the rupture must be controlled emergently. Options include:
1 Awake fibre-optic intubation. This is the safest course of action if time allows. Place the cuff of the ET tube beyond the rupture.
2 Emergency tracheotomy under local anaesthesia.
3 Rapid sequence induction if asphyxiation is imminent. Try to maintain spontaneous ventilation after suxamethonium wears off until the ET tube is below the tear.

◑ Tracheostomy, Elective

Anaesthetic Management of the Intubated Patient

1 Position the patient with a 1 L bag of fluid between scapulae. Have the neck extended and the head resting on head ring. Ensure that the patient is adequately paralysed.
2 Deflate the endotracheal tube cuff when the surgeon is just about to incise the trachea. If the surgeon ruptures the endotracheal tube cuff during the dissection, change to a bag ventilation technique which is easier to control than using the ventilator. If the leak is too large, ask the surgeon to 'plug' the tracheal stoma to improve the seal.
3 Increase the FiO_2 to 100% 5 min before the tracheal tube is inserted and ensure that the patient is adequately paralysed. There is an increased risk of tracheal fire when 100% O_2 is used. N_2O also supports combustion. However, the risk of airway fire must be weighed against the risk of desaturation if complications occur with tracheal tube insertion. Precautions against airway fire in this situation include:[16]
   a) Filling the cuff of the endotracheal tube with saline.

b) Ensuring there is no cuff leak.

c) Pushing the cuff of the endotracheal tube to just above the carina.

d) Advise the surgeon not to use diathermy when incising the trachea.

If a fire occurs:

a) Disconnect the endotracheal tube from the O_2 supply. O_2 flowing through a burning tube results in a blow torch effect. Pull the tube out of the patient.

b) Extinguish the fire e.g. cut large hole in a litre bag of N/S and pour an adequate amount over the fire to extinguish it.

c) When the fire is extinguished and the charred tube fragments are removed, reintubate the patient.

d) Evaluate the extent of fire injury by bronchoscopy and laryngoscopy. Use bronchial lavage to wash fire-related debris out of the bronchial tree.

e) Manage the patient postoperatively in the intensive care unit.

4 When the surgeon is ready to insert tracheal tube, pull the endotracheal tube back slowly under your direct vision until the tube is just cephalad to the tracheal stoma. This way, if there is a problem with tracheostomy tube insertion the endotracheal tube can easily be reinserted into the trachea.

◯ Tramadol Hydrochloride

Tramadol is an atypical opioid analgesic drug that is also useful for treating postoperative shivering. **See** *Shivering Postoperatively*. A synthetic 4-phenyl-piperidine analogue of codeine, tramadol has a mu opioid receptor agonist action and also blocks the neuronal reuptake of monoamine oxidase, noradrenaline and serotonin.[17] Tramadol has 10–15% of the potency of morphine parenterally.[17]

Dose

Adult PO, IM, PR Dose 50–100 mg 4–6 h max 400 mg/day. The oral route requires ≈ 20 min–1 h to have an effect which peaks after ≈ 2 h. In patients >75 years the max dose is 300 mg. If using sustained release tramadol (tramal sustained release) give 100–200 mg 12 h.

Adult IV/IM Bolus Dose 50–100 mg IV over 2–3 min or IM 4–6 h. For severe pain follow a 100 mg bolus with 50 mg boluses every 10–20 min to a max total dose of 250 mg.

Adult IV Infusion Dose Give an initial bolus dose of 100 mg over 2–3 min. Load 200 mg of tramadol in 500 mL of N/S. Run an infusion of 15 mg/h (= 37.5 mL/h). Reduce the rate after 6 h.

Adult Patient-controlled Analgesia Give an initial bolus dose of 100 mg over 2–3 min. Load 300 mg of tramadol in 60 mL N/S. Begin with a bolus dose of 20 mg with a 5 minute lockout.

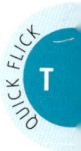

QUICK FLICK
T

Adult Epidural Dose 100 mg in 10 mL N/S epidurally can provide effective postoperative analgesia. This dose can be repeated as required to a maximum of 400 mg/day.[18]

Paediatric Dose 1–2 mg/kg PO, IM or IV dose 4–6 h.

Advantages

1 Tramadol has a relative lack of serious side effects compared with other opioids and non-steroidal anti-inflammatory drugs. There is a low potential for respiratory depression and dependence.[19]
2 The drug is well absorbed orally.
3 Tramadol does not cause spasm of the sphincter of Oddi.[20] Urinary retention and constipation are less likely than with other opioids.
4 Tramodol does not cause morphine effects or a withdrawal effect in patients on methadone.[21]
5 Tramadol is thought to be safe to use in labour, and is unlikely to cause birth defects during pregnancy.[21]

Disadvantages

1 Tramadol is mainly metabolised by the liver with 30% excreted in the urine as unchanged drug.[20]
2 Sixty per cent of tramadol's metabolites are excreted in the urine. Therefore use the drug cautiously in the presence of renal/liver impairment.
3 There is a risk of seizures if the patient is receiving drugs which lower the seizure threshold such as tricyclic antidepressants and monoamine oxidase inhibitors or if the patient has a history of seizures.[20]
4 There is a risk of serotonin syndrome if tramadol is given with a drug that increases serotonin levels in the CNS e.g. selective serotonin reuptake inhibitors such as sertraline, tricyclic antidepressants, moclobemide, venlafaxine and St John's wort.[22] **See** *Serotonin Syndrome*.
5 Tramadol can cause dizziness, nausea, confusion, drowsiness and headache. Nausea caused by tramadol is not antagonised by ondansetron.[21]
6 Rapid IV injection of tramadol may cause hypotension due to peripheral vasodilation.[23]
7 Tramadol analgesic effects may be reduced by concomitant administration of ondansetron.

◗ Tranexamic Acid

This is an anti-fibrinolytic, lysine analogue drug that decreases bleeding and transfusion requirements during cardiac surgery.[24] The drug acts by attaching to the lysine binding site on the plasmin molecule displacing plasminogen from fibrin.[25] A suggested dosage is 10 mg/kg loading dose then an infusion of 1 mg/kg/h.[26] Tranexamic acid is 6–10 × more potent than epsilon-aminocaproic acid, another lysine analogue drug. **See** *Epsilon-aminocaproic Acid*.

○ Transcutaneous Cardiac Pacing

See *Pacing, Pacemakers and Anaesthesia*.

○ Transfusion Related Acute Lung Injury (TRALI)

This condition is an acute immune reaction to blood transfusion leukocyte antibodies. The onset of this condition occurs 1–2 h after transfusion and peaks at about 6 h. This condition is characterised by:

1 non-cardiogenic pulmonary oedema
2 hypoxia
3 fever.

Treatment

There are no specific measures and treatment is supportive. Transfusion should be ceased and if the patient survives, recovery should occur within 4 days.

○ Transposition of the Great Vessels

More than a brief overview of this complex topic is beyond the scope of this manual. In this condition:

1 The aorta arises from the right ventricle.
2 The pulmonary artery arises from the left ventricle.
3 In malposition of the great vessels, there may be only one ventricle or both vessels may arise from the same one of two ventricles.

Transposition of the great vessels is incompatible with life unless some other defect allows mixing of the pulmonary and systemic circulations e.g. a VSD. Treatment for this condition includes:

1 *Atrial Switch Procedure* (Mustard or Senning procedure) in which venous return to the heart is redirected into the pulmonary circulation and pulmonary venous return into the systemic circulation at an atrial level. This involves a baffle inserted across the atrial septum and directing blood flow appropriately. The right ventricle provides the systemic circulation pump. Progressive right ventricular failure and tricuspid regurgitation are likely if the patient lives long enough. This procedure has been replaced by the arterial switch procedure.

2 *Arterial Switch Procedure*. In this procedure the aorta is transferred to the left ventricular outflow tract and the pulmonary artery to the right ventricular outflow tract. The coronary arteries must be reimplanted from the pulmonary artery to the root of the aorta. The left ventricle is the systemic circulation pump. The pulmonary valve acts as the aortic valve

and may leak and supravalvular pulmonary artery stenosis may occur. Also coronary artery stenosis may occur. Overall the results and long-term outcome from this procedure are excellent.

Anaesthetic Considerations for Repaired Transposition of the Great Vessels

1 If the neo-aortic valve leaks maintain a mild tachycardia.
2 Consider endocarditis prophylaxis for relevant procedures. *See Bacterial Endocarditis (BE) Prophylaxis*.

○ Transtracheal Jet Ventilation

Facilitated by a device such as a Sanders injector. This device consists of:

1 High-pressure tubing for attachment to the 'wall' O_2 outlet or other source of high pressure (50 psi) O_2.
2 The high-pressure tubing is attached to one end of the injector. The injector contains a regulator that reduces the O_2 pressure to about 30 psi.
3 This lower pressure O_2 is transmitted from the injector through another piece of pressure tubing which has a leur lock at its distal end. This leur lock can be attached to a cannula placed in the trachea. *See Cricothyroid Puncture and Cricothyrotomy*.
4 A button on the injector is used to release bursts of high pressure O_2.

Technique for Transtracheal Jet Ventilation

1 One person must concentrate solely on maintaining the cannula in place.
2 0.5 s 'bursts' of O_2 are usually sufficient to ventilate an adult. Look for chest inflation to help judge jet ventilation time.
3 There must be a pathway for exhalation gas otherwise air-trapping and lung hyperinflation will occur. Jaw thrust and oral/nasal airways may assist in expiration. A second cannula placed in the trachea is not effective in allowing expiration. If no pathway for expiration can be achieved proceed to cricothyrotomy.
4 Insufflation of the tissues is an ever present risk.

○ Transurethral Resection of Prostate (TURP)

The main challenges associated with TURP surgery are blood loss and TURP syndrome due to excessive absorption of glycine. The blood transfusion rate is about 6%.[27] Laser-assisted transurethral prostatectomy is revolutionising this procedure, making it safer and shortening hospitalisation times.

Anaesthesic Technique

A regional or general anaesthetic technique are equally satisfactory.[28] It is important that the patient does not cough as this makes surgery more

difficult. If regional anaesthesia is used, anaesthesia to T9 is required.[29]
An appropriate dose of heavy bupivacaine 0.5% is 3 mL for most patients.
It is very important to minimise the absorption of bladder irrigation fluid and
prevent hyponatraemia.

Methods of achieving these aims and other important aspects of
anaesthetic care include:

1 Limit the height of the irrigation bag to 60 cm above the prostate.[30]
   The bag should *not* be pressurised and frequent bladder emptying
   should occur. Ensure that only 1.5% glycine is used for bladder irrigation,
   not water.
2 Limit resection time to <1 h.[30]
3 Give prophylactic gentamicin 120–240 mg especially if the patient is
   chronically catheterised.
4 Only use N/S for IV fluid replacement and use minimal IV fluids.
5 Treat hypotension associated with spinal anaesthesia with vasopressors
   rather than large volumes of IV crystalloid solution.[31]
6 Erection can interfere with surgery. If persistent, spray the base of
   penis with ethyl chloride. If erection persists consider an injection
   of metaraminol 0.5 mg in 10 mL of N/S injected into the corpus
   cavernosum, with a tourniquet around the base of the penis.[32]

TURP Syndrome

This is due to excessive absorption of glycine and consists of:

1 *Hyponatraemia*, leading to a decreased level of consciousness and/or
   seizures. These cerebral effects are due to cerebral oedema due to the
   hypo-osmalality of the plasma. Severe reactions are usually associated
   with serum Na^+ < 120 mmol/L. For a description of ECG changes
   associated with hyponatraemia *see Electrocardiography*.
2 *Hypervolaemia*, resulting in problems such as pulmonary oedema.
3 *Ventricular tachycardia or fibrillation*, can occur if serum Na^+ falls to
   100 mmol/L or less.
4 *Visual disturbances, haemolysis* and *coagulopathy* may also occur.

Treatment of TURP Syndrome

1 Ensure adequate airway, ventilation and satisfactory pulse rate and mean
   arterial pressure. Notify the surgeon.
2 Cease glycine infusion and surgery as soon as possible.
3 Measure serum Na^+. If this is >120 mmol/L and the patient is
   asymptomatic treat with fluid restriction + frusemide and minimal N/S
   as sole IV replacement fluid.
4 If serum Na^+ <120 mmol/L and the patient is symptomatic give
   50–100 mL boluses of hypertonic saline over 1 h. Usually no more than
   300 mL will be required. Recheck serum Na^+ after each bolus. Rapid

correction of hyponatraemia may cause central pontine myelinosis (osmotic demyelination syndrome) which is usually fatal. Correct serum Na^+ to 120 mmol/L only, and do not increase serum Na^+ by more than 12 mmol/L per day. If hypertonic saline is not available consider boluses of sodium bicarbonate.[31]

5 Treat pulmonary oedema in the usual way:
   a) give O_2 therapy
   b) sit patient up and give frusemide 40 mg IV.
   See *Pulmonary Oedema*.

6 Treat seizures with midazolam boluses up to 10 mg and phenytoin if required. If status epilepticus occurs consider thiopentone and muscle relaxants with anaesthesia until serum Na^+ improves. ***See*** *Epilepsy, Status*.

Glycine Toxicity
Glycine can cause:
1 Transient visual disturbances/blindness. This resolves in 8–48 h and may be due to glycine acting as an inhibitory neurotransmitter at the retina.[33]
2 Decreased cardiac output.
3 Encephalopathy and seizures.
4 Hyperammonaemia (ammonia being a metabolite of glycine). This can cause nausea, vomiting and loss of consciousness. Consciousness returns after serum ammonia levels fall below 150 mmol/L.[33]

Laser Assisted Transurethral Prostatectomy[34]
Patients requiring TURP surgery have greatly benefited by the introduction of laser resection, using either holmium:yttrium-aluminium-garnet (YAG) laser or potassium-titanyl-phosphate (KTP) laser.

Advantages of Laser Resection
1 Less absorption of irrigant and N/S can be used.[35]
2 Blood loss is minimised especially with the KTP laser.
3 Patients do not need to cease anti-clotting/anti-platelet medication preoperatively.
4 Hospital stays of 1–2 days are feasible.
5 Very unfit patients can be anaesthetised with caudal anaesthesia only.[33]

Disadvantages
1 The procedure may take a little longer than conventional TURP.
2 The procedure is technically demanding and surgical time may be prolonged to allow time for training.
3 With the KTP laser the tissue is vaporised, hence this can only be used with non-malignant disease.

◗ Transversus Abdominis Plane Block

The abdominal wall derives its sensory innervation from the anterior divisions of the spinal segmental nerves (T7–T11). The transversus abdominis plane refers to the plane between the transversus abdominis and internal oblique muscles through which these nerves pass. In the midaxillary line the anterior divisions divide into a lateral and anterior cutaneous branches. The nerves can be blocked in this plane by a single injection or with bilateral injections for surgical wounds that cross the midline.

Indications
Abdominal surgical wounds, particularly from the symphysis pubis to around T8 level.

Technique
Although this block was originally described without ultrasound, the use of ultrasound makes this a very simple and safe procedure to perform. The steps are:

1 Position the patient supine. Obtain IV access.
2 Place the ultrasound probe over the lateral abdomen between the iliac crest and the rib margin. The long axis of the probe should be at 90° to the bed.
3 Visualise the three muscle layers (from the skin inwards): external oblique, internal oblique and transversus abdominis.
4 After sterilising and preparing the skin, insert a 100 mm needle using an in-plane approach (pointing towards the bed) so that the tip lies between the innermost and middle muscle layer. The needle tip should be approximately in the midaxillary line.
5 Inject LA e.g. ropivacaine 1% 20 mL for an ipsilateral wound, or bilateral injections of 20 mL ropivacaine 0.5% for a wound that crosses the midline. The injected solution should be visible as a lens shape between the muscle layers.

◗ Tricuspid Regurgitation and Ebstein's Anomaly

Topics Covered in this Section
▶ Tricuspid Regurgitation
▶ Ebstein's Anomaly

Tricuspid Regurgitation
Aetiology
Causes of tricuspid regurgitation include:

1 Functional due to dilatation of the right ventricle (RV). RV dilatation may occur with pulmonary hypertension and right ventricular volume overload due to aortic stenosis.
2 Rheumatic fever. There is usually tricuspid stenosis as well.

QUICK FLICK **T**

Pathophysiology

Tricuspid regurgitation causes right atrial volume overload which is usually well tolerated. Associated conditions such as pulmonary hypertension are more important to consider. **See** *Pulmonary Hypertension*.

Anaesthetic Considerations[36]

1 Provide antibiotic prophylaxis. **See** *Bacterial Endocarditis (BE) Prophylaxis*.
2 Maintain intravascular volume and CVP in the high normal range to maintain RV stroke volume.
3 Avoid high intrathoracic pressure.
4 Avoid factors which increase pulmonary vascular resistance. **See** *Pulmonary Hypertension*.

Ebstein's Anomaly

Description

This is a congenital condition characterised by the following:[36]

1 Malformed tricuspid valve leaflets that may be displaced downwards into the right ventricle.
2 The part of the right ventricle adjacent to the valve is atrialised and the remaining functional RV is thus small.
3 The tricuspid valve is usually regurgitant but may be stenotic.
4 There is usually an interatrial communication (80%) such as an ASD or patent foramen ovale through which there may occur right-to-left shunting of blood.

Clinical Features

The condition may cause a wide spectrum of effects from congestive cardiac failure in neonates to asymptomatic adults.

  Clinical effects include:

1 Heart murmur usually systolic.
2 Supraventricular and ventricular dysrhythmias Wolff Parkinson-White syndrome may occur in up to 20% of patients.[37]
3 Cyanosis.
4 Paradoxical embolism through the interatrial communication.
5 Congestive cardiac failure.
6 ECG usually shows tall wide P waves and first degree AV block.
7 Possible massive enlargement of the right atrium may occur. A cardiothoracic ratio on CXR of > 0.65 is a predictor of sudden death.[38]

Anaesthetic Management

Due to the rarity of this condition it is difficult to provide clear anaesthetic guidelines from the literature but the following is a guide:

1 Provide antibiotic prophylaxis. **See** *Bacterial Endocarditis (BE) Prophylaxis*.

2   Use appropriate monitoring (e.g. arterial line, CVP) depending on the severity of the patient's condition and the nature of the surgery. PA catheter insertion may provoke life-threatening dysrhythmias.[38] When inserting a central line ensure that the Seldinger wire and the tip of the CVP line stay within the SVC. CVP lines may increase the risk of bacterial endocarditis.[37]

3   Induction times may be prolonged due to pooling of induction drugs in the enlarged right atrium.[38]

4   Provide cardiovascular stability by maintaining preload, afterload and sinus rhythm. Tachycardia is poorly tolerated due to reduced filling of the small RV.

5   Factors which increase right-to-left shunt (if present) must be avoided. These include hypotension, raised intrathoracic pressure and pulmonary vasoconstriction. *See* *Pulmonary Hypertension*.

6   IPPV may cause increased right-to-left shunting due to increased intrathoracic pressure.

7   An opioid based 'cardiac' anaesthetic may help provide optimal CVS stability more effectively than volatile agents.

8   Avoid introducing any intravascular air due to the risk of paradoxical emboli.

Obstetric Implications

1   There should be close consultation between the anaesthetist, cardiologist and obstetrician.

2   The extra cardiovascular stress of pregnancy can precipitate symptoms or cause life threatening deterioration in patients with Ebstein's anomaly. This deterioration may include RV failure, worsening right-to-left shunting and worsening dysrhythmias.

3   In the absence of cyanosis and dysrhythmias, pregnancy tends to be well tolerated.[39]

4   Epidural anaesthesia has been used successfully in these patients for labour and delivery.[37,40] Establishment of the block should be done slowly and carefully with appropriate monitoring e.g. arterial line, central line, ECG monitoring.

5   Use epidural opioids to help minimise epidural LA requirements. Consider intrathecal opioids.

6   Do not use adrenaline containing LA solutions.

7   It is very important to minimise the risk of intravascular air due to the risk of paradoxical embolism. For example do not use a loss-of-resistance to air technique when siting the epidural.

8   Aorto-caval compression must be avoided.

9   SAB anaesthesia for CS is contraindicated in patients significantly affected by Ebstein's anomaly.[37]

10 Syntocinon should be used cautiously due to its vasodilating effects and prostaglandin $F_{2\alpha}$ is suggested as a possible alternative.[37] Ergometrine should be avoided due to its vasoconstrictive effects on the pulmonary vasculature.[37]

◑ **Trimetaphan**

This is a monoquaternary sulfonium derivative and acts as a ganglion blocker at sympathetic and parasympathetic ganglia. It does this by competing with acetylcholine at cholinergic receptor sites. It also has some direct vasodilating properties and causes histamine release.[41] It is used for its hypotensive effects.

Dose

Adults Mix 500 mg in 250 mL of 5% glucose. Give trimetaphan by infusion starting at a rate of 25 µg/kg/min and titrate to response. In a 70 kg patient = 50 mL/h. Can also give boluses of 1–4 mg (0.5–2 mL of above solution). Acts rapidly and effects wear off ≈ 30 min after cessation of infusion.

Problems with Trimetaphan Use

1 Do not use in asthma patients as it releases histamine.[41]
2 Trimetaphan inhibits plasma pseudocholinesterase and prolongs the action of suxamethonium.[42]

◑ **Tropisetron**

5-HT$_3$ receptor antagonist antiemetic drug.
Adult dose: 2 mg IV over at least 30 s once daily.

REFERENCES

1 Findlow D, Doyle E. Congenital heart disease in adults: Review Article. *Br J Anaesth* 1997; 78: 416–30.

2 Sasada M, Smith S. *Drugs in Anaesthesia and Intensive Care*, 2nd edn. Oxford University Press, Oxford 1997; 362–4.

3 Myles PS, Hendrata M, Bennett AM et al. Postoperative nausea and vomiting. Propofol or thiopentone: Does choice of induction agent affect outcome? *Anaesth Intensive Care* 1996; 24: 355–9.

4 Gowda RM, Misra D, Tranbaugh RF, Ohki T, Khan IA. Endovascular stent grafting of descending thoracic aortic aneurysms. *Chest* 2003; 124: 714–19.

5 Fuchs RJ, Lee WA, Seubert CN, Gelman S. Transient paraplegia after stent grafting of a descending thoracic aortic aneurysm treated with cerebrospinal fluid drainage. *J Clin Anesth* 2003; 15: 59–63.

6 Gelman S. The pathophysiology of aortic cross-clamping and unclamping. *Anesthesiology* 1995; 82: 1026–60.

7 Crawford ES, Crawford JL, Safi HJ et al. Thoracoabdominal aneurysms:

preoperative and intraoperative factors determining immediate and long term results in 605 patients. *J Vasc Surg* 1986; 3: 389–404.

8   DeBakey ME, Cooley DA, Crawford ES et al. Aneurysms of the thoracic aorta. *J Thorac Surg* 1958; 36: 393–420.

9   Galla JD, Ergin MA, Lansman SL et al. Use of somatosensory evoked potentials for thoracic and thoracoabdominal aortic resections. *Ann Thorac Surg* 1999; 67: 1947–52.

10 Safi HJ, Miller C. Spinal cord protection in descending thoracic and thoracoabdominal aortic repair. *Ann Thorac Surg* 1999; 67: 1937–9.

11 Ehrlich M, Grabenwoeger M, Cartes-Zumelzu F et al. Endovascular stent graft repair for aneurysms on the descending thoracic aorta. *Ann Thorac Surg* 1998; 66: 19–25.

12 Mallett SV, Cox DJA. Thromboelastography. *Br J Anaesthesia* 1992; 69: 307–13.

13 Oster DL, Chang S-P B. Thyrotoxicosis. In Yao F-S, *Yao and Artusio's Anesthesiology Problem-Orientated Patient Management,* 4th edn. Lippincott-Raven, Philadelphia 1998: 571–83.

14 Gupta A, Lawrence AT, Krishnan K et al. Current concepts in the mechanisms and management of drug-induced QT prolongation and torsade de pointes. *Am Heart J* 2007; 153: 891–9.

15 Fan CM, Ko PC-I, Tsai K-C et al. Tracheal rupture complicating emergent endotracheal intubation. *Am J Emerg Med* 2004; 22: 289–93.

16 Lim HJ, Miller GM, Rainbird A. Airway fire during elective tracheostomy. *Anaesth Intensive Care* 1997; 25: 150–2.

17 Lewis KS, Han NH. Clinical Review. Tramadol: a new centrally acting analgesic. *Am J Health-Syst Pharm* 1997; 54: 643–52.

18 Delikan AE, Vijayan R. Forum: Epidural tramadol for postoperative pain relief. *Anaesthesia* 1993; 48: 328–31.

19 Bamigbade TA, Langford RM. The clinical use of tramadol hydrochloride. *Pain Reviews* 1998; 5: 155–82.

20 Sasada M, Smith S. *Drugs in Anaesthesia and Intensive Care*, 2nd edn. Oxford University Press, Oxford 1997: 370–1.

21 Broome IJ, Robb HM, Raj N et al. The use of tramadol following day case surgery. *Anaesthesia* 1999; 54: 289–92.

22 Medicinal mishaps: serotonin syndrome. *Australian Prescriber* 2002; 25: 19.

23 Cossmann M, Kohnen C. General tolerability and adverse profile of tramadol hydrochloride. *Rev Contemp Pharmacother* 1995; 246–9.

24 Horrow JC, Van Ripper DF, Strong MD et al. Hemostatic effects of tranexamic acid and desmopressin during cardiac surgery. *Circulation* 1991; 84: 2063–70.

25 Levy JH. Novel pharmacologic approaches to reduce bleeding. *Can J Anesth* 2003; 50: S26–S30.

QUICK FLICK

T

26 Horrow JC, Van Ripper DF, Strong MD, Grunewald KE. The dose response relationship of tranexamic acid. *Anesthesiology* 1995; 82: 383–92.

27 Mebust WK, Holtgrewe HL, Crockett ATK et al. Transurethral prostatectomy immediate and postoperative complications. A co-operative study of thirteen participating institutions evaluating 3885 patients. *J Urol* 1989; 141: 243–7.

28 Monk TG. Anesthesia for urological procedures. *Audio-Digest Anesthesiology* 1998; 40: 5.

29 Hatch PD. Surgical and anaesthetic considerations in transurethral resection of the prostate. *Anaesth Intensive Care*, 1987; 15: 203–11.

30 Hahn RG. The transurethral resection syndrome. *Acta Anaesthesiol Scand* 1991; 35: 557–67.

31 Jensen V. The TURP syndrome. *Can J Anaesth* 1991; 38(1): 90–7.

32 Quinney N, Lomas I. Treatment of priapism during transurethral resection of the prostate. *Br J Hosp Med* 1995; 54(8): 393–4.

33 Yao F-SF, Malhotra V, Sudheendra V. Transurethral resection of the prostate. In: Yao F-SF, Malhotra V, Fontes ML, eds. *Yao and Artusio's Anesthesiology: Problem-Orientated Patient Management*, 6th edn.Lippincott Williams & Wilkins, Philadelphia, Pennsylvania 2008: 797–821.

34 Hanson RA, Zornow MH, Conlin MJ, Brambrink AM. Laser resection of the prostate: implications for anesthesia. *Anesth Analg* 2007; 105: 475–9.

35 Costello TG, Crowe H, Costello AJ. Laser prostatectomy versus transurethral resection of the prostate for benign prostatic hypertrophy: comparative changes in haemoglobin and serum sodium. *Anaesth Intensive Care* 1997; 25: 493–6.

36 Stoelting RK, Dierdorf SF. Valvular Heart Disease. In Stoelting RK, Diersdorf SF, eds. *Anesthesia and Co-Existing Disease*, 4th edn. Churchill Livingstone, Philadelphia 2002; 25–44.

37 Groves ER, Groves JB. Epidural analgesia for labour in a patient with Ebstein's anomaly. *Can J Anaesth* 1995; 42: 77–9.

38 Mason R. Ebstein's Anomaly. In *Anaesthesia Databook: A Perioperative and Peripartum Manual*, 3rd edn. Greenwich Medical Media Limited, London, 2001: 155–6.

39 Donnelly JE, Brown JM, Radford DJ. Pregnancy outcome and Ebstein's anomaly. *Br Heart J* 1991; 66: 368–71.

40 Linter SPK, Clarke K. Caesarean section under extradural analgesia in a patient with Ebstein's anomaly. *Br J Anaesth* 1984; 56: 203.

41 Mostellar JR. Deliberate hypotension. In: Duke J, Rosenberg SG, eds. *Anesthesia Secrets*. Hanley & Belfus, Philadelphia, Mosby St Louis, 1996: 465.

42 Ramanathan J, Bennett K. Pre-eclampsia: fluids, drugs and anaesthetic management. *Anesthesiol Clin North Am* 2003; 21: 145–63.

○ Ultrasound Guided Regional Anaesthesia

Due to space restrictions only a very brief introduction to this topic is possible.

Ultrasound Physics

Ultrasound consists of high frequency sound waves sent through tissues. Sound waves used for medical imaging have a frequency >2 MHz (human hearing is in the range of 40 Hz–15 KHz). Lower frequencies penetrate more deeply than higher frequencies. The sound waves are either absorbed, reflected or pass through the tissue (conducted) depending on the density of the tissue. The sound waves are generated by piezoelectric crystals, via electric currents applied to quartz crystals causing them to expand and contract. Returning sound also causes a current to be generated which can be transduced and displayed.

Technical Terms

1 *Short and Long Axis View* Refers to the orientation of the probe in relation to the nerve(s) being visualised. In the short axis view the probe is held perpendicular to the nerve so the nerve is seen end on (looks like a circle). In the long axis view the probe is held parallel to the nerve (so the nerve looks like a length of cord).

2 *In-plane/Out-of-plane* Refers to the needle approach either in line with the long axis of the probe (in-plane) or perpendicular to the long axis of the probe (out-of-plane).

3 *Gain Control* This control amplifies the returning signals. Increasing the gain improves the image but unfortunately amplifies artefacts as well. Adjust this until the best image is obtained.

4 *Power Control* Increasing the power increases the penetration.

5 *Compress/Dynamic Range/Greyscale Control* This control is used to get the 'best image'. Increasing the compression increases the whiteness of the image improving detail but ultimately leads to a 'snow-storm' image. Decreasing the compression makes the image more 'black and white' with loss of detail. The compression should be adjusted until 'enough' but not 'too much' detail is displayed.

6 *Hyper Echoic (Echo Dense)* Appear brighter on ultrasound e.g. nerves, bone, air.

7 *Hypo Echoic (Echolucent)* Appear dark on ultrasound e.g. CSF, blood. These substances reflect little sound.

8 *Colour Flow Doppler* The ultrasound machine is able to assign a colour to material moving away from the probe and material moving towards the probe. By convention BART is used **b**lue **a**way, **r**ed **t**oward.

Tips for Success

1 Obtain a good teacher of ultrasound guided nerve identification.
2 Practise diligently.
3 Use the nerve algorithm preset.
4 Use lots of ultrasound gel.
5 Use small deliberate movements of the probe.
6 Keep the tip of the needle visualised by 'jiggling' the needle. This deforms the tissues which are visible on the screen. Never advance the needle while 'jiggling'.
7 The tip of the needle can also be identified by injecting 1 mL of LA. The injected LA will be visible on the screen.

❯ Umbilical Vein Catheterisation

See Neonatal Resuscitation.

❯ Unfractionated Heparin

See Heparin (Unfractionated and Low Molecular Weight Heparins).

❯ Unifocal Atrial Tachycardia

See Supraventricular Tachycardias (SVT).

❯ Unwashed Shed Blood Transfusion

In this technique on-going blood loss from surgical wounds is collected during the postoperative period into a purpose built canister such as a Stryker Consta Vac CBC II. This blood is filtered and re-transfused without further processing. Some devices use an anti-coagulant. Studies have not indicated any clinically relevant side effects.[1] Blood should be returned to the patient within 6 h of the completion of surgery.

❯ Uterine Atonia, Postpartum

See Postpartum Haemorrhage.

❯ Uterine Inversion

This is an obstetric emergency associated with:

1 Severe haemorrhage/exsanguination.
2 Cardiovascular instability due to haemorrhage and vasovagal reflexes secondary to traction on the peritoneum.[2] There may also be traction on sympathetic nerves producing neurogenic shock.
3 Severe pain.

Treatment

1 An attempt should be made by the obstetrician to immediately push the uterus back to its normal position. However the constricted cervix may prevent this. Urgently transfer the patient to the operating theatre.
2 Resuscitate the patient with IV fluid volume replacement via large bore IV cannulas using crystalloid/colloid/blood as appropriate.
3 Provide analgesia for the patient's often severe pain.
4 Induce GA with a rapid sequence induction. **See** *Rapid Sequence Induction (RSI)*.
5 Provide uterine relaxation with increased inhaled concentration of volatile anaesthetic agent. If insufficient relaxation results give glyceryl trinitrate IV or sublingually as described for *Uterine Relaxation for Retained Placenta* below.
6 Rarely laparotomy may be required to replace the uterus.

⊙ Uterine Relaxation for Retained Placenta

Uterine relaxation may be required for a retained placenta, external version of the second twin and uterine inversion. Uterine relaxation can be obtained by giving an increased concentration of volatile inhalational anaesthetic agent during general anaesthesia. Rapid uterine relaxation can also be obtained giving IV glyceryl trinitrate (GTN) 50 µg boluses[3] or sublingual metered dose spray (e.g. 800 µg).[2]

Preparation of IV Glyceryl Trinitrate for Uterine Relaxation

Remove 1 mL from an ampoule containing 50 mg of glyceryl trinitrate in 10 mL (5 mg) and dilute to 10 mL with N/S. Take 1 mL (500 µg) from this solution and dilute to 10 mL resulting in a final concentration of 50 µg/mL. Give 1 mL boluses as required. The dose required is variable but 100–200 µg is usually effective.[4]

⊙ Uterine Rupture

The incidence of uterine rupture is about 0.05% of all deliveries with a maternal mortality of about 10% and a fetal mortality of about 20%.[5] In patients with a previous CS the incidence is about 0.6%.[5] Risk factors include uterine scar, use of oxytocics to augment labour, prolonged labour, previous uterine perforation (e.g. at D&C) and breech extraction.

Symptoms and Signs

1 Abdominal pain which is often atypical.
2 Acute fetal bradycardia or sudden profound fetal distress may be seen.
3 PV blood loss.
4 Cessation of contractions.
5 Hypovolaemic shock.

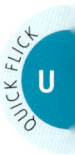

QUICK FLICK

U

6 Change in abdominal shape.

7 Haematuria.

Anaesthetic Management

1 Ensure adequate patient airway and breathing.

2 Replace the patient's intravascular volume with appropriate IV fluids (crystalloid, colloid, blood).

3 Immediate laparotomy is usually required.

4 General anaesthesia is usually required but, if the mother and fetus are stable, regional anaesthesia can be considered.[6]

See *Blood Loss Assessment and Initial Management*.

REFERENCES

1 Muñoz M, Cobos A, Campos A et al. Postoperative unwashed shed blood transfusion does not modify the cellular immune response to surgery for total knee replacement. *Acta Anaesthesiol Scand* 2006; 50: 443–450.

2 Dawson NJ, Gabbott DA. Use of sublingual glyceryl trinitrate as a supplement to volatile inhalational anaesthesia in a case of uterine inversion. *Internat J of Obstet Anaesth* 1997; 6: 135–7.

3 Peng ATC, Gorman RS, Shulman SM et al. Intravenous nitroglycerin for uterine relaxation in the postpartum patient with retained placenta (letter). *Anesthesiol* 1989; 71: 172–3.

4 Axemo P, Fu X, Lindberg B et al. Intravenous uterine relaxation. *Acta Obstet Gynecol Scand* 1998; 77: 50–3.

5 Lynch JC, Pardy J. Survey: Uterine rupture and scar dehiscence. A five-year survey. *Anesth Intensive Care* 1996; 24: 699–704.

6 Yap OW, Kim ES, Laros RK Jr. Maternal and neonatal outcomes after uterine rupture in labour. *Am J Obstet Gynecol* 2001; 184: 1576–81.

○ Vagal Manoeuvres

See *Supraventricular Tachycardias (SVT)*.

○ Vasa Previa

In this condition the fetal umbilical vessels, instead of attaching securely to the placenta, run unsupported through membranes overlying the internal os of the cervix. They then attach to the placenta (velamentous insertion) or to an accessory placental lobe. These unsupported vessels are very prone to tearing or occlusion during labour. Normal vaginal delivery is impossible and fetal death from haemorrhage is very likely once the membranes containing these vessels rupture. Management is elective CS in cases diagnosed prelabour (by colour-doppler sonography) and emergency CS in cases diagnosed during labour.

○ Vasopressin

Acts by causing vasoconstriction through activation of V_1 receptors. Also causes antidiuresis through its actions on V_2 receptors in the distal tubule of the kidney. This drug is useful:

1 For the treatment of vasodilatory shock associated with severe sepsis unresponsive to a noradrenaline infusion.
2 For the treatment of vasodilatory shock related to post-cardiopulmonary bypass unresponsive to a noradrenaline infusion.
3 For the treatment of uncontrolled bleeding oesophageal varices.
4 As an alternative vasopressor to adrenaline in the management of shock resistant VF.

Dose
For vasodilatory shock, administer as an IV infusion preferably through a central line. Mix 20 units (U) of vasopressin with 40 mL of 5% glucose run at 0.08–0.1 U/min = 10–12 mL/h. For VF cardiac arrest give 40 U as a single dose.

○ Vecuronium

NDNM blocking bis-quaternary aminosteroid analogue of pancuronium.

Dose
0.1 mg/kg IV with recovery occurring in about 30 min. Can also be given by infusion at a rate of 50–80 µg/kg/h.

Advantages

1 Vecuronium is very cardiovascularly stable and lacks the tachycardiac effects of pancuronium.
2 Low potential for histamine release.
3 May be lower risk of allergic reaction than rocuronium.

Disadvantages

1 Effects of vecuronium may be prolonged in renal and liver failure. About 25% of the vecuronium dose is excreted unchanged by the kidney, the rest is metabolised by the liver.
2 Must be reconstituted from powder form at the time of injection.
3 Slower onset than rocuronium.

▷ Veins of the Upper Limb

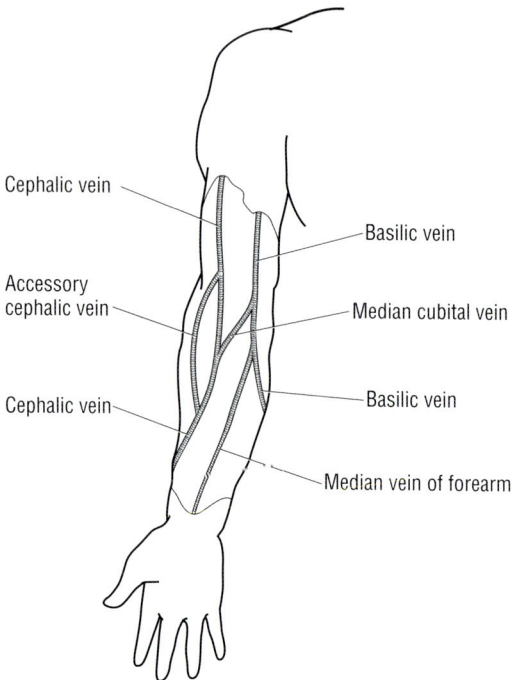

Figure V1 Veins of the upper limb

⊙ Valdecoxib

Long-acting oral COX-2 selective NSAID. Also available as a parenteral prodrug, parecoxib. **See** *Parecoxib*.

⊙ Venous Gas Embolism

See *Gas Embolism, Venous*.

⊙ Ventricular Ectopic Beats (VEBs)

VEBs are not life threatening if there is no underlying heart disease. VEBs after a myocardial infarction may precede ventricular fibrillation but treatment of VEBs is probably not beneficial (IV lignocaine is no longer recommended).[1] Ensure electrolytes are normal and treat any other possible underlying cause such as myocardial ischaemia. Beta blockers may be tried in patients who are symptomatic from VEBs.

⊙ Ventricular Ejection Fraction

See *Cardiac Investigations*.

⊙ Ventricular Fibrillation

See *Cardiac Arrest*.

⊙ Ventricular Septal Defect (VSD)

A VSD is the most common congenital heart disease (CHD). These can be multiple and difficult to repair fully. Small unrepaired defects may lead to increased risk of endocarditis and paradoxical embolism. Larger unrepaired defects can lead to increased right ventricular and pulmonary artery pressure and pulmonary hypertension. **See** *Pulmonary Hypertension* and *Eisenmenger's Syndrome*.

After VSD repair there is an increased risk of conduction abnormalities particularly RBBB, LAD and AV block which can progress to complete heart block.

⊙ Ventricular Tachycardia (VT)

Defined as >2 consecutive ventricular ectopic beats. Termed sustained ventricular tachycardia if the duration of the tachycardia is more than 30 s.[2] Subdivided into monomorphic and polymorphic VT.

Monomorphic VT

QRS complexes have the same morphology. It is the most common cause of broad complex tachycardia, but supraventricular tachycardia (SVT) with aberrant conduction can look similar. **See** *Broad Complex Tachycardia*. Always seek early expert cardiology assistance.

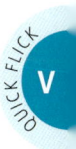

Treatment of Monomorphic VT in the Cardiovascularly Compromised Patient

1   If pulseless VT immediate non-synchronised DC shocks (**see** *Cardiac Arrest*).
2   If the patient has adverse signs defined as SBP < 90 mm Hg, chest pain, heart failure, or a heart rate > 150 bpm, cardiovert the patient under sedation or anaesthesia.[3] Use synchronised monophasic shocks of 100 J, 200 J, 360 J. If using biphasic cardioversion about half the energy of monophasic defibrillation is required.
3   If the initial cardioversion is unsuccessful give an antiarrhythmic drug. Use sotalol (possibly the drug of choice)[4] or amiodarone, and repeat cardioversion.
4   Identify and treat the cause of the VT if possible e.g. give IV potassium and magnesium if hypokalaemia is present.
5   Overdrive RV pacing may be effective.[5]

Treatment of Monomorphic VT in the Cardiovascularly Stable Patient

1   If the patient is cardiovascularly stable give sotalol 1–1.5 mg/kg IV over 5 min. Give a repeat dose of 0.5–0.75 mg/kg if needed. Alternatively use amiodarone 5 mg/kg IV over 30 min, then IV infusion of 10–15 mg/kg over 24 h.
2   Procainamide can be considered.
3   If pharmacotherapy unsuccessful perform R wave synchronised DC monophasic cardioversion 100 J under sedation or anaesthesia. If using biphasic cardioversion about half the energy of monophasic defibrillation is required.
4   Overdrive RV pacing may be effective.[4]

Polymorphic VT Treatment

1   If pulseless VT immediate non-synchronised DC shocks (**see** *Cardiac Arrest*).
2   If the patient has adverse signs as described above first decide if the Q-T interval is prolonged. If yes the patient may be suffering from torsades de pointes. **See** *Torsades de Pointes*. Look at the rhythm tracing for the distinctive pattern of torsades, a widening and narrowing pattern looking like a twisting motion.
3   If the Q-T interval is not prolonged treat as for monomorphic VT.

◖ Verapamil

Calcium channel blocking drug useful for the treatment of:

1   hypertension
2   angina

3 dysrhythmias such as supraventricular tachycardia (SVT), atrial fibrillation and atrial flutter.

Dose

Adult For the treatment of dysrhythmias give 1 mg IV increments to a maximum of 10 mg.

Problems with Verapamil/Contraindications and Interactions

1 Adenosine rather than verapamil is now the drug of choice for treating SVT. Several fatalities have occurred from giving verapamil to patients with broad complex tachycardia in the mistaken belief that an SVT rather than VT was occurring. Verapamil must never be given in the presence of an undiagnosed broad complex tachycardia.[6]

2 Patients given verapamil while receiving β receptor blocking drugs or inhalational agents may suffer severe bradycardias.[7]

3 Verapamil and dantrolene, in combination, may cause severe hyperkalaemia and resultant ventricular fibrillation.[8]

4 Verapamil is contraindicated in AF associated with Wolff-Parkinson-White syndrome, sick sinus syndrome and 2nd or 3rd degree heart block. It is also contraindicated in heart failure, cardiogenic shock and porphyria.[9]

REFERENCES

1 Wesley RC, Rash W, Zimmerman D. Reconsiderations of the routine and preoperational use of lidocaine in the emergent treatment of ventricular arrhythmias. *Crit Care Med* 1991; 19: 1439–41.

2 *Cardiovascular Drug Guidelines*, 2nd edn. Victorian Medical Postgraduate Foundation Therapeutics Committee, Melbourne 1995: 133.

3 Sanghavi S, Rayner-Klein J. Management of peri-arrest arrhythmia. *Br J Anaesth CEPD Reviews* 2002; 4: 104–12.

4 Ho DSW, Zecchin RP, Richards DA et al. Double blind trial of lignocaine versus sotalol for acute termination of spontaneous ventricular tachycardia. *Lancet* 1994; 44: 18–22.

5 Holt A. Management of Cardiac Arrhythmias. In Bersten AD, Soni N, Oh TE. *Oh's Intensive Care Manual*, 5th edn. Butterworth–Heinemann, Oxford 2003: 157–205.

6 *Cardiovascular Drug Guidelines*, 2nd edn. Victorian Medical Postgraduate Foundation Therapeutics Committee, Melbourne 1995: 119.

7 *Cardiovascular Drug Guidelines*, 2nd edn. Victorian Medical Postgraduate Foundation Therapeutics Committee, Melbourne 1995: 108.

8 Willis C. Acute Dysrhythmias. In: Parsons PE, Wiener-Kronish JP, eds. *Critical Care Secrets*. Hanley and Belfus, Inc, Philadelphia, Mosby-Year Book, Inc, St Louis 1992: 126–35.

9 Sambrook A, Small R. Antiarrhythmic drugs; antihypertensive drugs in pregnancy. *Anaesthesia and Intensive Care Medicine* 2003; 4: 266–72.

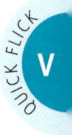

QUICK FLICK

V

W

◐ Warfarin

Synthetic coumarin derivative used as an anticoagulant for the treatment and prevention of venous and arterial thromboembolism. Acts by preventing the synthesis of Vitamin K dependent clotting factors II, VII, IX and X.

Dose
Adult Day 1 give 10 mg if <70 yrs old, 5 mg if >70 yrs old. Day 2 give 5 mg. Check INR on day 3 and dose patient depending on the following table.

Table W1 Day 3 dose of warfarin based on day 3 INR

INR	Dose
<2	5 mg
2–3	4 mg
>3	omit

If giving heparin or low molecular weight (LMW) heparin, overlap heparin with warfarin for at least 5 days and do not cease heparin or LMW heparin until the INR is in the target range. See table below.

Table W2 Therapeutic INR for various disease states

Condition	Desirable INR range
Prosthetic heart valve	2.5–3.5
Recurrent severe DVT/PE, Arterial thrombo-embolic disease	2.5–3.5
DVT, PE, valve lesions, prevention of thrombo-embolus after MI, AF, TIAs	2–3.0
Tissue heart valves for 3 months after insertion	2–3.0
DVT prophylaxis	2–2.5

Warfarin and Surgery
See *Anticoagulation Therapy and Surgery*.

Emergency Reversal of Warfarin
It is recommended to consult a haematologist in this situation. Rapid reversal of warfarin may be required for:

1 Emergency surgery in a patient who is therapeutically anticoagulated.
2 Major bleeding in a patient who is therapeutically anticoagulated or over anticoagulated.

The effects of warfarin can be rapidly reversed by:

1 Vitamin K 5 mg IV. INR will be reduced in 4–6 h.
2 Prothrombinex-HT. The dose depends on the INR (**see** *Prothrombinex-HT*):
   a) INR 2–3.9   25 U/kg.
   b) INR 4–5.9   35 U/kg.
   c) INR > 6   50 U/kg.
3 Fresh frozen plasma 5–8 mL/kg.
4 Recombinant activated factor VII 80 μg/kg IV.

Warfarin and Obstetric Patients

Use of warfarin in pregnancy is associated with a 30% fetal loss rate. Warfarin can cause nasal hyperplasia and bone stippling.

◗ Weights of Children, Average

Table W3 Average weights in children by age

Age	Estimated Wt
Neonate	3 kg
4 months	6 kg
1–8 years	(2 × age) + 9
9–13 years	3.3 × age

◗ Whole Blood

Defined as blood collected with an anticoagulant and without further processing. Platelets and white cells in whole blood become nonviable after a few days. There are few indications for whole blood such as neonatal exchange transfusions.

Leukocyte depleted whole blood has been filtered to remove most of the white cells. Its use is indicated:

1 For patients who have febrile non-haemolytic transfusion reactions.
2 To reduce the risk of HLA alloimmunisation in patients who are likely to have repeated transfusions.
3 To reduce the risk of transmission of white cell carried infections such as cytomegalovirus.

◗ Wolff-Parkinson-White (WPW) Syndrome

This is the most common ventricular pre-excitation syndrome, meaning the ventricular muscle is activated faster than should occur from normal conduction of atrial impulses. An accessory atrio-ventricular connection pathway enables atrial depolarisation to be conducted to the ventricles much faster than through the atrio-ventricular (AV) node leading to tachycardias or atrial fibrillation. Characteristic ECG findings are:

1 Short PR interval <3 mm (0.12 s).

QUICK FLICK

W

2 Slurred upstroke on QRS complex (delta wave).

3 QRS is prolonged (>0.12 s).

4 Secondary ST segment and T wave changes.

These patients are prone to the following dysrhythmias:

1 Paroxysmal supraventricular tachycardia (80%). In 85% the QRS complexes are narrow and in 15% they are widened.

2 Atrial fibrillation/atrial flutter (20%). These can be life threatening because ventricular rate can be very fast. QRS complexes are irregular and wide.

WPW may be associated with other abnormalities such as Ebstein's anomaly, hypertrophic cardiomyopathy and mitral valve prolapse.[1]

Treatment of WPW Syndrome Dysrhythmias

Regular Narrow Complex SVT

1 Seek expert cardiology advice early and if possible contact the patient's cardiologist. Find out what treatments have been used successfully in the past.

2 If the patient is cardiovascularly stable, aim to decrease the rate of AV node conduction. Try vagal manoeuvres such as carotid sinus massage.

3 If unsuccessful give adenosine (**see** *Adenosine*).

4 Verapamil can be used if adenosine is not effective.[1]

5 Use synchronised DC cardioversion with sedation or anaesthesia if the patient becomes unstable or the above treatment is not successful.

Atrial Fibrillation or Irregular Wide Complex Tachycardia Thought to be Atrial Fibrillation

There is usually marked variation in the width of the QRS complex and variability in the tachycardia. This dysrhythmia should not be treated by drugs decreasing AV node conduction. Do not use digoxin, verapamil, diltiazem, adenosine or β blockers as these drugs can lead to very fast ventricular rates due to rapid conduction down the accessory pathway.[1] This can in turn lead to degeneration into ventricular fibrillation. Treatment includes the following:

1 Procainamide is the drug of choice.[2] Give 50–100 mg every 2 min to a total dose of 1 g.[1]

2 Propafenone IV is very effective at slowing the ventricular rate.[1]

3 Use synchronised DC cardioversion with sedation or anaesthesia if the patient becomes unstable or procainamide is not successful.

4 Prior electrophysiological studies may have indicated which drugs are effective in individual patients. If possible discuss drug therapy with the patient's cardiologist.

Long-term Treatment of WPW

1. Radiofrequency ablation of the accessory pathway is the treatment of choice for symptomatic patients.
2. Chronic oral anti-arrhythmic therapy.

Patients with Asymptomatic WPW

Unless there is a family history of sudden cardiac death, it is unclear whether further investigation and treatment of these patients is justified. Some of these patients will go on to have symptomatic WPW.[1]

Wound Catheter Infusions of Local Anaesthetic

Continuous infusions of LA into surgical wounds via special catheters does significantly reduce postoperative pain. An example is the PainBuster Pain Management system consisting of:

1. A balloon filled with LA.
2. A filter.
3. Attached to the filter is a length of tubing which terminates with a constrictor to control the rate that LA is expelled by the balloon. The constrictor should be in contact with the patient's skin to keep it a constant temperature.
4. A second catheter is attached to the flow restrictor which is placed under the surgical wound by the surgeon. This catheter has multiple orifices to deliver LA evenly under the wound.

Infusion Rate

A suitable infusion rate is ropivacaine 0.2% 10 mL bolus then 10 mL/h for 48 h. Beaussier et al. argue that for abdominal wounds placement of the catheter between the peritoneum and the musculoaponeurosis layer is more effective than subcutaneous placement.[3]

Wrist Blocks

The median, ulnar and radial nerves can all be blocked at the wrist. For the distribution of these nerves in the hand ***see*** *Elbow Blocks*. Distal arm blocks are not recommended when a tourniquet is used except for short procedures.[4]

Technique

Median Nerve

Lies between the tendon of palmaris longus (roughly in the middle of the wrist) and flexor carpi radialis (just lateral to palmaris longus).

1. Mark the point 2 cm proximal from the most distal wrist crease, between these tendons.
2. Insert 25 G needle through to the deep fascia at this point and paraesthesia should be obtained at a depth of < 1 cm.[5]
3. Inject 5 mL of LA as the needle is withdrawn.

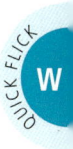

Ulnar Nerve

1. Insert the needle on the ulnar side of the ulnar artery (between the ulnar artery and flexor carpi ulnaris) to the ulnar styloid.
2. Inject 5 mL of LA as the needle is withdrawn.

Radial Nerve

1. Insert the needle just lateral to the radial artery 2.5 cm proximal to the wrist joint.
2. Inject 3 mL of LA, then inject a superficial ring of LA solution dorsally over the border of the wrist into the 'anatomical snuff box' area (between the extensor tendons of thumb).

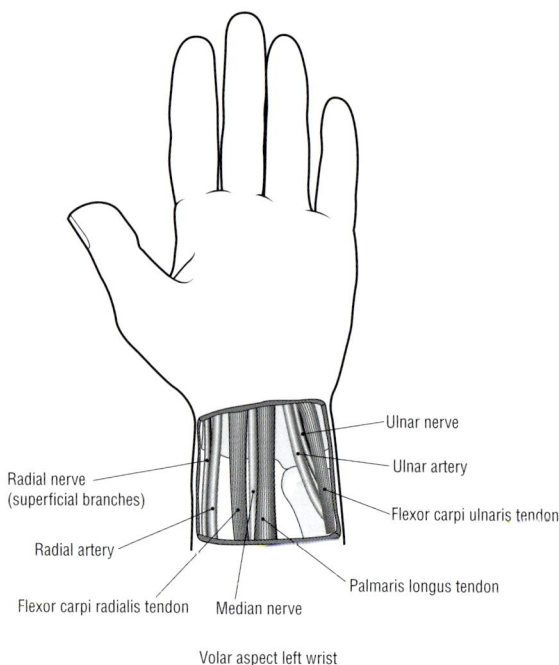

Volar aspect left wrist

Figure W1 Wrist anatomy for wrist blocks

REFERENCES

1. Al-Khatib SA, Pritchett ELC. Clinical features of Wolff-Parkinson-White syndrome. *Am Heart J* 1999; 138: 403–13.
2. Gerstenfeld EP, Beaudette SP, Mittleman RS, Becker RC. Supraventricular

Tachycardias. In Irwin RS, Rippe JM. *Manual of Intensive Care Medicine*, 3rd edn. Lippincott Williams and Wilkins, Philadelphia, 2000: 240–52.

3   Beaussier M, El'Ayoubi H, Schiffer E et al. Continuous preperitoneal infusion of ropivacaine provides effective analgesia and accelerates recovery after colorectal surgery. *Anesthesiol* 2007; 97: 461–8.

4   Delaunay L, Chelly JE. Blocks at the wrist provide effective anesthesia for carpal tunnel release. *Can J Anesth* 2001; 48: 656–60.

5   Bridenbaugh LD. The upper extremity: somatic blockade. In: Cousins MJ, Bridenbaugh PO, eds. *Neural Blockade in Clinical Anesthesia and Management of Pain*, 2nd edn. JB Lippincott Company, Philadelphia 1988: 387–416.

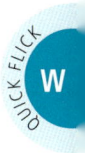

QUICK FLICK

W

X

○ Xenon

'Inert' noble gas with potent anaesthetic properties at atmospheric pressure. When using xenon for anaesthesia, nitrogen must be washed out of the lungs by getting the patient to breathe 100% O_2 for 5 min. This is because xenon must be used at an inhaled concentration of 60–70% for anaesthesia.[1]

Physical Properties and MAC

Blood:Gas Solubility Coefficient	0.115
Oil:Gas Solubility Coefficient	1.9
Boiling Point	−107.1°C
MAC	71

Indications

Xenon is a good choice of anaesthetic for patients with limited cardiovascular reserve. It has been used successfully for a patient with Eisenmenger's syndrome having laparoscopic cholecystectomy.[2]

Advantages

1 Xenon probably does not undergo biotransformation.
2 Rapid induction and emergence.
3 Not thought to be teratogenic.[3]
4 Does not trigger malignant hyperthermia.[1]
5 Xenon has minimal effects on the cardiovascular system.[1]

Disadvantages

1 Xenon is very expensive (AUS$60/L) as it must be prepared from air. Xenon's concentration in air is only 0.0000087%.[4]
2 Cerebral blood flow is increased if Xenon concentration > 60%.[1]

REFERENCES

1 Lynch C, Baum J, Tenbrinck R. Xenon anaesthesia. *Anesthesiology* 2000; 3: 865–8.
2 Hofland I G, Tenbrinck R. Xenon anaesthesia for laparoscopic cholecystectomy in a patient with Eisenmenger's syndrome. *Br J Anaesth* 2001; 86: 882–6.
3 Boomsma F, Rupneht, Veld AJ et al. Haemodynamic and neurohumoral effects of xenon anaesthesia. *Anaesthesia* 1990; 45: 273–8.
4 Shaw AD, Morgan M. Editorial: Nitrous oxide: time to stop laughing? *Anaesthesia* 1998; 53: 213–15.

Appendix 1: Drug Infusion Regimens Summary

Adrenaline
Mix 6 mg adrenaline with 100 mL 5% glucose, start infusion at 5 mL/h.
Titrate to effect.

Dobutamine
Mix 250 mg dobutamine with 100 mL N/S.
Dose range 0.5–40 µg/kg/min. For a 70 kg patient = 1–60 mL/h (usual range required 5–20 mL/h).

Dopamine
Mix 200 mg dopamine with 100 mL N/S. Dose range 1–20 µg/kg/min.
For 70 kg patient = 2–40 mL/h.

Esmolol
Presented as a solution containing 10 mg/mL. Give LD 0.5 mg/kg over 1 min then infusion 50–150 µg/kg/min.
For a 70 kg patient = 21–63 mL/h.

Isoprenaline
Mix 2 mg isoprenaline with 50 mL of 5% glucose. Start infusion at 5 mL/h.
Dose range for adults is 0.5–8 µg/min = 1–12 mL/h.

Glyceryl trinitrate
Mix 250 mg GTN with 500 mL 5% glucose.
In adults run at 10–400 µg/min = 1–40 mL/h.

Noradrenaline
Mix 6 mg noradrenaline with 100 mL 5% dextrose.
In adults start infusion at 5 mL/h and titrate to effect.

Phenytoin
Mix 15–18 mg/kg phenytoin with 100 mL N/S (not glucose). Infuse no faster than 50 mg/min.

Sodium nitroprusside
Mix 50 mg SNP with 100 mL 5% glucose. Dose range 0.3–6 µg/kg/min. For 70 kg patient run at 2.5–50 mL/h (up to 80 mL/h in an emergency).

▷ Appendix 2 Some Important Biochemical and Haematological Reference Ranges

Sodium	136–146 mmol/L
Potassium	3.2–5.5 mmol/L
Chloride	94–107 mmol/L
Carbon dioxide	24–31 mmol/L
Anion gap	12–20 mmol/L
Urea	2.5–6.5 mmol/L
Creatinine	60–125 μmol/L
Total bilirubin	2–21 μmol/L
Total protein	63–84 g/L
Albumin	35–53 g/L
Alkaline phosphatase	30–115 u/L
Gamma-glutamyl transpeptidase	8–43 u/L
Alanine aminotransferase	10–47 u/L
Prothrombin time	11–18 s
Activated partial thromboplastin time	25–36 s
White cell count	$4–11 \times 10^9$/L
Haemoglobin	13.0–18.0 g/dL
Platelets	$150–400 \times 10^9$/L (150 000–400 000/mm^3)
Blood glucose level	3.9–6.2 mmol/L
Troponin levels	0–0.05 μg/L no myocardial damage
	0.05–0.1 μg/L minor cardiac damage
	> 0.1 μg/L significant cardiac damage